TIMELESS SECRETS OF HEALTH & REJUVENATION

Also by Andreas Moritz

• • •

The Amazing Liver and Gallbladder Flush

Lifting the Veil of Duality

Cancer Is Not A Disease (New)

It's Time to Come Alive

Simple Steps to Total Health

Heart Disease No More!

Diabetes – No More!

Ending the AIDS Myth

Hear the Whispers, Live Your Dream

Heal Yourself With Sunlight

Sacred Santémony

Ener-Chi Art

All of the above are available at **www.ener-chi.com**, **www.amazon.com**, and other online or physical bookstores

TIMELESS SECRETS OF HEALTH & REJUVENATION

Unleash The Natural Healing Power That Lies Dormant Within You

---

BREAKTHROUGH MEDICINE FOR THE 21STCENTURY

Andreas Moritz

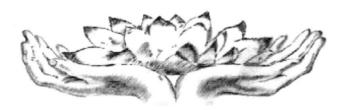

Your Health is in Your Hands

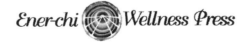

Ener-chi Wellness Press

For Reasons of Legality

The author of this book, Andreas Moritz, does not advocate the use of any particular form of healthcare but believes that the facts, figures, and knowledge presented herein should be available to every person concerned with improving his or her state of health. Although the author has attempted to give a profound understanding of the topics discussed and to ensure accuracy and completeness of any information that originates from any other source than his own, he and the publisher assume no responsibility for errors, inaccuracies, omissions, or any inconsistency herein. Any slights of people or organizations are unintentional. This book is not intended to replace the advice and treatment of a physician who specializes in the treatment of diseases. Any use of the information set forth herein is entirely at the reader's discretion. The author and publisher are not responsible for any adverse effects or consequences resulting from the use of any of the preparations or procedures described in this book. The statements made herein are for educational and theoretical purposes only and are mainly based upon Andreas Moritz's own opinion and theories. You should always consult with a health care practitioner before taking any dietary, nutritional, herbal or homeopathic supplement, or beginning or stopping any therapy. The author is not intending to provide any medical advice, or offer a substitute thereof, and makes no warranty, expressed or implied, with respect to any product, device or therapy, whatsoever. Except as otherwise noted, no statement in this book has been reviewed or approved by the United States Food & Drug Administration or the Federal Trade Commission. Readers should use their own judgment or consult a holistic medical expert or their personal physicians for specific applications to their individual problems.

ISBN: 978-0-9792757-5-3

- First edition (titled The Key to Perfect Health), November 1997
- Second Edition (titled The Key to Health and Rejuvenation), November 2000
- Third Edition (titled Timeless Secrets of Health and Rejuvenation), February and July 2005
- Fourth Edition/Revision (titled Timeless Secrets of Health and Rejuvenation), November 2007
- Fifth Edition (minor revisions), July 2009

Cover Artwork and Design: *Beyond the Horizon* (oil on canvas) by Andreas Moritz

Printed in the United States by Lightning Source, Inc.

Table of Contents:

Chapter 4:

Chapter 5:

Chapter 7:

Chapter 8:
Healing Secrets Of The Sun   260

Chapter 9:

Chapter 15:

What Doctors Should Be Telling You – 37 Health Threats To Avoid   465

"If it's never our fault, we can't take responsibility for it.
If we can't take responsibility for it, we'll always be its victim."
~ Richard Bach

INTRODUCTION

Good health is the most valuable possession you could possibly have. This simple truth applies as much to a newborn baby as to an elderly man, a mother, a doctor, the common person on the street, or the president of a country. Whenever your body becomes sick or does not perform up to what you think is normal, you may experience a state of discomfort, fear or depression that can only be remedied by restoring your body's former health and vitality. To truly feel comfortable within yourself and in your surroundings, you must be able to heal every kind of 'dis-ease' that you experience.

You are indeed capable of healing yourself. Your state of health is but a reflection of how you perceive yourself and your world. This naturally places the responsibility for your wellbeing where it belongs - in your own hands. Once you have achieved vibrant health, you will not just feel well. You will have become 'whole', perhaps, for the very first time in your life.

Timeless Secrets of Health and Rejuvenation can help unleash the tremendous power of healing that lies dormant within you and restore balance on all levels of the body, mind and spirit. Using you own healing powers establishes a permanent comfort zone or continuous sense of satisfaction which forms the basis for a creative, successful and rewarding life.

When you fall ill or your body ages abnormally fast, you may develop an urge to look for a remedy that promises quick relief. Today there is a medical drug or treatment for almost every illness. You are led to believe that if you only suppress or eliminate the symptoms of a disease, such as pain, you have also have eradicated the disease. This ill-founded belief seems to be deeply engraved in our minds. The medical industry plays a major role in re-enforcing it by offering us almost only symptom-oriented treatments. Of course, our own impatience to get well makes us perfect candidates for these fast-acting remedies. But each time we remove a symptom without attending to its cause, we further distance ourselves from regaining the balance required for continuous health and vitality. Consequently, good health remains but a dream, and we may resign ourselves to some degree of ill health, resorting to saying things like "Well, that's life!" or "We all have to die from something!"

Regaining your health is not about applying a magical quick fix; rather, it is a reconstruction process that affects every part of your life such as creativity, job, relationships, emotions, happiness, etc. It would be very simplistic to assume that a few vitamin pills, a new wonder drug, an operation, or even an alternative medical treatment could, on the spur of the moment, undo the effects of many years of neglect. The body may have had to endure much strain from not receiving proper nourishment or sufficient sleep and exercise for years on end. *Timeless Secrets of Health and Rejuvenation* is about setting the preconditions for the body to do what it knows best - creating and maintaining balance - regardless of age and previous health problems. You can find the key to bring balance into every aspect of your life by starting to take responsibility for your own health.

This book deals with the most down-to-earth issues of health, such as lifestyle, diet, nutrition, exercise, daily routine, exposure to sunlight, and the like, some of which are derived from Ayurvedic Medicine. Ayurveda, which literally means *Science of Life*, is the most ancient and complete system of natural healthcare. Apart from discovering Ayurveda's time-tested insights into the secrets of healing and longevity, you will also learn how to apply a number of highly effective and profound cleansing procedures that have seemingly miraculous effects on your physical, emotional and spiritual well-being. The simplified scientific knowledge and common sense used in this book generate the motivation for 'turning the key' of health and rejuvenation. The book also sheds light on the most common diseases and misunderstood medical practices today, of which everyone should be aware.

Concerning the improvement of personal health and well-being, we are being challenged to make a major shift in both our individual and collective attitudes to health and freedom. We must move away from the pre-programmed expectations of illness and aging toward the anticipation of continual youthfulness and vitality. The old saying that everyone has to age and die seems to be a repeatedly verified belief doctrine that most people in the world follow blindly without questioning its validity. Could it be possible, instead, that illness and old age occur *because* we believe they are an inevitable curse to which we all are subjected and with which we are doomed to live? If so, in order to fulfill the curse or belief, as happens with most self-fulfilling prophecies, we are setting the stage for its execution. Although quite unaware of this human drama, we actually allow ourselves to adopt various methods of self-destruction, through derogatory diets, lifestyle and behavior. Right from the early years of childhood, our parents, teachers and society have sentenced us to the 'fact' that the body has no choice but to deteriorate and eventually to die from old age or illness. It used to be that you would only see a doctor if you felt ill. Today, you must have a doctor regularly check on you before you are born and then for the rest of your life. The generally accepted belief that humans are fragile beings that need medical assistance from time to time, especially as they grow older generates a distinct feeling of being out of control, of being dragged down the dark corridor of time by a mysterious power called aging.

The feeling of not being in charge or control is one of the most common causes of physical and mental illness; most people call it 'stress'. The idea of being vulnerable and unsafe generates fear, which in turn triggers profound biochemical changes in the body. These changes become the physical 'reality' of ill health and aging. Through the intimate mind/body connection, every thought and feeling, to a greater or lesser degree, alters your experience of health and well-being. A bout of depression can paralyze your immune system, and falling in love can boost it.

If you are convinced that aging is natural and cannot be avoided, this will be the reality you will create for yourself. Likewise, you can draw on the same force that causes destruction in the body and direct it toward healing and rejuvenation. You can prove to yourself that growing old and becoming more prone to illness are merely the manifested projections of ignorance about the real nature of life. Disease and aging are *not* part of your body's genetic design. Even the so-called 'death-gene' which is in charge of terminating the lives of cells in our body according to their various predetermined life spans, is the one that keeps us alive. Without this gene we would all die from cancer within weeks. In this sense, controlled destruction is the giver of life, and life growing out of control, as is the case with cancer cells, can be the harbinger of death. New gene research suggests that we could grow as old we want to. There is nothing in the normal, original setup of our body that indicates it is causing its own aging or diseases. However, abundant evidence exists to show that aging and illness originate in the combined effects of fearful, negative mental attitudes, emotions, and excessive accumulation of toxic waste material in the body.

As the human race, we are about to recognize the vanity of participating in the *hypnosis of social conditioning* that keeps our mind veiled in the shadows cast by misinformation. Many of us have already begun to let go of the fears and doubts that keep us from realizing the tremendous powers that are patiently waiting for us to put them into action. To make a real difference in life, we need to employ our vast potential of energy, creativity and intelligence for the truly essential issues in life and for generating a profound sense of happiness. One of the keys to unleash our endless potential is the body itself.

The body is constantly engaged in turning over its cells, which in itself is a miraculous and extremely complex process, unmatched by anything man has ever created (*please note that whenever I use the terms 'man' or 'mankind', I am referring to both genders*). The numerous types of proteins that make up your genes and constitute the cells in your body are replaced every 2-10 days. Radioisotope studies show that 98 percent of the atoms that compose your body today won't be there in a year's time. This renewal process affects all parts of the body, including the blood, muscles, organs, fat, bones, nerves, and as recently confirmed, brain matter. With the continual replacement of all the cells, you should be able to have a new body and, consequently, a new lease on life, at least once every few years. In this book you will learn about the body's built-in mechanisms that can stop the clock of aging and make you younger and healthier the more years you add to your chronological age.

We are right in the middle of a tremendous global transformation that has already greatly influenced, if not shaken up, the very foundation of conventional medicine. The old division of body and mind into completely separate and independent entities is crumbling fast with the knowledge supplied by the more progressive wings of medical science such as *Psycho-Neuro-Immunology* or *Mind/Body Medicine*. The division of body and mind, which is based on the old and outdated paradigms of understanding human nature, has never really existed. Nevertheless, this false notion about the true reality of human existence continues to make man believe he is essentially a physical being. And to some degree, we all agree with that idea. Since today's study and practice of human health largely ignores the important role of the mind, feelings and emotions, those put in charge of taking care of our well-being stand little chance of guaranteeing us a reasonably satisfying state of health. As it will become apparent from reading this book, instead of eradicating disease from the surface of the earth, the purely symptom-oriented approach to health care has greatly diminished the probability of truly curing diseases and, in fact, has contributed to the occurrence of chronic diseases and death more than any other cause.

We are now beginning to recognize the inseparability of the body and mind. The breakthrough discoveries in the field of *mind/body medicine* have already helped thousands of people regain their health. Current scientific understanding shows that mind and body never exist as separate or independent entities. A hand can never write a letter unless the mind orders the hand to do so. You cannot even move your eyes to read these words unless your mind has given you the definite instruction to follow their sequence. The mind also must have the proper perception of the body and the will to maintain life. Consider, for example, a person with anorexia. Because the person's thoughts are distorted to believe that she is fat, the desire to eat is greatly diminished or stopped, causing the physical body to deteriorate or even die. Thus, the mind and body are intimately connected and dependent on one another. Our life is controlled by what I call 'super intelligent body/mind'. Without its supervising presence, the body's 60-100 trillion cells, with their over one trillion biochemical reactions per second each, would proportionally generate as much chaos and confusion as would be created in the case of the dissolution of the universe.

You can also experience the intimate relationship between mind and body when you get a stomachache from feeling upset, or when you faint after receiving a very distressing piece of information. Some people have literally turned gray overnight due to a traumatic event, and others blush when they feel embarrassed. Heart attacks can be triggered by a single bout of anger or intense anxiety, regardless of whether the coronary arteries are clogged or open. All thoughts and feelings are instantly translated into biochemical compounds within the brain and within every other part of the body, thereby altering physical appearance and performance. In fact, every bit of mental activity leaves us with a specific physical sensation known as emotion. Emotions are composites of both mental impulses and physical changes, and they express the totality of one's health at any given time.

Your endocrine system, which produces hormones in response to your mental experiences, is indeed your personal drug store and it comes free. Your inner pharmacy can make any drug you need, and you are the pharmacist who writes the appropriate prescriptions. Depending on your emotional response or reaction to a particular event or challenge, the drugs and their doses vary accordingly. They may include the stress hormones *adrenaline, cortisol* and *cholesterol*. When released into your bloodstream in response to anger, fear or rejection, for example, these hormones can save your life, but if secreted in an ongoing manner, they may damage the blood vessels and impair the immune system. Your happy emotions on the other hand manifest as *endorphins, serotonin, interleukin II* or other drugs that are related to the experiences of pleasure and satisfaction. If you produce enough of these chemicals, you may even be able to arrest the aging process.

Carefully controlled studies have shown that you can reduce your biological age by 10-15 years within ten days, provided your interpretation of your life experience undergoes rapid and positive changes. By contrast, you can also put on 20 extra years within a single day if you enter a state of hopelessness and depression. Hormones produce extremely powerful effects, both in a positive and negative sense. Yet even more powerful than hormones are the thoughts and intentions that trigger them.

For many years now, hospitals have been recording cases where cancer patients have experienced what is generally known as 'spontaneous remission'. A remission of a cancerous tumor or other serious illnesses may occur when the affected person suddenly enters a feeling of profound trust and unprecedented happiness. Others recovered from a terminal illness when they got 'addicted' to laughter. Our physical makeup is capable of providing formerly unknown and extremely powerful chemicals in response to a newly adopted perception of reality. This intrinsic ability of the human mind/body system can help evolve our hormonal system (endocrine system) to a much higher level of efficiency and bestow abilities to our body that are beyond our current level of understanding or imagination. The mind/body connection will be discussed at great length at the beginning of this book because it forms an essential part of the endeavor to improve our physical and mental health.

The journey to develop a permanent state of health and vitality has very little to do with treating disease, yet treating illness is the main focus of conventional medicine. True healing is about reestablishing the intimate connection that exists between a healthy body and a healthy mind. It would be foolish to try combating darkness in a room when all we need to do is to switch on the light. The darkness isn't the problem we need to get rid of. It is the missing light that creates the darkness. By lighting a candle in a dark room, the darkness disappears instantly. Likewise, disease disappears by the act of generating healthy, life-supporting effects in our body and mind. The bottom line is that good health remains an unrealistic dream when the focus is on disease. Blaming an illness for our lack of well-being, and treating it as if it were an enemy, forms the very basis of today's health crisis.

A basic natural law states that *energy follows thought*. If disease is your point of focus, or remains a point of reference and truth in your life, you are going to be stuck with it because disease thrives on negative energy. Over 90 percent of all diseases in our Western civilization are chronic by nature and there are no successful treatments available for these, at least not in the field of conventional medicine. The inadequacy of the modern medical system to deal successfully with chronic disease is rooted in the collective conviction that we need to get rid of the symptoms of disease in order to get our health back. If we instead focused our attention on setting the preconditions and restoring the mechanisms responsible for creating and maintaining good health, health would return quite naturally. It is not disease that needs attention, it is the patient who requires love, care, nourishment and the feeling of being complete again. The single most important experience that the unbalanced body/mind needs for healing is the experience of happiness which results when a person begins to take his health in his own hands and removes whatever congestion and imbalance that may exist in the body. This is a highly self-empowering process which is pleasing to the heart, body and soul.

A fascinating study showed that happy people are the least likely to catch colds, regardless of how often they are exposed to a cold virus. Also, people who are in love show a higher resistance to disease. To create a positive state of health can be a powerful happiness-generating event. Happiness returns spontaneously in a person who, suffering from a cold or a disease, starts to feel better again. Happiness and health are attractive to us; disease is not. Unhappy people can never be truly healthy, just as unhealthy people can rarely be truly happy. A person who suffers from cancer and learns to apply the methods of regaining his happiness described in this book may suddenly cure himself, but if he continues hating his mother, father or ex-spouse, then even these or similar therapies are bound to be unsuccessful in the long run. By focusing on disease or negativity in life, one remains trapped in unresolved and continuous cycles of anger and conflicts. This, in turn, will have a powerful immune-suppressive effect and prevent true healing from taking place. The focus on the destructive characteristics of a disease - widely known as symptoms of disease - cannot serve as a source of inspiration to bring about a real healing response and an ever-evolving state of health. There is, in fact, little to be gained from a fascination with disease, including its diagnosis. In contrast, there is everything to be gained from a fascination with health.

The human body has no built-in programs for sickness, but it has many programs to maintain a state of perfect equilibrium or balance, and if balance is lost, to return to it. It is the nature of the human being to be healthy, but it is up to us to set the preconditions for these programs to work efficiently. To repeat, healing is absent when happiness is absent. Bereaved persons, whose sense of joy has virtually become non-existent, demonstrate this most clearly. Widows rank among the highest in the risk groups for cancer. Sadness, because of the loss of a loved one, blocks a person's normal immune response to fight cancer cells, even though his or her T-cell count may be in the normal range. Major studies on heart disease have shown that lack of happiness and job satisfaction head the list of risk factors for heart attacks; they are far more endangering to our health than animal fats, alcohol and even cigarette smoking.

The main purpose of life is to increase happiness. Any action that deviates from our purpose and does not support this most basic principle of life is destined to fail or generate impediments - problems that are designed to lead us back to the path of happiness. This is as true for the field of health as it is for every other area in life. Most of the advice given in this book has an uplifting or a clarifying effect, thus providing a solid foundation for creating and maintaining good health. The *liver and gallbladder flush* described in chapter seven, which can remove hundreds of gallstones from these important organs within a few hours, can by itself trigger waves of utter wellness and eliminate deep-seated anger and frustration. The clearing of severely blocked ducts and channels of circulation in the body can have truly blissful effects and most certainly change one's priorities in life. With the continued improvement of your health, you may find yourself entering a state of completeness where the pieces of the puzzle of life will naturally fit into their designated places.

As you read about the various ways of improving your physical health, try to remember that they are closely tied to your mental and emotional well-being. If you suffer from a particular illness like cancer, heart disease or AIDS, apart from dealing with the physical aspect of the imbalance, you will also need to attend to its mental and emotional counterparts. Disease is not something that you just 'catch'. Instead, it is something you create by repeatedly setting up the same limitations that prevent your body and mind from being in their naturally balanced states.

You don't need to receive permission from anyone or from any government agency to improve your health because this is your natural birthright. The advice given in this book is not meant for curing diseases because it is not disease that needs curing; it is the suffering person who needs to become whole, happy and vital again. You can never really cure a disease because disease only occurs when health is no longer being created or when you are no longer in tune with your inner purpose, your natural sense of joyful existence, and the world around you. However, once you have allowed balance to return to your body and mind, disease will disappear by itself, just as the darkness of the night disappears with the light of the day.

Most of the data and research that I mention in this book is based on what are generally considered 'reliable' sources, such as published papers and scientific journals. But although I have cited scientific research studies throughout the book to clarify and illuminate basic insights, it is my opinion that medical research in itself cannot serve as a reliable source of truth and reality. In fact, most medical research has been used to serve vested interest groups, such as the pharmaceutical industry, to manipulate the masses into submission and expose them to potentially fatal treatments. All research is unaltered by the changing factors of time, the unaccountable subjectivity of the researchers and those being researched, as well as the intended objectives of the research.

In my view, scientific research should not be used in an exclusive manner to formulate a particular truth because it is very easy to employ research studies as a means of manipulating opinions and beliefs. In the United States, the FDA withdraws about 150 pharmaceutical drugs from the market each year because of the harmful and dangerous side effects they generate in numerous consumers. These are the same drugs that the FDA had approved several years earlier, on the basis of the rigorous 'scientific' testing procedures that are employed in all clinical studies today. Take the example of the arthritis drug VIOXX, or other painkillers, including CLELEBREX, ALEVE, and BEXTRA. Isn't it astounding that these poisonous, expensive drugs could have passed all the supposedly rigorous, scientific safety tests and been sold to millions of unsuspecting arthritis sufferers, just to find out years later that they sharply increase the risk of heart attack and stroke? Could there be double standards for 'rigorous testing' in the field of medical research: one for 'before' and one for 'after' introducing these drugs to the market? How many thousands of people needed to die (death dramatically raises the stakes for expensive law suits) before the drug producer Merck 'volunteered' to withdraw the drug from the market? Likewise, how can powerful antidepressants be given to unhappy children, when it has been demonstrated that these drugs increase the risk of suicide? These are questions that reflect physics' 'uncertainty principle' which turns the use of medical drugs into a gamble with one's life. The stamp of scientific approval is perhaps one of the most dangerous tools employed by the medical industry today.

I am often asked to supply the exact references for those studies I sometimes refer to, but doing so would place too much credence and reliance on something that is so heavily flawed and unreliable. I suggest that you take any statement or argument you are not sure about into your heart and ask your body how it feels. (A *body-testing* procedure is described in chapter one) Most likely, you will receive a definite answer from your body, which will signal either weakness or strength, or any other form of discomfort or comfort, depending on the input. This book is about enhancing your intuitive and cognitive abilities, rather than presenting mere book knowledge to satisfy intellectual needs. The secrets of health and rejuvenation constitute not a foreign body of knowledge we need to introduce from outside. *You* are the source of these secrets, and the timeless healing wisdom contained in this book is here to show you how to discover and apply these secrets for your own benefit as well as that of mankind.

CHAPTER 1

Solving the Mind/Body Mystery -
And the Magic That Occurs When You Do

Mind Over Matter

The united force of your body, mind and spirit continually seeks to provide you with nourishment, vitality and happiness. The body uses food, water and air to renew and sustain itself. The mind chooses a task that keeps it creative and active. The spirit looks for ways to expand by generating waves of love, peace and freedom and to share happiness with the world as a means of gaining fulfillment.

A delicious meal prepared by a loving parent or spouse can nourish your mind, body and spirit alike. Enjoying one's food can be a spiritual experience, just as much as it can be a physical and a mental one. Being totally 'present' while eating not only triggers powerful pleasure hormones but also provides a sense of union between you, the food you eat and the process of eating. Enjoying the company of a dear friend or family member at the meal further enhances your sense of joy and satisfaction just as a beautiful piece of music soothes not only the spirit but also relaxes the mind and body.

Everything that you do and experience - physically, mentally and emotionally - has a profound bearing on your entire being. Each one of your thoughts, feelings and emotions causes profound changes in your body, mind and spirit. Think of the consoling and loving words you once received from a dear friend while you felt desolate and low.. Did you feel encouraged and uplifted by your friend's presence and words? Did you notice how your body, perhaps bent over, tired and uptight, suddenly began to feel more relaxed and energized? The depressed look on your face turned into a grateful smile and you said, "Thank you, I feel so much better now." On the other hand, can you think of an instance in your life when you received a very distressing phone call, such as a loved one being involved in an accident? The fear that gripped you at that moment had a paralyzing effect on you. But, seconds later, a friend brought you the blessed information that your loved one had escaped unscathed and was well and healthy. Quite immediately, the state of shock ceased and was replaced by a deep sense of peace, joy and relaxation, and your physical strength returned. The sudden good news elevated your feelings and brought the smile back to your face. One split second was enough to trigger a profound internal transformation that changed everything from within you. For a brief moment you experienced a state of utter illness and despair, followed by another moment of perfect health. Unwittingly, you discovered the ultimate causes of illness and wellness.

A German professor of medicine, Dr. Ryke Geerd Hamer, was able to prove that every physical illness, such as cancer, is triggered or preceded by the effects of an unresolved conflict in the life of a patient. After twenty years of research and therapy with over 31,000 patients, Dr. Hamer finally established firmly, logically and empirically, how biological conflict-shock results in a cold cancerous or necrotic phase and how, if the conflict is resolved, the cancerous or necrotic process is reversed to repair the damage and return the individual to health. According to Dr. Hamer, disease, or what he calls "the meaningful biological program of nature," is divided into five biological events, all of which can be identified, measured and observed. These events are part of a system that makes possible a definite (not just statistically probable) prediction of disease progression and development.

A biological conflict-shock - called a DHS (Dirk Hamer Syndrome) causes the appearance of a focus of activity in the brain - called an HH (Hamerschenherd). An HH is composed of a set of concentric rings that can be seen in a computerized tomography scan (CT) centered on a precise point of the brain. The location of the focus depends on the nature of the shock-conflict or conflict contents. As soon as the HH appears, the organ controlled by that specific brain center registers a functional transformation. This transformation can manifest as a growth, as tissue loss or as a loss of function.

The resolution of the conflict would naturally remove these concentric rings in the brain and stop or reverse the symptomatic occurrence of what we generally refer to as 'disease'. This is not difficult to understand. For example, the calm and reassuring words and loving care by a friend can trigger such powerful biochemical responses in your body that your posture changes, your physical expression relaxes and your mood improves. Research informs us that all of our thoughts, feelings, emotions, desires, intentions, beliefs, realizations and recognitions are instantly translated into *neuropeptides* or *neurotransmitters* in the brain. These hormones serve as chemical messengers of information. The messages they deliver determine how your body functions.

Scientists have already located over a hundred different *neuropeptides,* and many more are believed to exist. A nerve cell or neuron produces and uses these peptides to transmit information to another neuron. This form of transmission, which often is referred to as 'firing', magically occurs in each of the millions of neurons in our brain, and at the exact same moment. Immediately after the transmission ends, the peptides are neutralized by enzymes, erasing all physical evidence of that thought or feeling. Yet you have stored the information in the memory bank of your consciousness. If need be, you will be able to recall or remember it.

This simple example shows that your brain is not the ultimate authority of your body. How do the millions of neurons know which type of neurotransmitter they need to make for each specific thought, right at the moment of its occurrence? What causes their simultaneous 'firing' throughout the brain? And more astonishing, how does one neuron know what the other neuron thinks when there is no direct physical connection between the two? This mystery is now becoming increasingly perplexing. In recent years, scientists have discovered that these chemical messengers are not only made by brain cells, but also by all the other cells in the body. This raises the question whether we think only with our brain cells or also with other cells in the body. There is indeed enough scientific evidence to show that skin cells, liver cells, heart cells, immune cells, etc. all have the same remarkable ability to think, emote and make decisions as brain cells.

The cells of our body are equipped with receptor sites for these peptides, which explains why every cell knows what every other cell does or thinks. There cannot be any secrets between cells. Every instruction given or received somewhere is felt as an instruction everywhere. By utilizing these biochemical pathways, the body can translate a strong emotion of fear into chemical messages that order your adrenal glands to trigger the secretion of the stress hormones *adrenalin* and *cortisol*. Once these hormones are released into your bloodstream in sufficient amounts, your heart starts pounding and the blood vessels that supply your muscles with blood begin to dilate. This preprogrammed defense strategy of the body makes it physically possible for you to run away from a perilous situation or to avoid, for example, being run over by a car. However, this effect, known as the *fight or flight response*, constricts important blood vessels in the body, such as the major arteries in the internal organs, and elevates the blood pressure. If such stress responses occur on a regular basis, they can impair digestive and eliminative functions and cause considerable damage to the entire body.

Most people assume that only the adrenal glands can secrete *adrenalin,* but this is not so. Each cell in the body produces this stress hormone, although in proportionally lesser quantities. After the initial burst of energy and physical strength resulting from an adrenalin shot, all the cells in your body may suddenly turn 'jittery' and your body starts shaking. You may feel as if you have lost all your energy in the process. Without your conscious control you have actually practiced 'mind over matter'.

Testing Your Mind/Body Response

At this point, I recommend you learn a simple muscle test derived from the healing method of *Behavioral Kinesiology.* This test will demonstrate to you that at each moment your thoughts, intentions, desires, etc. exert total control over your body. I will refer to this test several times in this book whenever it may be useful to find out whether a particular food, medicine, beauty product, situation, environment, or even a particular desire is conducive to your health or not.

Everyone practices 'mind over body' at all times. However, most of us do it unconsciously. The main purpose of this test is to bring this intimate relationship of the mind and body to the surface of your awareness and truly experience it in a very concrete and conscious way. Whenever you apply the muscle test, you will reawaken the inner wisdom of your body and strengthen your natural instincts, trust and intuition. Eventually, you won't need to apply the test anymore to know what is and what isn't beneficial for you. To conduct the test, find yourself a partner. Follow these simple steps for muscle testing:

1. Both of you need to stand. Your <u>left</u> arm should hang down relaxed by your side, while your <u>right</u> arm is extended in a horizontal position, with your elbow stretched. (If you are left-handed, use your left arm for testing)

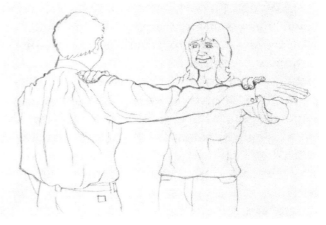

2. Next, ask your partner to stand in front of you. Look at a neutral place, such as a door or a wall, and try not to think of anything or anyone. Ask your partner to place his/her <u>right</u> hand on your right shoulder to keep your body posture in a stable position, and his/her <u>left</u> hand on top of your right arm, just over your wrist (see **illustration 1 of 2 on the right**).

3. Now, ask your partner to press down on your arm, while you try to resist the pressure. Instruct your partner to do this quickly and firmly, but not in a jerky manner, and not longer than about three seconds. The idea is to maintain the pressure only as long as it takes him/her to notice your arm's strength of resistance. Pressing longer will make the muscle weak and produce a faulty test result.

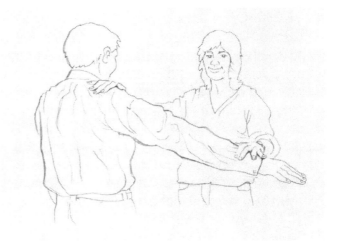

4. Your arm muscle should be testing strong in this neutral state. (Please note that a particularly negative thought, an expectation, physical illness, or being under the influence of shock, alcohol, or drugs may substantially distort the outcome of this muscle test)

5. Next, keep your right arm outstretched, while you try to think of a situation, person, past experience, etc. that would make you feel angry, nervous, or uncomfortable in some way. At the same time, repeat Step 3. You will notice you are not able to resist the pressure applied to your arm, and your arm muscle will immediately give in and become weak. (see **illustration 2**)

Then try to think of someone you love or care about and ask your partner to test your arm muscle once more. Your arm muscle will be strong again.

You may repeat Step 5 of the test while listening to hard rock music, watching a violent movie, or looking at fluorescent light. To test whether a particular shampoo, toothpaste medical drug or food item is suitable for you, place any of these items into one of your hands while you ask your partner to test the muscle of your other arm. Note: If you are left-handed, it is better to test your left arm and place the tested item in your right hand. If these items are not available, merely think of them as he tests you on these products, one at a time.

It may be necessary for you to experiment with this technique on each other for a while before it becomes second nature to you. It is necessary to have an open and unbiased mind when you conduct the test. Don't try to influence or manipulate the outcome in any way, for this may lead to false results. Remember that every thought influences the body in a specific way. Ask any questions you may have that can be answered with a 'yes' or with a 'no'. This may even concern important decisions you need to make, journeys to take, or foods to eat, etc. Once again: to test food items, it may be enough to just look at or think of the food while applying the test.

If you don't have a partner to test you, you may use your whole body as a testing device. Stand in a relaxed manner and repeatedly say the word 'yes' to yourself. This should move or swing your body forward. Now repeat the word 'no' and you find your whole body moving backward. Thus, by asking a question or holding a food or substance close to your chest, you will either swing forward or backward, depending on the body's response to it.

The body's own biofeedback system always works - it never lies. The muscles will respond to a particular stimulation either with weakness or with strength, so long as the test is conducted properly. If even a so-called 'health food' contains something that your body cannot process or digest properly, this feedback system will immediately inform you about it, simply by receiving the appropriate messages from your body cells. A fearful thought, disruptive noise from the street, or the picture on the television news of a killed person is transmitted to your body cells, too. Your body's response is completely accurate and reflects the exact quality of the information passed on to you. However, the way you perceive a situation, challenge or threat may not be as clear to you at all times. Be aware that subconscious desires or aversions can change testing results.

Generally speaking, the cells in your body can detect the frequencies of incoming substances and check whether they are useful or harmful for you at any given time. A cola soft drink gives off different frequencies than an apple. The concentrated phosphoric acid, artificial flavors and sweeteners, large quantities of refined sugar (mostly fructose corn syrup) and other chemicals contained in cola soft drinks are very destructive for biological life forms. So the body's cells will consider them to be poisonous and go into a stress response. Their energy production, measured by the amount of ATP molecules they make, begins to drop abruptly as a result of this response. This practically means that the tissues in the body get increasingly cut off from the routes of energy supply and, hence, become weakened. In practical terms, this situation forces all the organs, glands, blood vessels, nerves and muscles to subsist on minimal energy, which *jeopardizes* the normal functioning of the body. Obviously, the weakening of the arm muscle during the muscle testing procedure occurs in direct response to a perceived external or internal threat or conflict.

Note: You can obtain more detailed information on the procedure from a good book on applied kinesiology. Some circles of kinesiology practitioners are of the opinion that the arm-muscle test is not accurate and cannot be used as a tool for measuring the mind-body response. This would, however, imply that the arm muscles are not directly influenced by the frequencies of information we generate or are exposed to. In other words, the arm muscles would not be included in the internal network of communication. This defies the very principles of physiology and mind/body medicine. Inaccuracies occur only when the rules of the test are not followed exactly and when hidden desires manipulate the results. Eventually, you want to rely only on what your heart tells you. Concentrating on your heart while asking a particular question will usually generate some feeling, some 'knowingness', or even a verbal answer. The first response or impulse tends to be the one to go by.

Stress - And a Shrinking Thymus

The thymus gland, which regulates the activation of *T-cells* (circulating immune cells, also called white blood cells), is the first organ that is affected by stress. *T-cells* help the body to identify and remove cancer cells and other invading agents. The weakening influence on the thymus gland may be caused by such factors as news of negative events, dehydration or the consumption of nutritionally poor and processed foods or beverages. All of these reduce *T-cell* activation by thymus hormones and leave the body without sufficient defenses against the spread of cancer cells and other causes of disease.

The thymus gland shrinks when it is exposed to stress. It is well known that following a serious injury, surgery or sudden illness, millions of white blood cells are destroyed, and the thymus gland shrivels up to half of its normal size. Looking at video footage of Adolf Hitler, a child abuser or a wanted terrorist may be enough to stress your thymus gland significantly. The next time you read a magazine or watch a movie, ask a friend to test your arm muscles while you view the different pictures. You will find that some of these pictures make your muscles strong, whereas others make them weak. (Of course, if you were completely infused with love and compassion versus fear and judgment, you would not suffer such a stress response at all.[1])

Your thymus gland has to deal with massive amounts of negative influences, considering the almost daily exposure to radio, television, newspapers, junk food, chemicals in foods and beverages, indoor and outdoor pollution, and people with negative attitudes etc. that you encounter. Even advertisements that show people smoking cigarettes or drinking alcoholic beverages have a weakening effect on your thymus.

Most people are not aware how much of their life energy is drained by exposing themselves to stressful situations. Regularly spending time in unhealthy environments like smoke-filled rooms or experiencing energy-depleting influences such as driving at night or eating while tired can simply overwhelm the body. When there is no energy left to function normally, one becomes nervous or begins to panic. The most common expression you hear people say when this happens is: "I feel so tense today" or "I am utterly stressed out". Stress is nothing but an experience of constant exhaustion of the thymus gland caused by negative or weakening influences in life. Stress ceases to affect us when we stop exposing ourselves to such influences and corrects the damage that has been caused by them in the past. You can positively strengthen and recharge your thymus and entire body through uplifting and encouraging activities, eating nutritious foods, listening to relaxing music, and spending more time in

---

[1] To learn how to develop such a life, please refer to the book *Lifting the Veil of Duality* and the method of *Sacred Santémony* by the author.

natural surroundings than indoors or in front of the television set. Whether you choose to weaken or strengthen your body, in both cases you are practicing "mind over matter."

Placebo - The True Healer?

The placebo effect works in a similar way. *Placebo* is a Latin word which translates as: "I shall please". If something pleases you, it automatically triggers the release of pleasure hormones in your body, which means that in the event of an illness, you are likely to experience a healing response. In the field of medicine, the placebo effect is a phenomenon described as a measure for testing the efficacy of new drugs or therapies. **Note:** Shutting down or suppressing a symptom of disease has nothing to do with healing it. There are three possible explanations of why and how healing takes place.

1. **A particular non-suppressive treatment triggers a curative response by the body**

2. **The healing power of nature is at work.** This includes especially the immune system's natural response to stop and eliminate disease-causing factors. While this principle (of the body healing itself) applies to the majority of all medical cures, this 'secret ally' of all doctors is hardly ever introduced to patients. The human organism rarely receives praise for the extraordinary abilities it displays when dealing with infections and physical injury. The body's own remarkable healing ability is behind *every* success in the healing profession. In many instances, healing occurs *despite* the side effects that so often arise from the use of medical drugs or invasive procedures. If the body's healing response remains absent, not even the most advanced medical technology or expertise will have any value.

3. **The placebo effect triggers the healing response**

Orthodox medicine originally defined the placebo as an inert substance that, for psychological reasons only, is administered to satisfy or please a patient. However, this definition is no longer considered accurate or sufficient. The placebo effect can occur as a result of administering substances that are *not* inert, just as much as it can be triggered by procedures or pills that do *not* include medication. The placebo effect implies that the patient's belief in a 'drug', which may just be a sugar pill or snake oil, has the power to stop pain and even cure a disease. A basic feeling of trust in a particular treatment or even the doctor can also act like a placebo. A research study is not considered valid or scientific unless it includes a placebo that is applied to a control group.

When the success rate of the drug or treatment is higher than the success rate of the placebo, then the drug has passed the test for effectiveness. In the past, the placebo has even been used to study coronary bypass techniques and cancer radiation treatments. In the case of a number of coronary bypass studies, the surgeons opened the chests of the heart patients in the placebo group and immediately stitched them back up again, *without* actually performing a bypass operation. After surgery, all the patients were informed that their operation had been a success. Some of the placebo group patients confirmed that they experienced relief of chest pain. A number of the heart patients who received the actual bypass surgery also reported relief of pain. If the 'success' rate in the bypass group is higher than in the placebo group, then the bypass operation is considered to be an effective method to relieve chest pain.

An early carefully controlled study with patients suffering from angina pectoris showed that 5 out of 8 patients who had genuine surgery and 5 out of 9 patients who only received a sham operation felt much better afterward. Two of the patients with sham operations even experienced a remarkable increase in physical stamina and endurance. A group of highly skeptical researchers repeated the same experiment with another group of 18 patients. Neither the patients nor the examining cardiologist knew who had actually received the surgery. The results were that 10 out 13 patients with real surgery and 5 out of 5 patients with the sham operation had improved significantly. This experiment demonstrated that the placebo effect combined with the body's healing response might actually be the real power behind successful surgery. Surgery, just like every other treatment, can work as a placebo for the patient; and it seems to have no significant advantage over the placebo. It would, however, be very unwise to have a sham operation and continue with a detrimental lifestyle. The survival rates with sham operations are not more than two years, and with normal surgeries they are not much longer, unless the patient makes major changes to his diet and lifestyle.

When the Placebo Becomes Your Medicine

The mechanics of placebo healing is centered in the belief of the patient that a drug, an operation, or a treatment program is going to relieve his pain or cure his illness. Deep trust or a sure feeling of recovery is all that the patient has at his disposal to initiate a healing response. Utilizing the previously described powerful mind/body connection, the patient may release natural *opioids* (morphine-type painkillers) from areas of the brain that are activated by certain thought processes. The corresponding *neurotransmitters* for pain relief are known as *endorphins*. Endorphins are about forty thousand times more powerful than the strongest heroin.

A patient who develops a cancerous growth may start producing extra amounts of *Interleukin II* and *Interferon* to destroy the tumor cells. Being products of the DNA, the body can make these anti-cancer drugs in every cell and eradicate cancer in a moment (spontaneous remission), provided the patient knows how to trigger their release. The triggers are trust, confidence and happiness, and are the same triggers that can cause a placebo response. To buy these drugs on the pharmaceutical market, you will have to spend up to $40,000 per course of treatment. The 'success rate' with the administered drugs is less than 15 percent, and their side effects are so severe that they can destroy the immune system and sow the seeds for future diseases, including cancers (see the section on 'Cancer - Who Makes It?' in Chapter 10). A 15 percent success rate is typically less than what a normal placebo effect would achieve.

Your body is capable of manufacturing every drug that could possibly be produced by the pharmaceutical industry. Synthetically derived drugs only 'work' because the cells of the body have receptors for some of the chemicals contained in the drugs. This means that the body is capable of making these chemicals too, otherwise these receptors wouldn't exist. The body knows how to make them with the utmost precision, in the correct dosage, and with perfect timing. The body's own drugs cost us nothing, and they have no harmful side effects. Pharmaceutical drugs, on the other hand, are very expensive and much less specific and accurate. In addition, the side effects they produce usually end up being more severe than the ailments for which they are used. What makes matters worse is that an estimated 35-45 percent of all prescriptions have no specific effect on the disease for which they are prescribed. The bottom line is that the majority of positive results are directly caused by the body's own healing response or triggered by the placebo effect. They have nothing to do with the medical treatment itself.

The Placebo in Action

Medical doctors have the status and power to inspire in their patients the confidence to believe that, for their condition, they are receiving the most suitable and best treatment available. The hope to find relief and to get better may be the main motivation behind a patient's visit to the doctor. Also, the doctor is likely to believe that his prescription will produce the desired effect, that is, relieve his patient's symptoms. The combined belief of the doctor in his treatment and the trust of the patient in his doctor can produce a 'medicine' that is capable of transforming even a useless treatment or a non-specific drug into a dynamo of healing. This can very well lead to a definite improvement of the treated condition, and in some cases, to a complete cure. This medicine, though, is nothing other than the placebo effect.

If the doctor is convinced that the treatment of the patient's illness will be successful, the patient's perception of the doctor's confidence is much more likely to produce a placebo response than if the doctor is doubtful about his approach. Dr. K. B. Thomas from Southampton, England has shown that a doctor doesn't even need a prescription to help his patients. Dr. Thomas selected 200 patients who were suffering from various symptoms such as headaches, stomach pains, back pains, sore throats, coughs and fatigue. First he divided the patients into two groups. The patients in group one received a clear diagnosis and a 'positive' consultation, during which the doctor assured them that they would soon recover. He told the second group that he wasn't completely sure what was wrong with them and asked them to come back again in case there was no improvement. Then he divided each group into two subgroups, of which one received a prescription that was a placebo. After two weeks, 64 percent of the patients with the 'positive consultation' had improved considerably compared to 39 percent of the patients who received uncertain advice. Of those patients who received a prescription (placebo), 53 percent had improved, whereas among those without a prescription, 50 percent had improved. This experiment demonstrates that a medical doctor can have a more powerful healing effect on his patient than a prescription drug.

This example may also explain an unusual phenomenon: doctors who really believe what they are doing is best for their patients - although it may defy the logic of scientific understanding - achieve much better results, and their patients do well. If a doctor can inspire a patient to believe that he is going to improve, he has done a much better job than any sophisticated treatment may be able to accomplish. A leading article in the medical journal *Lancet* asked why it should be wrong to give a placebo when the essential modern therapeutic means have no better effects than placebos. It should be the primary aim of medical training to produce a warm-hearted, honest and optimistic doctor who listens to his intuition and feels both compassion and love for his fellow human beings. Medical students should be tested for these basic human characteristics. Those students who are unable to pass this test should be prohibited from practicing medicine. The doctor's very presence can work as medicine. What kind of therapy he uses may indeed prove to be of secondary or complementary value. Thus, the doctor as a living placebo-provider can be more powerful than his treatment, without harmful side effects.

The current trend by large proportions of the population to seek alternative practitioners is not so much based on *what* they offer to a patient, rather, it is a matter of *how* they make their patients feel. The fact that alternative therapists use mostly natural methods and compounds for their treatments makes natural therapies more acceptable to the patient than medical treatments. It also makes their approaches more humane and potentially more powerful as placebos.

We all have a preprogrammed natural instinct to know what is good and useful for us, although many people have managed to subdue it. This gut feeling senses a healing effect from pure, fresh foods, healing herbs and other natural remedies. An herb from the Himalayan mountains or a piece of ginger is more likely to trigger a placebo response in us than the synthetic fat *Olestra* or a pharmaceutical drug used to reduce blood pressure. Natural things are naturally pleasing to the body and mind.

A naturopath has become a symbol for natural healing. Even if his methods may not be very effective, the symbol may still be powerful enough to trigger a good placebo response.

In every medical treatment, the placebo is actually the main determinant of the degree of success the treatment has. The results of every controlled study ever done confirm this statement. If any other treatment administered in the medical system proved to be as effective and consistent as the placebo effect, it would most certainly have been heralded as one of the biggest medical breakthroughs of all times. However, the placebo effect is never or only rarely mentioned in medical textbooks. This is unfortunate because the placebo plays at least as important a role in the process of healing and recovery as an expensive drug or sophisticated medical machinery.

A typical example of this is the drug *digitalis*, which has been used by doctors for over 200 years to treat heart disease, despite the fact that its long-term benefits and safety have never been proven. A major three-year double-blind control study (*New England Journal of Medicine,* 1997) conducted by *The Digitalis Investigation Group* showed that out of 3,397 heart patients who received digitalis, 1,181 patients had died by the end of the study period. Compare this with the 1,194 who died out of 3,403 patients who had received a placebo, and it becomes clear that *digitalis* is no better than a sugar pill in preventing death through heart disease. Still it remains the preferred treatment (over the placebo). Is it possible that those individuals in the digitalis group who didn't die during the course of the study actually survived not because of taking *digitalis* but because of the same reasons the individuals in the placebo group survived? Most likely so, given the almost identical mortality figures. As shown by this study, *digitalis's* only value was to trigger a placebo effect, just as the dummy drug did. In other words, any benefits of the drug besides being a trigger for the placebo response are non-existent.

During medical training, every would-be doctor has to face the unpleasant fact that drugs themselves cannot induce a healing response. A drug may work in only 35 percent of the people who receive it. The rest of them may have either no results or become worse because of the drug's side effects. Doctors also know that a patient has a much greater chance of improving with a certain drug if they *guarantee* an improvement. They have learned that a patient can get better by merely looking at a medicine. However, this effect depends more on the imaginative power and the trusting nature of the patient than it does on the medicine itself.

The Miracle of Spontaneous Healing

Although modern medicine has virtually stumbled over the healing mechanism of the body, it still has not recognized it as such. Almost all of the scientific studies conducted on the thousands of drugs and treatments applied by medical doctors throughout the world included the placebo effect. Although the placebo effect is a purely subjective response by the patient or the subject being tested, it somehow became an essential factor for medical research to be considered objective and reliable. Nevertheless, the placebo effect, which represents the body's own healing mechanism, has never been the subject of research. After all, you cannot patent the placebo healing response and make money from selling it. Instead of learning about the body's healing mechanisms, all the attention has been focused on testing medical drugs or procedures as profitable modalities for the treatment of symptoms of disease. Since these drugs or treatments cannot heal anything - only the body can - they have nothing in them to encourage healing *except* the potential to act as a placebo. Considering the fact that suppression of symptoms has nothing to do with cure, these approaches can be only of secondary value, if indeed they have any value at all.

Moreover, it is erroneous to assume that the improvement of symptoms following a particular treatment must necessarily result from that treatment. Treatments have no healing powers of their own and remain ineffective unless they are able to work as triggers for the placebo or healing response by the body. In addition, treatments geared merely toward getting rid of the symptoms of disease with no regard to its causes, have nothing to do with real healing. Bringing temporary relief to the symptoms may be very desirable for the patient and gratifying to his doctor, but in the long-term, such an approach makes it increasingly difficult for the body to heal itself. Oftentimes, this leads to chronic illness. True healing occurs because of the existing mind/body connection, the removal of internal congestion, and the body's own inherent healing power.

The body's powerful healing mechanism was clearly demonstrated in a classic study on three groups of patients, all of whom suffered from bleeding ulcers in their stomachs. The patients in each group were informed that they would be tested for a new drug that could stop the bleeding of their ulcers. One group received the new drug, the second group was given a drug that increased bleeding, and the third group was given inert placebo pills. Most of the patients were desperate individuals who hoped that the new drug would help them get rid of their agonizing health problem. The results astounded the researchers. The bleeding stopped in patients from all the groups, even in those who received the drug that was supposed to increase bleeding. Could the belief in the new wonder drug have been powerful enough to override the high toxicity of a bleed-inducing drug?

Obviously, in response to their thoughts and feelings of hope and trust, the patients' bodies not only produced special drugs that effectively stopped the bleeding of their ulcers, but they also neutralized the poisonous substances contained in the drug that was meant to induce bleeding.

Thousands of different studies tell of the amazing effects of the placebo response. In another classic study conducted in 1950, pregnant women who suffered from severe morning sickness were given syrup of *ipecac*, which is an effective compound to induce vomiting. The women were told that *ipecac* was a powerful new cure for nausea. To the amazement of the researchers, the women ceased vomiting.

Another intriguing experiment was conducted with the help of medical students. 56 students received either a pink or a blue sugar pill, and they were told that the pills were either tranquillizers or stimulants. Only 3 of the 56 students reported that the pills had no effect on them. Most of the students who received the blue pills assumed that they were tranquillizers and 72 percent of them felt sleepy. Furthermore, the students who took two blue pills felt sleepier than did those who took only one pill. By contrast, 32 percent of the students who ingested the pink placebo pills reported that they were less tired, and one-third of the students stated that they had side effects ranging from headaches, numbness, and watery eyes to stomach cramps, intestinal pains, itching in the extremities and difficulty walking. All responses by the students, except for three of them, were caused by their imaginative beliefs.

The implications of these and similar experiments could have revolutionized the entire medical approach to disease. Unfortunately, the law prohibits the sale of 'drugs' that contain nothing but inert substances. Without such a law, many people could have become their own best healers, using only their trust in a drug that, in reality, isn't a drug at all. On the other hand, if placebo sales were made legal, anyone could make a dummy drug and sell it as a real one. But then who is to decide which one is more effective? A former president of the Royal College of Physicians in London once estimated that only 10 percent of all diseases could be manipulated effectively by modern methods of treatment, including the administration of drugs. Disease manipulation does not necessarily mean that drugs have a curative effect. Actually, most of them merely suppress symptoms, and they are costly. By contrast, a placebo is very cheap or even cost-free. And it has no harmful side effects.

Healing Is Up to the Patient

Most medical researchers know that the patient's mental and emotional state can make the crucial difference whether an administered drug or treatment program is effective or not. If a patient is experiencing depression, anxiety, negative stress, trauma or an emotional crisis, the prescribed treatment will have a much lower chance of success. This fact may explain why pharmaceutical drugs have such meager success rates, on the average, only about 35 percent. The majority of people find no improvement with these drugs, and many report harmful, and sometimes, devastating side effects. Any scientific experiment that tests a medical drug against a placebo, or anyone taking such a drug should, therefore, incorporate or consider the following four crucial points:

1. Are there fewer subjects in the experimental group suffering from depression, anxiety or trauma than in the placebo group?
2. Would the experiment end differently if the control group received the real drug and the experimental group the placebo?
3. Would the results of the experiment be the same if the researchers assigned to administer the drug to the different groups were asked to switch the placebo and drug groups?
4. Would any pharmaceutical company risk repeating the same experiment, but with different subjects, if this could lead to significantly altered or even contrary results?

It is important to realize that a particular drug or treatment may produce different results in different people and can, therefore, not be considered objectively testable for efficacy. A drug may not work for a particular patient unless he 'allows' it to work. The patient's state of mind, which includes his emotions and subconscious acceptance or resistance to healing, plays the main role in determining how successful the treatment will be for him. The type of therapy he receives may, in fact, play a secondary role. The renowned researcher, Dr. Herbert Benson from Harvard University, once stated: "Most of the history of medicine is the history of the placebo effect." In other words, the ability to cure a disease rests solely with the patient.

Any existing or past trauma, sadness, depression, anger, or unresolved conflict can lead to unconscious programming of the patient's cells to shut down their receptor sites to both internally produced and externally supplied drugs. This may render any medical intervention useless, if not harmful. It is well known that if a patient is in shock, for example, he cannot be treated or undergo surgery. The same principle applies, although to a lesser degree, to a patient's subjective condition when he receives a treatment, for example, to heal a cancerous tumor. With a general drug failure rate of 65 percent, it is obvious that drugs *do not* do the trick. Rather, it is the recipient of the drugs who determines whether healing takes place or not. True healing requires trust in yourself, your body, and a profound conviction that you deserve to be healthy. Once the body receives the go-ahead signal from you - the conscious being that you are - you will spontaneously invoke a healing response, and your body will take care of the necessary details.

The various levels of trust and belief that different patients place in the potency of a drug may be responsible for the wide range of responses witnessed by doctors around the world. A higher degree of trust can actually increase the placebo's effect from a 25 percent to a 75 percent efficacy! For example, the healing rate for duodenal ulcers among placebo groups in controlled clinical studies ranges from 20 percent to 70 percent. Unless researchers also study the psychological state of the subjects, it is highly unpredictable who will respond positively to a placebo. Some patients report relief of pain after they have been injected with sterile water. An average of 3 to 4 out of 10 surgery patients with serious wounds (caused by ulcers) experience significant pain reduction after they have been injected with a salt solution. No reliable methods in modern medicine exist that can determine or guarantee which patients will respond to a placebo. It is equally impossible to predict how well a patient will respond to a real drug treatment or surgery. Indeed, the subjective state of the patient plays a major, if not the determinant, role in curing an illness.

It is well known that wounds may or may not produce pain, depending on whether the wounded person considers his injury a 'good' or 'bad' wound. According to doctors' reports, many soldiers who were wounded on World War II battlefields did not even require painkillers when they felt that their injuries would help them get into the safety of a hospital and then back home. To them, the injury was the best thing that could have happened to them. On the other hand, a similar serious wound afflicted in civil life through an accident can cause tremendous pain and trauma if it is associated with loss of health, mobility, and financial resources. This suggests that our interpretation of a given situation determines the effect it will have on our lives.

Is Today's Medical Practice Trustworthy?

To conduct double-blind control studies in order to establish whether a particular drug or treatment is useful is a very dubious and misleading practice. Because of the highly elusive and undetermined subjective state of the tested patients, these studies, which are considered the backbone of medical science, may in fact produce very unrealistic, contrived results and outright fraudulent results. Yet they are presented to the public as 'proof' for the reliability of scientific research and medical applications. All this is changing now since recent disclosure of flawed and bad research in medical journals, such as omitting crucial data concerning the arthritis drug Vioxx, or publishing two papers by the South Korean researcher Dr. Hwang Woo Suk, who fabricated evidence that he had cloned human cells.

"Journals have devolved into information-laundering operations for the pharmaceutical industry," say Dr. Richard Smith, the former editor of BMJ, the *British Medical Journal*, and Dr. Richard Horton, the editor of The Lancet, also based in Britain. The journals have a vested interest in keeping the drug giants happy. Industry advertisements is what keeps the journals alive (and also the mass media). In addition, drug companies pay the journals large sums of money for reprints of articles reporting findings from large clinical trials that involve their products. Some journals fail to retract known cases of fraud for fear of lawsuits. Editors may 'face a frighteningly stark conflict of interest' in deciding whether to publish such a study, said Dr. Smith. It is often easier to just let fraudulent data slip through their fingers or minds in the hope that nobody will find out. Fraud has also slipped through in part because editors have long been loath to question the authors. The peer-review system of medical journals, which is supposed to be the iron-gate for keeping away fraudulent medical studies, is now more than questionable, given the recent disclosures of flawed published studies.

There is more reason to be cautious about taking medical research too seriously. In 1994 and 1995, researchers at the Massachusetts General Hospital surveyed more than 3,000 academic scientists and found that 64 percent of them had financial ties to drug corporations. According to the report, which was published in the *Journal of the American Medical Association* (JAMA), 20 percent of the 3,000 researchers actually admitted that they had delayed publication of research results for more than 6 months, to obtain patents and to 'slow the dissemination of undesired results'. "Sometimes if you accept a grant from a company, you have to include a proviso that you won't distribute anything except with its OK. It has a negative impact on science," says Nobel Prize-winning biochemist Paul Berg.

Furthermore, a major research report by the Office of Technology Assessment (OTA), an arm of the United States Congress, came to the most startling conclusion of all. The 1978 report stated: "Only 10 to

20 percent of all procedures currently used in medical practices have been shown to be efficacious by controlled trial." In its October 1991 issue, the prestigious *British Medical Journal* (BMJ) confirmed this report by stating that about 85 percent of all medical procedures and surgeries are scientifically unproven. In other words, 80 to 90 percent of the common medical treatments available to the general population have no scientific backing, and it is doubtful whether they are justified at all. These findings fall in line with World Health Organization (WHO) statistics, which confirm that 90 percent of all diseases prevalent today are not treatable with orthodox medical procedures. Yet, the official medical system claims to have the ultimate authority over treating these diseases. Many doctors actually believe that most of what they practice is based on pure science.

However, it would be erroneous to generalize these findings. Some very successful methods in modern medicine are unmatched by any other form of treatment. They concern mainly acute health conditions caused by accidents, including burns, fractures, heart attacks, certain life-threatening infections, as well as matters of hygiene. The high success rate of medical treatment in these areas is a truly remarkable and exemplary achievement.

For the other 90 percent of diseases, which the WHO recognizes as untreatable by regular medical approaches, modern research techniques have so far failed to produce any breakthrough results. These illnesses comprise the typical chronic ailments, including heart disease, arthritis, diabetes, cancer, etc. Chronic disease is the combined effect of one or several causal factors that are rarely, if ever, considered or recognized in the treatment programs of conventional medicine. With regard to a chronic illness, and contrary to an accidental injury, for example, it is simply not enough to attempt to fix its symptoms. Conducting reliable studies on chronic diseases is therefore virtually impossible, unless of course, crucial factors such as diet, lifestyle, state of mind, emotions, existence of conflict and the like were incorporated in the testing procedures.

It seems that none of the researchers even consider the fact that the healing mechanism, which is triggered by a patient's strong belief in a drug, takes place not only in the placebo control group but also in the main experimental group. It is not very scientific to declare that a new medical drug produces a higher rate of improvement than a placebo when the placebo effect - the patient's trust in the drug - is at work in both groups. The very fact that the placebo effect has to be included as an essential part of every study shows that the subjective state of the patients in both groups remains the major determining factor in the outcome of the experiment. If the placebo group has a success rate of 35 percent and the drug group has a success rate of 40 percent, it is obvious that at least 35 percent of the drug group's success is attributable to the placebo effect and the drug itself causes only 5 percent improvement. Its true success rate of perhaps 1-3 percent (after eliminating other factors of influence such as mental and emotional states) does not justify giving the drug to millions of unsuspecting patients. Yet it is nevertheless advertised and sold as an effective treatment of disease. Obviously, medical research cannot be considered objective or scientific.

Why Some Heal and Others Don't

There is no simple or magical method to make a patient believe in the treatment he receives. The success of the placebo response depends mainly on the patient's psychological condition and whether he has a good reason to believe in his doctor. The following points describe three major categories of personality, which may determine your success in overcoming a serious or life-threatening illness:

1. You feel depressed about everything in your life. You blame others and circumstances for your suffering. You are not happy when others are satisfied and joyful because this increases your feeling that something is missing in your own life. Seeing people being happy makes you feel worse. You lack enthusiasm and self esteem, and your outlook on life is rather dismal. You get angry even without a specific reason. Many times you feel you don't like yourself and you even put yourself down in front of others. You frequently say things like: "Whatever I try doesn't work for me" or "I knew from the beginning that the medicine wouldn't help me". You were unhappy and disappointed during much of your life, and you try not to remember your past. You give up easily and justify your failure by saying, "It's too difficult" or "Nobody cares about me anyway". You feel you are a victim of some kind, and you behave like one. You look for sympathy for your plight, but become angry when you don't receive it. You feel life does not have much to offer, and you see no real purpose in living. You prefer to hang out with friends who also feel as depressed as you do.

2. You are a fighter and you are not willing to give up. Your determination seems to get you through periods of pain and agony. You desperately want to live, and you frequently say things like, "I am going to beat this" or "I am not going to allow this to get me down". However, deep inside you are scared, and you are afraid of not being successful. You often feel lonely and create doubts in your mind. Hope is a big word for you. You hang on to hope as if it were a lifeline.

3. You are easygoing and relaxed. You feel that your disease is not a coincidence or even a reason to become upset or angry. You are not afraid of illness because you interpret it as the body's healing response and an important sign or lesson that may enforce major changes in your life, some of which you were not willing to make before. You are not in a desperate hurry to get rid of the disease and prefer to go through the rough periods consciously. Your attitude toward the disease is not a negative one, even though it makes you uncomfortable temporarily. You listen to the 'messages' your body is sending you, and you learn from them. You accept responsibility for somehow having created this situation yourself, but you don't have feelings of guilt or self attack. The idea that you give meaning to everything in your life - positive or negative - is not a theoretical concept but a practical way of life for you. You feel gratitude toward yourself and others for having arranged your life the way it is at this present moment. You believe in a higher purpose in life and trust that you are taken care of in one way or another. Each and every moment is a precious opportunity for growth and learning about life and self-empowerment. Death is not a frightening issue for you because you know that life doesn't end with physical death, and that there is a special purpose in dying as well. You are involved in practices such as meditation, energy healing, and bodywork, including, Shiatsu, Reflexology, massage, Tai Chi, Yoga and other forms of physical exercise. You feel that the disease will disappear by itself once you have learned the accompanying lesson(s) and are ready to embrace the necessary changes initiated by this illness.

As you may have guessed, persons who are in category 3 or have similar personality traits are better candidates for the placebo effect or for healing themselves than those in categories 1 and 2. A person in category 3 has no reason to believe that a medicine or a treatment will not work. He simply knows within himself that because the reason for the illness is actually a positive one, whatever the outcome, he is going to benefit from it. If one approach to healing does not work for him, he won't feel disappointed but will have enough motivation to look for alternative solutions. If nothing from the outside seems to heal his illness, he is likely to realize that he is has to do it from inside. He already knows, or will come to realize, that the ultimate healer lies within. Not many sick people fall into this category; they are actually the type of people who rarely fall ill.

While a person in category 2 has a good chance of recovery due to his positive attitude, he may nevertheless undermine the placebo effect by reserving a slight doubt in the back of his mind, "just in case…." Trying to think positively is basically motivated by his fear and is, therefore, not good enough to trigger a sufficient healing response. He may be sending out two contradictory signals to his *body/mind*: "Yes, I am going to feel better with this new drug!" and "But I will need to have a backup plan just in case it doesn't work for me". The positive attitude is mitigated or negated by the fear-based doubt. Doubt or fear is a form of energy. If fear motivates or drives your thoughts and actions, this fear brings about exactly what you are afraid of.

A person in category 1 has hardly any self-esteem and spends all his energy accusing others or blaming karma or bad luck for his deplorable situation. He is incapable of triggering the placebo response. Hence he may remain chronically ill unless he begins to value himself and reevaluate his life. Many times, disease manifests itself as a test to find out how much we value ourselves. You can only have as much faith in a drug, a medical treatment or even God as you have in yourself. Self-doubt blocks the healing energies to work for you. A person with low self-esteem lacks self-trust. And trust in oneself is the necessary element to trigger the placebo response, which is needed to truly cure any disease (versus just removing symptoms).

This connection also works when the healing response is triggered by an external source such as another person, like a therapist or a healer. The success that hands-on healing or prayer can have for a sick person is the result of a two-way process but largely depends on the patient's receptivity, deserving ability, and acceptance. If he believes that he deserves to be healed, his body and mind become more receptive to the healing energies, which may include those generated through prayer and loving thoughts. For an increasing number of people, natural forms of healing are much more likely to trigger a placebo or healing response than standard medical procedures, which explains the current tremendous interest in alternative or complementary forms of medicine.

The Paradigm Shift

A definite shift is taking place among medical doctors in the United States and other industrialized nations from the specialized areas of practice toward a more holistic approach to health and healing. Many MDs are becoming disillusioned with their limited field of expertise, which mainly consists of conducting blood tests, giving EKGs, using scalpels, or prescribing pills for diagnosed symptoms of illness. A significant number of U.S. medical schools are now adding courses on holistic and alternative medicine, subjects that were considered taboo in medical circles not long ago. As mentioned before, modern high-tech medicine cannot be applied to chronic diseases. Medical attention is indispensable during situations of crisis when organs have failed, when injuries caused by accidents require surgery or when someone is fighting a life-threatening infection. The vast majority of illnesses, however, are chronic in nature. They include high blood pressure, heart disease, multiple sclerosis, rheumatoid arthritis, diabetes, depression, and other acute disorders that become chronic, including cancer and AIDS.

Patients are becoming increasingly disenchanted with the endless high-tech scans and tests provided by modern medicine. They offer none of the personal care and encouragement which an ill person, in need of a positive placebo effect, so badly needs. This feeling of alienation and helplessness drives many into the hands of alternative practitioners who spend more time with their patients and offer them approaches that include self-help programs like meditation, yoga, dietary advice, and natural remedies. In 1997 Americans made 627 million visits to practitioners of alternative medicine and spent $17 billion of their own money to pay for alternative therapies, including cancer treatment. It is estimated, by none other than the Harvard Medical School, that one out of every two persons in the United States between the ages of 35 and 49 used at least one alternative therapy in 1997. In Australia, 57 percent of the population now use some form of alternative treatment. In Germany 46 percent do, and in France 49 percent do. In addition, a daily increasing number of medical practitioners are turning 'alternative'. **Note:** Going 'alternative' does not necessarily mean you are better off than using conventional methods of therapy. Up to 30 percent of people who visit an alternative practitioner claim to be "very dissatisfied" by the treatment they receive, and up to 24 percent of people using an alternative treatment have reported some adverse reaction to their treatment.

Consumer demand and the economic crisis of the medical system are probably the main reasons that increasing numbers of medical practitioners have turned to low cost treatments and even to prayer and spirituality. Particularly in the United States, where insurance fees for malpractice are exorbitant, physicians are increasingly interested in attending to their patients' spiritual needs. By building more personal relationships with their patients, a doctor lowers his risk of litigation considerably. This may also restore the doctor's image as an infallible caretaker, a role that used to be the rule rather than the exception. The doctor's role as a friend and guide during the difficult times of sickness can, in fact, be a very crucial element in leading a patient to recovery.

The shift from a conventional doctor to an alternative doctor or to one who really cares, however, may not be sufficient to invoke a healing response. Exercising your will and desire to take your health into your hands and to take responsibility for everything that happens in your life is perhaps the most powerful method of healing there is. It tackles the original cause of almost every illness i.e. feeling inadequate, unworthy or not being in control (although most people believe these feelings result from being ill). The most profound and continuous guarantee of good health is the taking of responsibility for your own health and life. This includes the search for and application of natural ways to improve the body, as much as avoiding those factors and influences that cause it harm. Once you know what causes disease, you will be able to rebalance the situation and lay the foundation for optimal health. The following chapters provide an in-depth understanding about ways you may be contributing to your own ill health, aging and disabilities and show you how you can stop and reverse this process for good.

CHAPTER 2

The Hidden Laws Behind Sickness and Health

Disease is Unnatural

The main conclusion we can draw from the study of health and healing is that a natural way of living can prevent disease from arising. Illness results when we deviate from this way of life. It manifests itself when the body tries to neutralize and eliminate accumulated harmful substances and fluids. To restore health, we need to assist the body in removing these toxins; a nutritious diet and a natural program of health care will prevent them from accumulating again.

Disease is the occurrence of a toxicity crisis, which is the body's attempt to return to a balanced condition called homeostasis. This healing or toxicity crisis occurs when toxins in the body have reached a certain level of concentration, which, in this context I refer to as 'tolerance'. I consider toxins to be internally produced or externally supplied substances that have deleterious effects on the body's organ systems, individual organs, tissues, cells, and subcellular units. Toxins may include chemical food additives, environmental pollutants, trapped metabolic waste products, and poisons generated by bacteria that decompose undigested foods in the gut. Once the body's tolerance level for toxins has been reached, it signals pain or other forms of discomfort. This stimulates the organs and systems of elimination, such as the skin, respiratory system, liver, large intestine, kidneys, lymphatic system and the immune system into defensive action. The liver, lungs, colon, kidneys, skin and lymphatic glands may temporarily become congested as the body tries to remove these toxins. The immune response may include the mobilization of immune cells and antibodies that help to reduce the level of toxicity to below the limit of tolerance (see **illustration 3**). During this reactive stage of the toxicity crisis you may feel weak or worn out because the body utilizes every ounce of energy it can get to clear itself of the toxins. Under normal circumstances, physical strength, appetite and good mood will begin to return several days after this healing response. This may give you the impression that your health is back to normal, whereas in many cases you may only have passed the symptom level of the toxicity crisis.

Unless you eliminate the factors that have led to their buildup, the toxins are likely to accumulate again and cause another toxicity crisis. Since the immune system becomes progressively weaker with each new crisis, the likelihood of fully recovering one's health and vitality diminishes, too. The final outcome of repeated cycles of toxicity crises is chronic illness.

Over one hundred years ago, chronic diseases were, indeed, quite rare. At the beginning of the 20th century, only 10 out of 100 people suffered an ongoing illness. Today, chronic diseases make up over 90 percent of all health problems. Nowadays, the general population and doctors alike tend to believe that it is both correct and beneficial to get rid of the symptoms of a disease by any means possible. In most cases, the methods used consist of drugs and surgery. Although their application conveniently bypasses the need to detect and attend to the causes of these symptoms, which are simply indicators of toxicity in the body, the net result of such an approach is the depression of the body's vital organs and systems. Since the body is thus denied the opportunity to remove accumulated toxins, the next time it occurs, it will last longer or be more severe than the first time.

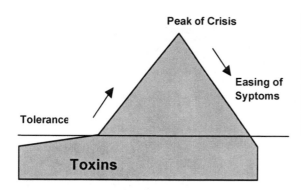

Toxins gradually rise to the level of tolerance where they produce symptoms of discomfort or disease, i.e., a toxicity crisis. Once the peak level of the crisis has been reached, symptoms begin to ease and the condition reverses.

Illustration 3: The Toxicity Crisis

This causes further wear and tear on the immune system and makes a person susceptible to develop exacerbated forms of acute and chronic illnesses. The well-known physician Dr. Henry Lindlahr made this profound and astute observation: "The greatest part of all chronic disease is created by the suppression of acute disease by drug poisoning."

Most of us have made the collective 'agreement' that once a sick person recovers after taking medicine, his improvement must 'obviously' be the result of the medicine. However, this assumption may be erroneous. Healing always takes place *in* the body and is controlled *by* the body. If for any reason, the body can no longer heal itself, even the most powerful medicine cannot achieve what the body's faltering healing system has failed to do.

Disease manifests itself when the body's natural healing responses are weakened or suppressed. The body has a constant tendency to return to its normal state of equilibrium, which is perhaps the real power behind healing any condition. Sometimes the belief in a particular treatment or medicine (placebo) can serve as a trigger for the body to restore equilibrium - an effect that is often wrongly attributed to the treatment rather than to the energies of trust and perseverance that it may be generating in the patient.

The body's maintenance of perfect balance is seriously undermined by energy-depleting influences. A chain smoker, for example, who has developed arteriosclerosis (hardening of arteries) and heart muscle weakness due to constant exposure to carbon monoxide and nicotine, stands very little or no chance of being cured if he continues to smoke. Stockbrokers and professional gamblers have a very high risk of developing heart disease because they suffer constant shocks in their line of work. Taking them away from their jobs by hospitalizing them is often enough to help them regain their health. The suggestion that the medical treatment they receive is responsible for their improvement, however, is more than misleading. They recover because their main source of stress is gone.

The Symptom of a Disease Isn't the Disease

Although you may think you have found the best medicine for your particular health condition, you will not truly be healed unless you stop creating or maintaining its causes. The law of cause and effect applies to everything in life. You may succeed in stopping the symptoms of an illness, but this will only force your body to push the toxic substances into its 'deeper' structures, including the tissues of the organs, joints and bones. Since suppressing toxins makes them 'disappear' from the network of general circulation, the body's ability to tolerate them seems to improve temporarily. This, of course, gives you the leeway to hold on to even more toxins without developing any obvious signs of ill health. If the first lines of the body's defense system were still intact, the body would readily deal with this buildup of toxins by manifesting a cold, a fever or an infection. You would actually feel quite ill. If none of these occur, however, you may believe that you are doing quite well, health-wise, and you are able to get on with your life in the usual manner. Then suddenly, without much warning, an even larger wave of toxicity is unleashed. A typical example of such a crisis is the sudden heart attack or stroke. Many victims of such an attack claim that they have always been "perfectly healthy".

Most serious and life-threatening diseases usually begin with minor problems, such as a simple irritation of the mucus lining in the stomach. This can be caused by overeating, abrasive foods and beverages, or emotional stress. If one's food is too heavy or difficult to digest, the stomach passes some of its hydrochloric acid upward into the esophagus, which gives rise to the sensation of 'heartburn'. A whooping 60 million Americans experience heartburn at least once a month. Over 16 million are plagued by it daily.

Contrary to common belief, heartburn or acid reflux is not caused by too much stomach acid, but by too little of it. Because of an insufficient supply of hydrochloric acid, food remains undigested in the stomach for too long, causing stomach upset. As the acid makes its way into the esophagus, it starts to digest the lining of this delicate structure - hence, the burning sensation.

You can easily test whether *your* digestive problems are related to too little stomach acid. Eat some fresh ginger with a pinch of salt or cayenne pepper before your meal. This will stimulate acid production. If that doesn't help, a common acid supplement called *betaine hydrochloride* (HCI) may work. (Avoid HCI, however, if you have an ulcer) If either of these methods alleviates your symptoms, you will know that your heartburn problem is due to too little stomach acid. To improve digestive functions on a permanent basis, and to solve the problem of low stomach acid, cleanse your liver and intestines and avoid foods that are difficult to digest, such as meat and fried or processed foods. (See later chapters for details) When food is not digested properly, vitamins and nutrients aren't absorbed, leaving you susceptible to a host of degenerative diseases.

If the **irritation** of the stomach lining occurs more frequently because of regular consumption of coffee, soft drinks, sports drinks, sugar, chocolate, meat, nicotine, alcohol, drugs, and other unhealthful items, it may lead to a fully developed **inflammation**. Unless the person's lifestyle and diet are altered to eliminate these irritating substances, an **ulcer** will form. Incapable of removing the daily generated metabolic waste, cellular debris and toxic food particles from the area of the ulcer lesions, the stomach cells can no longer perform their normal activities. While suffocating in such an unnatural and toxic environment, the body must take recourse to unusual survival mechanisms. The most affected stomach cells may be forced to alter their genes through what is known as 'cell mutation'. It may seem that these mutating, 'out-of-control' cells have lost their awareness of being an integral part of the body. However, just like everything the body does, the alteration of the genetic programs of these cells serves a useful purpose, that of removing and absorbing some of the acidic metabolic waste products and other harmful material. This *symptom of disease* is called **cancer**, which is just another name for the body's herculean effort to deal with the constant irritation and poisoning of its cells. Thus, stomach cancer is a natural response to a continuous irritation of stomach cells.

Most currently used medical treatments target only the symptoms of disease, as if they were the disease itself. The prevailing concept is to remove the symptoms in the hope that the disease will disappear as well. In many cases, the use of sophisticated diagnostic tools can precisely identify the symptoms of a disease, which could be a stomach ulcer, cataract of the eyes, stones in the gallbladder, or a tumor in the uterus. The 'treatment' may consist of cutting out the 'culprit', along with the affected organ in far too many cases. The patient is sent home under the impression that he has been cured. Not being aware of what has caused his problems in the first place, his body may turn into a living time bomb. To date, the purely clinical approach of diagnosis has not been able to identify the causal factors for over 80 percent of all diseases. This is perhaps the biggest drawback of today's medical system.

Searching for the root causes of illness is not a focus in medical training. Hence, we cannot blame medical professionals for the current crisis in medical care. In addition, doctors are often pressured by their patients to act as 'legalized drug pushers' or 'symptom hunters'. Many patients practically demand that their doctor remove their symptoms of ill health quickly and by any available means, so they can get on with their lives. They don't realize that this behavior drives them ever closer to another, more intensified toxicity crisis. Added to this dilemma, the side effects that accompany most existing treatments are often so severe that it is questionable whether they are justified at all. This is particularly true when they are used for relatively minor problems.

Miraculous Infection

The following saying sums up the infection myth: "To declare that bacteria and viruses cause all disease is tantamount to declaring that flies cause all garbage." The truth is that microbes actually help cure disease, or at least prevent its escalation. Infection represents one of the body's most extraordinary processes of self-defense. During this rescue mission, the immune system fights off invading bacteria or viruses that have been 'invited' by the host's weakened condition and by the presence of harmful waste material. This engagement of the immune system via an infection is vital to restoring the body's functions. Although these two phenomena appear to be contradictory, they are not. Both are necessary for healing to occur. The germs break down weak, injured or dead cells and waste material that a congested body is no longer able to eliminate, and the immune system deals with the toxins these germs produce when they do their job. The immune system is also essential for keeping germ activity under control and removing these microbes when they are no longer needed.

Doctors usually try to combat bacterial infections with antibiotic drugs. They believe that the bacteria involved in an infection are harmful, but this viewpoint is very incomplete and potentially life-endangering. Germs are naturally 'lured' to the scene of a weak organ or injured parts of the body when the body's own cleansing and healing systems are overwhelmed. Infectious bacteria or viruses naturally avoid areas that are clean and healthy, for there is nothing for them to do or live on. For this reason, germs alone cannot be held responsible for causing disease. This simple truth is confirmed by the fact that if 100 people are exposed to the same cold or flu virus, for example, only a fraction of them will actually get infected. Modern medical research has never really pointed out or tried to understand what makes one person immune to a particular virus and another susceptible to it. Otherwise, we all would have been taught long ago how to stay healthy or how to recover our health if we have fallen ill.

The germ theory of disease upon which almost the entire modern medical system is based, was postulated by the French chemist Louis Pasteur in the latter part of the 19th century. Although Pasteur admitted on his deathbed that his theory was wrong, the whole world had already accepted and begun to perpetuate the myth of the germ theory of disease. Pasteur finally realized that germs cannot cause infection without an underlying reason. He acknowledged that it is rather the cell environment or milieu that determined what types of germs and how many of them attached themselves to the cells of organic matter. This is what a contemporary of Pasteur, Antoine Beauchamp, had discovered and taught long before Pasteur came to the same realization at the end of his life. Beauchamp felt that the ecology of the blood and tissues played the critical role in deciding whether disease conditions would manifest or not.

In 1883 Beauchamp boldly declared: "The primary cause of disease is in us, always in us." We are all exposed to microbes in our body 24 hours a day, throughout our lifetime. In fact, we have more microorganisms in our body than we have cells. Some are dependent on oxygen; others are not. Basically, some microorganisms help us to digest our food and manufacture important substances like vitamin B12, while others help to break down waste materials, such as fecal matter. Without them we would 'drown' in a pool of garbage. Obviously, to survive we need both types of microorganisms, and we breed them inside the body. Beauchamp's work demonstrated that if the acid/alkaline balance (pH) of the body tipped toward acidity, the body produced more 'food' for the destructive germs to feed upon, and the risk of becoming sick increased.

In his experiments, Beauchamp was able to prove the existence of *pleomorphism*, primitive microbes which exist in every person's blood and cells. These can alter their form to appear as different germs. Hence, primitive, harmless microbes live in a strong and healthy alkaline pH but morph themselves into bacteria when the pH changes to become mildly acidic. These bacteria, in turn, become fungi when the pH rises to a level of medium acidity. Finally, fungi become viruses when they are exposed to a strong acid pH. The body's pH moves from alkalinity toward acidity when acidic metabolic waste products, dead cell material, blood proteins, and toxins are trapped and accumulate in the body's fluids and tissues. The result is a toxicity crisis, which is nothing other than the body's attempt to return to a more alkaline state.

Infection is one of the body's most effective means of getting over a toxicity crisis, unless the immune system has already been compromised to a point of no repair, as was common during the Middle Ages when the plague killed millions of malnourished and immune-deficient people. Microbes get out of control only when the level of toxicity in the body is extremely high. In such a case, short-term medical intervention would be justified. The treatment should, however, be accompanied or preceded by cleansing the body from toxins and waste material. Suppressing an infection with prescription drugs can have severe consequences that sometimes may show up years later as heart disease, rheumatism, diabetes, or cancer. This also applies to painkillers - the most commonly used medication in the world today.

Painkillers - The Beginning of a Vicious Cycle

"Drugs never cure disease. They merely hush the voice of nature's protest, and pull down the danger signals she erects along the pathway of transgression. Any poison taken into the system has to be reckoned with later on even though it palliates present symptoms. Pain may disappear, but the patient is left in a worse condition, though unconscious of it at the time."
~ Daniel. H. Kress, M.D.

Taking painkillers, unless it is absolutely necessary for extremely painful conditions, is an act of suppressing and destroying the healing intelligence of the body. When ill, the body may require pain signals to trigger the appropriate immune response for the removal of toxins from a localized area and to prevent the individual from further harming himself. Pain is *not* a disease and should therefore not be treated as one. Pain is the body's natural response to congestion and the subsequent dehydration and malnourishment of the cells and tissues. It occurs in the presence of toxic material and is often accompanied by infection. In most cases, a pain signal occurs when one of the brain's first aid hormones, called *histamine,* is secreted in large amounts and passes over the pain nerves near or alongside a congested area.

The body also uses *histamines* to reject foreign materials such as viral particles or toxic substances and to direct other hormones or systems in the body to regulate water distribution. The latter function of histamine is very important, for where there is a buildup of toxins, there is also an acute water shortage (dehydration). When the pain signal becomes suppressed, however, the body is confused over how it should deal with the congestion and subsequent increase of toxicity. Painkillers also prevent the body from learning about the progressive condition of cellular dehydration. In addition, in order to process painkillers, the cells of the body have to give up even more of their precious water.

Usually, the intensity of pain rises with the concentration of toxins and materials such as blood proteins trapped in the fluid surrounding the cells. This liquid substance is called interstitial fluid or connective tissue, and it is drained by the lymphatic system. When the lymphatic system is congested due to digestive problems or other reasons which I will explain later, the escape route for these blood proteins and toxins is closed. To prevent the immediate destruction of the cells by these highly acidic and reactive proteins and toxins, the body surrounds them with water. This in turn causes further obstruction and prevents the proper oxygenation of the cells. Pain directly results from this lack of oxygen. Research published in December 1964 by one of the earlier journals of the American Medical Association, *Today's Health*, proved that blood proteins naturally leave the bloodstream and enter the connective tissues, but if not instantly removed by the lymphatic system, they can cause disease and death in as little as 24 hours.

The body certainly knows about this danger and acts accordingly. The brain produces the perfect amount of natural painkillers, i.e. endorphins (endogenous opioids), in order to keep the pain tolerable but still strong enough to maintain a powerful and active immune and cleansing response. Synthetically derived painkillers on the other hand cause an electrical short circuit of the pain signal. The brain and the immune system, though, need to receive this signal to be able to attend to the endangered area. The sudden suppression of pain can be likened to cutting the wires of an alarm system that is protecting a house. When a burglar enters this house, nobody will notice it. By cutting off its communication with the brain, the body is unable to remove all the trapped toxins and blood proteins, and their destructive effect may go unnoticed. What is so disturbing about taking pharmaceutical drugs, such as pain medication, is that they need blood proteins to carry them to their destinations. Since the blood proteins are trapped in the connective tissues of an organ, these drugs become trapped there, too. This causes the serious side effects and frequent deaths for which these drugs are so well known. The pharmaceutical industry, of course, does not want you to know that by taking their drugs you are gambling with your life.

Pain medications not only keep the body ignorant about a particular physical problem, they also sabotage its healing efforts. The regular use of painkillers suppresses endorphin production in the brain, thereby causing drug dependency. This also lowers the body's tolerance level for pain, making even minor problems of congestion very painful. Some people have abused their bodies in this way to such an extent that they suffer from excruciating chronic pain, although the causal problem may actually be only a minor one. When painkillers are no longer effective enough, some people may even wish to take their lives to obtain the desired relief.

If you have been on painkillers for arthritis or other painful conditions but now know that taking drugs such as Vioxx, Aleve, Celebrex, and aspirin dramatically increases your risk of heart attack and stroke, you may want to switch to natural alternatives until you have eliminated the root causes of your pain (as this book recommends that you do). According to the *New England Journal of Medicine*, "anti-inflammatory drugs (prescription and over-the-counter medications which include Advil, Motrin, Aleve, Ordus, aspirin, and over 20 others) alone cause over 16,500 deaths and over 103,000 hospitalizations per year just in the U.S." The amount of five major painkillers sold at retail establishments rose 90 percent between 1997 and 2005, according to an Associated Press analysis of statistics from the Drug Enforcement Administration.

Even the smallest amount of aspirin triggers at least some degree of intestinal bleeding. Regular use of aspirin has serious consequences. Nearly 70 percent of those taking aspirin daily show a blood loss of ½ to 1 ½ teaspoons per day, and 10 percent lose as much as two teaspoons per day. A recent study published in the *Annals of Internal Medicine* showed that use of NSAIDs such as aspirin and ibuprofen increased the risk of high blood pressure (HPP) by nearly 40 percent. Similar use of acetaminophen was found to increase HBP risk by 34 percent.

The following list provides you with alternative solutions to pain management without interfering with the body's own efforts to heal itself:

- **Boswellia (*Boswellia serrata*)** is an Ayurvedic herb. It alleviates pain and improves mobility in people with arthritis. It also has **anti-carcinogenic, anti-tumor, and blood lipid lowering activities.** Dosage: 1,200 to 1,500 mg of a standardized extract containing 60 to 65 percent boswellic acids two to three times daily.
- **Bromelain,** an enzyme derived from the pineapple stem, has anti-inflammatory effects. Dosage: 500 mg three times daily between meals.
- **Cayenne (*Capsicum annuum*) cream.** For pain relief, apply to the affected area two to four times daily.
- **Devil's claw (*Harpagophytum procumbens*)** may improve knee and hip pain. Dosage: 1,500 to 2,500 mg powdered extract daily, or 1-2 ml of the tincture three times a day. Do not take devil's claw if you have a history of gallstones, heartburn or ulcers.
- **Evening primrose, black currant and borage oils** reduce joint inflammation. Dosage: Up to 2.8 g of Gamma Linolenic Acid (GLA) daily. Avoid any refined oils or margarine.
- **Fish oils** to reduce joint inflammation and promote joint lubrication. Dosage at least 1.8 mg of DocasaHexanenoic Acid (DHA), an omega-3 fat and 1.2 mg of Eicosapentaenoic acid (EPA), an omega-3 fat.
- **Ginger (*Zingiber officinale*)** tea made with fresh ginger. Eat fresh ginger before and with meals, take 1 to 2 grams of ginger powder in capsule form two or three times daily, or use 1 to 2 ml of the tincture two or three times daily.
- **MSM (Methylsulfonylmethane) - organic sulfur -** has natural anti-inflammatory properties. Dosage 2,000 to 8,000 mg daily. Start on a small dosage and build up gradually.
- **SAM-e (S-adenosylmethionine)** prevents the loss of water in cartilage, which keeps the joint more flexible. Dosage: 600 to 1,200 mg daily for two months, followed by 400 to 800 mg daily as a maintenance dosage.

Caution: If you take any of the above, be sure to avoid non-steroidal anti-inflammatory drugs (NSAIDs) such as aspirin or ibuprofen to avoid adverse reactions.

Besides taking supplements, there are of course, other options for pain relief that you may wish to explore. These include dietary adjustments, exercise, physical therapy, stress management, massage therapy, acupuncture, acupressure and yoga.

Stimulants Make Strong People Weak

All stimulants are 'sweet' when ingested but 'bitter' in their effects. You can become addicted to them without even recognizing your dependency. If you are used to drinking a few cups of coffee a day, try this: Go on a 'coffee fast', which means having no coffee for an entire day, and observe how you feel as the day progresses. After a few hours you may notice a dull sensation in your head and a feeling of weakness and lack of energy throughout the body. Some people develop headaches in the afternoon; others yawn and feel downcast. These effects may seem to be due to the absence of coffee in your diet that particular day, but it actually reveals the weakening impact the coffee has been having on your heart. You may argue, "But drinking coffee is normal, everyone does it." Most people in the industrialized nations will also fall seriously ill at some stage in their lives. For example, one in every two people in the U.S. will develop cancer at some stage of his or her life. This is now considered to be an almost 'normal' experience, too.

Stimulants, as contained in coffee, tea and cigarettes, seem to be welcome and fast-acting substances for those who feel the need for a boost of energy, to wake up their mind or to feel more buoyant and alive. But since these stimulants have no real energy on their own, where is the energy boost coming from? Obviously, the body provides it. Stimulants are nerve toxins that trigger a powerful defense reaction in the body. When you smoke a cigarette or drink a cup of coffee or power beverage, the resulting boost in energy occurs because of this immune response. Therefore, the experienced increase in physical energy is actually an energy loss for the body.

Many people now drink decaffeinated coffee in the belief this protects them against the addictive effects of caffeine. *Consumer Reports* recently tested cups of decaf coffee ordered at six of the most popular coffee shops in the United States. A regular cup of coffee has from 85 to 100 milligrams of caffeine, while decaf coffee has from 5 to 32 milligrams of caffeine (about the same amount contained in 12 ounces of Coca-Cola Classic). In addition to still getting a significant amount of caffeine, drinking three cups or more of decaffeinated coffee may cause an increase in harmful LDL cholesterol by increasing a specific type of blood fat linked to the metabolic syndrome, according to a study presented at the American Heart Association's Scientific Sessions 2005. Decaffeinated coffee is made from more acidic beans than regular coffee. These strong acids have shown to increase the incidence of heartburn, osteoporosis, Glaucoma and rheumatoid arthritis. Decaf coffee can, in fact, quadruple the risk of developing rheumatoid arthritis in three months, compared with people who drink regular caffeinated coffee or tea. In other words, if you feel you cannot do without coffee, it is far better to drink a properly brewed cup of real, unprocessed coffee (or better, this healthy coffee described below).

There are other causes of energy depletion, such as overeating or ingesting unnatural foods. Natural food, although it has a stimulating effect, provides balanced doses of physical energy and helps to support all functions in the body. This kind of natural stimulation maintains physiological balance or homeostasis. Eating too much of any kind of food, on the other hand, causes over-stimulation, and so does regular snacking. Excessive sexual activity, overworking, stress and fear also cause continuous over-stimulation. Thus, the body, in an attempt to deal with the increased demands placed upon it, begins to over-secrete its own stimulants. These are the stress hormones *adrenalin, cortisol, epinephrine, cortisone, endorphins, prolactin*, etc., which are needed to sustain the body's most essential activities. Yet, abusing the stress response day after day and thereby wasting the body's energy resources take their toll on both the body and the mind.

One of the undesirable side effects of excessive *adrenalin* secretion, for example, is a constriction of important blood vessels, including those that supply the intestines. This greatly diminishes the body's ability to digest food and eliminate harmful waste products. Consequently, destructive bacteria begin to decompose the waste matter while producing powerful toxins. Many of these toxins enter the lymph and blood. Toxins have a strongly stimulating influence on the body, which may drive a person into a mode of hyperactivity. The body's energy reserves become depleted further, and a toxicity crisis or acute illness becomes unavoidable. The toxicity crisis can weaken the body to such an extent that it is hardly able to perform. Thus, the body allocates energy only to those functions that are absolutely vital. Given this condition, feeling faint, nauseous or weak is perfectly natural. This helps the body to preserve energy and use it to break down the toxins and eliminate them from the area of congestion. If the energy-depleting causes are discontinued, the body will regain its balance. But if they are not, the body may enter one crisis after another until the person falls seriously ill. Through constant over-stimulation, even a strong and healthy person may eventually become weak, frail and chronically sick.

Healthy Coffee: This is good news for coffee drinkers who just like drinking coffee, but without its unpleasant and harmful side effects. WholeFoodFarmacy.com has come up with a coffee that is made from real coffee beans, but that does not give you that typical burning sensation or the jitters. It actually is a health drink that has many benefits, such as boosting immunity. Their coffee is a delicious, mountain grown, fair trade, organic coffee that is roasted to perfection. The whole coffee beans are then proprietarily infused with 4 unique, ancient, renowned mushrooms. These mushrooms are Cordyceps Sinensis, Ganoderma Lucidum (Reishi), Agaricus Blazei, and Coriolus Versicolor. Known for their immune building potential, these mushrooms render an even more immediate enjoyment. You may even drink it to relax or before bedtime.

Our Constant Need for Cleansing

The body is continually involved in a process of self-renewal. Each day of your life, the body is challenged to build 30,000,000,000 new cells (anabolism), but in order to maintain homeostasis, it also must destroy the same amount of old cells. The breaking down of dead, worn-out cells leaves behind a massive amount of cellular debris, which is instantly taken up and removed by the lymphatic system. The waste can only be removed if there is enough water available to transport it through and out of the body. However, if the body has been weakened through constant over-stimulation, overeating or sleep deprivation (all of these have dehydrating effects), the cleansing process becomes inefficient, and toxic compounds begin to accumulate in the lymph vessels. Some of these toxins seep into the bloodstream, which could cause blood poisoning. To prevent such an event and to keep the blood as pure as possible, the body tries to dump many of the toxins in the connective tissue (the fluid surrounding the cells). Since the lymphatic system, which is responsible for removing most cellular metabolic waste products, dead cell material and acidic blood proteins from the connective tissue is already congested, the cell environment cannot be cleaned up properly and becomes increasingly toxic. The cell environment's pH moves toward higher acidity. When the connective tissue cannot accommodate any more toxins, they begin to invade the blood vessels and also the cells of organs. The first cell groups to become affected with toxins are also the first to be deprived of regular supplies of water, oxygen and nutrients, and hence, the first to signal a toxicity crisis. A toxicity crisis reflects the accumulation of too many acidic compounds (acidosis), including lactic acid, uric acid, ammonia, urea, blood proteins, and of course, toxins of various kinds.

Although only one organ or part of the body may develop a symptom of acidosis, such as an ulcer, occluded blood vessels or a tumor, in reality, the whole body has fallen ill. To deal with this precarious situation, all the systems and organs team up to fight for the body's survival. They do this by diverting energy from the digestive system, muscles and other areas toward the afflicted part. This concerted action provides the immune system with enough energy and resources to counteract the threat imposed on the body by high concentration of toxins. Consequently, during the course of the immune response, the afflicted person may feel very weak, tired and ill. This, however, is *not* the time to interrupt the body's healing efforts or to stimulate it in any way (through drugs, food, TV, excitement, or any other activity). What the body needs is rest.

During a toxicity crisis most people tend to panic and go to a doctor, who immediately attempts to suppress the symptoms of the body's healing response, which mistakenly is called disease. After a few such interventions, which usually consist of medication, the condition may begin to turn from acute to chronic.

The incidence of chronic illness began to increase dramatically with the onset of medical intervention via such treatments as drugs, surgery, and radiation. All of these interfere with the body's own healing responses. Although medical intervention has saved the lives of many people who have been afflicted with acute illnesses such as a stroke or heart attack, it has had little impact on chronic diseases. These diseases are likely to remain chronic unless the mainly *symptom-oriented* approach of treatment becomes *cause-oriented*.

Symptoms of Disease are like Sand in the Hand

Symptoms of disease are highly changeable, if not unpredictable. The causes of disease remain obscure to most medical practitioners and their patients. A stomach catarrh, or inflammation of the mucous membrane, for example, may initially show up as an irritation and then become an ulcer. Next it may be perceived as a hardening of tissue and, eventually, be diagnosed as cancer. The course and intensification of pathological symptoms (signs of disease) may vary from person to person, and relatively few people develop the cancer stage. However, the previous stages can be equally life threatening. As a matter of fact, many more people die from acute digestive problems than from cancer and coronary heart disease.

A stomach catarrh may be accompanied by various kinds of complaints, including stomach upset, nausea, vomiting, gastritis, and cramping of the stomach. In truth, two people suffering from gastritis never have exactly the same symptoms. One of them may be a very nervous person and his symptoms of gastritis may include headaches and insomnia. The other may suffer an epileptic attack. As the stages of the disease become more pronounced, some, but not all afflicted patients, develop anemia as a result of ulceration and putrefaction of cell proteins. A number of people form hemorrhoids when stomach ulcers begin to occur. Others suffer from stomach congestion, where the food is practically stuck and vomited every second or third day.

Modern medicine views each set of symptoms as different types of disease, each of which requires a separate approach or treatment by a specialist. This makes medical diagnosis and treatment so complex that even doctors are confused as to what measures to take to help their patients. Each new variation of disease produces different symptoms in different people, and the specialists are unable to identify the common cause of the various complaints. Since doctors aren't trained to search for the cause of the complaints, they tend to treat the various symptoms as if they were separate diseases. To them, the initial stomach pain seems to have no connection with the inflammation of the catarrh; the thickening of the stomach lining is dissimilar to a stomach ulcer; an ulcer is certainly not a malignant tumor; and the tumor just appears out of the blue.

A physician may be able to stop initial pain in the stomach with an antacid or a painkiller, and when the catarrh occurs, he may prescribe anti-inflammatory drugs. As the growing ulcer becomes unbearable, a surgeon may decide to cut it out. When the cancer appears, an oncologist may prescribe chemotherapy, radiation, or surgical removal of the tumor and parts of the stomach. Yet none of these symptoms are diseases in themselves; all of them are caused by something else, and without dealing with that something else, the disease will continue to appear in other, seemingly unrelated forms and variations. Symptoms are like sand in the hand. They are fleeting and inconsistent. Only those trained to connect symptoms with their causes can reveal the true nature of disease. Clearly then, it is *not* in the best interest of the patient merely to receive treatment for the symptoms of his chronic ailments. Addressing the underlying cause is crucial for genuine healing to occur.

Searching for the Cause

Not many people try to find out why their stomach becomes irritated or in what ways they may have contributed to their own illnesses. Instead, they feel they are doing all they can to become well by simply treating the symptoms of their illness as they manifest one by one. Unfortunately, even by removing the final stage of the symptom of disease, which in the above case is a cancerous tumor, the physician has done nothing to address the cause of the very first symptom of disease, stomach pain. Eating irritating foods and bottled salad dressings or having too much refined salt or hot chili may have caused the pain. Others causes may include feeling emotionally upset, smoking, drinking too much alcohol, regular intake of coffee, soft drinks, or artificial sweeteners, overeating, liver congestion, or not drinking enough water.

The latter is probably the most common, yet the least known cause of stomach problems and many other illnesses. I am using the example of stomach disorders to describe the basic mechanisms leading to disease. Most stomach pains are signals of advanced dehydration of the mucus lining. Consisting of 98 percent water and 2 percent water-holding scaffolding, the mucus layer serves as a natural buffer of protection against stomach acids. The cells below the mucus layer secrete sodium bicarbonate, which is kept there to neutralize any of the hydrochloric acid that may pass through the mucus lining. The resulting chemical reaction between the two chemicals produces salt from the sodium bicarbonate and chlorine from the hydrochloric acid. Consumption of foods that require the secretion of large amounts of hydrochloric acid, such as meat, fish, eggs, cheese, and other high protein foods, thus causes high salt production inside the stomach. This alters considerably the water-holding properties of the scaffolding material of the mucus lining. Regular consumption of such foods in large amounts leads to an intensified acid neutralization, and subsequently, to an accumulation of salt deposits in this layer. This causes 'erosion' which will allow the acid to reach the stomach wall, and the result is the well-known pain of *dyspepsia*.

As long as the mucus barrier is properly hydrated through regular water intake, and protein and fat consumption is moderate, any salt deposits are washed away. In addition, sodium bicarbonate is retained, and the hydrochloric acid is neutralized before it even has the chance to penetrate the mucus layer. Thus, there can be no better acid barrier to the stomach wall than water. Yet the stomach pain, which in most cases is rather a thirst pain, is usually combated with antacids and other medications. These drugs, however, do not offer efficient protection against the natural action of the hydrochloric acid. Most people with stomach ulcers and severe abdominal or dyspeptic pain, experience almost instant and total relief of their discomfort after drinking 1-2 glasses of water. Caffeine-containing beverages such as most soft drinks, tea or coffee, on the other hand, have a diuretic effect, and draw water from the protective stomach lining. One cup of coffee or an alcoholic drink can easily bring on a painful attack.

The stomach pain is the first signal to tell a person that something is off balance with regard to his eating habits or the hydrating of his body. The suppression of this pain through drugs usually prevents the patient from finding out what is causing it. Thus, the ignorance about the mechanism of water metabolism - mistaking the thirst pain for a disease, which is a gross misdiagnosis - can be held responsible for the suppression of the initial symptoms of discomfort that could eventually end up as cancer. Most cancers are the result of repeatedly suppressing mild symptoms of illness such as a cold, pain, infection, or headache and treating them as if they were real diseases.

The purely clinical approach to treatment focuses on the progressive stages of pathological symptoms and keeps producing new findings that promise a cure for each of these problems. In 1982, a bacterium was discovered by Marshall and Warren, which supposedly causes more than 90 percent of duodenal ulcers and up to 80 percent of gastric ulcers. The microbe is a spiral-shaped gram-negative bacterium known as *Helicobacter pylori* (H. pylori).

The link between H. pylori infection and subsequent gastritis and peptic ulcer disease has been documented through studies of human volunteers, antibiotic treatment studies and epidemiological studies. This well-established link, however, does not reveal much about which one of the two is the cause and which is the effect. This stomach bug may just as well be a 'byproduct' of ulceration rather than its cause. Such a scenario would not be unusual since bacteria automatically appear wherever there is dead matter, as occurs in ulcerated tissue. The antibiotic drugs omeprazole and amoxycillin, now prescribed for stomach ulcers, together with secretion inhibitors, destroy the bug, and the ulcers disappear. This, of course, brings great relief to many sufferers. Why do the ulcers disappear? Bacteria produce toxins which prompt the body's inflammatory response (ulceration). However, inflammation is not a disease but the body's way to heal itself and prevent a much more serious condition than an ulcer (see explanation below). Most people would be inclined to conclude that the ulcers are caused by the bug. However, once the antibiotics and acid inhibitors are discontinued, the bug and the ulcers may return. According to research, H. pylori colonizes the stomach in about 50 percent of all humans, and once you have it, you have it for life.

In countries with high socio-economic standards, infection is considerably less common than in developing countries where virtually everyone may be infected. If H. pylori causes stomach ulcers, why doesn't everyone in the developing world have them? Instead, stomach ulcers are much more common in the industrialized world. Although most people in the world have H. pylori bacteria in their stomach right from early childhood, in most of these individuals, H. pylori infection is asymptomatic. Only 10-15% of infected individuals will at some time experience peptic ulcer disease. The main question we need to ask is not whether an individual who suffers from a stomach ulcer is infected with H. pylori, but why this bacterium is more active or proliferates in some individuals rather than in others. And why does it return after the ulcer has been 'cured' by the drug treatment? In other words, there must be another reason for the ulceration than simply the presence of a particular bacteria that half of the people on this planet share.

In reality, the prescription drugs have no curative effects at all because the afflicted person depends on their continual or occasional intake. What they do 'accomplish', however, is to destroy all kinds of bacteria in your gut, including those that help you break down toxins and undigested foods which have accumulated in the stomach, particularly in the lower part, called the *antrum*. Interestingly, the chronic infection linked with stomach ulcers is always initiated in the antrum. The H. pylori bacteria naturally return to the gut when the antibiotics are no longer there to destroy them. Why would they do that? To do their job. It is their function to go to places where dead, damaged cells and toxins need to be broken down and removed. If you eat too much food, not all of it can be digested. The presence of undigested food in the stomach is a cause of continuous irritation and toxicity. In addition, certain foods and food combinations are so difficult to digest that they stay in the stomach too long, thereby overstimulating acid secretions. All this damages, weakens or destroys stomach cells. A proliferation of H. pylori bacteria occurs in direct response to the damage caused by inappropriate foods and eating habits.

To reiterate, these bugs can be found everywhere and in everyone, yet only a few people develop stomach ulcers. Why do H. pylori 'cause' a gastric ulcer in 1 out of 20 people and not in the other 19, although the bacterium is found in all of them? Similarly, a trapped nerve can be seen as a cause of disease in the body, but not every trapped nerve results in disease. Instead of looking for an external culprit for such a problem, wouldn't it be far more important to find out *why* some trapped nerves produce pathological changes and others don't? Why does the same frightening situation cause a panic attack or an infarct in one person and not in another? Could it be possible that these external 'causes' of disease may simply serve as a trigger to ignite the high toxicity bomb already present in a person's body, thus leading to a toxicity crisis, which is commonly known as 'disease'?

Conventional medicine erroneously assumes that removing a symptom or infectious bacteria also removes the health condition. However, in reality, the removal of the symptoms creates a far more serious and life-threatening situation. Increasing evidence, for example, suggests that the disappearance of H. pylori, the bacterium present in peptic ulcers, may actually be contributing to the obesity epidemic. H. Pylori regulates the production of leptin and ghrelin. Leptin is a protein hormone with important effects in regulating appetite, body weight, metabolism and reproductive functions. Ghrelin, a circulating growth hormone-releasing peptide derived from the stomach, stimulates hunger and food intake. Destroying H. pylori in the stomach, can upset the balance of these hormones and lead to spiraling effects of weight gain and injury to all organs and systems in the body. The saying that a little knowledge is a dangerous thing certainly applies to the symptom-oriented approach of conventional medicine.

Note for sufferers of stomach ulcers: Licorice has traditionally been used as an excellent medicine for peptic ulcers. However, the licorice compound glycyrrhetinic acid has been found to elevate blood pressure in some people. Hence, a procedure was developed to remove this compound from licorice and form deglycyrrhizinated licorice (DGL). The result is a very successful anti-ulcer agent without any known side effects.

According to numerous studies, DGL stimulates and/or accelerates the factors that protect against ulcer formation, including the increased production of mucin, the protective coating in the stomach and intestines. Study participants have found DGL to be an effective anti-ulcer compound. Several head to head comparison studie, have shown that DGL is more effective than Tagamet, Zantac or antacids in both short term treatment and maintenance therapy of gastric and duodenal ulcers. DGL also has been effective in reducing the need for H. pylori proliferation, perhaps because of the removal of toxic harmful compounds feeding these germs. DGL must mix with saliva to be effective in healing peptic ulcers. It may promote the release of salivary compounds that stimulate the growth and regeneration of stomach and intestinal cells. Don't use DGL in capsule form, as this has not been shown to be effective. DGL in chewable tablet form is available through most supplement suppliers.

The salt-ulcer link: H. pylori becomes more virulent in the presence of higher salt concentrations according to a study presented at the conference of the *American Society for Microbiology*. Researchers discovered that in the presence of salt, H. pylori is more likely to produce proteins that cause it to be more dangerous to humans, and more likely to produce ulcers.

"Apparently H. pylori closely monitors the diets of those people whom it infects," said lead researcher Dr. Hanan Gancz of the Uniformed Services University of the Health Sciences in Bethesda, Maryland. "We think that when there are high levels of salt in the stomach environment, H. pylori over-produces [the factors that] enable it to survive, which in the long term increases the risk of illness."

Gancz also pointed out that doctors have long been aware of a link between high salt intake and increased risk of gastric cancer.

It is not clear from the study whether the increased risk of developing stomach ulcers and stomach cancer also applies to the consumption of unprocessed full-spectrum sea salt, versus refined, bleached table salt. If you suffer from a stomach ulcer, try reducing your salt intake, especially if you are a Pitta type (see details about body types in Chapters 5 and 6).

Defying a Hopeless Prognosis

Jenny was only 25 years old when she came to me with progressive Crohn's disease, a chronic inflammatory condition of the alimentary tract. There was chronic patchy inflammation with edema of the full thickness of the intestinal wall, causing partial obstruction of the lumen. She had been told that her condition was irreversible and would eventually lead to her death. Jenny was heading toward internal suffocation. Despite the various treatments she had received - all of which consisted of painkillers, antibiotics and strong anti-inflammatory drugs, including cortisone - her condition worsened progressively. Since there were no signs of improvement, her doctors increased the dosage of the drugs at regular intervals. Her face and body were covered with spots that she scratched to bleeding point during the night. She had several other symptoms, including strong menstrual cramps, headaches and severe lower-back pain.

After examining Jenny through the methods of Ayurveda pulse reading and eye interpretation (iridology) and listening to her medical history, I pointed out to her that her intestinal troubles were caused by what she was eating. Jenny consistently consumed highly acid-forming foods and beverages that had strong irritating effects on the intestinal lining and led to major blockages of the liver's bile ducts with intrahepatic gallstones. (See Chapter 3 for details) In addition, the strong prescription drugs she ingested every day interfered with her body's attempt to rid itself of the accumulated undigested, harmful foods. Besides impairing the immune system, the poisonous compounds of the prescription medicines had also removed large quantities of minerals and water from her tissues and cells. All medications have diuretic effects. Without enough water, which is the principal means of transport and healing in the body, the body faces a situation of crisis, namely, body drought or dehydration.

The severe congestion of her liver and intestinal tract and the general dehydration of Jenny's body caused most of her chronic complaints, including the pain in her head, back and lower abdomen. The medicines led to a massive buildup of toxins and harmful bacteria in the intestines, as they had wiped out nearly the entire population of her gut's friendly, probiotic bacteria. Being a lively young person who lived in a nightlife society (Cyprus), she had very little sleep during nighttime hours. Her irregular sleeping habits and subsequent chronic fatigue made it difficult for her digestive system to cope with any type of food, which further increased the toxicity in her intestinal tract.

I suggested a series of cleansing and rehydration procedures, along with a diet that corresponded to her natural body type and physical condition, as well as a number of changes in her lifestyle that would help rebalance her disturbed biological rhythms. In addition, I advised her to have emotional clearing sessions to deal with the underlying patterns of fear and insecurity she had experienced since early childhood.

One month later, a checkup with her doctor revealed that the disease had 'disappeared' and so had all her skin problems and other symptoms. Twelve years later, she is still as healthy and radiant as can be. She is now married and has two beautiful, healthy children. What I have learned from this and similar cases is a simple understanding of healing that can be applied to almost every disease. I have summarized this in the following statement:

"The symptoms of a disease cannot be the cause of the disease; they are its effects. Therefore, a disease cannot be cured by merely removing its symptoms. The most effective way of dealing with disease is to remove any energy-depleting factors that can interfere with the body's ever-present effort to return to its natural state of balance or equilibrium. Overeating, poor nutrition, lack of sleep, not drinking enough fresh water, use of pharmaceutical drugs and stimulants, etc. all deplete the body's energy reserves and render it susceptible to a toxicity crisis that may involve bacterial, viral or fungal infections. On the other hand, cleansing the body from accumulated waste material and establishing a healthy diet and lifestyle, set the preconditions for the body to heal itself."

Trusting in the Nature of Your Body

Almost every so-called disease is a toxicity crisis that results from accumulating toxins to the level of intolerance (the disease phase). The body is left with no choice but to find an outlet for these toxins. A toxicity crisis may be accompanied by various symptoms such as a headache, a cold, joint pain, a skin rash, bronchitis or other types of infections. Any of these symptoms indicate that the body is attempting to rid its most congested parts of harmful toxic substances. Once the immune system has lowered toxicity to below the level of tolerance, which may differ from person to person, the symptoms begin to disappear again (the healing phase). All of life moves in cycles, and there is no exception to this law. One of the most unfortunate side effects of medical intervention is that it prevents the natural cycle of disease and healing to be completed. This is how the well known physician Henry Lindlahr poignantly summarized this basic medical truth: "The greatest part of all chronic disease is created by the suppression of acute disease by drug poisoning." Being satisfied with merely suppressing symptoms leaves us with many diseases today for which the causes remain obscure. The healing phase that naturally follows a toxicity crisis never even has a chance to occur.

If a simple cold is not allowed to take its natural course, the next time you suffer a cold and try to suppress it, it may turn into a chronic catarrh. Further interference with the body's healing efforts can turn the catarrh into pneumonia. Pneumonia can be fatal if the elimination of toxic secretions is undermined through suppressive drugs. Likewise, a recurring migraine may one day become a mental breakdown; high blood pressure can turn into a heart attack; and a stomach catarrh may develop into a cancer.

If we would allow a toxicity crisis to go through its natural stages of development and resolution, and if we also stopped depleting the body's energy resources, disease would rarely arise, and it would not become necessary to fight it when it did. A toxicity crisis may, however, lead to serious complications if the ill person prevents his body from successfully clearing out any waste products or noxious substances that have congested his eliminative organs or systems for some time. These include the liver, colon, kidneys, lymphatic system, skin and lungs.

Patients who take the seemingly more effective, fast and convenient 'shortcut' of medical intervention to restore their health may remember their illness with apprehension while continuing to live with a subconscious fear of a possible recurrence. But those who are cured by their body's natural healing powers are more likely to recall their illness as an experience of great emotional and physical release, which greatly increased their self-confidence and well-being. Having recovered their health by trusting and supporting their body's own healing ability, they may also have made a quantum leap in personal development. Many patients report that their natural recovery from an illness led to major improvements in their attitude toward life in general and their relationships with others.

A toxicity crisis can be a unique opportunity to balance out old *karma* and bring about positive changes on the physical, emotional and spiritual levels of life. By entrusting your own body with the healing process, a new sense of freedom begins to dominate your awareness, and old fears and anxieties start to dissipate. The tactic of *fighting a disease until the end* is not only unnecessary but also reinforces the false belief system that true healing occurs only rarely or is a matter of *luck*. Research has confirmed quite the contrary: Over 80 percent of all illnesses disappear completely on their own. This, of course, is due to the body's innate healing capabilities.

To assist the body's healing efforts while going through a toxicity crisis, it is important to take a natural purgative, colonic irrigation or at least an enema each day to release accumulated toxic waste in the intestinal tract. It is also good advice to keep one's feet warm, get complete rest, and avoid watching television (due to its stimulating and dehydrating effects). Eating food during the crisis can interfere with the healing process, since this uses up the energy the body tries to direct toward eliminating toxins. But drinking plenty of warm water helps with the much needed cleansing and rehydration process in the body. Also recommended is a warm bath before bedtime and, in case there is pain, a hot bath as often in the day as is comfortable. To aid the healing process, regular exposure of one's body to fresh air and natural sunlight can be very beneficial too, as both have strong immune-stimulating effects. These and similar measures greatly help the body to overcome a toxicity crisis within the shortest possible time. Trusting in the body and not being afraid of it play a key role in one's recovery.

All serious diseases are 'innocent' in the beginning. Most of them start off as simple colds, headaches, stomach pains, indigestion, intestinal cramps, fatigue, stiffness of joints, skin trouble, and similar minor ailments. These seemingly 'insignificant' complaints can turn vicious when 'cured' too quickly. They can never really be cured by symptom-oriented approaches of treatment because each minor toxicity crisis that is suppressed adds more toxins to the system and depletes constitutional stamina and vitality. In addition, if the causes of these relatively small complaints are not removed on time, more serious impairment of the body's functions may result. This may be the starting point of a long-lasting illness. The following section deals with the four most common factors that contribute to the development of a more intensified toxicity crisis or disease.

CHAPTER 3

The Four Most Common Causes of Disease -
And the Ancient System that Frees You from Each One

1. <u>Gallstones In The Liver and Gallbladder</u>

Many people believe that gallstones can be found only in the gallbladder. This is a commonly made yet false assumption. Most gallstones are actually formed in the liver, and comparatively few occur in the gallbladder. (**Illustration 4a**) You can easily verify this assessment by giving yourself a liver flush. It matters little whether you are a layperson, a medical doctor, a scientist, or someone whose gallbladder was removed and, therefore, is believed to be stone free. The results of the liver flush[2] speak for themselves. No amount of scientific proof or medical explanation can make such a cleanse any more valuable than it already is. Once you see hundreds of green, beige-colored, brown or black gallstones floating in the toilet bowl during your first liver flush, you will intuitively know that you are on to something extremely important in your life. To satisfy your possibly curious mind, you may decide to take the expelled stones to a laboratory for chemical analysis or ask your doctor what she thinks about all that. Your doctor may either support you in your initiative to heal yourself, tell you this is just ridiculous, or warn you against it. However, what is most significant in this experience is that you have taken active responsibility for your own health, perhaps for the first time in your life.

Not everyone is as fortunate as you are. An estimated 20 percent of the world's population will develop gallstones in their *gallbladder* at some stage in their lives; many of them will opt for surgical removal of this important organ. This statistical figure does not account, though, for the many more people who will develop gallstones (or already have them) in their *liver*. During some thirty years of practicing natural medicine and dealing with thousands of people suffering from all types of chronic diseases, I can attest to the fact that each one of them, without exception, has had considerable quantities of gallstones in his or her liver. Surprisingly, only relatively few of them reported to have had a history of gallstones in their gallbladder. Gallstones in the liver are, as you will understand from reading this book, the main impediment to acquiring and maintaining good health, youthfulness and vitality. Gallstones in the liver are, indeed, one of the major reasons people become ill and have difficulty recuperating from illness.

The failure to recognize and accept the incidence of gallstone formation in the liver as an extremely common phenomenon may very well be the most unfortunate oversight that has ever been made in the field of medicine, both orthodox and holistic.

---

[2] When I refer to the *liver flush*, it includes flushing of the gallbladder as well.

Relying so heavily on blood tests for diagnostic purposes, as conventional medicine does, may actually be a great disadvantage with regard to assessing liver health. Most people who have a physical complaint of one kind or another may have perfectly normal liver enzyme levels in the blood, despite suffering from liver congestion. Liver congestion is among the leading health problems, yet conventional medicine rarely refers to it, nor do doctors have a reliable way to detect and diagnose such a condition. Liver enzyme levels in the blood become elevated only when there is advanced liver cell destruction, as is the case, for example, in hepatitis or liver inflammation. Liver cells contain large amounts of enzymes. Once a certain number of liver cells are ruptured, their enzymes will start showing up in the blood. When detected through a blood test, this increased count of liver enzymes indicates abnormal liver functions. In such an event, however, the damage has already occurred. It takes many years of chronic liver congestion before liver damage becomes apparent.

Standard clinical tests almost never reveal the occurrence of gallstones in the liver. In fact, most doctors don't even know they grow there. Only some of the most advanced research universities, such as the prestigious Johns Hopkins University, describe and illustrate these liver stones in their literature or on their websites. They refer to them as 'intrahepatic gallstones'.[3]

By understanding how gallstones in the liver contribute to the occurrence or deterioration of nearly every kind of illness, and by taking the simple steps to remove them (for details, see Chapter 7), you will put yourself in charge of restoring your own health and vitality, permanently. The implications of applying the liver flush for yourself - or, if you are a health practitioner, for your patients - are immensely rewarding. To have a clean liver equals having a new lease on life.

The following are a few examples indicating the extreme importance of a healthy, clean liver:

- Almost every illness is either directly or indirectly caused by congestion of the liver bile ducts and gallbladder.
- Trapped, toxic bile is the source of most digestive problems.
- Congested bile ducts in the liver can turn harmless chemicals into cancer-causing substances - and then scatter them throughout the body.
- A poorly functioning liver can block 70 percent of the blood flow to the heart.
- The liver is responsible for mental clarity and emotional stability.
- The liver can spill proteins into the lymphatic system, setting off a myriad of immune system reactions - from allergies to autoimmune diseases, and from colds to cancer.
- The liver's enzymes can turn the body's own steroid hormones into either beneficial or deadly hormones. The latter can give a person cancer of the reproductive organs.

The liver is the largest gland/organ in the body. It weighs up to three pounds, is suspended behind the ribs on the upper right side of the abdomen, and spans almost the entire width of the body. Being responsible for hundreds of different functions, it is also the most complex and active organ in the body.

Since the liver is in charge of processing, converting, distributing and maintaining the body's vital 'fuel' supply (for example, nutrients and energy), anything that interferes with these functions must have a serious, detrimental impact on the health of the liver and the body as a whole. The strongest interference stems from the presence of gallstones.

---

[3] On the Internet, search for *Johns Hopkins Medical Institutions*. Then locate *Digestive Disease Library*, click on *Biliary Tract*, choose *Cholangiocarcinoma*, go to bottom of page, and click *on Next Section*. Repeat more times; then scroll down to the last illustration on that page.

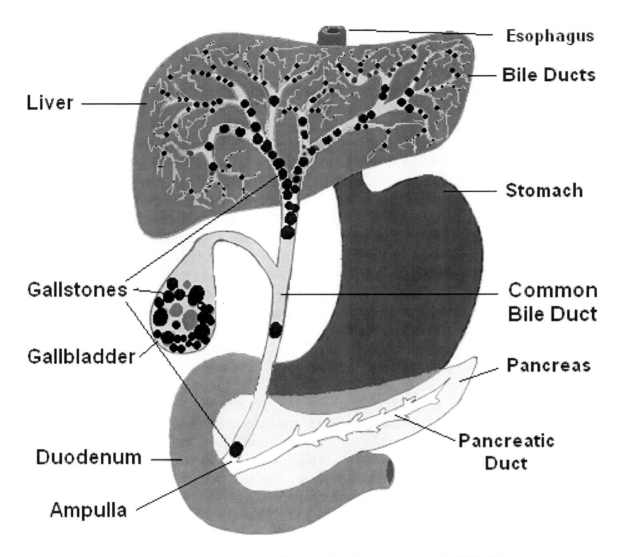

Liver

Esophagus

Bile Ducts

Gallstones

Gallbladder

Stomach

Common
Bile Duct

Pancreas

Duodenum

Pancreatic
Duct

Ampulla

Illustration 4a: Gallstones in the Liver and Gallbladder

Besides manufacturing cholesterol - an essential building material of all organ cells, hormones, and bile - the liver also produces hormones and proteins that affect the way the body functions, grows and heals. Furthermore, it makes new amino acids[4] and converts existing ones into proteins. These proteins are the main building blocks of the cells, hormones, neurotransmitters, genes, and so forth. Other essential functions of the liver include breaking down old, worn-out cells, recycling proteins and iron, and storing vitamins and nutrients. Gallstones are a hazard to all these vital tasks.

In addition to breaking down alcohol in the blood, the liver also detoxifies noxious substances, bacteria, parasites, and certain components of pharmaceutical drugs. It uses specific enzymes to convert waste or poisons into substances that can be safely removed from the body. In addition, the liver filters more than one quart of blood each minute. Most of the filtered waste products leave the liver via the bile stream. Gallstones obstructing the bile ducts turn the bile toxic and lead to high levels of toxicity in the

---

[4] Right from a newborn's first breath, the body produces amino acids and proteins from the nitrogen, carbon, oxygen, and hydrogen molecules contained in the air.

liver and, ultimately, in the rest of the body as well.. This development is further exacerbated by one's intake of pharmaceutical drugs, normally broken down by the liver. The presence of gallstones prevents their detoxification, which can cause 'overdosing' and devastating side effects, even at normal doses. It also means that the liver is at risk for damage from the breakdown products of the drugs on which it acts. Alcohol that is not detoxified properly by the liver can seriously injure or destroy liver cells.

One of the liver's most important functions is to produce bile, about 1-1.5 quarts per day. Liver bile is a viscous yellow, brown or green fluid that is alkaline (versus acidic) and has a bitter taste. Without sufficient bile, most commonly eaten foods remain undigested or partially digested. For example, to enable the small intestines to digest and absorb fat and calcium from the food you eat, the food must first combine with bile. When fat is not absorbed properly, it indicates that bile secretion is insufficient. The undigested fat remains in the intestinal tract. When undigested fat reaches the colon along with other waste products, bacteria break down some of the fat into fatty acids or excrete it with the stool. Since fat is lighter than water, having fat in the stool may cause it to float. When fat is not absorbed, calcium is not absorbed either, leaving the blood in a deficit. The blood subsequently takes its extra calcium from the bones. Most bone density problems (osteoporosis) actually arise from insufficient bile secretion and poor digestion of fats, rather than from not consuming enough calcium. Few medical practitioners are aware of this fact and, hence, merely prescribe calcium supplements to their patients.

Apart from breaking down the fats in our food, bile also removes toxins from the liver. One of the lesser known but extremely important functions of bile is to cleanse the intestines. Bile also stimulates intestinal peristalsis, responsible for healthy, regular bowel movements. Poor peristalsis is a leading cause of constipation.

When gallstones in the liver or gallbladder have critically impeded bile flow, the color of the stool may be tan, orange-yellow, or pale as in clay, instead of the normal greenish-brown.

Gallstones are a direct product of an unhealthy diet and lifestyle. If gallstones are still present in the liver or gallbladder even after all other disease-causing factors are eliminated, they pose a considerable health risk and may lead to illness and premature aging. For this reason, the subject of gallstones has been included here as a major risk factor or cause of disease. The following sections describe some of the main consequences of gallstones in the liver and gallbladder on the different organs and systems in the body. When these stones are removed, the body as a whole can resume its normal, healthy activities.

When The Liver's Bile Ducts Become Obstructed...

The most common but rarely recognized health problem today is blockage of the liver's bile ducts through gallstones (**Illustrations 4b & c**). If you suffer any of the following symptoms, or similar conditions, you most likely have numerous gallstones in your liver and gallbladder:

- Low appetite
- Food cravings
- Digestive disorders
- Diarrhea
- Constipation
- Clay-colored stool
- Hernia
- Flatulence
- Hemorrhoids
- Dull pain on the right

- side
- Difficulty breathing
- Liver cirrhosis
- Hepatitis
- Most infections
- High cholesterol
- Pancreatitis
- Heart disease
- Brain disorders
- Duodenal ulcers

- Nausea and vomiting
- A 'bilious' or angry personality
- Depression
- Impotence
- Other sexual problems
- Prostate diseases
- Urinary problems
- Hormonal imbalances
- Menstrual and

- menopausal disorders
- Problems with vision
- Puffy eyes
- Any skin disorder
- Liver spots, especially those on the back of the hands and facial area
- Dizziness and fainting spells
- Loss of muscle tone
- Excessive weight or wasting
- Strong shoulder and back pain
- Pain at the top of a shoulder blade and/or between the shoulder blades
- Dark color under the eyes
- Morbid complexion

- Tongue that is glossy or coated in white or yellow
- Scoliosis
- Gout
- Frozen shoulder
- Stiff neck
- Asthma
- Headaches and migraines
- Tooth and gum problems
- Yellowness of the eyes and skin
- Sciatica
- Numbness and paralysis of the legs
- Joint diseases
- Knee problems
- Osteoporosis
- Obesity
- Chronic fatigue
- Kidney diseases

- Cancer
- Multiple Sclerosis and fibromyalgia
- Alzheimer's disease
- Cold extremities
- Excessive heat and perspiration in the upper part of the body
- Very greasy hair and hair loss
- Cuts or wounds that keep bleeding and don't want to heal
- Difficulty sleeping, insomnia
- Nightmares
- Stiffness of joints and muscles
- Hot and cold flashes

People with chronic illnesses often have several thousand gallstones congesting the bile ducts of the liver. Some stones may have also grown in the gallbladder. By removing these stones from these organs through a series of liver flushes and maintaining a balanced diet and lifestyle, the liver and gallbladder can restore their original efficiency, and most symptoms of discomfort or disease in the body can start subsiding. You may find that any persistent allergies will lessen or disappear. Back pain will dissipate, while energy and well-being will improve. Ridding the liver bile ducts of gallstones is one of the most important and powerful procedures you can apply to improve and regain your health.

Gallstones - A Constant Source Of Disease

The majority of gallstones in the liver consist of the same 'harmless' constituents that are found in liquid bile, with cholesterol being the main ingredient. A number of stones consist of fatty acids and other organic material that has ended up in the bile ducts. The fact that the majority of these stones are just congealed clumps of bile or organic matter makes them more or less 'invisible' to x-rays, ultrasonic technologies, and even *computerized tomography* (CT).

The situation is different with regard to the gallbladder, where up to about 20 percent of all stones can be made up entirely of minerals, predominantly calcium salts and bile pigments. Whereas diagnostic tests can easily detect these hardened, relatively large stones in the gallbladder, they tend to miss the softer, noncalcified stones in the liver. Only when excessive amounts of cholesterol-based stones (85–95 percent cholesterol), or other clumps of fat, block the bile ducts of the liver may an ultrasound test reveal what is generally referred to as 'fatty liver'. In such a case, the ultrasound pictures reveal a liver that is almost completely white (instead of black). A fatty liver can gather up to 20,000 stones before it succumbs to suffocation and ceases to function.

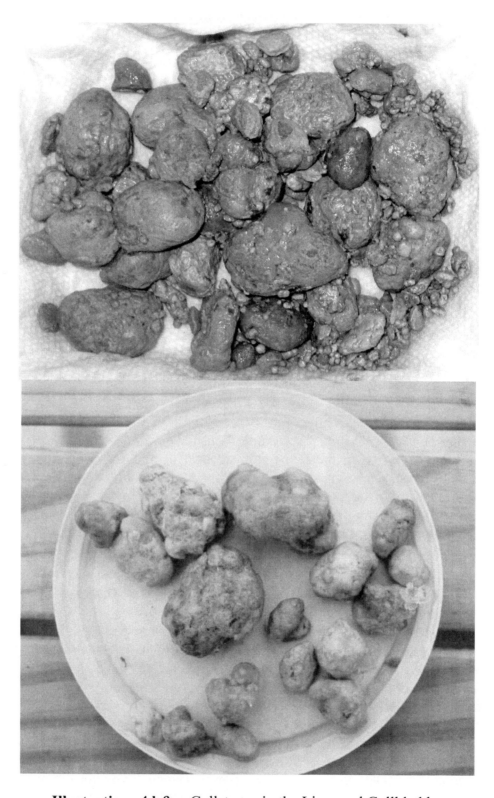

Illustrations 4 b&c: Gallstones in the Liver and Gallbladder

The gallstones found in the liver come in all shapes and colors. Most of them are bright-colored or dark-green; yet some others can be white, red, black or tan-colored. They result from overeating, an unhealthy diet and lifestyle, as well as stress and repressed anger. As the stones grow in size and become more numerous, the liver cells are compelled to reduce bile production. Normally, the liver produces well over a quart of bile each day. This is the required amount to properly digest food in the small intestine. When the major bile ducts are blocked, barely a cup or less will find its way to the intestinal tract. The restricted bile secretions not only impair digestion but also prevent the liver from excreting toxins and propelling the stones out of the bile ducts. Hence bile becomes toxic. Some of the toxic bile is backwashed into the blood, thereby affecting all vital organs, including the brain. This also affects blood circulation in the liver. The walls of the liver's blood vessels (sinusoids) become increasingly clogged up. Consequently, *Low Density Lipoproteins* (LDL and VLDL, also called *bad cholesterol*) are increasingly prevented from leaving the bloodstream, hence the rise in blood serum cholesterol.

Since gallstones are porous, they can pick up or absorb toxins, bacteria, viruses, parasites and cysts that are passing through the liver, like fishing nets collect fish. The stones can become a constant source of infection, supplying the body with an ever-increasing number of fresh bacteria. The attempt to permanently cure intestinal bloating, cystitis, Candida, stomach ulcers, infectious diseases or any of the above conditions is likely to fail if the bacteria-harboring gallstones are not removed from the liver.

On occasion, one or several gallstones get stuck in the *cystic duct* - in the vessel that links the common bile duct with the gallbladder - or in the *common bile duct* itself. In this case, the wall of the duct undergoes strong spasmodic contractions in order to propel the stones onward. The contractions of the duct wall can cause excruciating pain throughout the abdomen, in the back and also in the legs and arms.

When the gallbladder is packed with gallstones, it also may go into extremely painful, spasmodic muscle contractions, a condition known as a gallbladder attack. Gallstones can trigger strong reactions of irritation and inflammation of the walls of the gallbladder and the cystic and common bile ducts. There may be superimposed microbial infection. Today, over 20 million Americans suffer gallbladder disease, and each year about one million of them opt for an expensive gallbladder operation.

If a person has his gallbladder removed surgically, he may feel tremendous relief from the acute painful attacks, and his digestion is likely to improve for a short while. This is due to comparatively more bile being available for the digestive process. The disadvantage is, however, that bile now comes in small trickles throughout the day, rather than in large amounts when it is needed to digest a meal. Bile causes injury to the intestinal walls unless it is mixed with food. In addition, since the patient still has all the stones left in his liver, the digestive troubles are most likely to return or get worse. Excessive weight gain is common. Other existing health problems such as pain, asthma, bursitis, heart disease, and arthritis become intensified as well.

If gallstones become stuck in the *ampulla of the bile duct*, where the common bile duct from the liver and gallbladder joins the pancreatic duct, jaundice and acute pancreatitis usually develop. This condition can eventually lead to cancerous tumors in the pancreas and to a number of other diseases.

Gallstones of any kind, size and number can be easily and safely removed through the liver and gallbladder flush described in *Employing Nature's Healing Powers,* Chapter 7, or in my book *The Amazing Liver & Gallbladder Flush.* The first positive effects that are commonly noticed soon after the liver flush are pain relief and regained or enhanced energy, vitality and general well-being. Although liver flushes can be done by people of any age, including children over 10 (many children today have gallstones in the liver) and the elderly, I recommend doing the flush only after having followed the general guidelines for creating a healthy body for at least four to six weeks, as is described in the following chapters. The colon and kidney cleanses outlined in Chapter 7, *Employing Nature's Healing Powers*, are an ideal preparation for a liver flush, too.

During a series of liver flushes, I passed about 3,000 small pea-sized green stones, hundreds of chickpea sized and a dozen large ones of up to one inch (2.5 centimeters) in diameter. Subsequent flushes during the following 5 years showed that my liver was completely clean. The effects of each flush were often dramatic and added more and more benefits to the previous one(s). The overall results were that my energy and vitality increased by at least three-fold, all discomfort, stiffness and pain in the body, particularly in the back, ceased and digestion and elimination normalized. Speaking for myself, the liver flush is the best thing I have ever done for my physical and mental well-being.

You may wonder why in mainstream medicine there is no medical knowledge or reference that deals with gallstones in the liver. The reason for this extremely important missing link is that the theories of modern medicine tell you that gallstones can only be formed in the gallbladder, and not in the liver. The 'experimental evidence" supporting this theory is mainly based on taking x-rays or ultrasound scans, which can detect only the few stones in the gallbladder that may have grown to a certain size and are calcified (mineral stones). Most diagnostic tools used today are not able to detect the hundreds or thousands of non-calcified, hardened bile deposits in the liver and recognize them as intrahepatic gallstones, as Johns Hopkins University does. As already mentioned, ultrasound scans can reveal fatty deposits in the liver only when an excessive number of oversized stones (20,000 or more) are congesting the liver bile ducts (fatty liver).

If you had a fatty liver and went to the doctor, she would tell you that you had excessive fatty tissue in your liver. It is less likely, though, that she would tell you that you had *intrahepatic gallstones* (stones obstructing the liver's bile ducts). As mentioned before, most of the smaller stones in the liver are not detectable through ultrasound or CT scans. Nevertheless, careful analysis of diagnostic images by specialists would show whether some of the smaller bile ducts in the liver were dilated because of obstruction. A dilation of bile ducts caused by larger and denser stones or by clusters of stones may be detected more readily through *magnetic resonance imaging* (MRI). However, unless there is an indication of major liver trouble, doctors rarely check for intrahepatic stones. Unfortunately, although the liver is one of the most important organs in the body, its disorders are underdiagnosed all too often. Even if the early stages of a fatty liver or gallstone formation in the bile ducts were easily recognized and diagnosed, today's medical facilities offer no treatments to relieve this vital organ of the heavy burden it has to carry.

The presence of gallstones in the liver can easily be verified by anyone suffering from a chronic illness, including those whose gallbladder has been removed. By performing a liver flush, the body will release plenty of non-calcified, bile-coated stones. These stones are identical to the green non-calcified stones found in a surgically removed gallbladder. When cut through their middle part, both these 'types' of gallstones bear typical age marks, similar to those seen in cut tree trunks. Proper analysis would reveal their age and the kinds of toxins, chemicals and bacteria the body had or has to deal with most. Sweeping the liver clean eliminates thousands of bits of poisonous substances that have helped form the stones and plague the thousands of liver bile ducts. Cleansing the liver bile ducts from gallstones is one of the most important and powerful procedures you can do to regain or improve your health.

Note: For further details on how cleansing the liver and gallbladder can make all the difference in the treatment of disease and can improve your health and vitality, please refer to *The Amazing Liver and Gallbladder Flush*. It will teach you how to remove painlessly up to several hundred gallstones at a time. (The procedure is also provided in Chapter 7 of this book.) The size of the stones ranges from that of a pinhead to a small walnut, and in some rare cases, a golf ball. The actual liver flush takes place within a period of less than fourteen hours and can be done conveniently over a weekend at home. Chapter 1 explains in detail why the presence of gallstones in the bile ducts, both inside and outside the liver, can be considered the greatest health risk and the cause of almost every major or minor illness. In

Chapter 2, you will be able to identify the signs, marks, and symptoms that indicate the presence of stones in your liver or gallbladder. Other chapters deal with the possible causes of gallstones and what you can do to prevent new ones from occurring. In Chapter 4, you will learn the actual procedure to rid your body of gallstones. Chapter 6 "What Can I Expect from the Liver and Gallbladder Flush?" covers some of the possible health benefits of this profound self-help program. In addition, you will find out what others have to say about their experiences with the liver flush. The frequently asked questions section, Chapter 8, deals with many queries you may have about the flush. To reap the maximum benefit from this procedure, I strongly encourage you to read the entire book before starting with the actual liver flush.

2. Dehydration

The human body is composed of 75 percent water and 25 percent solid matter. To provide nourishment, eliminate waste, and conduct all the trillions of activities in the body, we need water. Most modern societies, however, no longer stress the importance of drinking water as the most important 'nutrient' among nutrients. Entire population groups are substituting water with tea, coffee, alcohol and other manufactured beverages. Many people don't realize that the natural thirst signal of the body is a sign that it requires pure, plain drinking water. Instead, they opt for other beverages in the belief that this will satisfy the body's water requirements. This is a false belief.

It is true that beverages such as tea, coffee, wine, beer, soft drinks, sports drinks and juices contain water, but they also contain caffeine, alcohol, sugar, artificial sweeteners or other chemicals that act as strong dehydrators. The more of these beverages you consume, the more dehydrated your body becomes because the effects they create in the body are exactly opposite the ones that are produced by water. Beverages containing caffeine, for example, trigger stress responses that at first have strong diuretic effects, leading to increased urination. Beverages with added sugar drastically raise blood sugar levels. Any beverage that provokes such a response coerces the body to give up large quantities of water. Regular consumption of such beverages results in chronic dehydration, which plays a part in every toxicity crisis.

There is no practical or rational reason to treat an illness (toxicity crisis) with synthetic drugs or even with natural medications and methods unless the body's need for hydration has been met first. Drugs and other forms of medical intervention can be dangerous for the human physiology largely because of their strongly dehydrating effects. Most patients nowadays are suffering from 'thirst disease', a progressive condition of dehydration. Some parts of the body may be dehydrated more than others. Unable to remove toxins from these parts due to insufficient water reserves, the body is faced with the consequences of their destructive effects (toxemia). The lack of recognition of the most basic aspects of water metabolism in the body more often than not becomes a 'diagnosed' illness, when it is really the body's urgent cry for water. What doctors generally refer to as disease, is largely an advanced condition of dehydration and the resulting inability of the body to rid itself of waste materials and toxins.

Recognizing Dehydration

Those who have lived for many years without proper water intake are the most likely to succumb to the buildup of toxins in the body. Chronic disease is always accompanied by dehydration and, in many cases, caused by it. The longer a person lives on a low water ration and/or on a high ration of stimulating beverages or foods, the more severe and long-lasting will be the toxicity crisis. Heart disease, obesity, diabetes, rheumatoid arthritis, stomach ulcers, hypertension, cancer, MS, Alzheimer's, and many other chronic forms of disease are preceded by years of 'body drought'. Infectious agents such as bacteria and viruses cannot thrive in a well-hydrated body. Drinking enough water is, therefore, one of the most important disease-prevention measures you can take.

Those who do not drink enough water, or who unduly deplete their body's water reserves through overstimulation for a period of time, gradually lower the ratio of the volume of water that exists inside the cells to the ratio of the volume of water that is found outside the cells. Normally, the water ratio inside cells is higher than the one found in the cell environment. Under conditions of dehydration, the cells may lose up to 28 percent or more of their water volume. This certainly undermines *all* cellular activities, whether the cells in question are those of the skin, stomach, liver, kidney, heart or brain. Whenever there is cellular dehydration, metabolic waste products are not removed properly. This causes symptoms that resemble disease, but they are really just indicators of disturbed water metabolism. Since more and more water begins to accumulate outside the cells in order to dilute and help neutralize the toxic waste products that have accumulated there, the dehydration may not be apparent to the afflicted person. He may, in fact, notice that he begins to hold on to water in his legs, feet, arms and face. His kidneys may also begin to hold on to water, markedly reducing urinary secretion and causing the retention of potentially harmful waste products. Normally, cellular enzymes signal to the brain when cells run low on water. Enzymes in dehydrated cells, however, become so inefficient that they are no longer able to register the drought-like condition. Subsequently, they fail to convey the emergency situation to the brain, which would normally push the 'thirst alarm button'.

Demetria, a 53-year-old Greek woman, consulted me to find relief for the painful condition of gallbladder disease. Her skin was dark gray, indicating a high concentration of toxins in her liver and throughout her body. Seeing how dehydrated (and swollen) her body was, I offered her a glass of water. She said: "I never drink water, it makes me sick!" I told her that her natural thirst signals were no longer working due to cellular dehydration, and that without drinking enough water, her body could not return to balance. It was obvious to me that her body would use any amount of water she drank to instantly remove some of the toxins lurking in her stomach, giving rise to nausea. In her case, any therapy *other than drinking water* would have been a waste of her time and money. Demetria's difficult condition required that she begin sipping small amounts of hot, ionized water every half hour (see directions in 'General Guidelines' of Chapter 6) to help remove these toxins until she was able to drink larger portions of regular water.

A dehydrated person may also be suffering from a lack of energy. Because of a shortage of water inside the cells, the normal osmotic flow of water through the cell membrane becomes severely disturbed. Similar to a stream running down a mountain, the movement of water into the cells generates 'hydroelectric' energy, which is subsequently stored as ATP molecules (the main source of cellular energy). As a rule, the water we drink keeps the cell volume balanced, and the salt we eat maintains the balanced volume of water that is kept outside the cells and in circulation. This generates the perfect osmotic pressure necessary for cellular nourishment and energy production. In a dehydrated state, the body fails to sustain this vital mechanism, thereby leading to potentially serious cell damage.

The Pain Connection

Another major indicator of dehydration in the body is pain. In response to an increasing shortage of water, the brain activates and stores the important neurotransmitter *histamine,* which directs certain subordinate water regulators to redistribute the amount of water that is in circulation. This system helps move water to areas where it is needed for essential metabolic activity and survival when facing such a shortage, as may occur during a drought. When histamine and its subordinate regulators for water intake and distribution move across pain-sensing nerves in the body, they trigger strong and continual pain. These pain signals may manifest, for example, in rheumatoid arthritis, angina, dyspepsia, low back problems, fibromyalgia, neuralgia, migraine, and hangover headaches. They are necessary to alert the person to attend to the problem of a widespread or localized form of dehydration.

Taking *analgesics* or other pain-relieving medications such as *antihistamines* and *antacids* can cause irreversible damage in your body. They not only fail to address the real problem (which may be dehydration), but they also cut off the connection between the neurotransmitter, histamine, and its subordinate regulators, such as *vasopressin, Renin-Angiotensin (RA), prostaglandin (PG),* and *kinins*. Although the action of pain-killing drugs can relieve localized pain for a while, it also precludes your body from knowing the priority areas for water distribution. This can greatly confuse your body's internal communications systems and spread chaos throughout the body. *Antihistamines* - oftentimes referred to as allergy drugs - effectively prevent the body's *histamines* from ensuring balanced water distribution.

The problem worsens once the body has reached a certain pain threshold. In addition to jeopardizing the water-regulating mechanisms, these painkillers become ineffective because the brain takes over as a direct center for monitoring pain perpetuation (unless, of course, the body is properly hydrated again). If your body produces lasting pain for no apparent reason (not caused by an injury), before drawing any other conclusions, you should interpret this as the body's cry for water and its attempt to remedy an unbalanced condition. Prescription pain medication suppresses the body's primary signal of dehydration. Pain killers 'short-circuit' the body's emergency routes for water supply; they also sabotage proper waste elimination and sow the seeds of chronic illness.

There is enough documentation to show that pain medications may have fatal side effects. They can cause gastrointestinal bleeding, which kills thousands each year. The morphine-type compounds these legal drugs contain can also lead to serious, life-altering addictions. When the famous radio host, Rush Limbaugh, announced on his radio program that he was addicted to pain medication, his life was in shambles. But he is not alone in this. There are millions of people who initially started off by taking an 'innocent' Advil for the occasional headache, but ended up being unable to live without strong painkillers. Once you start using dehydrating medications like these, you will mostly likely develop the same kind or even worse pain over and over again.

The most recently documented and widely popularized side effects of pain killers, such as Vioxx, Celebrex and the over-the-counter drug Aleve (Naproxen), should tell you that there *are* no safe painkillers. These drugs were found to increase the risk of heart attacks and strokes by at least 50 percent. Aspirin and other 'harmless' drugs belong to the same class of painkillers as the above. Today, there are millions of heart disease sufferers who, out of ignorance and misguided trust in the medical system, the FDA and the pharmaceutical industry, believed that taking a little innocent baby pill wouldn't do them any harm. The revelation that this little pill could destroy their heart or damage their brain if they took it for more than 10 days may be no less than shocking. But how many people listen to such warnings if all they want is to 'get rid of that annoying pain'?

Taking a 'harmless' little pill that makes you feel better within a matter of minutes and allows you to get on with your life may feel like the right thing to do. And, if the pain medicine tastes delicious, the 'miracle drug' couldn't possibly do you any harm, or could it? *Tylenol Extra Strength* 'cool caplets', the latest craze among painkilling medications, makes these dangerous drugs appear harmless. It's both a breath mint and a pain reliever. But is it really a sound idea to add the temptation of flavoring to a pain-reliever that, by the FDA's own admission, plays a role in at least 100 reported (a fraction of the real figure) unintentional deaths each year? This may change now that the scandals surrounding drug approval and the revelations concerning shoddy research are increasingly being exposed, or will it? If you were to ask people on the street if they considered acetaminophen to be a completely benign medication, most would respond with a "yes." That totally undeserved reputation may only be reinforced when mint flavoring is added to the mix.

Once you decide to end a drug addiction, life is not going to be easy. Those who are able to afford a rehabilitation treatment can choose a rapid anesthesia detox for about $5,900. To become truly rehabilitated, though, they will need to deal with the underlying causes of the pain that originally led them to take addictive drugs. The bottom line is this: The body's natural pain signal is a perfectly normal response to an abnormal situation - simple dehydration. In many cases, the body's blood vessel walls, liver bile ducts, lymphatic ducts, kidneys, intestinal tract, and other organs of elimination are so congested that chronic dehydration becomes inevitable. To restore health, the body needs to be cleansed and nourished properly, which is the main theme of this book.

Most people have no real understanding of what pain is. They rarely perceive it to be an important part of the body's healing efforts. Pain is always a sign of resistance to what moves or flows naturally. The resistance can occur either as a result of some physical obstruction, such as constipation or lymph congestion, or from an emotional resistance to a particular person or situation. Once recognized, the causes of resistance can usually be resolved. Fighting pain tends to lead to more pain, whereas releasing the resistance lessens the pain. Even if you experience some pain while supporting the body through cleansing, rest and good nutrition, the pain actually helps to accelerate the healing. If you stay with the pain, rather than suppressing it with drugs, you will find that it will decrease naturally in a matter of hours or a few days. Trying to combat every ache or pain with painkillers, on the other hand, is an addiction that causes much fear and more pain in your life. Feeling one's pain with an attitude of acceptance removes all kinds of fear from your life. In addition, the pain experience itself will stimulate the secretion of the body's own natural painkillers and healing hormones - the endorphins. Overall, once you have identified and dealt with the causes of the pain, it is just a matter of time before the pain disappears altogether.

Of course, in the rare case that the pain becomes simply unbearable, the use of painkillers may be unavoidable. At the same time, the pain-afflicted person should get on a hydration and cleansing program, as well as end any dehydrating influences in his life.

'Body Drought' - The Strongest Type of Stress

The human brain, working round the clock, requires more water than any other part of the body. Typically, the brain contains about 20 percent of all the blood that circulates through the body. It is estimated that brain cells consist of 85 percent water. Their energy requirements are not only met by metabolizing glucose (simple sugar), but also by generating 'hydroelectric' energy from the water drive through cell osmosis. The brain depends greatly on this cell-generated source of energy in order to maintain its hugely complex processes and efficiency.

Water deficiency in the brain tissue cuts down the brain's energy supply, and thereby subdues many of its vital functions - a situation most people call depression. With a lower than normal level of brain energy, you are unable to meet your physical, personal and social challenges and subsequently succumb to fear, anxiety, anger and other emotional tribulations. You may feel drained, lethargic, stressed and depressed. Chronic fatigue syndrome (CFS), for example, is mostly a symptom of progressive brain dehydration that results from the inability to readily remove all metabolic waste matter and cellular debris from the brain and other vital parts of the body. What CFS sufferers refer to as 'brain fog' is actually an accurate description of the congestion that occurs in the brain. CFS is not a vicious disease that somehow gets hold of a person for no apparent reason. It may disappear quite spontaneously when the afflicted person stops stimulating the brain with such things as caffeine, tobacco, medication and animal products and begins a consistent program of cleansing, hydrating, and nourishing the body. [For more information on Chronic Fatigue Syndrome and Fibromyalgia Syndrome (FMS), please see the articles page on the author's website, www.ener-chi.com.]

The Stress Response

When dehydrated, the body has to put up the fight of a lifetime - similar to the one experienced during a famine or a 'fight or flight' situation. It responds to such a crisis by mobilizing several powerful hormones, *including adrenalin, endorphins, cortisone, prolactin, vasopressin, and Renin-Angiotensin (RA)*. Endorphins, for example, help us to withstand pain and stress and allow the body to continue most of its activities. *Cortisone* orders the mobilization of stored energies and essential raw materials to supply the body with energy and basic nutrients during the crisis. This hormone actually allows the body to feed off itself, a situation that is warranted during a famine. Of course, this is also very stressful and potentially dangerous for the body, as can be seen by such emotional expressions as "I cannot cope anymore" or "this is really eating at me." Many patients with rheumatoid arthritis, multiple sclerosis (MS) or other degenerative diseases take *cortisone* drugs, which often give them a boost of energy and morale for a relatively short period of time. The 'success; of the drug, however, only lasts for as long as the body can tap into any energy and nutrient reserves still left. Once the body has used up its emergency provisions, it will barely function anymore, and the symptoms of disease will worsen considerably.

Constriction of blood vessels

When the cells in the body are under-supplied with water, the brain's pituitary gland produces the neurotransmitter *vasopressin*, a hormone that has the ability to constrict blood vessels in areas where there is cellular dehydration. During dehydration, the quantity of water in the bloodstream is reduced. *Vasopressin*, as its name suggests, squeezes the vascular system, i.e. the capillaries and arteries, to reduce their fluid volume. This maneuver is necessary to continue having enough pressure in the vascular system to allow for a steady filtration of water into the cells. This gives vasopressin a hypertensive property. High blood pressure is a common experience among people who are dehydrated. (For more information on hypertension and heart disease, see Chapter 9.) A similar situation occurs in the liver's bile ducts, which begin to constrict in response to water shortage in the body. Gallstone formation is a direct result of dehydration.

Drinking alcoholic beverages suppresses the secretion of vasopressin and thereby increases cellular dehydration. If alcohol consumption is excessive, cellular dehydration may reach dangerously high levels. The typical 'hangover' that occurs after alcohol abuse is nothing but an extreme state of dehydration of the brain cells. To survive the alcohol-induced 'drought', the body has to secrete more stress hormones, among them the addictive endorphins. With regular consumption of alcohol, i.e. having a drink every day for several months or years, dehydration increases even further, and endorphin production becomes an addictive occurrence. This may lead to alcoholism, a disease that has devastating consequences on a person's personal and social life.

Water Retention and Kidney Damage

The Renin-Angiotensin (RA) system becomes activated whenever there is a shortage of water in the body. This brilliantly designed system is used to direct the body to hold on to water wherever possible. It instructs the kidneys to inhibit urination and tightens the capillaries and the vascular system, particularly in areas that are not as vitally important as the brain and the heart muscles. At the same time, it stimulates an increase in the absorption of sodium (salt), which helps the body to retain water. Unless the body returns to its normal level of hydration, the *RA system* remains activated. But this also means that the pressure of the blood against the walls of the blood vessels remains abnormally high, thereby causing the damage that is known as cardiovascular disease.

Hypertension and the retention of urine in the kidneys may lead to kidney damage. Conventional treatments for this condition consist mostly of diuretic (urine-forming) drugs and restricted salt consumption. Both can have severe drawbacks. Diuretic drugs, which are used to normalize blood pressure, as well as reduced salt intake, strongly undermine the body's emergency measures to save the little water it has left for normal cellular activities. The resulting stress response causes a further increase in dehydration, and the vicious cycle is complete. Many of the kidney transplants performed today are a result of chronic dehydration, which is caused by something as simple as not drinking enough water, consumption of alcohol, eating foods high in animal protein, or overstimulation of the nervous system.

The Caffeine and Alcohol Drama

The caffeine contained in such beverages as tea, coffee, soft drinks and most power drinks, not only stimulates and stresses both the central nervous and immune systems, but also acts as a powerful diuretic. For every cup of coffee or tea you drink, your body has to relinquish up to three cups of water to remove the toxic caffeine. Iit cannot afford to give up this water without suffering some sort of damage. The caffeine-containing soft drink beverages work in a similar way. Caffeine, being a nerve toxin, stimulates the adrenal glands to secrete stress hormones and to trigger a strong immune response that may give you the false impression that this newly found energy and vitality was somehow provided by the consumed beverage.

The secret behind these stimulants is that the immune reaction mobilizes enough energy for you to feel perked up and clear-headed, at least for as long as your body remains stimulated. To remove the caffeine from the blood, the body is forced to take water from its cells. This results in cellular dehydration and temporary thinning of the blood. Because the thinning of the blood makes you feel good, you won't notice the imminent danger of dehydration. The dehydrating effect of the caffeine in soft drinks is ample reason to avoid them. Unfortunately, caffeine is not the only culprit in soft drinks.

Soft Drinks May Seriously Harm Your Health

New evidence confirms that soft drinks cause serious cell damage. Research from a British university suggests a common preservative found in drinks such as Coca-Cola, Fanta and Pepsi Max has the ability to switch off vital parts of DNA - a problem more usually associated with aging and alcohol abuse. This can eventually lead to cirrhosis of the liver and degenerative diseases such as Parkinson's. The findings reveal serious consequences for the hundreds of millions of people worldwide who consume carbonated beverages. They also reopen the debate about food additives, which have been linked to hyperactivity in children.

The biggest concern centers on the safety of E211, known as sodium benzoate, a preservative used for decades by the $150 billion global carbonated drinks industry. Sodium benzoate derives from benzoic acid. It is used in large quantities to prevent mold from forming in soft drinks such as Sprite, Oasis and Dr Pepper. This common preservative is also added to pickles and sauces.

In the past, sodium benzoate had already been identified as an indirect cause of cancer. When mixed with the additive vitamin C in soft drinks, it produces benzene, a carcinogenic substance. Now, Dr. Peter Piper, professor of molecular biology and biotechnology at Sheffield University, England, has released the results of his research on the impact of sodium benzoate on living yeast cells in his laboratory. Professor Piper discovered that benzoate damaged an important area of DNA in the 'power station' of cells known as the mitochondria. He told *The Independent* on Sunday, May 27, 2007: "These chemicals have the ability to cause severe damage to DNA in the mitochondria to the point that they totally inactivate it: they knock it out altogether. The mitochondria consumes the oxygen to give you energy and if you damage it - as happens in a number of diseased states - then the cell starts to malfunction very seriously. And there is a whole array of diseases that are now being tied to damage to this DNA - Parkinson's and quite a lot of neuro-degenerative diseases, but above all, the whole process of aging."

While referring to outdated tests done by the U.S. Food and Drug Administration and the World Health Organization, Professor Piper said: "The food industry will say these compounds have been tested and they are completely safe. By the criteria of modern safety testing, the safety tests were inadequate. Like all things, safety testing moves forward and you can conduct a much more rigorous safety test than you could 50 years ago."

It is obvious that the government is not going to take a stand against the powerful food and beverage industry. It is up to everyone to protect themselves and their families against the careless policies and practices of those in charge of public health. Not allowing your children to drink soft drinks is one of the most important things you can do for their safety and good health. The same applies to sport drinks which, according to a report issued by the University of Californian in Berkeley, can raise body weight a stunning 13 pounds each year if only one 20-ounce bottle is consumed each day.

A new study conducted at Boston University School of Medicine (released August 2007) shows that drinking as little as one can of soda - regular or diet - per day is associated with a 46 percent increased risk of metabolic syndrome which plays a major role in heart disease and diabetes. According to the study, other harmful side effects of soda, both diet and regular, include:

- A 31% greater risk of becoming obese.
- A 30% higher risk of having a larger waist linc.
- A 25% higher risk of developing high blood triglycerides or high blood sugar.
- A 32% greater risk of having low levels of good cholesterol.
- A trend toward an increased risk of high blood pressure.

Over the long term, the effects of the acidity, sugars, artificial flavors and sweeteners, and such preservatives as E211 contained in soft drinks can be devastating to the body. It would take 32 glasses of water at an alkaline pH of 9 to neutralize the acid from just one 12 oz. cola or other soda. In response to ingesting a cola, apart from risking dehydration, the body will have to use up reserves of its own stored alkaline buffers, mainly calcium from the bones, teeth and DNA. This raises the body's alkalinity levels in order to maintain proper blood alkaline pH levels. Once these reserves are exhausted, your life is at risk. There are enough acids in one soda to kill you, if your body didn't possess a mechanism to neutralize them. How long it takes before your body succumbs to the acid attack and suffers an acidosis depends upon how soon your mineral buffers are depleted. Acidic blood levels are a leading cause of death!

Caffeine, which is a major component in most soft drinks, removes water from the body faster than the body can absorb it again, thereby generating constant thirst. People who frequently drink soft drinks are never really able to quench their thirst because their bodies continually and increasingly run out of cellular water. Some college students drink as many as 10-14 cans of cola a day. Eventually, they confuse their bodies' never-ending thirst signal with hunger and begin to overeat, causing swelling and excessive weight gain. Apart from its diuretic action and its addictive effects on the brain, regular caffeine intake overstimulates the heart muscles, causing exhaustion and heart disease.

Alcohol's diuretic effect on the body is similar to that of caffeine-containing beverages. For example, drinking one glass of beer results in the body forfeiting up to three glasses of water. As mentioned before, a hangover is the result of alcohol abuse, which causes the brain to suffer severe dehydration. If this occurs repeatedly, a large number of brain cells become damaged and die. As a result, many important brain functions slow down or become suppressed. Recovery is possible to a certain extent if alcohol consumption is discontinued. To properly rehydrate the body, please carefully follow the directions in *Drinking Water - The Greatest Therapy*, Chapter 6.

Watch what kind of water you drink

Now that you may be convinced that water is perhaps the best and most natural beverage for your body, the next challenge is to find a source of water that doesn't make you sick. Chlorine in your drinking water can certainly make you sick, according to a gigantic Finnish study of 621,431 individuals living in 56 towns. The researchers were able to determine that women who were exposed to chlorinated water had a 48 percent increased risk of bladder cancer, a 38 percent increased risk of rectal cancer, a 90 percent increased risk of esophageal cancer and an 11 percent increased risk of breast cancer. Men were not affected as much as women. Adding chlorine to drinking water causes a chemical reaction that results in the formation of a cocktail of carcinogens.

Some of nature's most valuable and essential anti-cancer and disease-preventive phytochemical nutrients, which are commonly found in natural foods, have been discovered to form deadly cancer-causing substances when consumed or combined with chlorinated tap water. This has recently been confirmed by a joint study undertaken in Japan by research scientists at the National Institute of Health Sciences and Shizuoka Prefectural University. These deadly compounds have been named MX, which stands for 'unknown mutagen'. Just think of how many people eat, for example, vegetables but also drink chlorinated tab water with their meal. The main concern is that once eliminated from the body, large amounts of these poisons are infiltrating our wastewater treatment and water recycling systems.

It is very disconcerting that especially the fresh plant foods we wash with chlorinated water generate these toxins. Eating these foods and drinking chlorinated water at the same meal certainly exacerbates the situation. The deadly cancer-causing agents this combination produces are extremely toxic in infinitesimal amounts. Thus, only very little chlorine is required to bring about a powerful destructive effect. All this creates the need for implementing new water treatment methods which do not use chlorine for cities and households. You may not be able to get your government to switch over to a healthier and more effective water treatment system, but you can certainly do this for yourself and your family.

There are many simple filtration systems that don't cost you much but can make a huge difference to your health. They are readily available in stores and on the Internet, and almost every new refrigerator comes with one already built into it. Just filtering out chlorine and some other contaminants is of tremendous benefit.

The following are some of the options you have: more sophisticated and more costly water treatment systems, such as the H20 Concept 2000. Its unique technology removes pesticides and herbicides from the water and leaves your drinking, shower, and pool water as fresh and clean as pure mountain water. The H2O Concept 2000 uses electrical impulses to break calcium bicarbonate and magnesium bicarbonate into calcium carbonate and magnesium carbonate, with the byproduct being CO_2. The CO_2 is dispelled at the faucet in minuscule amounts. Calcium carbonate and magnesium carbonate are the soluble forms of these two minerals. In their soluble states these minerals cannot adhere to the inner surfaces of pipes, the water heater coil, or glass surfaces and faucets. The H2O Concept 2000 will significantly reduce any existing scale over time. Although quite pricey at the beginning, this system saves money in the end (see *Product Information)*. It is virtually maintenance-free.

Another excellent whole house water filtration system is the ECOsmarte (search the Internet). It uses dual ionization and oxygen electrodes to remove chemicals in both well and city water. It is a great alternative to water softening and reverse osmosis systems because it filters out calcium and bacterial debris while also controlling hard water scale build-up within the water pipes. Puritec is another company that offers a wide range of good filtration systems for every budget and need.

Much less pricey, yet very effective and excellent for people who are not only interested in proper hydration, but also want to cleanse the body from toxins, are water ionizers. (See Chapter 7 for details.)

The most commonly used methods to remove chlorine and numerous other contaminants from your drinking (and, ideally, shower) water are filtration and reverse osmosis systems. Although these can also be pricey, they are still an affordable option if you consider the cost of suffering through a bout of cancer. To help replenish some its lost minerals, you could add a few grains of basmati rice and a pinch of unrefined salt to the water.

Distilled water, which is produced when water is boiled, evaporated and the vapor condensed, is the closest to natural rainwater. It is excellent for hydrating the body cells, but unlike rainwater, it is lifeless (stripped of its life force). As in the case of reversed osmosis water, adding 3-4 grains of basmati rice and/or a pinch of unrefined salt to one gallon of distilled water gives back some of the lost minerals; exposing it to direct sunlight for an hour or placing a clear quartz crystal in the water for an hour helps somewhat to re-energize it.

Distilled water is free of dissolved minerals and, therefore, has the special property of actively absorbing and removing toxic substances from the body. Studies validate the benefits of drinking distilled water when one is seeking to cleanse or detoxify the system for short periods of time.

Despite its potential benefits, distilled water can be harmful if taken for prolonged periods. Distilling water can lead to the loss of electrolytes (sodium, potassium, chloride) and trace minerals such as magnesium - deficiencies that can cause heart beat irregularities and high blood pressure. Cooking with distilled water may pull the minerals out of foods, thus lowering their nutritional value.

When exposed to the air, distilled water actively absorbs carbon dioxide and becomes more acidic. Drinking distilled water regularly, therefore, may increase the overall acidity in the body. This was confirmed by the U.S. Environmental Protection Agency which stated: "Distilled water, being essentially mineral-free, is very aggressive, in that it tends to dissolve substances with which it is in contact. Notably, carbon dioxide from the air is rapidly absorbed, making the water acidic and even more aggressive. Many metals are dissolved by distilled water."

Regular consumption of cola beverages and other soft drinks are harmful to the body because of their high content of sugar, artificial sweeteners, coloring, and other acidic chemicals. Studies have consistently shown that heavy consumers of soft drinks discharge large amounts of calcium, magnesium and other trace minerals into the urine. However, one major ingredient of these beverages, distilled water, may be another major factor involved in the loss of minerals in the body.

Although distilled water draws poisons out of the body, it is best to use it for only about 10 days at a time. Discontinue its use when you feel weak or otherwise unwell. It is best to avoid using distilled water as your general drinking water.

Prill beads are another form of water treatment. Although they cannot replace a water filter, they still cleanse the water and make it 'thinner'. This has a positive effect on the blood, lymph and basic cellular processes. Prill beads can be found in the U.S. though the Internet.

Of course, the old-fashioned method of boiling your drinking water for several minutes causes the chlorine to evaporate.

Finally, another inexpensive way to get rid of most chlorine in water is to use vitamin C. One gram of vitamin C will neutralize 1ppm (part per million) of chlorine in 100 gallons of water. This is particularly useful if you want to lie in the bathtub without suffering the irritating effects of chlorine on your skin and in your lungs.

To summarize, these are some facts you may want to remember or pass on to others:

- An estimated 75 percent of Americans are chronically dehydrated.
- In 37 percent of Americans, the thirst mechanism is so weak that it is mistaken for hunger. According to research at the University of Washington, drinking just one glass of water shut down midnight hunger for almost 100 percent of the dieters involved in the study.
- Slight dehydration will slow down your metabolism by 3 percent.
- Not drinking enough water is the #1 cause of daytime fatigue.
- Research indicates that 8-10 glasses of water a day could significantly ease joint and back pain for up to 80 percent of sufferers.
- A mere 2 percent drop in body water can trigger fuzzy, short-term memory trouble with basic math problems and result in difficulty focusing on the computer screen or printed page.
- Drinking 5 glasses of water daily decreases the risk of colon cancer by 45 percent. The same amount of water can slash the risk of breast cancer by 79 percent and the risk of bladder cancer by 50 percent.

Warning about plastic bottles: Try to stay away from water or other beverages contained in plastic bottles, especially the soft types. Many people now have large numbers of phthalates (plasticizers used to make plastic flexible, also used in the cosmetics industry) accumulated in their body. Plastic products are water and fat-soluble. The body's natural way of protecting itself against toxic chemicals, such as those seeped from plastic bottles, is to store them in fat cells and connective tissues. This survival response can lead to weight gain and unsightly cellulite in women.

An estrogen-like compound widely used in plastic products is thought to be causing serious reproductive disorders, according to a statement by several dozen scientists, including four from federal health agencies. The compound, bisphenol A (BPA), is one of the most-produced chemicals in the world, and almost everyone has traces of it,or more, in their bodies. The statement, published online by the journal Reproductive Toxicology, was accompanied by a new study by researchers from the National Institutes of Health finding uterine damage in newborn animals exposed to BPA. The researchers indicated that such damage is a possible predictor of reproductive diseases in women, including fibroids, endometriosis, cystic ovaries and cancers. Earlier studies linked low dose BPA to female reproductive-tract disorders, early-stage prostate and breast cancer, as well as decreased sperm counts in animals.

BPA is found in polycarbonate plastic baby bottles, large water-cooler containers and sports bottles, microwave-oven dishes, canned-food liners, and some dental sealants for children.

The disastrous impact plastic has on the environment is difficult to determine. Currently, there are more plastic particles in the oceans than there is plankton. Plastic particles seep into the ground water from landfills; and rivers and streams carry them to the seas and of, course, back into our bodies through the water we drink and the fish we eat. To make a difference, drink only filtered water and try to use glass, ceramic, wooden, stainless steel or other natural containers and utensils whenever possible.

3. Kidney Stones

The kidneys truly are the body's 'master chemists'. They not only remove waste products and excess fluids from the body via the urine, but they also maintain a critical balance of salt, potassium and acid - not a small feat for such relatively small organs. The kidneys produce a hormone - erythropoietin (EPO) - that stimulates the production of red blood cells. Other kidney hormones help regulate blood pressure and calcium metabolism. The kidneys even synthesize the hormones that control tissue growth. When the kidneys become damaged, other organs suffer as well.

The main responsibility of the kidneys is to keep the blood pure and healthy and to maintain proper fluid balance in the body. To accomplish this enormously complex feat, the kidneys need to constantly monitor normal blood volume and filter out the right quantity of urine. There are many interfering factors that could disrupt this mechanism and cause congestion in the kidneys. These factors include overstimulation, dehydration, fatigue, overeating, consuming highly processed foods, gallstones, blood pressure disturbance, digestive disorders (especially constipation), prescription or narcotic drugs and vitamin supplements. (See more on these subjects in later chapters.)

When the kidneys are not able to separate the necessary amounts of urine from the blood, part of the urine keeps circulating around the body, thereby depositing urinary waste products in the blood vessels, joints, tissues and organs. This implies that fluids and waste products are trapped in the body and begin to accumulate. The ultimate result is potentially extreme swelling and symptoms of uremia (an overload of toxic byproducts) or kidney failure. Many skin diseases, strong body odor, sweating of the palms and feet, water retention, lymph congestion, abdominal swelling, rapid weight gain, weakness, high blood pressure and other disorders, are all indications of toxic blood caused, to a large degree, by the presence of obstructive urinary deposits, such as sand crystals and stones, in the kidneys.

Stones in the kidneys start off as tiny crystals and can eventually become as large as an egg. The tiny crystals are too small to be detected by x-rays, and since they do not cause pain, they are rarely noticed. Yet they are big enough to block the flow of liquid through the tiny kidney tubules. Crystals or stones are formed in the kidneys when urinary constituents, which are normally in solution, are precipitated. Precipitation results when these particles occur in excessive amounts or when urine becomes too concentrated. The crystalline particles or stones usually have very sharp edges or angles. Once released by the kidneys along with the urine, they may cut and wear away the inner surface of the urinary canal (ureter) during their passage to the urinary bladder. This can cause severe pain in the loins and/or lower back. There may even be blood in the urine, pain running down the legs, numbness in the thighs and difficulty in passing urine.

Most crystals or stones originate in the kidneys, although some may also be formed in the bladder. If a large stone enters one of the two ureters, urinary discharge becomes obstructed. This can lead to serious complications, such as kidney infection or failure. Regardless of where in the kidneys the blockage occurs, it restricts their ability to remove and regulate water and chemicals, causing these delicate organs to suffer injury. The kidneys' various functions may be affected separately, so urine output may seem to be normal despite significant kidney disease.

The Types of Stones and Their Effects

The most common solutes involved in the formation of crystals and stones are oxalates, phosphates, urates, uric acid and the amino acids cystine and cysteine. Eight varieties of crystals or stones can be formed from these solutes, for various reasons.

Foods or beverages that contain large amounts of oxalic acid cause oxalate stones. A cup of regular tea (not green or herb tea) contains about 20 mg of oxalic acid, which is far too much for the kidneys to excrete. Initially, the body uses calcium to neutralize the acid. By doing so, oxalic acid turns to calcium oxalate. If tea drinking becomes a regular habit, any excessive calcium oxalate in the kidneys is deposited in the form of tiny crystals. Chocolate, cocoa beverages and chocolate ice cream are also high in oxalates. Anyone who has consumed or now consumes these foods on a regular basis may be growing oxalate stones in the kidneys, especially children whose kidneys are still very small and delicate. Also, if you ingested over 200 mg of Vitamin C per day, some of it would be converted into oxalate. Except for a tiny amount that is actually used by the body, the rest would be excreted in the gut and urine. Vitamin C is not as harmless as many believe it is, especially in its synthetic and isolated form.

Uric acid crystals make up another type of kidney stone. Uric acid is a waste product that is formed from purines in food. Foods with the highest purine content are:

- Tea
- Beef
- Bacon
- Calf tongue
- Carp
- Chicken and Chicken soup
- Codfish
- Duck
- Goose
- Halibut
- Sardines, canned
- Liver

- Kidneys
- Heart
- Meat extract, broths
- Salmon, canned
- Gravies
- Scallops
- Herring
- Smelt
- Roe
- Liver sausage
- Meat soups
- Perch
- Pike

- Pork
- Rabbit
- Mutton
- Shellfish
- Trout
- Turkey
- Veal
- Yeast
- Sweetbread
- Anchovies
- Lentils

As you can see from the list, protein foods derived from animals and fish make up the bulk of uric acid-generating foods. Once the proteins are broken down in the liver, the uric acid is passed on to the kidneys for excretion with the urine. If the kidneys are unable to remove all the uric acid, its concentration in the blood rises. As a result, the extra uric acid is deposited first in those areas of the body that have the poorest circulation and oxygen supply, that is, the toes of the feet or fingers of the hands. These deposits of uric acid and other harmful substances in the toes and fingers can make the joints rigid, stiff and unbending. (Check particularly the small toes of your feet, which show the condition of the bladder.)

Naturally, wherever waste products are stored inside or outside the body, specialized bacteria will also be present to help break them down. Accordingly, any deposits of uric acid in the body attract certain aerobic bacteria to decompose this waste product into ammonia. If the bacteria feeding on the uric acid crystals invade these waste-saturated tissues in sufficient numbers, inflammation and pain result. Gout and arthritic conditions are the most common symptoms of this involuntary 'cleansing response'. The uric acid crystals in the toes are made from the same material as the uric acid stones in the kidneys.

A similar situation may occur in the heels. Heel spurs are due to deposits of uric acid and various phosphates. The uric acid attracts bacteria, leading to pain, and the phosphates are responsible for causing rigid and hard structures. Swelling or edema around the foot or ankle, caused by poor kidney and adrenal functions, may accompany this condition.

As discussed earlier, the kidneys and adrenal glands regulate water and salt levels throughout the body. If their functions are subdued due to stones in the kidneys, your body may thus be holding water in the feet, legs, abdomen, face, arms and organs.

Many kidney stones are formed as a result of insufficient water intake and the consumption of foods or beverages that have dehydrating effects, including meat, artificial sweeteners, sugar, alcohol, tea, coffee and sodas. Also, smoking cigarettes or watching television for too many hours has a dehydrating effect on the body and causes urine to become overly concentrated. This increases the precipitation of urinary constituents.

Eating lots of strongly acid-forming foods, such as meat, fish, dairy products, baked goods, candy, sugar and the like, forces the body to release many of its valuable minerals, thereby altering the pH (acid/alkaline balance) of the urine. This not only causes mineral deficiencies in the body, especially in the bones and teeth, but also turns the normally acidic urine filtrate alkaline. In alkaline urine, other substances may be precipitated, including phosphates.

Phosphate stones are formed, in particular, from eating too many foods that are high in phosphate and low in calcium, such as meat, processed breakfast cereals, breads, pasta and nuts, as well as all carbonated beverages. To neutralize the highly acidic phosphate, which could easily burn the delicate kidneys, the body leaches extra amounts of calcium from the bones and teeth and uses whatever magnesium it can obtain from such foods as green vegetables. As mentioned earlier, it takes over two gallons of water to neutralize the acidity of one can of soda. So be kind to your kidneys and substitute water for any soda you may be in the habit of drinking.

The presence of phosphates generates an acidic environment in the body, which literally dissolves bones, leading to osteoporosis and shrinkage of the body frame. It also causes tooth destruction, coronary heart disease, digestive disorders, cancer, and any other diseases that are related to calcium deficiency. A person who eliminates more than 150 mg of calcium with his or her urine in a 24 hour period - an emergency measure taken by the body to combat excessive acidity - is in the process of rapidly dissolving the bones. Some of the calcium combines with the phosphates, forming various calcium phosphate crystals, which can lead to hardening of the arteries and common arthritis.

Please also be aware that excessive sodium chloride (table salt) in the diet predisposes a person to kidney stones. In addition, for every gram of sodium chloride that your body cannot get rid of, your body uses 23 times the amount of water to neutralize the salt, which can lead to fluid retention, unsightly cellulite, arthritis, gout, rheumatism and gallstones. This is primarily an issue for people who mostly dine on prepared foods (90 percent of Americans), which are loaded with table salt (very toxic). The average American eats 4,000 to 6,000 mg of sodium chloride each day. Unrefined salt does not have the same effect, though. In fact, real salt it is an essential nutrient without which the body would become seriously ill. For more information, see the section on unrefined salt in Chapter 7.

Why Do a Kidney Cleanse?

More than twenty million Americans suffer from kidney problems. These problems include urinary tract infections (UTIs), kidney stones, kidney cancer, polycystic kidney disease (PKD), nephrotic syndrome and genetic disorders. The kidneys make a tremendous effort in their attempts to keep the blood clear of toxic substances such as lead, cadmium, mercury and other heavy metals (although these are difficult to pass). The kidneys also maintain fluid and electrolyte balance and regulate the pressure that the heart creates to force the blood through their filtering system. Kidney stones greatly undermine these vital functions, which may further increase the chance of accumulating heavy metals in the body and raise its general level of toxicity. This may lead to infection, high blood pressure, heart disease, brain disorders, cancer and many other imbalances.

The following signs indicate the presence of crystals and stones in the kidneys or bladder:

- A dark or whitish color under the eyes.
- Puffy or swollen eyes, particularly in the morning.
- Deep wrinkles under and around the eyes.
- Tiny whitish, tan-colored or dark lumps under the eyes, which can be felt or made visible when stretching the skin outward toward the cheekbones.
- Overlapping of the upper eyelid.
- Chronic pain in the lower back.
- Swelling of feet and legs.
- Constant fear or anxiety.

A number of herbs can effectively dissolve kidney stones within a period of three to six weeks. (See 'The Kidney Cleanse' in Chapter 7, *Employing Nature's Healing Powers*) Regardless of whether someone has been diagnosed with kidney stones or not, doing a kidney cleanse once or twice a year has tremendous curative and preventive benefits. The kidney cleanse not only improves overall physical health, but also reduces stress, fear and anxieties.

4. What Makes You Weak Also Makes You Ill

Flu epidemics were rare 100 years ago. When they did occur, only the very poor and frail became seriously ill or died. Now, there is a flu epidemic every year, and some of them can last all year round. The theory that the flu strikes only during the fall (typically November, lasting through the winter months December, January and February) is scientifically incorrect. If someone has the flu in April, he just calls it 'a cold', despite the fact that the April and November flu versions share the same virus.

For clarification purposes, the story was a entirely different in 1918, when 20-40 million people, mostly young adults, died during the 'Spanish flu' pandemic. This pandemic, however, wasn't a natural cleansing event so typical for the now yearly flu epidemics. The 1918 outbreak was directly linked with the Great War (World War 1). The influenza A virus strain of subtype H1N1 behind the flu pandemic was unusually severe and deadly. What made it that way? At no time in history was the world exposed to such massive and 24-hour pollution created by the fumes and smoke resulting from continuous bomb and grenade explosions, the burning of entire cities, the effects of mustard gases and other biological weapons by Germans. Nobody remained uninfluenced by it.

The pollution created in Iraq today will affect every part of the globe within 24 hours, as the earth rotates around its axis. In fact, part of the exhaust produced by a single car driven in Beijing this moment will end up in your lungs tomorrow. This is a scientific fact. Pollution isn't an isolated phenomenon and it wasn't back in 1918.

The flu spread even to the Arctic and remote Pacific islands. Viruses constantly adjust to the conditions of the environment. This is known as viral mutation. Extreme and sudden changes from a fairly clean atmosphere before World War I to the most heavy polluted atmosphere in human history also created a sudden extreme viral behavior. Viruses are meant to keep the ecological balance intact, or help restore it when it is upset.

Many of the 1918 pandemic victims were healthy young adults, in contrast to most influenza outbreaks which predominantly affect juvenile, elderly, or otherwise weakened patients. The young adults had the strongest immunity and, therefore, developed exaggerated immune reaction to the virus, known as 'cytokine storm' (a condition when the immune activates too many immune cells in a single place in response to a new and highly pathogenic invader). The very young and the elderly are not capable of generating such powerful immune responses. A repeat of the 1918 is very unlikely unless we experience yet another catastrophic event, such as a nuclear or biological war that would suddenly raise global pollution levels to another extreme level. Gradually increasing pollution levels may certainly increase the incidence of flu outbreaks, but will unlikely trigger such extreme viral behavior as occurred during the Great War.

Today's 'normal' flu epidemics affect a lot more people and are accompanied by much stronger symptoms than ever before. The viruses that afflict us now and a century ago are still very much the same. What has changed dramatically among the general population, though, is the natural resistance of most people to viral attacks. Today, our natural immunity to these germs is many times lower than it was just 100 years ago. Tooth decay and depleted vision among young people are very common now. Numerous new and rapidly growing epidemics are now proliferating, a phenomenon unheard of just two centuries ago. They include millions of people suffering from diabetes, heart disease, cancer and obesity - the latter being the most common cause behind illness and death.

The fact that our modern societies are plagued with so many chronic illnesses shows that entire generations possess weak constitutions, caused mainly by stress, unhealthy diets, and harmful lifestyles. People who lived a hundred years ago and enjoyed good hygienic conditions were much less prone to develop chronic illnesses than we are today. Heart disease, for example, which is today's leading cause of death, rarely killed anyone at the beginning of the 20th century.

Our time is characterized by overstimulation, which has a strong, energy-depleting effect on the body. The following are but a few of the many possible factors that lead to a depletion of our physical energy:

- Watching television too often and for too many hours
- Emotional stress and trauma
- Time constraints and the pressure of having too much to do
- Excessive noise, air, water and soil pollution
- Constant exposure to artificial lights
- Pharmaceutical drugs
- Coffee, tea, alcohol and soda beverages
- Sugar, sweets and chocolate
- Meat and junk food
- Overeating
- Sleep deprivation
- An irregular lifestyle/daily routine
- Excessive sex
- Too little water intake

This list is by no means complete, but it gives you a sense about the wide range of weakening influences that we are generally exposed to in today's modern world. All of these factors lead to the retention of potentially toxic waste products in the body. Toxins are formed in the body when metabolic waste products and debris from old, worn-out cells (totaling over 30 billion cells each day) are no longer eliminated properly. If they remain in the body, they become subject to bacterial attack and are met with a dramatic increase in free radical activity. Free radicals are generated in the body to oxidize and destroy as much of the accumulated waste and weak or dead cells as possible. The resulting toxins generated by this act of self-preservation act as stimulants. They stimulate the body into action to eliminate them from the system.

Under normal circumstances, i.e. if the body's life force or vital energy is strong and efficient, the body can do this without getting overtaxed or being harmed. Through balanced periods of rest and activity, it spontaneously returns to its state of equilibrium. But when the body is exposed to too much stimulation and is unable to rebalance itself, its 'batteries' can no longer fully be recharged. With 'flat batteries', the physical engine is unable to rid itself of all the metabolic and cellular waste generated minute by minute, day after day, and year after year. As a result, much of the waste and its resulting toxins spread throughout the body. Wherever they occur in extremely high concentrations, they provoke a toxicity crisis. Such a crisis indicates that the body's resistance to disease (immunity) has dropped to a level of low efficiency.

When the body is forced to hold on to too many toxins, it is also more prone to infection. If an infection is treated through suppressive methods rather than supportive ones, chronic illness may result. Chronic illness predisposes one to accelerated aging and premature death. Each time an infection is suppressed, the subsequent congestion in the deeper-lying structures of the body increases the workload of the heart, making it increasingly weak and stressed. Heart disease, which is the prevalent killer in most countries of the industrialized world, could largely be prevented if we didn't suppress immune responses such as the common infection.

When a virus or bacterium, normally rendered harmless by the immune system, infects a person who is filled with toxins, the infection itself proves that the immune system was already compromised prior to the infection taking hold. For as long as an energy-depleting influence is maintained and toxicity and dehydration continue to impair immunity, even the most powerful antibiotics won't be able to stop the infection permanently. As already mentioned, bacteria, viruses and fungi are not the real causes behind infections, although this is what the patient is told. Infectious germs cannot thrive in a healthy, clean environment. To do their work, which is to dispose of waste and destroy dead or damaged cells, they need to be in a fertile environment - a terrain that offers them a job worth their while.

We have been led to believe that the most common and dangerous bacteria and viruses to humans either already dwell within our bodies or live in our immediate surroundings such as the foods we eat, the air we breathe, the bathrooms we use, the door handles we touch, the pets we cuddle, or the hospitals we visit. What we are not told is that these microorganisms can strike only as long as the body is congested and unable to remove its own toxic waste.

A patient who is trapped in the vicious cycle of infection-antibiotics-infection-antibiotics can break it and prevent further episodes of infection through a program of cleansing and resting. Both of these are required to help the body eliminate accumulated toxic waste. Before starting on a cleansing protocol though, I encourage people to identify any existing sources of energy-depletion in their lives and to replace these with energy-increasing ones.

Today even many young people are suffering from chronic diseases, and unless they make some drastic changes in their lives, they will find it difficult to ever be truly healthy. The body cannot heal if it keeps accumulating new toxins faster than it can dispel them.

A friend of mine, a physician at the general hospital on the Mediterranean island of Cyprus, was involved in a research study on 721 secondary school children in Cyprus (1995). He told me that the majority of the children his research team studied already had signs of hardened arteries. Another study showed that 52 percent of primary school children in Cyprus are overweight or obese and have elevated levels of blood cholesterol. This is quite a surprise, given the fact that not so many years ago, the Mediterranean countries had some of the best health records in the world. This doctor also told me that almost every child in Cyprus had at least once or twice received a course of antibiotics to suppress an infection. Such a practice was unheard of in Cyprus before the 1970s.

Almost every modern country in the world is now reaping the deadly consequences of unhealthy habits and inappropriate medical treatments. The United States spends about 1.5 trillion dollars each year on health care, and projections indicate that this amount will double in less than ten years. Retail pharmacies filled 3 billion prescriptions in 2000. Sadly, we don't get much in return for all this money and drug use. Instead, the U.S. ranks as only the 37th healthiest nation in the world. France tops the list. [The French are very health conscious. The use of herbal remedies is widespread. Their health care system is free for all citizens, and doctors receive bonuses for keeping their patients healthy and teaching them how to stay that way.]

Almost all prescribed drugs have a suppressive effect. This means that they interfere with the body's attempt to break down the very toxins that make it susceptible to disease-causing agents. To regain its balance, the body has to create a toxicity crisis, or disease. The current trend is toward chronic illness among today's youth, even in countries that have had excellent health records until recently. This trend is so pronounced today that, should it continue unabated, almost all resources of future governments will be spent on 'sickness care'. Michael Moore's famous documentary movie, *Sicko*, released in June 2007, made an excellent presentation about that trend, although it fell short on telling us how to become and stay healthy. Unless people like you and me take responsibility for our health and begin to practice real, personalized 'health care', the disturbing trend toward chronic disease at younger and younger ages will continue.

Illness Is A Toxicity Crisis

A toxicity crisis indicates a condition caused by the presence of bacterial toxins or other harmful substances in the lymph, blood and tissues. It only occurs when the body has a pressing need to return to the state of balance, or homeostasis. The body has a built-in mechanism that allows it to remove toxic, harmful substances in a much shorter time than it takes to accumulate them. By interfering with this process (called 'disease'), we disrupt the body's vital cleansing efforts and become vulnerable to external, destabilizing influences or agents. A vaccine or medicinal drug, for example, can readily become a trigger for damaging an organ or a system in the body. The weakest, most congested organ in the body is mostly likely to be the first to malfunction. Any attempts to treat the diseased organ without removing the underlying causes will not only fail to restore the organ's full health and vitality, but most likely will actually contribute to further complications.

Further on in this book you will learn why it is a potentially dangerous practice, in most cases, to treat merely the symptoms of disease using such common medical protocol as giving blood transfusions to people with low hemoglobin levels, treating the testicles for impotence, or cutting out ulcers and tumors. The use of prescription drugs, which contain nothing to remove the toxins in the blood, lymph, and tissues, may even kill a patient. This is because no doctor really knows for certain the toxicity and congestion level in the body of his patient, which to a great degree determines the intensity of the body's reaction to the drug and the gravity of its side effects. In an otherwise healthy person, the additional poisons that infectious germs generate during an infection normally remain in the body only for as long as the toxicity crisis lasts. Provided we support the body in its cleansing efforts by giving it plenty of rest and enough water to drink, this natural self-healing process, falsely called 'infectious disease', naturally eliminates all traces or effects of toxicity that can result from the microbial activity. The situation is completely different in someone whose health has already been compromised.

As you would expect, you can only reap what you have *sown* in the past, but you certainly have a choice about *what* you sow now and in the future. Unless you live in an impoverished country or circumstances are highly antagonistic to living a healthful life, you can now begin to make positive and educated choices with respect to taking care of your basic needs. Oftentimes, though, people feel they are unable to let go of unhealthy habits or a detrimental lifestyle, usually because of unfulfilled desires, feelings of inadequacy or a habit of putting themselves down.

The body has a hard time remaining healthy when it is abused by overstimulation of the mind, body and senses. Such constant strain can deplete your energy resources faster than they can be replenished. The permanent energy deficiency that results from such overuse of resources is the main cause of discomfort and disease in the body. Although most people now know how unhealthful and potentially dangerous are such practices as smoking cigarettes, overeating, drinking alcohol excessively, not sleeping enough and eating heavy meals in the evening, many seem unable to change their self-abusive ways. The inability to let go of a harmful addiction indicates that the blood carries large amounts of impurities and the liver is unable to remove these (mostly because of bile duct congestion). Both of these conditions can be dealt with effectively through a series of liver flushes, as described in this book and in *The Amazing Liver & Gallbladder Flush*. As the liver performs more efficiently again, the body's natural instincts begin to re-awaken and a sense of satisfaction and emotional stability returns. The enhanced sense of well being and resultant vitality makes it much easier to quit smoking and working too many hours, or to stop eating junk food and living on coffee.

Symptoms of ill health can occur in a variety of intensities and with numerous modifications. Trying to locate the cause of an illness in its effects or via its symptoms is nearly impossible. Stomach ulcers, appendicitis, tonsillitis, arthritis, congested arteries, cancer and most other illnesses merely indicate the presence of various sources and degrees of toxicity. It is becoming more and more evident that congestion and an increase in the acidity of the body's fluids and tissues starve cells of basic nutrients, thereby weakening and damaging them. The above 'diseases' all share one common element - an inflammatory response induced by the body itself. Inflammation does not just happen out of the blue, and it certainly is not a disease. It occurs only if and when the body decides that it is necessary to destroy weak or damaged cells that are contaminated with pathogenic material or toxins. The body does not choose an inflammatory response because it intends to destroy itself. Instead, such a response is its most efficient way to save itself from acidosis (extreme toxicity) or septic shock. The poisons generated by rotting cells (flesh) inside the body would quickly kill the patient if the body did not initiate an inflammatory response to dispose of them. Not knowing the true mechanisms of healing, doctors and patients alike tend to blame the body for making the 'mistake' of interfering with and preventing the seemingly uncontrolled decomposition of some of it parts. Inflammation is the body's genuine and intentional effort at self-preservation. It is an integral and necessary part of almost every disease process, or shall I say, healing response.

This following is the definition of inflammation given by *Wikipedia*, the free online encyclopedia: "Latin, *Inflammatio*, to set on fire, is the complex biological response of vascular tissues to harmful stimuli, such as pathogens, damaged cells, or irritants. It is a protective attempt by the organism to remove the injurious stimuli as well as initiate the healing process for the tissue. Inflammation is not a synonym for infection. Even in cases where inflammation is caused by infection it is incorrect to use the terms as synonyms: infection is caused by an exogenous pathogen, while inflammation is the response of the organism to the pathogen. In the absence of inflammation, wounds and infections would never heal and progressive destruction of the tissue would compromise the survival of the organism." For this very reason, the current medical model, which is centered on suppressing inflammation, is unsuitable for the treatment of the most common diseases. Suppressing the symptoms of illness though prescription drugs or other medical procedures undermines the inflammatory responses the body requires to heal and save itself.

Most diseases are inflammatory responses by the body. These include allergies, age-related frailty, arthritis, asthma, Alzheimer's disease, atherosclerosis, cancer, chronic fatigue syndrome, congestive heart failure, dementia, depression, diabetes, heart attack, inflammatory bowel disease, kidney disease, lupus, macular degeneration, osteoporosis, periodontal disease, obesity, skin disorders, stroke. Normally, the body's natural response to injury, irritation or invasion would never lead to such extreme illnesses. However, our modern environment bombards us with stresses that trigger the inflammation response too often. When overwhelmed with constant irritation, inflammation in the body takes on a life of its own and becomes a permanent condition. This type of chronic inflammation occurs silently, and symptoms may become apparent only until a tumor shows up or the heart fails. During both an active and silent inflammation response, the body produces more white blood cells, which start to burrow deep into the walls of blood vessels, causing further damage and irritation. To prevent total destruction, your body responds by plugging up all those tears and injuries with LDL cholesterol (see chapter 9).

To diagnose and treat any of the above-mentioned illnesses as separate diseases, not only confuses and misleads the patient, but also causes a myriad of complications. Over eighty percent of people who fall ill recover on their own, without any medical intervention. Accordingly, it is more than likely that disease is actually a toxicity crisis that most people's bodies are able to resolve naturally. Once the amount of toxic waste has reached a peak level of tolerance or point of saturation, an appropriate immune response (inflammation) begins to occur. This healing process (falsely labeled disease) helps to reduce the degree of toxicity to below the point of tolerance, simply by neutralizing and removing the toxins, trapped metabolic waste products, and cellular debris, as well as the microbes that feed on them. For this reason, the symptoms of illness begin to vanish by themselves if the toxicity crisis is allowed to take its natural course. Thus, a headache, cold, tonsil infection, gastritis or stiffness in the neck and shoulders, all appear and disappear again in their own time, unless, of course, we interfere with and don't support the body's healing efforts. The occurrence of illness and recovery correspond to the cycles of building up and breaking down the underlying congestion and toxicity that has accumulated in the body.

If your doctor's treatment turns out to be successful, you will most likely thank him for having cured you. On the other hand, if you get well without any external help, you might say you were just very fortunate. Healing, though, does not take place in either case. What most people call 'healing' is actually the body's ceaseless, and if necessary, reinforced effort to eliminate metabolic waste, dead cells, chemical toxins, heavy metals, billions of dead bacteria, and other harmful waste materials. To heal is to be whole. Wholeness or health is the spontaneous occurrence of balance, which occurs naturally when the body removes all the daily-generated waste products and cellular debris and by giving it the nourishment it requires. Creating health is but an ongoing, daily process of regeneration because the elimination of waste materials and the uptake of nutrients will never stop for as long as we are alive. There may be nothing more mysterious about health and healing than maintaining the fine line of balance that exists between these two basic processes.

Illness is like darkness; neither of them actually exists. Darkness is merely the absence of light. By turning on the light, darkness disappears because it has no cause or power of its own. Symptoms of disease cannot be mistaken to be the disease, which makes them equally unreal. They only appear to be real in the absence of health, just as darkness appears to be real only in the absence of light. It is not wise to fight what is not there. Rather it is much more advantageous to do everything possible to keep one's body clean, relaxed, nourished and energized.

Are We Poisoning Our Children With Food?

Most of us were brought up with the belief that disease is caused by external things. Few people know that germs can only 'germinate' in a dead and toxic medium or environment. Parents who see their children go through one infectious illness after another are especially concerned about giving their offspring every possible protection against infectious diseases. Immunization seems to be one way of safeguarding their children's lives. If their child still happens to 'catch' an infection, antibacterial or antiviral drugs are generally considered the best treatment option.

Being so used to blaming external pathogens (disease-causing factors) such as bacteria or viruses for an infection, not many people even consider the possibility that their health problems may have something to do with the food they eat. Could it really be possible that children (and also adults) who suffer from repeated infections are, in fact, only reaping the consequences of being poisoned by such unhealthful products as soft drinks, ice cream, chips, processed chocolate products, candy, 'light' foods, 'fast' foods, processed breakfast cereals, frozen meals, canned foods, and bottled salad dressings? [There is more on this subject in Chapter 13.]

Over 40,000 different food items now occupy the shelves of modern grocery stores. Ninety-eight percent of them have nothing to do with what nature intended a human being to eat. Our digestive system has no way to make use of foods robbed of their natural, intrinsic life energy or manipulated and processed to a point of uselessness, regardless of the wonderful ingredients listed on their product labels. If foods are made in a laboratory, as most of them are, you can no longer consider them food. Instead, they have turned into poison. With their immune systems impaired by large amounts of these man-made, acid-forming foods and the chemical additives they contain, children barely stand a chance of fighting off the normally harmless germs that are part of our natural environment.

The situation is worsened if children haven't been breastfed long enough to build up their natural immunity. Many infants are still being fed commercial formulas, and these contain rancid (oxidized) cholesterol which results from the milk-drying process. The solid foods that most mothers introduce during the first year of a baby's life are generally sterilized during the canning process, resulting in a total degradation of their original life force. Rancid fat/cholesterol is a cancer-producing substance and the cause of many diseases, including allergies and . Several years ago, the British government discovered that nine brands of commonly used infant formula contained potentially harmful chemicals. Formula made with cow's milk is a product that has been chemically altered in a laboratory. The same applies to both soy-based and protein hydrolysate formulas. There is nothing natural about these foods. Just imagine what feeding lifeless, factory foods to human infants must do to them! How many infants are regularly seen by doctors because of various illnesses? Giving formula to a baby poses a major health risk, particularly because his immune system has not yet fully developed, leaving the infant unable to defend himself against these chemically altered, unnatural foods.

The food that most closely resembles breast milk is coconut milk. Many people in tropical parts of the world have raised healthy children on coconut milk when breast milk was not an option. Unless raised on breast or coconut milk, nearly every child will suffer from some ailment or another. (See further details on the major health risks of cow's milk and its products in Chapter 13.)

In addition, an entire cocktail of contaminants and noxious substances may be present in a child's drinking water, as well as in the indoor and outdoor environment. These may easily suppress the just developing immune system of the child, making him susceptible to a whole range of illnesses. All of this has a great influence on how well a growing child will be able to navigate through the many physical, mental and emotional challenges he may have to meet in his life.

Today's younger generation is sicker than any generation has ever been before. Schools and colleges feed our children cheap, low-nutrition foods, and the situation at home is not much better. Many diseases that used to strike only the adult population are now commonly found among young people. Would you have believed even 25 years ago that hardening of the arteries, high blood pressure, Type 2 diabetes and obesity would one day be as common among children as they are today? Childhood obesity increased from 5 percent in 1964 to about 20 percent today - and it is rising. Children spend an average of 5 to 6 hours a day on sedentary activities, including watching television, using the computer, and playing video games. Today's children are bombarded and brainwashed with well-crafted TV ads from fast-food chains and other purveyors of high-fat, high-sugar meals and snacks. When one totals the sugar intake of the average American, including refined sugar, high fructose corn syrup and artificial sweeteners, the shocking intake is 142 pounds a year, or roughly 2 ½ pounds per week, according to a report by CBS Broadcasting on June 17, 2007. This figure has risen 23 percent in the last 25 years and is a major cause of soaring rates of obesity and diabetes. Children make up a large proportion of the sugar-consuming population.

A recent study reported that two-to-six-year-olds who watch television are more likely to choose food products advertised on TV than children who do not watch such commercials. All of this has produced a generation of children who are at high risk for obesity-associated medical conditions. Doctors report a surge in young adolescents who are developing Type 2 diabetes - which can lead to heart disease, high blood pressure, kidney disease, stroke, limb amputations, blindness and, of course, a diminished quality of life and shortened life span.

The consumption of foods that are of no use to the body is a major cause of disease, including infection. Meat or other flesh foods belong in that category. When you eat meat, your body can extract only a fraction of the meat's constituents, and the rest has to be disposed of in different ways. A large portion of the undigested meat protein is broken down by the meat's own cellular enzymes and also by bacteria present within the intestinal tract. Since decomposed meat cells consist of degenerated and coagulated[5] protein, their putrefaction results in the release of *putrescine* and *cadaverine*[6], which are deadly and highly irritating cadaver poisons. Other carcinogenic chemicals, such as *heterocyclic amines* (HCAs), are formed from the cooking of muscle meats such as beef, pork, fowl and fish. (See also Chapter 6 on vegetarianism.) Research conducted by the National Cancer Institute (NCI) as well as by Japanese and European scientists indicates that heterocyclic amines are created within muscle meats during most types of high temperature cooking. Such powerful poisons alone are enough to leave the body vulnerable to any kind of infection.

In most hospitals, both young and older patients are given meat, such as sausages, eggs, fish and poultry to eat, sometimes on the day after the patient has undergone surgery or other invasive treatments. These procedures cause the digestive system to be at its weakest. The patients' already strained digestive and immune systems are unable to handle these additional toxins, while also trying to eliminate as much fecal waste from the bowel as possible. Many hospital patients suffer from constipation because of drug treatments, lying in bed all day, or eating constipating foods, such as meat and potatoes. Congested bowels are a highly fertile ground for microbial infection, which is more likely

---

[5] Heating animal proteins hardens and destroys them. This is called coagulation. For example, a raw egg, which is liquid to begin with, becomes hard when boiled or fried. Its proteins lose their natural thee-dimensional structure, which makes them practically useless for the body.
[6] Colorless, foul-smelling ptomaines, produced by the breakdown of amino acids in living and dead organisms. Putrescine and cadaverine were first described by the Berlin physician Ludwig Brieger in 1885. The two compounds are largely responsible for the foul odor of putrefying flesh, but also contribute to the odor of such processes as bad breath and bacterial vaginosis.

to occur in the hospital environment where germs are present in larger quantities. In essence, hospitals and their diet plans pose a serious danger to people who are already ill.

The life of a sick child may depend on whether he is able to remove most of the decomposing substances in his intestines before they are absorbed into the bloodstream and lymphatic system. If gallstones obstruct the liver bile ducts (now quite common among children, too), the liver is no longer able to remove all the toxins that enter the blood via the bowel; hence 'food poisoning' occurs. Most so-called epidemics are in fact forms of food poisoning or chemical poisoning. They occur among people with high levels of toxicity and low immunity, meaning, those who are *already* ill. Instead of giving hospital patients easy-to-digest liquid foods to eat, they are most often given solid, concentrated foods, such as meat, pork, eggs, etc. This will merely deplete the little energy they have left in them. This energy must now be used to attend to the newly ingested food, when the body should be using its energy stores to overcome the toxicity crisis. An immune system that has already been compromised by a massive influx of toxins is no longer able to effectively ward off bacteria, parasites or viruses. In fact, these germs become the body's last resort to deal with the toxic load.

A child who is fed meat, eggs and dairy products, including milk, as well as junk food (low in, or void of, nutritional value) is much more likely to develop digestive problems and children's diseases such as diphtheria, smallpox or septic fever, than a child who eats fruits, salads, vegetables, grain foods, nuts and drinks plenty of fresh water. Most parents feel responsible for the health and safety of their children. By becoming more conscious of their own eating habits, they will automatically want to give their children the best and most nutritious foods and beverages available. This can contribute greatly toward creating a generation of healthy young people who will be known for their absence of illness.

The Basic Disease Process

The body is made up of cells that are turned over at regular intervals, at a rate of about 30 billion a day. Each day, cellular enzymes face the task of breaking down 30 billion old, worn-out cells that can no longer properly absorb and utilize oxygen and other nutrients. This results in the generation of large amounts of cell debris. Moreover, each of the 60-100 trillion cells making up the body generates metabolic wastes that need to be disposed of without delay. These excretions are substances left over from metabolic processes, which cannot be used by the organism. (They are not needed nor do they have lethal effects.) These include the nitrogen compounds urea, uric acid, ammonia, lactic acids (from anaerobic exercise) CO_2, phosphates, sulphates, indoles, food additives and the like. Under normal conditions, the lymph and blood swiftly remove these waste materials from the fluid that surrounds the living cells (connective tissue). In addition to these excretions (by-products of cell metabolism), the blood dumps blood plasma proteins (including albumins, globulins, fibrinogens, and regulatory proteins) into the connective tissue. If these naturally occurring wastes and blood proteins are not removed promptly, they begin to accumulate in areas of the body that are not suited for such a purpose. Eventually, congestion occurs and the body needs to employ more drastic measures of self-preservation. According to research done in 1961, trapped plasma proteins can actually kill a person within 24 hours. Once stored waste has reached a certain limit or threshold, it seriously impairs the functions of the affected parts of the body— the intestines, liver bile ducts, gallbladder, appendix, tonsils, reproductive organs and kidneys, to name some major ones. To avoid the danger of damage to healthy cells, or organ and system failure, the body begins to employ oxygen free radicals, enzymes and destructive bacteria (putrefaction-causing) and fungi to help break down the mixture of dead cells and metabolic waste. Toxins are unavoidable byproducts of this healing attempt by the body. At this stage of the healing process (called 'disease'), the immune system becomes engaged, trying to remove both the waste matter and the toxins, as well as any weak and damaged cells. This response is commonly known as 'inflammatory disease'. Inflammation is now increasingly recognized as the common, most immediate cause of every acute and chronic disease process. But, as described above, inflammation and infection are not diseases, but basic survival attempts initiated by the body. Various organs and systems in the body are designed to deal efficiently with the daily-generated waste products.

- The liver breaks down cellular components and detoxifies drugs, alcohol and noxious substances.
- The lungs remove the highly acidic metabolic waste product, carbon dioxide, and other toxic gases.
- The kidneys and bladder remove excessive blood plasma, as well as uric acid, urea, ammonia and other waste matter delivered by the liver.
- The colon excretes fecal matter, mucus, dead bacteria and parasites.
- The hair and nails remove proteins, excessive mineral salts, pigments and oil.
- The skin, being the second largest organ of elimination, eliminates sweat, and yes, 40-60 percent of all the waste in the body.
- The lymphatic system, which has to continuously circulate and purify the 18 liters (19 quarts) of waste-loaded lymph fluid contained in the body, plays a major role in the detoxification process.

All of this activity, of course, requires copious quantities of water. When the body becomes dehydrated, the blood becomes overly concentrated (thick) and subsequently draws water from nearby cells. Although the blood is made thinner through this maneuver, the connective tissue surrounding the cells, and the cells themselves, loses precious water required to excrete and remove metabolic waste. The result is congestion, which hinders the waste matter from leaving the body. (To go on a hydrating program, refer to the guidelines in the section, *Drinking Water - The Greatest Therapy of All*, in Chapter 6.) In contrast, a well-hydrated body is capable of both nourishing itself and detoxifying its tissues. This ensures that the body's equilibrium, or balance, is maintained at all times. In a well-hydrated state, the various activities in the body can be conducted in a flawless manner because there is no congestion or holdup anywhere.

In their naturally occurring amounts, body wastes have a slightly stimulating effect. This helps to maintain the functions of elimination. However, if the body's energy is depleted and immunity is subdued due to an excessively stimulating diet and lifestyle or insufficient water intake, the continuously necessary process of detoxification and waste removal becomes disrupted.

All major diseases are caused and preceded by some form of obstruction. An obstruction in the liver, for example, is most likely due to gallstones in the bile ducts (intrahepatic gallstones). It affects the nutrient supply, metabolism and energy distribution throughout the body. A constipated colon causes the backwashing of waste, thereby flooding the body with toxins. A kidney stone can lead to the retention of urine and raise the pressure of the blood against the arteries; hypertension is the result. Lymphatic blockage leads to lymph edema, heart congestion, cancer, obesity, arthritis, and almost every chronic illness. The various types and intensities of the toxicity crisis (disease) result from the various degrees and locations of congestion in the body. In truth, though, if one part of the body is sick, the entire body is sick. It is simply not possible to divide such systems as the cardiovascular, immune, lymphatic and nervous systems into segments that don't influence one another in an immediate and profound way. The severity of disease is largely determined by the amount of toxins, gallstones, kidney stones, fecal matter and metabolic and cellular waste the body has accumulated.

The basic remedy for the most common diseases is as follows:

- Stop all unnecessary 'energy leaks' and allow your body to get enough rest
- Clear up the blocked bile ducts of the liver
- Remove kidney stones/grease
- Clean the passages of the gastrointestinal tract
- Take in enough fresh air, clean water, natural sunlight and nutrient-rich food
- Move your body regularly

All of these are necessary to sustain bodily functions, including the elimination of daily-generated metabolic and cellular waste products. The following list provides you with an overview of possible factors that have congesting effects on the liver, produce kidney stones, dehydrate the body and sap its energy.

⇒ Not drinking enough water
⇒ Drinking iced beverages, especially when the body is hot
⇒ Overeating
⇒ Insufficient nourishment
⇒ Highly processed and refined foods
⇒ Ill-combined foods (such as meat and potatoes; fruit and cereal)
⇒ Coffee, tea, alcohol and other stimulants
⇒ Carbonated beverages
⇒ Tobacco, narcotics
⇒ Pharmaceutical drugs, such as statins, steroids, antibiotics or painkillers
⇒ Irregular daily routine
⇒ Insufficient sleep
⇒ Watching too much television
⇒ Exhaustion, strain, stress
⇒ Environmental hazards
⇒ Pollution, both indoor and outdoor
⇒ Anger, rage, envy, greed, fear, jealousy, egotism, anxiety and other such negative feelings
⇒ Lack of harmony and happiness
⇒ Extreme and excessive habits
⇒ Sedentary lifestyle
⇒ Overstimulation of the senses
⇒ Injuries

Any of these or similar causes of depleting energy in the body and mind can lead to a serious buildup of toxicity in the body's fluids, and thus, trigger a toxicity crisis (acute illness). The crisis is necessary to mobilize the immune system, find an outlet for the toxins and return the body to a state of equilibrium or balance. If the causes remain intact, however, and continue to weaken the body further, it is left with no other choice than to develop a continual toxicity crisis, which is known as chronic disease. The following chapter deals with the part of our body where toxins are most likely to be produced first.

CHAPTER 4

Where Most Disease Begins -
And the Real Secrets to Prevention

More than 56 million Americans report symptoms of gastroesophageal reflux disease,
20.5 million suffer from gallstones, 14.5 million from peptic ulcer, and 3.1 million from
constipation. Millions more don't report digestive trouble but suffer from Irritable Bowel Syndrome.

To comprehend the fundamental reasons we become weak, age or fall ill, we must first understand the purpose and activities of the digestive system. The digestive system represents not only the physical 'engine' of the body, but also the center of emotions and the seat of the subconscious mind. If you wish to understand and deal with the most influential, yet least tangible, basis of any physical illness, you have to include its mental and emotional aspects. Although the body and mind appear to be separate entities, each with a completely different purpose, they are intrinsically one, and they function as one unit. All events on the physical level, like eating food, cell metabolism, removal of waste or exercising the body, occur at the same time on the mental and emotional planes as well. Accordingly, you cannot keep an emotional or mental experience secret from the body.

If you are diagnosed, for example, with a certain illness, such as cancer, and you happen to take the diagnosis seriously, the biochemical impact of this sudden threat against your life (diagnosis) can cause you to die. This gripping fear of survival is enough to instantly stop the secretion of the body's natural anticancer drugs - interleukin 2 and interferon - and dramatically reduce the production of its healing hormones, including endorphins and growth hormones. At the same time, the fear induces a strong stress response (causing the release of stress hormones) that can last as long as the conflict or threat does. Both of these changes in the body's biochemistry practically prevent the body from healing itself. In other words, while being gripped by the fear of death from cancer or any other disease that threatens health and happiness, the diagnosis becomes a self-fulfilling prophesy. What most people don't know is that the diagnosis of disease is often more harmful than the disease itself. I would like you to keep this in mind the next time you feel tempted to check out: "What's wrong with me?"

What applies to the diagnosis of disease also applies to other conflict situations, such as the loss of a loved one or the painful end of a relationship. It is important for you to understand the true reasons behind emotional trauma[7] and illness. Once you know that disease is actually the body's attempt to end these underlying issues of conflict and imbalance, the fear of the unknown (of what disease really is) disappears and you can start supporting the healing process instead of sabotaging it.

---

[7] For details, see the author's book 'Lifting the Veil of Duality'.

The mechanisms behind the disease process are obscure to most, even to the majority of medical practitioners. Very little is known about the true origins of chronic diseases prevalent today. You may be aware of the risks that can contribute to an illness from which you are suffering, but how diseases manifest - from cause to effect (symptom) - remains elusive unless you begin to see the body and mind from a more holistic viewpoint. Understanding how the digestive system works, and in what ways it can lead to illness in the body and mind, can be of tremendous help on our journey of healing. [Whenever I refer to disease or illness I actually mean 'toxicity crisis', which is the body's natural healing response to an unnatural situation.] To provide you with a clearer and more comprehensive picture of the disease process, I have included some of the basic insights of *Ayurvedic Medicine*, which is the most ancient and complete system of natural health care. Once you know how to 'create' illness, you will also know how to reverse it. Such is the purpose of this chapter.

AGNI - The 'General' Of Digestion

Whenever food enters your mouth and touches the taste buds located on the surface of your tongue, your salivary glands begin secreting saliva. Saliva is needed to lubricate the food and to predigest cooked starches. At the same time, your pancreas and small intestine receive instructions to prepare for the release of the appropriate kinds and amounts of digestive enzymes and minerals necessary to help break down the food into the smallest nutrient components.

The first and most common cause of digestive trouble is swallowing food too quickly. This eating habit indicates anxiety, impatience and nervousness. Eating too quickly reduces saliva production in the mouth cavity, which is a major cause of tooth decay. One of the functions of saliva is to keep the mouth and teeth protected against harmful substances and irritating microbes.

There are other reasons why masticating food properly is so essential for our wellbeing. According to fascinating research conducted at the Gifu University in Japan, chewing actually improves memory by reducing the release of stress hormones. Magnetic resonance imaging (MRI) has demonstrated that the hippocampus, which helps control blood levels of stress hormones, is stimulated by the act of chewing. As a result, the simple act of chewing properly lowers both stress and stress hormones. So chewing your food well can actually reduce anxiety levels.

The Japanese researchers also found that when teeth were missing or in a state of disrepair, people tended to chew less. Subsequently, this led to increased stress hormone levels. The conclusion from this study is that good dental health and the ability to chew properly appear to be important factors in preserving our memory as we age and in protecting ourselves against the harmful effects of stress.

After passing through the esophagus, the food enters the stomach. If the food contains carbohydrates (complex sugars and starches as found in vegetables and grains), the salivary enzymes continue to digest these foods for about an hour before the stomach begins to secrete its gastric juices. If the food is swallowed too quickly, these foods remain mostly undigested and begin to ferment.

Gastric juice is composed of hydrochloric acid, enzymes, mineral salts, mucus and water. The action of the acid kills many of the harmful microbes and parasites that are naturally present in fresh produce, meat, fish, dairy products and other foods. The hydrochloric acid also breaks down some of the harmful substances that may accompany the food, such as certain food additives or chemicals. Special enzymes begin to act upon proteins that may be present in the food. Once saturated with enough acid, the food is forced in small jets into the duodenum.

The duodenum is a hollow jointed tube connecting the stomach to the jejunum, which is the central of the three divisions of the small intestine. It represents the first and shortest part of the small intestine, and it is where most chemical digestion takes place. It is called the cap because on an x-ray it looks a bit like a cap. Thereafter, the duodenum makes a C-turn going from the right to the left side of the abdomen. Bile from the liver and secretions from the pancreas come through the *ampulla of Vater* to mix with food in the duodenum. The pancreatic juices contain digestive enzymes, minerals and water to help break down starches further. The bile, which is forced into the duodenum via the common bile duct, aids in the digestion of fats and proteins. The duodenum participates in this very important part of the digestive process by releasing specific hormones and digestive juices. Ayurveda calls the entire activity in this section of the digestive system *AGNI*, or 'digestive fire'. AGNI 'cooks. the food further in order to make its nutrients available for the cells and tissues at a later stage (see **illustration 5**).

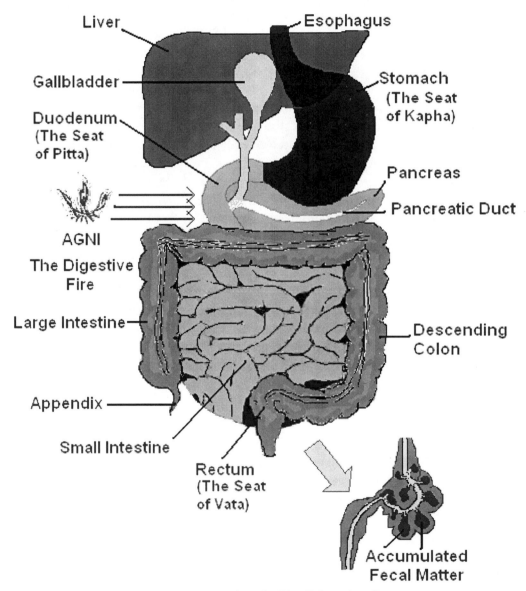

Illustration 5: The Digestive System

The small intestine has a total length of approximately 6 meters (18 feet). It is responsible for the absorption of nutrients, salt and water. On the average, approximately 9 liters (9.5 quarts) of fluid enter the jejunum (upper part of the small intestine) each day, a major portion of which is composed of digestive juices. The small intestine absorbs approximately 7 liters (7.4 quarts), leaving only 1.5 to 2 liters to move on to the large intestine. The absorptive function of the small intestine is brought about by an intricate array of cells within its lining (intestinal folds and villi) that absorb and secrete salts and nutrients as well as water in order to maintain normal salt and water balance within the body. In a healthy person, the absorptive function is so efficient that with a natural, balanced diet, over 95 percent of ingested carbohydrates and proteins are absorbed.

Specific sections of the small intestine perform specific functions. For example, the duodenum plays an important role in coordinating how the stomach empties and at what rate bile needs to be secreted into the intestine to optimize the digestive process. The duodenum is also a major site for the absorption of iron. The jejunum is a major site for the absorption of the vitamin, folic acid, while the end of the ileum (lower part of the intestine) is the most important site for the absorption of vitamin B12 and bile salts. The blood takes up all the nutrients and moves them to the liver for further processing.

The ingested food can be broken down into its basic nutrient components and made available for the complex metabolic processes in the body only when AGNI, the digestive fire, is strong. AGNI is fueled by bile, without which none of the other digestive juices would be sufficiently effective to break down food into its nutrient components. Bile is alkaline. When food that is saturated with hydrochloric acid enters the small intestine, it first needs to be mixed with bile before digestive enzymes can act on the food. An intestinal pH-value of high acidity would block enzyme secretion and become a major stumbling block for the proper digestion of food. Furthermore, in order for them to become activated, pancreatic enzymes must combine with bile before passing through the *ampulla of Vater*. To make this possible, the common bile duct and the pancreatic duct combine to form one short duct before joining the duodenum. As long as bile secretion from the liver's bile ducts and the gallbladder remain unimpeded by gallstones, good digestion is almost guaranteed, provided that the ingested food is fresh and wholesome.

The combination of nutritious food and strong AGNI forms the ideal partnership to help the body make sufficient amounts of amino acids, fatty acids, minerals, vitamins, glucose, fructose, trace elements and other vital substances available to all its parts. This, in turn, produces healthy blood, vital tissues and a youthful body. The quality of the blood and the tissues of the body, including those that make up the skin, mostly reflect the condition of the liver and the small intestine.

Toxic Body, Toxic Mind

If AGNI is depleted because of the reasons explained below, even the most wholesome foods can become harmful for the body. Low AGNI means that much of the ingested food will remain undigested. Undigested food cannot pass through the intestinal walls into the bloodstream, but must be processed in a different way. The food becomes a target for destructive bacteria and starts fermenting and putrefying. These destructive bacteria produce toxins and poisonous gases that can be strongly irritating for the intestinal lining, thereby reducing the digestive ability even further. Since less and less food is absorbed and utilized by the body, more and more waste is generated, which increasingly congests the gastrointestinal tract. At this stage, food turns into poison. Today, one-third of the Western world's population has been diagnosed with intestinal problems, yet the true figure is much higher when one considers all the undiagnosed cases. It is estimated that over two-thirds of Westerners are afflicted with some kind of intestinal trouble.

The small intestine, having the diameter of a large toe, is the most hidden organ in the body and has no direct connection to the outside world (unlike the colon and the stomach). The mental counterpart of this 'unseen' part of our body is what we may refer to as the seat of the 'unconscious'. The stored memories and hidden beliefs of the unconscious mind exert a strong influence over our thoughts, emotions, desires and behavior. Isn't it interesting that traditional medicine considers the origin of *Irritable Bowel Syndrome*, which is the general term used for most intestinal diseases, to be psychosomatic, that is, caused by the mind? In other words, if you feel frequently upset, angry, worried or simply unhappy, you are prone not only to suffer from 'mental indigestion' but also from physical indigestion. Imbalances of the small intestines are characterized by holding on to things in our insides, regardless of whether these are undigested food or unresolved emotional conflicts.

The cerebral cortex of the brain, which controls thought, is intimately connected with the digestive process. Hence, not only foods, but also thoughts need to be properly 'digested' or processed in order to become useful for us, and not to cause us any harm. Undigested thoughts have a poisonous effect on the body as a whole and, particularly, on the digestive system. Fear, anger, shock, trauma, anxiety and similar negative emotions may be locked up in the cellular memory of the intestines for a long time and without any obvious indications of their presence. Once they have reached a certain degree of concentration, they may suddenly erupt and alter one's personality in a negative sense; this can have a detrimental effect on the body as well. It is interesting to note that one of the brain's most powerful happiness hormones is also produced in the digestive system. In fact, 95 percent of serotonin is made in the digestive system (to regulate digestive functions), and only 5 percent is produced in the brain. A lack of happiness diminishes serotonin secretions and thereby weakens digestion of food.

The mind/body connection also works in the reverse order. When you eat highly processed, refined and denatured foods and/or when you eat while your AGNI is low (indicated by poor appetite), you begin to accumulate toxic waste in your intestines. The presence of toxins in the intestinal tract may give rise to nervousness, hyperactivity, nervous laughter or any other emotionally volatile condition. As a generalization, it can be said that toxins in the intestines are the physical counterparts of negative thoughts. Through the mind/body connection, negative thoughts and feelings translate into poisons and vice versa. Normally, the immune system, two-thirds of which is located in the intestines, takes care of both physical and mental toxins (negative thoughts and feelings). The immune system acts as both our physical and mental healing system. However, the immune system can easily become overtaxed when it is overly exposed to non-nutritious foods and negative thoughts (often called stress). You may already know that the thymus gland, which is part of the immune system, can shrink to half its size or less when you are under stress. This may make you susceptible to disease, ranging from a simple cold to cancer.

The 'Useless' Appendix and Its Amazing Role

In a general sense, those parts of the immune system and the lymphatic system that are located in the intestinal tract help to detoxify anything harmful that may come along with the food you eat. Through highly sophisticated processes, these systems are able to separate useful nutrients from unusable waste matter. Some potentially harmful waste products or natural food toxins such as plant-antibodies enter the lymphatic ducts for detoxification and elimination. Most of the nutrient elements are passed through the walls of the small intestine into the bloodstream, which carries them to the liver for further processing, distribution and cell metabolism. Other more specific nutrients, though, can only be absorbed through the walls of the large intestine. These nutrients are meant for nourishing and maintaining the nervous system. Any nutrients, minerals, water and waste products that are not removed by the small intestines now enter the ascending colon, just above the appendix.

In traditional Indian and Chinese medicine, the appendix is known to play a vitally important role. It breeds large quantities of friendly, probiotic bacteria and supplies them to the colon and other parts of the gut in order to neutralize any harmful substances. The strategic location of the appendix allows these useful microorganisms to blend with the fluid fecal matter as it begins its passage through the large intestine. More than 400 strands of beneficial bacteria live in the human gastrointestinal tract. By attaching themselves to the lining of the gut, they can elbow out potentially troublesome bacteria, such as *Candida Albicans*. Balanced populations of the friendly, probiotic bacteria in the gut effectively prevent vaginal and urinary tract infections. They also discourage tumors, particularly cancerous growths in the colon, either by emitting protective chemicals or by inhibiting the production of compounds that nurture cancers. A diminished population of probiotic bacteria, as caused for example by antibiotics, alcohol or junk foods exposes the gastrointestinal lining numerous toxins. This leads to an overstimulated immune system and, thereby, causes asthma, allergies and eczema.

Until very recently, doctors believed that the appendix has no real use or function. In 2005, 321,000 Americans were hospitalized with appendicitis. Removal of the appendix is one of the most commonly performed surgeries. Now, researchers comprised of surgeons and immunologists at Duke University Medical School say the appendix is there to protect the gut, which is not a small job by any means. This worm-shaped organ outgrowth acts like a bacteria factory, cultivating good germs, according to their study, published in the Journal of Theoretical Biology, October 2007.

Apparently, according to the 'new' discovery (which Ayurveda has known for 6,000 years), the function of the appendix seems related to the massive amount of bacteria populating the human digestive system. Most of the trillions of bacteria in the human body are beneficial and help digest food. But sometimes the flora of bacteria in the intestines die or are purged or are overtaken by destructive bacteria. Given the high number of congested colons and inflamed appendixes, this is a common phenomenon today. The appendix "acts as a good safe house for bacteria," said Duke surgery professor Bill Parker, a study co-author. Also, the worm-shaped organ outgrowth acts like a bacteria factory, cultivating the good germs, Parker said. The appendix's job is to reboot the digestive system.

For all practical purposes, and supported by the cleansing action of the bile from the liver, the appendix's job is to keep the colon neat and clean. If large quantities of undigested and decomposed foods reach this part of the intestines, congestion occurs. The intestinal congestion is followed by microbial infestation (through destructive bacteria), which can lead to thickening of the protective mucus membrane and ulceration of the intestinal wall. If microbial growth increases further, the appendix may become inflamed and even burst (**illustration 6**), undermining proper performance of the colon in the future. Removing the appendix can have long-term consequences for colon health and, as explained below, the health of the entire body. In most cases of an inflamed appendix, fasting for a few days and cleaning out the colon (colema, colosan, or colonic irrigation) can save it.

As opposed to the more continuous peristalsis of the small intestines, fecal contents are propelled into the large intestine (now commonly referred to as the 'colon') by periodic mass movements. These mass movements occur one to three times per day in this final section of the gastrointestinal tract. Once they have reached the rectum, the fecal matter stretches the nerve endings in the rectal walls and causes a reflex urge for a bowel movement.

The large intestine no longer breaks down food in this stage of digestion. It simply absorbs vitamins that are created by the bacteria inhabiting the colon. The large intestine is essential for absorbing water and compacting the feces.

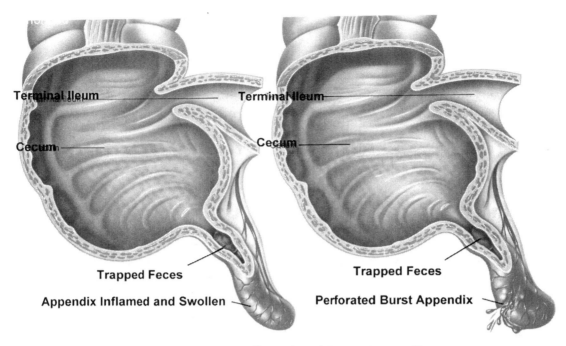

Terminal Ileum

Cecum

Trapped Feces

Appendix Inflamed and Swollen

Terminal Ileum

Cecum

Trapped Feces

Perforated Burst Appendix

Illustration 6: Inflamed and Burst Appendix

The whole digestive and eliminative process - from the ingestion of food to the bowel movement - should ideally take approximately 20-24 hours, depending on the types of food eaten and also on the time of day when the food was consumed. (See the following chapters for details.) However, in the majority of the population, the passage of food through the large intestine alone takes 25 hours or more. This condition is called constipation. I have had numerous patients who reported having a bowel movement only once every 2-5 days. In extreme cases, there was only 1 movement per week or 10 days. On the other hand, many people have bowel movements 3-4 times per day, and in some extreme cases, there may be up to 16 loose evacuations; these individuals cannot keep food in the body longer than 3 to 12 hours. Since most of the ingested food is not digested properly, it decomposes through the help of destructive bacteria. This is so irritating to the intestinal wall, that the body discharges it as fast and as often as possible. Consequently, waste eliminations are far too excessive and frequent.

Having regular bowel movements once or twice a day by itself does not necessarily indicate good digestion either. It's the quality of the eliminated waste that counts. The following are descriptions of the main problems that arise from poor digestion and inadequate elimination.

Internal Pollution

Most intestinal problems occur because of eating harmful foods. The following foods or cooking processes have strongly irritating effects on the protective mucus lining present throughout the alimentary canal, from the mouth to the anus: devitalized, processed, radiated, refined, deep-fried, microwave-cooked and canned foods. Highly acid-forming foods such as meat, fish, poultry, eggs, cheese, refined sugar, table salt, chocolate, candy, commercial fruit juices, coffee, alcohol, carbonated beverages and oral hallucinogenic and pharmaceutical drugs also irritate the intestinal lining. Since the body has no real interest in or capacity to digest and utilize something that is potentially harmful to the blood and cells, many of these products undergo biochemical transformations, known as fermentation and putrefaction. The colon alone can be home to over 700 different species of bacteria that normally help with proper waste disposal. However, when this process includes the fermentation and putrefaction of large amounts of improperly digested food, the naturally present destructive microorganisms proliferate and produce excessive amounts of toxic substances that may irritate or injure the intestinal lining. For all practical purposes, the intestinal lining serves as an internal skin, designed to protect the blood from becoming poisoned. Our life is in danger when this internal skin is injured.

Regular exposure of our 'internal skin' to such acidifying and irritating components as the phosphoric acid and other chemical additives contained in colas, for example, can lead to suppurating wounds and the perforation of the intestinal walls. I often see this type of damage as advanced tissue erosion while examining the iris (iridology) of regular soft drink consumers. As a natural side effect of repairing such internal wounds, pus is formed. Pus is decayed cell-matter containing plenty of bacterial organisms. Toxins released by the bacteria or fungi may cause further tissue damage and lead to poor organ function. These toxins also trigger a vigorous inflammatory response by the body, which can cause pain and obstruction, as is commonly found in *Crohn's disease* and *ulcerative colitis*. If removal of the pus from the wound is obstructed, it may turn septic and seep into the bloodstream, causing septic shock and, possibly, death. To avoid such a scenario, the body may allow polyps and cancerous tumors to form, which help siphon off some of these deadly poisons and keep them away from the blood for as long as possible. (See also chapter 10 on the real causes of cancer)

Blaming bacteria for causing an infection reflects great ignorance about the workings of natural processes both in the body and in the environment. As mentioned before, infection is not caused by bacteria, but by the presence of toxic substances and the resulting cell damage that attracts these organisms.

So-called deadly bacteria, which are involved in the most serious infections, can be found almost everywhere. They naturally live on such common places as your hands, lips, hair, cups, cutlery, door handles, toilet bowls, bathroom floors and kitchen sinks, but only a tiny fraction of the population gets sick because of them. These germs are totally harmless for us unless unhealthy habits or the suppression of the symptoms of disease (which always suppresses the immune system) 'turns' them into deadly weapons. Immunization serums, for example, contain highly toxic substances that are meant to heighten your immune response, but instead, they tend to weaken it. The ever-present bacteria in our environment may mingle with the serum and cause such side effects as shock, convulsions, brain damage and death. (More details on the effects of vaccination programs are in chapter 13) The bacteria are totally innocent unless they are given something spoiled to 'eat'. Dogs and cats lick them from their wounds, and once in contact with their mouth and stomach secretions, they are digested and rendered harmless. We are also equipped with more weapons than we need to deal effectively with any kind of bacteria. Healthy people kill off all bacteria and parasites before they have even a remote chance to do them any harm.

The story, however, is very different when waste products from undigested food linger in the intestinal tract longer than they should, sometimes for as long as weeks, months or even years. Food that is eaten either too quickly, in between meals, late at night, or wrongly combined, lowers AGNI, the digestive fire. Anger and fear also lower AGNI. The deadly microbes, normally neutralized and kept in check by the probiotic bacteria and the immune system in the gut, are given the green light to spread freely throughout the digestive tract. After they find a fertile breeding ground in the human sewer plastering the intestinal walls, the harmful bacteria dramatically increase in number in order to deal with the waste. While attacking the waste, these microbes produce large amounts of toxins. They literally turn everything they find into poison. Among the poisons generated are 'cadaverine'[8] and 'putrescine'.[9] These result from putrefying proteins, the same as those produced from decomposing cadavers.

---

[8] A colorless, viscous, toxic ptomaine, $C_5H_{14}N_2$, having an offensive odor, formed by the action of bacilli on meat, fish, and other proteins, including breakdown of living and dead organisms.

The release of these toxins prompts the intestinal lining and the intestinal lymph system, which harbor most of the body's immune cells, to absorb and neutralize the toxins. Yet the constant influx of toxins eventually becomes overwhelming, which causes lymph edemas to occur, especially in the *cysterna chyli* vessels and the *thoracic duct* (**illustration 7**). The obstructed lymph flow leads to swelling of the abdomen and subsequent lymphatic congestion in other parts of the body.

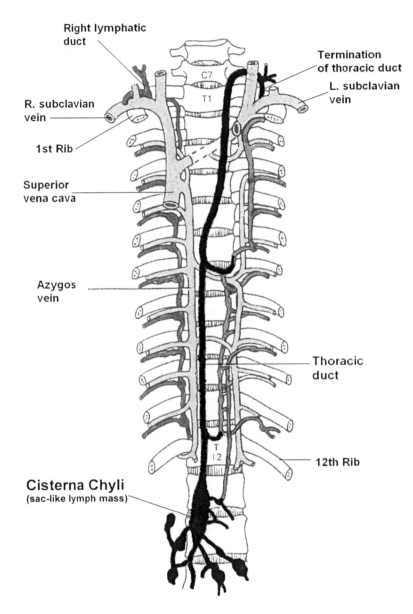

Illustration 7: The Body's Largest Lymphatic vessels

---

[9] An organic chemical compound $NH_2(CHH_2)_4NH_2$ (1,4-diaminobutane or butanediamine) formed by and having the smell of rotting flesh. Other foul-smelling chemical compounds include *methyl mercaptan* and *butyric acid*. Butyric acid is also found in rancid butter, parmesan cheese, and vomit.

The swelling or inflammation of the intestinal lining and the intestinal lymph is an emergency measure the body takes to prevent the absorption of toxins into the bloodstream. If these poisons made their way into the bloodstream, they could endanger the affected person's life (septic shock).

In its desperate attempts to prevent the blood from being poisoned, the body begins to harden the afflicted tissue. This is the first stage of ulcerative processes. If the unhealthy habits continue, more and more layers of hardened mucus are added, forming a thick crust around the troubled areas. This creates further rigidity of the intestinal tract, which in turn begins to obstruct blood circulation in the intestinal wall and to slow down intestinal motion (peristalsis). Consequently, food tends to remain longer in the body than it normally would. In due time, the food begins to decompose, produce smelly gases and lose moisture. This turns it into a sticky mass, which may become dry and hard. If large numbers of bacteria invade this mass, diarrhea may result. First, constipation and diarrhea may alternate, and if the condition persists, more frequent bowel movements and chronic diarrhea may occur.

Should We Kill Intestinal Parasites?

First, you can never live completely without parasites. We ingest them with our food and water, or by other means. Some always survive the assault by gastric juices. It is important to remember that parasites have no real interest in doing business in a healthy, clean intestinal tract because they would simply not be able to survive there in the long run. Instead, they proliferate in filthy, polluted environments. Parasites dig themselves into the tissues of intestinal walls that have absorbed toxins and receive poor circulation and nourishment.

Poor digestion is the main cause of parasitic infection, not the other way round. However, once infested by them, digestive trouble tends to worsen. The problem is that for every parasite you kill, you will have another one to deal with the following day. Parasites can multiply as quickly as you can think thoughts. Why would you want to kill them and then have the burden of eliminating billions of parasite corpses, many of which would remain trapped in the waste that feeds them? A good number of these dead parasites may end up in the lymphatic system and blood. The liver tries to filter them out and remove them via the bile ducts. Once parasites (dead and alive), have entered the bile ducts, they are engulfed by bile and thus become a cause of intrahepatic gallstones (gallstones inside the liver).

A better solution, although not quite as fast as killing them, is to improve digestive functions through a combination of liver/colon cleansing and adjustments to one's diet and lifestyle. This will help the body's immune system to take care of this problem step-by-step, rather than all at once. The assault on parasites can backfire and lead to recurring parasitic infections, while overtaxing the immune system. Killing bacteria through the use of antibiotics is not any different. Suddenly, a massive amount of dead bacteria floods the body, which merely sets the stage for a repeat infection and lots of harmful side effects. Dead bacteria become food for other bacteria. This is just one of the reasons antibiotics are a major indirect cause of infection and numerous degenerative diseases. (See more details in Chapter 16)

In some extreme cases, the killing of parasites is advisable to save, or prolong a person's life (if that is desirable). Such individuals tend to suffer from a near total impairment of the immune functions and an inability to cleanse the liver and colon. It is also helpful for those who have very large, snake-sized worms in their intestinal tract. The most important point to remember is this: When you try to kill parasites or other destructive organisms, be certain that you also remove the poisons/toxins that attract them into your body. There are a number of parasite cleanses using herbal remedies, such as wormwood, green hull walnut tincture and clove or similar formulas that also have detoxifying effects. Cleansing both the liver and colon while doing this is also helpful because it reduces the impact that the 'die-off' may have on your blood and lymph. Such methods of parasite cleansing, however, can take a long time and may be only partially successful, with one exception that I know of.

The mineral substance - sodium chlorite - may have the most balanced and immediate effects among all parasite cleansers. The main requirements for successful elimination of disease-related microorganisms are as follows:

1. Neutralize the toxins and poisons that weaken the immune system and feed the parasites.

2. Strengthen the immune system to remove these microorganisms and keep them at bay.

3. Kill off harmful parasites, viruses, bacteria, fungi, molds and yeast, all the same time.

The product *Miracle Mineral Supplement* (MMS) is a stabilized oxygen solution of 28% sodium chlorite (not 'chloride') in distilled water. When a small amount of citric acid solution, consisting of either vinegar, lemon or lime juice, is added to a few drops of MMS, chlorine dioxide is created. When ingested in this form, the chlorine dioxide instantly oxidizes harmful substances such as parasites, bacteria, viruses, yeast, fungi and molds within a matter of hours. At the same time, it boosts the immune system at least tenfold. By doing so, MMS has been shown to remove, for example, any strands of the malaria and HIV viruses from the blood within less than 24 hours in nearly every person tested. MMS has also been used successfully for many other serious illnesses, including Hepatitis A, B and C, typhoid, most cancers, herpes, pneumonia, food poisoning, tuberculosis, asthma, and influenza. (For more information see *Miracle Mineral Supplement* (MMS) in chapter 7)

AMA - The Main Cause of Congestion in the Body

In an unhealthy intestinal tract, mucus, toxins and fecal matter combine to create what Ayurveda calls *AMA* or *mucoid fecal matter*. The intestines begin to lose their natural shape as they try to accommodate the extra waste (**illustration 9**). Left with no other choice, they create protrusions that are filled with layers of obstructive AMA.

AMA is a breeding ground for parasites and microbes, as well as for cancer cells. The intestinal immune system tries to destroy as much of the destructive material as possible but eventually succumbs to the overload of toxins. This occurs when septic poison starts seeping into the bloodstream. Appendicitis, diverticulitis, colitis, polyps, colon strictures, hernias, Crohn's disease, amoebic dysentery and tumors are but a few of the symptoms directly related to the buildup and absorption of poisonous waste products in the intestines (**illustrations 9a-c**).

Consequences of an Overloaded Colon

The structural changes that the intestines must undergo to accommodate the excessive mass of waste are truly extraordinary. The can affect the health of many other organs in the body. (**illustration 8**)

One particular autopsy revealed a colon 23 cm in diameter, filled with layer upon layer of encrusted old, undigested food intermixed with hardened mucus, leaving less than 1 cm in diameter for passing stool (**illustration 10**).

An ever-increasing number of men and women have accumulated 40 pounds or more of such waste material in the colon alone. Such a condition can be recognized by an enormously extended waistline. In the United States, 65 percent of the population is overweight or obese. Weight problems usually occur first in the colon, and then in the other parts of the body. This waste accumulation may lead to a *prolapsed transverse colon* (**illustration 9a**), which in turn puts a great deal of pressure on the organs of the lower abdomen, including the urinary bladder, prostate or female organs. As a result, these organs may become dislocated, which causes them further structural and functional damage.

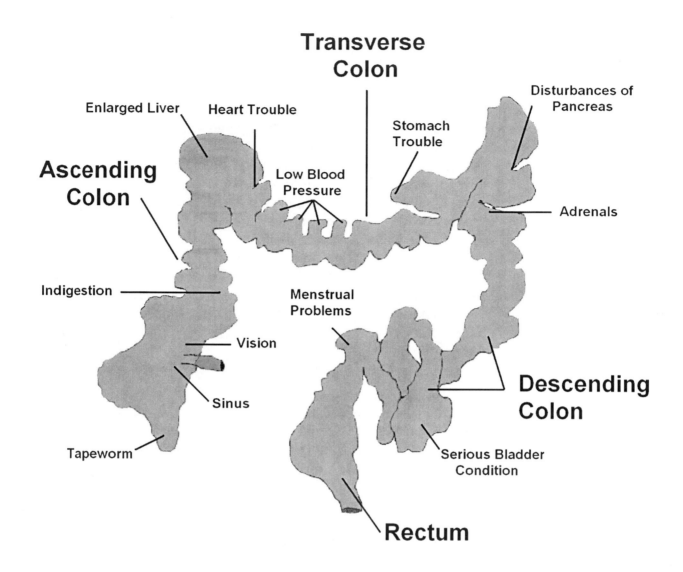

Illustration 8: Abnormally shaped colon

Waste deposits attract a lot of destructive bacteria, which produce toxins as a byproduct of their waste-decomposing activity. As some of these toxins start seeping through the colon walls into the blood, lymph and surrounding organs, more serious complications than just 'waste gain' begin to arise. Migraines, headaches, neck and shoulder pain, bloating, premenstrual tension, irregular menstruation, abdominal cramps, ovarian cysts, emotional instability, sexual disorders, kidney and bladder infections, reduced mental abilities, as well as cancer, are but a few of the complications related to an overloaded colon. In fact, chronic illness that is not linked with impaired colon functions is rare indeed. The bowel is a seat for major neural reflex points, which closely connect this organ with every part of the body (**illustration 11**). To whichever part of the colon AMA becomes attached, its corresponding part in the body becomes afflicted with symptoms of discomfort and disease.

For example, if the middle part of your transverse colon is chronically congested and weakened, you are likely to develop sinusitis. Likewise, if someone has accumulated toxic waste in the bent area of his ascending/transverse colon (right colic flexure), the functions of his right lung are subdued.

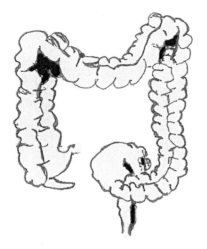
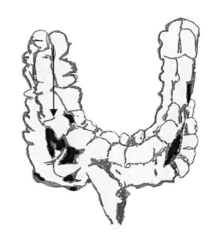

Normal Colon   **Prolapsed Transverse Colon**

Illustration 9a: Abnormal conditions of the colon

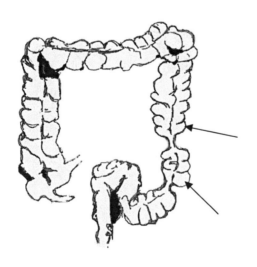
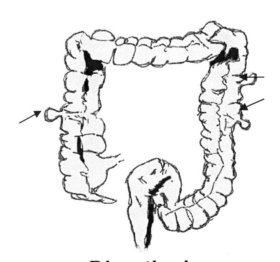

Strictures   **Diverticula**

Illustration 9b: Abnormal conditions of the colon

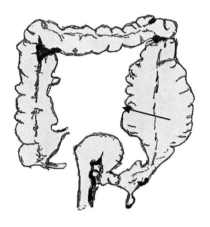 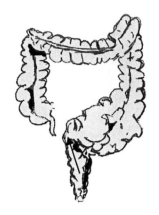

Colitis   **Ballooned Sigmoid Colon**

Illustration 9c: Abnormal conditions of the colon

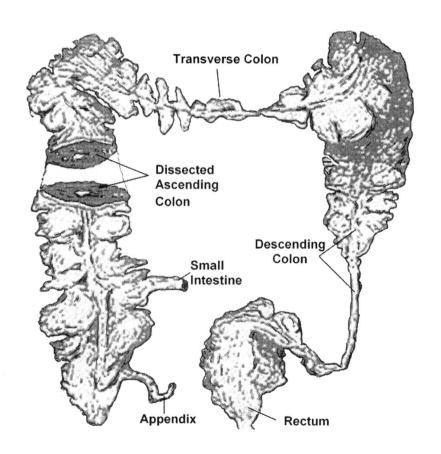

Illustration 10: X-ray of an overloaded colon

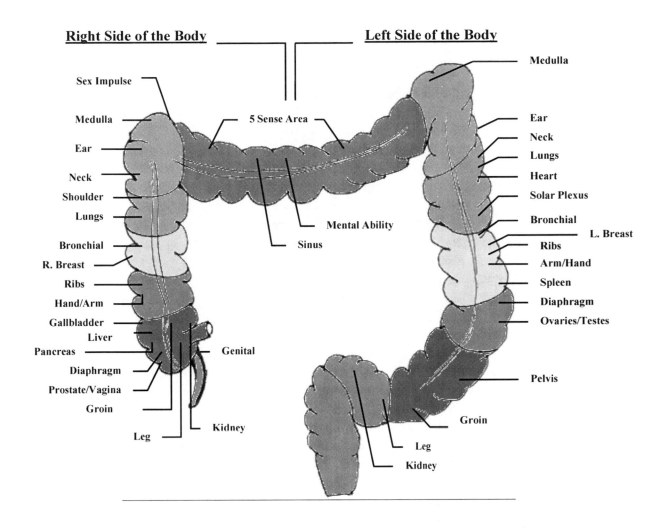

Right Side of the Body _____ **Left Side of the Body**

Labels (right side, top to bottom): Sex Impulse, Medulla, Ear, Neck, Shoulder, Lungs, Bronchial, R. Breast, Ribs, Hand/Arm, Gallbladder, Liver, Pancreas, Diaphragm, Prostate/Vagina, Groin, Leg, Kidney, Genital

Labels (center): 5 Sense Area, Mental Ability, Sinus

Labels (left side, top to bottom): Medulla, Ear, Neck, Lungs, Heart, Solar Plexus, Bronchial, L. Breast, Ribs, Arm/Hand, Spleen, Diaphragm, Ovaries/Testes, Pelvis, Groin, Leg, Kidney

Illustration 9: Bowel Reflex Points

When the right colic flexure becomes constricted or spastic, the shoulders become rounded, the sex impulse diminishes and migraines may occur. Many people, women in particular, suffer from migraines without ever realizing where they come from. When irritating substances are present in the nearby area of the *medulla-colon reflex point*, nerve impulses pass to the *medulla oblongata* at the base of the head, stimulating its vital centers. One of these centers controls the constriction and dilation of blood vessels. Initial pain causes the constriction of blood vessels, whereas severe pain causes blood vessel dilation, a fall in blood pressure and fainting. This results in poor circulation, especially in the hands and feet. Up to 80 percent of women in the industrialized world suffer from mild or severe forms of migraine because of colon dysfunction, of which constipation is the most common cause. Migraines may also be caused by other forms of congestion in the body, such as bile duct blockage, kidney stones, thickening and weakening of blood vessel walls, and so forth.

A note for migraine sufferers: A new study shows that patients who suffer from chronic migraine headaches may find great relief from butterbur or the butterbur root extract, *Petadolex*. The study was conducted in nine clinics in the U.S. and Germany and coordinated by researchers at the Albert Einstein

College of Medicine in New York. According to the study report, subjects who took 75 mg of this herbal product per day for four months saw a 50 percent or greater reduction in the frequency of their migraine attacks. The only side effect reported was occasional burping. Other earlier German studies confirm this finding. Petadolex can be purchased through many Internet sources.

Research also shows that riboflavin reduces migraine frequency. Natural foods that contain good amounts of riboflavin include leafy green vegetables, avocados and grains. Alcohol consumption and oral contraceptives tend to cause riboflavin deficiency. Ionic magnesium (see ionic minerals in *Product Information* at the end of the book) is also greatly beneficial. Since these nutrients need to be absorbed by the digestive tract, having a clogged colon can lead to deficiencies. Supplementing these nutrients while cleansing the intestinal tract can effectively reduce or eliminate the cause of migraines.

You may also be able to stop headaches by stimulating your body's natural painkilling ability. By applying pressure on a nerve just under your eyebrow, you can cause your pituitary gland to release painkilling endorphins. You can also release endorphins by drinking a glass of water with 2-5 teaspoons of cayenne pepper, although not everyone can muster that amount of pepper. The brain releases endorphins when the cayenne pepper hits your stomach lining. In addition, you may put a cold compress on your forehead or behind the neck, massage the ears, earlobes and the crown of your head.

Headache sufferers should check any medication they are taking for side effects. Prescription drugs are the single most common cause of headaches in older people. The risk is higher if you take multiple medications. In addition, common migraine triggers include acidic, processed foods and beverages such as soft drinks, sugar, chocolate, dairy products, fish, meat, eggs, peanuts and other nuts.

Other vital centers of the *medulla* include the *cardiac center,* which controls the rate and force of cardiac contractions; the *respiratory center,* which controls rate and depth of respiration; and the *reflex center,* which initiates the reflex actions of vomiting, coughing and sneezing. Congestion of the colon can lead to disorders in any of these vital areas.

If toxic waste accumulates underneath the lung reflex point in the first section of the descending colon, heart problems may begin to occur. An accumulation of toxic waste in the lower part of the ascending colon irritates the reflex points of the liver and gallbladder and can lead to contractions of the bile ducts and the formation of gallstones.

A stiff neck on the right side indicates that the movement of fecal matter in the ascending colon is very sluggish, leading to toxic overload and irritation of the bowel. Stiffness on the left side of the neck shows that you suffer from a similar problem in the descending colon. If you also experience stiffness or pain in the top parts of the left and right shoulder, it shows that your transverse colon is affected, too. A thorough colon cleanse can rectify the situation and bring relief to these areas. (See colon cleanse procedures in Chapter 7)

The Spreading of Symptoms

Through excessive stimulation or irritation of the *bowel neural reflex points,* symptoms of discomfort and disease start spreading to other parts of the body, and intestinal toxins begin to seep into the lymph and bloodstream. As a result, other organs of elimination and detoxification, such as the liver, kidneys, skin, lungs and the lymphatic system, may also become congested and overtaxed, which causes further debilitation and weakness.

The blood and lymph fluids are meant to eliminate the body's own 'natural' waste products, generated through the constant metabolic activity of its 60-100 trillion cells and the daily turnover of more than 30 billion cells. To break down, detoxify and remove such an astronomical number of old, worn-out cells in addition to the large amount of metabolic waste products that are generated every single day is an enormous feat the body is challenged to perform without ever getting a break. But when the intestinal tract is congested and harmful waste begins to overload the eliminative organs, the body has no other choice but to develop a toxicity crisis to save itself.

The liver is the first organ to receive the flood of toxins coming from the congested intestinal tract. When exposed to these toxins, the bile flora, which consists of beneficial bacteria, begins to alter, and intrahepatic stones are formed in the bile ducts. The stones trap the toxins to prevent them from doing further harm. But the stones also hinder bile secretions, and subsequently render AGNI, the digestive power, weak and inefficient.

Now, the vicious cycle is complete. Low AGNI leads to further intestinal congestion and ever-increasing toxicity in the liver. The liver is the body's primary blood-detoxifying organ. It removes toxins, waste products, bacteria, viruses and chemicals, via its bile ducts, with the intention to take these into the small and large intestine for excretion. Under healthy conditions, this is not a problem. But when the bile ducts are clogged with gallstones, these harmful substances remain in the blood, thereby forcing them to accumulate in the connective tissues of organs and systems in the body, including the brain and nervous system. It is not difficult to imagine that this will both weaken and prematurely age these organs and systems and also cause them to be chronically diseased eventually or even to fail.

Medical intervention, which usually does not include any cleansing procedures, may greatly interfere with the body's waste-eliminating efforts. Pain-reducing medication often leads to further pain and even death. The 'improvement' of the cough in pneumonia through drugs can be fatal, too. Removing a gallbladder that is filled with gallstones does not resolve the underlying problem because the major bile ducts of the liver continue to be blocked. Is it at all surprising that medical intervention fails to significantly improve chronic diseases? The reputable medical journal *New Scientist* announced on the cover page of one of its more recent issues that 80 percent of the medical procedures used today have never been properly tested. Nobody really knows what effects they actually have on patients. So many factors contributing to disease cannot be treated away simply by taking a few drugs or having surgery (more about this in *What Doctors Should be Telling You*, Chapter 16).

Moreover, the stress, tension and exertion that are so often an integral part of man's incessant drive for success, money and power, can deplete the vital energy of the body and lower the effectiveness of all the organs and cells to such a degree that they begin to suffocate in their own waste. Added to this dilemma, external influences such as drastic weather conditions, a change of seasons, traveling to other countries and midlife transition can sap the remaining energy the body needs to muster to adapt to these changes. While undergoing emotional duress, all of these factors combined may suddenly become a trigger for a serious health condition. It is for these or similar reasons that so many people have respiratory trouble in polluted cities during the summer periods or catch colds during the change of seasons. They may be suffering from low physical energy and a depleted immune system long before they actually fall ill.

When the cells and tissues in the body are no longer being supplied with adequate nourishment, water and oxygen, the aging process accelerates rapidly. Cancer and all other forms of continuous toxicity are, in most cases, a culmination of many years of overuse or 'underuse' (sedentary lifestyle) of the body, mind and senses, as well as incomplete elimination of waste matter from the body. What we need most in today's health care system is to encourage a balanced lifestyle right from the beginning of a person's life. This will help everyone to maintain the vital energy of the body on a continual basis. Vital energy is made available throughout the body by *Vata* - the principal power of movement in the body.

Vata - The Power of Movement

Ayurvedic medicine has always had a very thorough understanding of the human body and its intricate functions. Thousands of years ago, Ayurveda proclaimed that the main cause of ill health and premature death is located in the bowel. The ancient healers considered the large intestine to be an extremely important part of the body due to its vital roles. These include the synthesis and absorption of certain essential nutrients for the nervous system and the elimination of waste matter. When you think of it, without the internal motion (Vata) of fluids, waste and nutrients, the body would be dead.

Vata translates as 'air' or movement, and as such, is present throughout the body. Think of your body as a network of different canals, tubes or vessels through which it transports food, air, water, blood, lymph and waste. The nervous system, circulatory system, lymphatic system, digestive tract, bronchi and lungs, bile ducts, hormonal pathways, and cellular ducts are all part of this enormously complex network, sustained by the movement and power of Vata. Diminished or excessive motion in the body makes it ill, whereas balanced motion keeps it healthy and strong. So you can easily imagine that the most commonly found symptoms of 'dis-ease' such as pain, nervousness or fatigue, naturally occur when such motions become uneasy or difficult. If Vata (movement) is excessive, hyperactivity and hypertension may result; if Vata slows down and comes to a halt, constipation or bile duct blockage may occur. Congestion of the coronary arteries, blood vessel walls, lymph nodes, urinary ducts, prostate gland, uterus, sinuses, thyroid gland and other areas of the body all result from disturbed Vata activity. The blocked flow of Vata is responsible for the hundreds of diseases that conventional medicine tries to treat away with drugs or medication without giving due attention to what causes the congestion.

Vata, which is one of the three principal forces (doshas) that control all the functions in the body, is especially and most directly in charge of proper bowel activity. Vata's primary seat is in the colon. If the large intestine is clear of obstructions, Vata is able to perform its important activities throughout the rest of the body. This guarantees that all the systems function at their best. On the other hand, a buildup of fecal matter and hardened layers of mucus (AMA) in the large intestine drastically slows down Vata's eliminative functions in the colon and also in the rest of the body. Similarly, the accumulation of gallstones in the liver and gallbladder hinder Vata's transportation of bile and thus impairs AGNI, the digestive fire. Congestion in both of these important parts of the body directly and indirectly increases the retention of harmful substances in the intestinal tract. Consequently, healthy cells which constitute the intestinal tract, no longer have enough 'space' to breathe. Cut off from their life support system, many of them simply die off and are replaced with residues of toxic, undigested food. Other, more resilient cells, mutate into cancer cells.

Important Note: Sitting on a Western style toilet seat forces one to strain, making waste elimination difficult and incomplete. Human beings were designed to perform their bodily functions in the squatting position, as seen in all native populations. In order to be squeezed empty, the colon needs to be compressed by the thighs. Furthermore, for complete elimination of the fecal mass, the puborectalis muscle must be relaxed and the ileocecal valve from the small intestine needs to be closed. By ignoring these requirements, the sitting toilet makes it nearly impossible to empty the colon completely. In the sitting position, the puborectalis muscle forces the rectum out of its natural position and "chokes" it. Thus, Vata becomes blocked. This leads to fecal stagnation and the development of hemorrhoids, appendicitis, polyps, ulcerative colitis, irritable bowel syndrome, diverticular disease and colon cancer. On the other hand, squatting relaxes the puborectalis muscle and straightens the rectum. Infants of every culture instinctively adopt this posture to relieve themselves. As research has shown, if they don't get 'retrained' to sit on Western style toilet bowls, they rarely develop these intestinal disorders, unless their dietary and lifestyle habits are unbalanced. (For additional information on squatting and how to resolve this predicament, see the beginning of chapter 6)

Solving the Mystery of Back Problems

The accumulation of intestinal waste also affects the normally very strong muscles of the ascending, transverse and descending colon. One of their functions is to assist the body in maintaining a normal body posture. Insufficient blood and nutrient supply to the muscle cells that make up the large intestine causes them to become loose and weak. A prolapsed transverse colon as shown in **illustration 9a** is already enough to significantly distort one's posture. The spinal column is forced to cave in to help the rest of the body adapt to the collapsing structures of the colon.

The main sections of the gastrointestinal tract are affixed to the spinal column. So when the large intestine, for example, is forced to accommodate waste material beyond the daily normal amount, the weight of this load may pull the lower spine forward (see **illustration 12**). Since the resulting distortion of the spinal curvature puts an unequal distribution of body weight onto the spine, this generates several stress points, particularly in the area of the spine that lies closest to the rectum. It is at these stress points that the increase of body weight is most pronounced. This can lead to major lower back problems. The abnormal change of curvature in the lower back (note this gentleman's posture in the illustration before he underwent intestinal cleansing) also forces the upper back and neck areas to undergo major abnormal displacements. In many cases, the neck now curves forward, and the head is no longer sitting on the shoulders. These conditions can create chronic pain in the neck and shoulders. Please note that after intestinal cleansing, this man's body posture returned to normal.

Physical movement becomes increasingly difficult once the spinal structure has been altered in this or other abnormal ways. Consequently, lifting heavy objects or bending to the floor can cause muscle spasms and back pain for days and weeks, and it can even dislocate discs. In many cases, the enlarged colon puts pressure on the kidneys and urinary ducts (ureters) and displaces them. This may lead to retention of irritating and inflammation-causing urinary deposits, which is the main cause of the excruciating pain in the lower back that plagues so many millions of people. Prostate health and sexual performance may also be affected.

Another very common cause of back problems is gallstone formation in the liver and gallbladder. AGNI, the digestive fire, is fueled by bile. A person who accumulates toxic waste in the colon is also very likely to have gallstones in the liver and gallbladder. The two disorders go hand in hand. As the gallstones grow in size and number, the liver and gallbladder become enlarged and exert increasing pressure on the surrounding organs and parts of the body. The liver spans almost the entire width of the body. When this already large organ becomes even more enlarged, it restricts the movement of the diaphragm and reduces the breathing capacity of the lungs. The restricted breathing forces the lungs to hold back abnormal amounts of the acidic gas, *carbon dioxide*. To protect themselves against the extra acid, the lungs respond by producing more mucus than they normally would. This leads to lung congestion. If this situation is not resolved at the causal level, more and more mucus, dead cells and metabolic waste accumulate both in the lungs and bronchi. Eventually, the lungs become so enlarged that they push out the back, and in some more severe cases, also the chest. The back and shoulders become more hard and rounded, as is so often seen among the elderly and middle-aged, but now also among teenagers. All this may be accompanied by pain in the upper back, neck and shoulders.

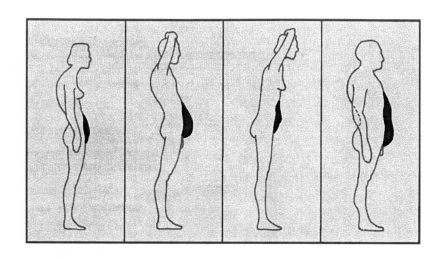

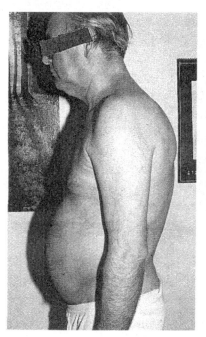
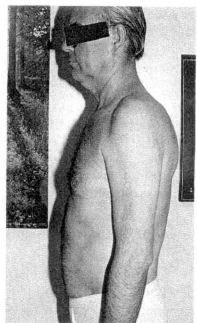

Before and After Intestinal Cleansing

Illustration 12: Abnormal Body Postures
In the diagram at the top, please notice the link between the black areas of waste matter and the changed spinal curvature). This is also shown in the lower photos.

The accumulation of gallstones in the gallbladder can give rise to hundreds of different symptoms in the body. Most of these have been discussed in greater detail in my book, *The Amazing Liver & Gallbladder Flush*. In this context, if the gallbladder, which is attached to the back of the liver, is packed with gallstones, the body needs to adapt its posture to the increasing pressure that the gallbladder exerts against the surrounding tissue and the spinal column. The result is *spinal scoliosis,* a common phenomenon among both the young and the old. The right shoulder may drop and the left shoulder may become raised. In some cases, even the left rib cage may begin to protrude. There may also be pain between the shoulder blades and a strong, dull ache in the middle/upper back area while standing upright for a while. The right shoulder and arm may become stiff. Frozen shoulder and tennis elbow are clear indications that gallstones are present in the liver and gallbladder.

If gallstones get stuck in one of the major bile ducts, there is strong, sharp pain around the area of the right shoulder, which may spread toward the entire back region. At that stage, due to spasmodic pain attacks, breathing becomes increasingly difficult. All of this can produce permanent back problems. [I personally suffered from most of these conditions (including a difficult spinal scoliosis) and over 40 gallbladder attacks, all of which disappeared completely after I cleansed my liver and gallbladder of a total of 3,500 stones.]

Over 60 percent of Americans are estimated to have back problems. About the same percentage of Americans are overweight, which basically means that their digestive systems are malfunctioning. If you also suffer from back pain and consider having surgery, you ought to be aware of the fact that more than two thirds of back pain sufferers who receive surgery for their condition end up with more pain than before. Unless the chunks of toxic waste are removed from the colon, gallstones removed via cleansing from the liver and gallbladder, and the kidney/ureters cleansed, the causes for back pain are likely to continue or worsen. The symptoms linked with these obstructions are not limited to the back. The congestion in these organs can also lead to a disruption in the flow of energy through the spinal nerves, contributing to problems in the legs, such as poor circulation, numbness, pain, and varicose veins.

Another major cause of back problems is dehydration, caused by stimulating (diuretic) foods, such as meat, coffee, tea, soft drinks, power drinks, alcohol, and by inadequate intake of fresh drinking water. Imagine that the water stored in the core of the spinal column supports over 75 percent of the weight of the upper body! Both restricted water supply and accumulated waste in the intestinal tract decrease the volume of spinal water and deplete the water contained in the disk cartilage and surrounding back muscles. Both may also lead to thinning of the intervertebral disks and, thereby, to muscle spasms. The shortening of height among the elderly, which is so often attributed to 'normal' aging, has actually nothing to do with aging, but is due to simple dehydration because of the reasons outlined above.

Back problems remain serious and complex problems only for as long as the most basic needs of the body are not met. Unless a back injury has occurred because of an accident, back problems can be permanently resolved; and even among most injuries, there can be significant improvements. The following are simple solutions to the most complex back problems:

1. Give the body sufficient amounts of water to drink
2. Remove accumulated waste materials from the intestinal tract
3. Eliminate all gallstones from the liver and gallbladder
4. Dissolve kidney stones (if not sure you have any, cleanse the kidneys anyway)

The following chapters provide you with detailed directions to that end. Successfully tackling the root causes of chronic back pain can mean a new lease on life for millions of people.

When the 'River' Takes a U-Turn

While digesting a major meal, beneficial bacteria in your intestines generate 10 liters or more of different kinds of gases (Vata). These gases help to stimulate and facilitate the peristaltic motion necessary to transport food and waste. Once this task has been accomplished, these gases are absorbed by the blood, which takes them to the lungs for elimination. However, if the colon is congested with old undigested foods, these gases become trapped inside the bowels. Hence, the natural downward movement of Vata slows down, comes to a halt, and is reversed eventually. Instead of eliminating all the waste matter via the rectum and anus, Vata quite literally takes a U-turn and moves parts of the toxic mass of fermented or putrefied food in the upward direction.

An impediment in any section of the intestinal tract acts like a dam that hinders the flow of food, waste, and gases, as well as blood and lymph. To understand this, you may imagine a river that is held up by a dam. As the water begins to back up, it causes extensive flooding.

The most severe form of obstruction is known as constipation. Constipation slows the passage of ingested foods through the gastrointestinal tract, which causes them to putrefy and ferment. Putrefaction occurs when intestinal microbes invade the proteins, peptides, and amino acids of eggs, fish, meat, milk and cheese. Poorly digested carbohydrates, such as wheat, beans, and fruits and vegetables, are broken down by fermenting bacteria. Decomposed foods contain a variety of toxic waste products, including hydrogen sulfide, ammonia, histamines, indoles, phenols and scatoles. Hydrogen sulfide and ammonia can damage the liver. Histamines can contribute to allergic disorders such as atopic dermatitis, urticaria (hives) and asthma. Indoles and phenols are considered carcinogenic, that is, they can cause cancer. Constipation leads to the backwashing of toxic compounds, many of which enter the lymphatic system. The rest of them escape either upward and downward or simply accumulate wherever they can in the intestinal tract.

The toxic waste products impart an offensive odor to human feces. Through the reversed Vata pressure, minute toxins, harmful bacteria, mucoid fecal matter and some of the harmful gases are forced all the way into the upper parts of the digestive tract, which causes something of a 'traffic jam'. This chaos can be felt as flatulence or intestinal bloating, cramps or feeling full. Flatus is comprised of over 250 gases, of which hydrogen is the most common.

As the internal pressure extends further upward, more and more toxins end up in the lymphatic ducts responsible for draining the gastrointestinal tract from normally-occurring metabolic waste matter, dead cell material and natural food toxins, such as antibodies. This generates *lymph edema* in the relatively large *cisterna chyli* vessels (**illustration 7**) located in the mid-section of the abdomen (belly button area), noticeable by a further extension or ballooning out of the abdomen. Collecting more toxins in the cisterna chyli vessels than they are able to neutralize or remove, is, in my opinion, one of the principal causes for nearly every chronic illness, including obesity, heart disease, diabetes, arthritis, Alzheimer's disease and cancer.

Lymph edema in the cisterna chyli vessels cause major obstructions in the thoracic duct, which is the body's largest lymphatic duct, responsible for draining nearly 90 percent of the body's daily-generated acidic metabolic waste products, dead cells and other toxic material. Wherever in the body this 'garbage' isn't readily taken up by the lymphatic system, it ends up poisoning the tissues and organs. When the body starts taking measures to protect itself against death through acidosis, most people tend to seek the help of a doctor, who will determine that this (survival attempt of the body) is a 'disease'. What the doctor probably won't realize is that the body does not stop trying to relieve itself of the toxic burden, even if a treatment successfully shuts down the symptoms of the 'disease'.

Whatever waste does not end up in the lymphatic system continues its journey through the ascending route. The continuous upward stream of waste particles, toxins, and microbes now passes into the duodenum, and sometimes even through the *ampulla of Vater* into the common bile duct. Just like water in a sinking ship, this AMA material may actually seep into every nuke and cranny of the upper body, including the pancreatic duct and the pancreas itself. Congestion in the pancreatic duct, apart from inhibiting the release of pancreatic enzymes, may cause pancreatic infection and even diabetes.

All this aggravates AGNI, the digestive fire. Lymph drainage from these organs becomes progressively more difficult, and the digestive system is heavily stressed and burdened with the task of keeping itself functional. As the digestion of food weakens further, the amount of trapped fecal matter in the colon, as well as toxins in the blood and lymph don't just affect how the body looks and feels, they make it increasingly difficult for the internal organs to function properly. The liver tries to cope with the rising level of toxins in the blood by making new gallstones. Gallstones in the liver's bile ducts can be considered a living time bomb. Food, instead of providing the body with energy and nutrients, is now increasingly converted into fat and toxin-filled waste. The body starts to deteriorate a little more each day.

The Dynamic Force of Pitta

The small intestine is mainly controlled by the energy of *Pitta* - the second bodily humor (dosha). Pitta, which in Sanskrit means 'bile', controls AGNI and therefore, digestion and metabolism. Pitta ensures that food is properly digested, absorbed and converted into the basic building compounds needed for the growth of new cells and tissues. Once Pitta-dosha becomes disturbed at its main seat where the gallbladder and pancreas are joined with the duodenum, all metabolic processes in the body are subsequently disrupted. Consequently, the assimilation and metabolism of nutrients becomes insufficient, and the body suffers the effects of malnourishment, even if the person eats well. Being overweight indicates that the body has reached this stage of intestinal dysfunction.

If Vata continues to act in its reversed mode, intestinal toxins and waste fragments, as well as portions of the bile released by the gallbladder and enzymes released by the pancreas, are pushed further toward the stomach. A continued diminished availability of bile and digestive enzymes can lead to obesity, which is a condition of advanced cellular starvation, as well as to heart disease and cancer.

Kapha - Cohesion, Structure and Stamina

The third principal force that controls the human body is Kapha. Kapha stands for cohesion, structure, stamina and strength. Its main seat is in the stomach and chest. Kapha controls the digestive juices and forms the connective tissue (the interstitial fluid surrounding cells), muscles, fat, bones and sinew. It also lubricates the joints, generates the mucus lining in the mouth, throat, lungs, stomach and intestines, and holds the body together. Without the cohesive properties of Kapha, the body would be a pool of disconnected cells scattered on the ground.

Kapha becomes aggravated when the reversed movement of the Vata force reaches the *pyloric sphincter* - the valve that connects the stomach with the duodenum. Reflux of bile from the gallbladder, as well as toxins and microbes from the intestines, and in some rare cases, even feces, may extend the walls of the duodenum and push through the *pyloric sphincter* into the stomach. Occasionally, this may trigger spasmodic constrictions and pain. The backed-up bile and AMA material may cause a number of stomach disorders. The stomach problems may vary according to the different toxins and microbes involved. Other aggravating factors may also be present, such as stress. Of course, the types and quantities of food being consumed also affect the symptoms and severity of the disorder. In most of these conditions, the stomach responds by secreting large quantities of mucus to protect its walls and the blood against the influx of these irritating substances. Mucus is one of the body's most effective means to absorb and 'digest' AMA.

If the situation continues, the stomach lining may become injured and dehydrated in places, exposing it to the destructive action of hydrochloric acid. The stomach cells begin to absorb toxic hydrogen ions. This, in turn, increases the cells' internal acidity, disrupts their metabolic processes and triggers inflammatory responses. This is known as acute gastritis, which may become chronic and lead to peptic ulcers and the growth of cancerous tumors. The disruption of Kapha in this part of the body can greatly undermine psychological balance and happiness. It is usually accompanied by a 'strange' feeling in the gut and by emotions of insecurity and nervousness.

Disturbing the Doshas

Symptoms include:

- Bad breath
- Frequent colds
- Coughing
- Bronchitis
- Asthma
- Pneumonia

- Lymph congestion
- Low immunity
- Hay fever
- Allergies
- Any Chronic illness

The reverse movement of Vata in the intestines displaces both Pitta-dosha (in the middle part of the body) and Kapha-dosha (in the stomach and chest). The more the toxins start backing up in the gastrointestinal tract, the less efficient the lymph drainage from the organs located in the pelvic area becomes . Eighty percent of the lymphatic system is associated with the intestines, making this area of the body the largest center of immune activity. This is no coincidence. The gastrointestinal tract is actually the part of the body where most disease-causing agents are generated and neutralized. Any lymph edemas or other kinds of obstruction in this important part of the lymphatic system can lead to potentially serious complications elsewhere in the body.

Wherever a lymph duct is obstructed, there must also be an abnormal accumulation of lymph fluid surrounding the area of the obstruction. Consequently, the lymph nodes located in such an area can no longer adequately neutralize or detoxify the following things: dead and living phagocytes[10] and their ingested microbes, dead or worn-out cells, cells damaged by disease, products of fermentation, pesticides in food, inhaled or ingested toxic particles, cells from malignant tumors and the millions of cancer cells every healthy person generates each day. Incomplete destruction of these hazardous substances can cause the associated lymph nodes to become inflamed, enlarged and congested with blood. Infected material may enter the bloodstream, causing septic poisoning and acute illnesses. In most cases, though, the lymph blockage occurs slowly, without any symptoms other than the swelling of the abdomen, hands, arms, feet or ankles, or puffiness in the face and eyes. This is often referred to as 'water retention', a precursor to or accompaniment of chronic illness.

---

[10] A phagocyte is a cell that ingests and destroys foreign matter such as microorganisms or debris via a process known as phagocytosis.

Continuous lymphatic obstruction usually leads to chronic toxicity. As explained before, almost every chronic illness results from congestion in the cisterna chyli vessels (**illustration 7**) which are situated in front of the second lumbar vertebra. This sac-like lymphatic mass collects lymph from the two lumbar lymphatic trunks, right and left, and the intestinal lymphatic trunk. In other words, all the lymph from the lower limbs, the walls and viscera of the pelvis, the kidneys and suprarenal glands, the deep lymphatics of the greater part of the abdominal wall, as well as the stomach, pancreas, spleen and the lower and front part of the liver, has to pass through the cisterna chyli to be filtered and detoxified. This is an enormous amount of lymph traffic for this central station in the middle of your body to deal with every day. It passes the lymph and chyle (a milky fluid consisting of lymph and emulsified fats, or free fatty acids formed in the small intestine from the digestion of fats) into the *thoracic duct*.

The thoracic duct is the common trunk of all the lymphatic vessels of the body, excepting those on the right side of the head, neck and thorax, the right arm, the right lung, right side of the heart and the convex surface of the liver. In the adult it varies in length from 38 to 45 cm and extends from the second lumbar vertebra to the root of the neck. It conveys the greater part of the lymph and chyle into the blood. Its large and small branches reach all the major parts of the upper body.

Eventually, the thoracic duct gets overburdened by the excessive influx of toxic material and becomes clogged up, too. The same fate befalls its numerous branches, those responsible for draining lymph from the surrounding areas, including parts of the lungs, bronchi, heart, thyroid, head, upper back and other areas of the upper body. Since the thoracic 'sewer canal' has to remove most of the body's daily-generated cellular waste and other harmful materials, a blockage there causes the backwashing of waste even in relatively distant parts of the body.

When the daily-generated metabolic waste and cellular debris are not removed from an area of the body for a certain period of time, symptoms of disease start to manifest themselves. The following are but a few examples of illness indicators that are directly related to chronic lymph congestion:

Obesity, ovarian cysts, uterine fibroids, enlargement of the prostate gland, rheumatism in the joints, enlargement of the heart, congestive heart failure, congested bronchi and lungs, enlargement of the neck area, stiffness in the neck and shoulders, backaches, headaches, migraines, dizziness, vertigo, ringing in the ears, earaches, deafness, dandruff, hair loss, frequent colds, sinusitis, hay fever, certain types of asthma, thyroid enlargement, eye diseases, poor vision, swelling in the breasts, breast cancer, kidney problems, lower back pains, swelling of the legs and ankles, scoliosis, brain disorders, memory loss, stomach trouble, enlarged spleen, irritable bowel syndrome, hernia, polyps in the colon and many others.

Normally, all lymphatic waste is detoxified in the lymph fluids (contained in the lymph nodes and lymph vessels) before it enters the blood. The thoracic duct extends vertically in the chest and curves posteriorly to the left *carotid artery* and left *jugular vein* at the C7 vertebral level to empty into the junction of the left *subclavian vein* and the *jugular vein* below the clavicle, near the shoulders. The subclavian vein enters the *superior vena cava* which leads directly into the heart.

In addition to blocking proper lymph drainage from the above-mentioned organs or parts of the body, congestion in the cisterna chyli and the thoracic duct permits toxic materials to be passed into the heart and its arteries. This unduly stresses the heart. It also allows toxins and disease-causing agents to enter the general blood circulation and spread to other parts of the body. Rarely is a disease not caused by some degree of lymphatic obstruction. For the most part, lymph blockage has its origin in poor digestive functions and congested liver bile ducts. Lack of physical movement also plays a role. Unlike the circulatory system, the lymphatic system has no central pumping device to push the lymph fluid throughout the body. Instead, proper lymph flow mostly depends on breathing and adequate muscular movement.

If the reverse motion of Vata continues uncorrected, noxious substances, gases and harmful bacteria from the lower parts of the intestines are further brought upward through the alimentary tract. The bacteria acting to decompose this waste begin to produce toxic, putrid gases, commonly referred to as 'bad breath'. Some of the gases may also enter the blood, which takes them to the bronchial system and lungs, causing irritation to their protective mucus lining. The offensive odor that results from bacterial decomposition of damaged or dead cells is nearly impossible to mask with mints or chewing gum.

The failure of the congested lymphatic system to efficiently remove metabolic waste material from the respiratory organs can cause a variety of symptoms. If trapped toxins in the bronchial system, for example, begin to mingle with germs that naturally reside there, the body will first try to remove some of them through the mucus formed during a cold or a cough. However, if such release efforts are subdued via medication or rendered ineffective by the ingestion of congesting foods or stress, the mucus lining begins to thicken further. This causes breathing difficulties, bronchitis and eventually, asthma. Pneumonia and other respiratory infections result when certain microbes, which are permanent and normally harmless residents in the lungs, find fertile ground in the congested environment and begin to spread. The bronchial system and the lungs attempt to remove some of the excessive mucus, which was formed in response to the irritation, by coughing it up into the throat. Chain smokers also experience this problem after awakening in the morning.

The supply of oxygen and water to the lungs, heart, liver, kidneys, stomach, intestines and other parts of the body becomes increasingly scarce as lymphatic congestion worsens. Consequently, the body can no longer guarantee proper elimination of carbon dioxide and other metabolic waste products, as well as cellular debris, from the tissues and organs.

If the body keeps moving AMA higher up in its efforts to eliminate the backed-up toxins, some of them may become deposited in and around the thymus gland, which is responsible for activating immune cells. Congestion of the thymus weakens the body's natural defenses against cancer, bacteria, parasites and viruses. If a nose catarrh occurs, it is extremely unwise to treat it as a localized disorder. A cold is a toxicity crisis, which represents the body's need to rid itself of toxins that have already spread everywhere. If head colds or the flu occur frequently, the mucus membranes may become hypersensitive to dust and pollen, which can cause sneezing attacks, bronchial spasms and constant watering of the eyes - typical symptoms of hay fever.

All toxins have a dehydrating effect because the body's cells have to give up precious water to remove them - water they cannot afford to do without. Allergies and asthma indicate that the body has increased its production of *histamine*, the neurotransmitter responsible for regulating water metabolism and water distribution, as well as antibacterial and anti-viral activities. In a well-hydrated body, foreign agents such as bacteria, viruses, chemicals and proteins as found in pollen, are neutralized quite easily without the need to raise *histamine* levels to an exaggerated level. *Histamine* activity becomes exaggerated when the body becomes dehydrated, which may occur due to the presence of toxins or insufficient water consumption. In the latter case, the body may become oversensitive to all sorts of allergens, including the potassium in orange juice.

In asthmatics, the exaggerated release of *histamine* promotes bronchial constriction. Once their dehydrated bodies receive their normal daily amount of water[11] and existing toxins, including those

---

[11] To stop the body's histamine response to dehydration, which constricts blood flow and reduce your need for water, all you may need is water. So the next time you have an asthma attack, instead of drugs, try drinking 2 or 3 glasses of water. It could stop your reaction almost immediately. (And make sure to drink at 6-8 glasses of water a day.)

produced from fermented and putrefied intestinal waste, as well as gallstones from the liver, are removed, *histamine* production decreases. Thus, bronchial constriction begins to lessen or disappear. In some extreme cases, though, to stop an allergy permanently, it may also be necessary to 'delete' the very memory of the immune cells that leads them to produce antibodies upon contact with the normally harmless allergens (foreign agents). To fully restore the body's balance, it may be necessary to neutralize all existing allergies, including the hidden ones, to foods, pollen, dust, chemicals, metals, and the like. (For details see Chapter 7: *Employing Nature's Healing Powers*)

If the body continues to accumulate toxins faster than it is able to remove them, it will eventually become 'tolerant' of them. In other words, you can 'get used' to drinking alcoholic beverages, smoking, eating too much and wearing yourself out, without developing any signs of major discomfort. This only means that the body has ceased to respond to the buildup of toxins. In this case, the body is no longer able to put up a 'good fight' and may undergo no further toxicity crises. Colds and fever now fail to come. This, however, is the time when the real trouble begins.

Unable to remove the toxic deposits, the body becomes severely congested. Hence, the normal signals of intact self-defense mechanisms can no longer occur and fail to alert the person about the imminent danger of permanent damage. This is the beginning of chronic disease. What would have been an occasional head cold before may now turn into chronic bronchitis, pneumonia, a stomach ulcer, chronic cystitis, syphilis, Alzheimer's disease, Multiple Sclerosis (MS), fibromyalgia (FMS), heart disease, cancer or any other illness. To diagnose and treat a cancerous tumor as an isolated, separate disease event is as illogical as blaming the water-deprived leaves of a plant for causing it to wither and die. Putting water on the leaves instead of its roots makes no sense, and it doesn't save the plant. Those who keep suppressing their bodies' cleansing mechanisms, such as an infection or a simple cold, hurt themselves more than they know. They sow the seeds for a vicious cycle of ill health. Supporting the body in its efforts to remove toxins through natural cleansing and immune-strengthening approaches, such as taking MMS, Pau D' Arco or Olive Leaf Extract (see chapter 7), is much more beneficial than trying to interrupt or stop the body's own relief efforts. MMS (also see www.ener-chi.com), for example, breaks down toxins into harmless components while strengthening the immune system and killing any infectious agents, all at the same time.

When Vata 'Hits the Head'

Symptoms include:

- Cardiac Arrhythmia
- Weight loss
- Muscle wasting
- Hot flushes
- Weight gain
- Nervousness
- Mental stress
- Thyroid problems
- Protruding eye balls

- Metabolic disorders
- Ear infection
- Meningitis
- Deafness
- Throat, teeth and sinus problems
- Eye trouble, headaches
- Hair loss
- Loss of Memory

When the 'river of toxins' flows into the upper parts of the body, it eventually reaches such sensitive areas as the thyroid gland. Blood flow and lymph drainage become impaired. Blood congestion, which is characterized by thickening of the blood, prevents hormones from reaching their target places in the body in sufficient amounts and on time. Consequently, the glands go into hypersecretion (overproduction) of hormones. If the thyroid moves into a hyperactive mode, the overall metabolic rate of the body increases. The body's cells become hyperactive and demand an ever-increasing amount of nutrients.

Given the congestion in the abdominal cisterna chyli vessels and the thoracic duct, the lymphatic ducts that drain metabolic waste from the thyroid into the thoracic duct fail to do so adequately. When lymph drainage from the glands is insufficient, they become congested. Lymph nodes may start swelling up and the thyroid becomes enlarged. This brings about hyposecretion (lack) of hormones.

Diseases related to imbalances of the thyroid gland include toxic goiter, Graves' disease, cretinism, myxoedema, tumors of the thyroid and hypo-parathyroidism, which reduces calcium absorption and causes cataracts. Behavioral disorders and dementia may also have their origin in thyroid imbalances. The failing detoxification of the thyroid gland results in *thyrotoxicosis.*

High toxicity in the thyroid gland often causes *cardiac arrhythmia,* which is a serious heart condition, one from which I suffered when I was a child. The heart simply becomes overstressed as it tries to supply extra oxygen and nutrients to the hyperactive body cells. Related symptoms include abnormal weight loss, muscle wasting and weakness, excessive heat production, redness of the chest, neck and face, and hyperactivity of the nervous system. The latter condition causes nervousness, physical restlessness and mental stress. In many cases, the eyes begin to protrude due to deposits of excess fat, degenerate proteins, fibrous tissue and other harmful material both inside and behind the eyeballs. The internal pressure in the eyes can cause staring, rigidity of eye movement and other vision problems.

If lymph congestion occurs, particularly in the thyroid gland of a Kapha body type (see section on body-types in chapter 5), the resulting low production of thyroid hormone decreases his basic metabolic rate, leading to weight gain and slowing mental activity. In this case, the body may feel cold, even when the environmental temperature remains high. In Vata and Pitta body types, hair loss may result.

Ear problems usually occur when, due to lymphatic congestion, metabolic toxins are not properly being drained from the chest and head areas. Other noxious substances stemming from the gastrointestinal tract may also be forced up into the auditory (Eustachian) tubes. If this coincides with an upper respiratory tract infection, microbes may move from the chest area into the ear canals and cause painful ear infections and the accumulation of pus (dead, decomposed cells). If wrongly treated (through pharmaceutical drugs) tumor formation, meningitis and other brain disorders, and even hearing loss may result. If you experience any liquid coming from your ears or discover a swelling near the ears, you need to start some cleansing procedures immediately. (See chapters 6 and 7.) **Note**: For short-term relief, the ancient technique of *ear coning* or *ear candling* can help drain old wax, fungus and toxic residues from the ears and open the lymph ducts for improved drainage. Placing several drops of urine into the ears also helps to clear up some of the congestion.

If at this stage of imbalance, the body is still fairly hydrated and is not interfered with, it will provide extra amounts of fluids and mucus to prevent toxins from entering the bloodstream. Any form of intervention in this very delicate area of the body should be handled with the utmost care, as it may damage the sense organs of sight, hearing, smell, taste and touch.

Most people think that problems such as tooth decay, tonsil infections, earaches, vertigo, tinnitus, sore throat, stiffness of the neck and shoulders, hair loss, a hoarse voice, broken speech, headaches, nasal and sinus congestion and so on, are accidental occurrences that don't need to be taken very seriously. Yet, these 'minor' complaints may indicate major imbalances in the digestive system. They can be the harbingers of eventually life-threatening circulatory problems, heart attacks, strokes and even brain tumors. An epidemiological study, conducted by the Centers for Disease Control and Prevention and published in the journal *Stroke,* found that greater tooth loss is associated with a higher risk for heart attack and stroke. Observing a group of 1,056 patients, a combined team of doctors and dentists with the Oral Infections and Vascular Disease Epidemiology Study (INVEST), reported in the journal *Circulation* that people with high levels of periodontal bacteria also had thicker internal linings of their carotid arteries - a major risk factor for stroke. Most recently, researchers from the Coronary Event and Periodontal Disease study (CORODONT) reported in the *Annals of Internal Medicine* that high levels of periodontal bacteria were related to a higher incidence of heart disease among the 789 CORODONT participants. If the flow of toxins out of the body reverses and begins to affect the organs and systems of the upper body, the seemingly insignificant symptoms caused by these poisons may lead to chronic illnesses or even death.

A continuous influx of toxins in the nasal area can cause an enlargement of the nasal bone or cartilage. Toxins act as strong stimulants and can increase growth factors, leading to excessive tissue growth. In this case, hay fever may result. Sinus headaches, weak eyesight, sore and swollen or puffy eyes, and general headaches are directly related to a buildup of toxins caused by lymphatic obstruction and the backwashing of waste from the intestines. The names that describe the various symptoms are not relevant. However, it is important to know that all these symptoms are indications of the body's attempts to eliminate toxins that have accumulated at various locations. The obstruction of Vata activity, i.e. the movement of air, water, lymph, blood, waste, or any other material through the body, is the common factor in every toxicity crisis (disease).

The crisis occurs when none of the three *doshas* are capable of conducting their assigned functions properly. Forced from their respective abodes, the normally benign doshas, Vata, Pitta and Kapha, become vitiated and destructive. By suppressing or combating the various symptoms of discomfort or disease, the doshas become even more unbalanced. The use of pharmaceutical drugs, which only aim to relieve the symptoms of disease, may cause long-term damage to the physiology and ought to be used solely as a last resort.

Any successful approach to healing must be based on balancing the three *doshas* - Vata, Pitta, and Kapha. Once settled in their respective, rightful places, they ensure that the body operates with the best possible precision and efficiency. All channels of circulation remain clear, digestion stays strong, and the elimination of waste matter is smooth, complete and frictionless. This allows the body to provide continuous nourishment to all its cells and tissues. The result is uninterrupted health and youthfulness throughout life.

Skin Diseases? Mirror, Mirror...

Several dozen skin disorders have been identified to date. However, like a mirror, each reflects the condition of the blood and the inner organs and systems. The most well known skin problems include acne, pruritus, the various forms of dermatitis, staphylococcal diseases of the skin, erysipelas, folliculitis, furuncles (boils), carbuncles, hidradenitis suppurativa, yeast infections, candidiasis (Candida), scabies, pediculosis, creeping eruption, warts, rosacea, hypertrichosis, alopecia, pseudofolliculitis barbae, keratinous cyst, psoriasis, lichen planus, toxic epidermal necrolysis, erythema multiforme, granuloma annulare, pemphigus, ichtyosis, keratosis pilaris, calluses, corns, pressure sores, hypopigmentation (vitiligo), hyperpigmentation, moles, skin tags, lipomas, angiomas, pyogenic granuloma, seborrheic keratoses, basal cell carcinoma, squamous cell carcinoma, malignant melanoma, Paget's diseases, Kaposi's sarcoma, stretch marks, wrinkles, liver spots, varicose veins, 'spider' veins, shingles, venereal disease, herpes, and others.

The skin is the largest organ of the body, weighing 7-12 pounds. It is vitally linked with every part of the body and serves as a reflector of the internal state of the organism. The skin can be 'read', giving important clues about conditions of the blood, lymph and the various organs and systems of the body. 'Reading' the skin is one the most accurate forms of diagnosis available. If the skin becomes diseased, it is unwise to treat it on the surface. Drug patches, salves, shots, chemical applications, cosmetic treatments, sprays and X-rays can be extremely harmful and often exacerbate existing skin disorders. Instead, attention should be given to what is causing them.

The outer skin continues over the lips and up to the nostrils, proceeding into the innermost parts of the body. This forms the inner skin, which lines the orifices (exits and entrances) as well as the entire gastrointestinal tract. The outer skin's texture, color and appearance may reflect a nutritional deficiency or glandular malfunction. With any external skin inflammation (skin disease) there is an inflammation of some part of the inner body. Inflammation is not a disease, but an appropriate healing response by the body to rid itself of harmful, irritating substances. As long as the internal inflammation or imbalance continues, the outer skin will continue to suffer from diseases (unless the symptoms are suppressed with drugs or other measures).

Whenever Vata's functions in the body are impaired, the organs of elimination become overtaxed and must be relieved by passing harmful, foul waste into the skin for excretion. Once all excretory organs have been restored to normal and regeneration has been achieved, previously ugly, pimply, coarse, puffy and gross-looking skin will once again assume its natural luster and beauty. Rashes or other eruptions will fade away, and even coarsening and wrinkling of the skin will smooth out and vanish.

Color changes, blemishes, pimples, blackheads, blisters, boils, roughness, thickness, dryness, excessive oiliness, over-tenderness, hardness and loss of elasticity, all indicate internal pollution and act as a constant reminder for the affected individual to improve internal hygiene. The body's main routes of excretion are the liver, kidneys, lungs, bowels, lymphatic system and skin. If the amount of toxins and poisons to be voided are unusually large, then the skin is called upon to assist with this elimination, but will consequently suffer inflammation. Unhealthy-looking skin speaks volumes about the struggle the body is going through, physically, emotionally and mentally. If the skin lacks healthfulness, it means that the entire mind/body system needs attention. Most 'infectious skin diseases', are simply efforts by the body to eject poisons and cleanse itself. The specific rashes on the skin (for example, scarlet fever, measles, chickenpox, smallpox, etc.) are simply testimony to the underlying toxicity crises within the body.

Skin diseases are a visible and valuable indication of the condition of the whole body. The severity of skin inflammation is linked with the amount and types of toxins the skin must remove to unburden the other organs of elimination. The skin disease is merely evidence of the body throwing off toxic debris by passing it through the skin. Healthy skin must excrete more than 1 pound of waste each day. When the body dumps more than that into the skin in order to protect the vital organs, some of the waste ends up lodged in the skin tissues, resulting in skin irritation and inflammation.

Some people are more prone to skin disorders than others. This is largely determined by an inherited weakness of certain internal organs, such as the liver, kidneys, lungs, or intestines. In my own case, my mother suffered three bouts of hepatitis before I was born, hence my liver was weak and started developing gallstones from a very early age. (Since I cleansed my liver, it has been healthy and vital.) An inherited weakness, however, is not responsible for the fact of disease; that is determined by the individual. Because of stress, an unbalanced diet and lifestyle, and an overexposure to toxins, the weakest link in the hereditary chain determines which organ, tissue or function will give way first. This in turn determines what kind of skin problem develops, such as boils, pimples, rashes, itching, bumps, warts, moles, lesions or tumors. All of these skin problems are the result of toxins in the blood and lymph trying to escape the body via the skin. Congestion in the organs of elimination and errors in diet and lifestyle are the primary causes of dry or oily skin, atrophy of the skin, blotchy complexion and pimples. Besides making the appropriate changes to one's diet and lifestyle, regular sunbathing of every part of one's body and face heals acne and nearly every skin disease quickly. (Also see chapter 8, *'Healing Secrets of the Sun'*)

CHAPTER 5

28 Proven Secrets for Returning to Abundant Health

"The ultimate cause of human disease is the consequence
of our transgression of the universal laws of life."
~ *Paracelsus*

The Wonders of Our Biological Rhythms

Although it may not be apparent to a layperson, the human body is largely run by 'biological rhythms'. All organs, systems and cells are controlled by exact, cyclic patterns of rest and activity, which we can aptly call the 'universal laws of life'. The following are a few examples of the biological rhythms that follow these laws:

- Normal menstrual cycles repeat themselves every 27 ½ days.
- The stress hormones *adrenaline* and *cortisol* are naturally released into the bloodstream during the early morning hours to promote physical activity.
- Immunity and iron concentrations in the blood reach low levels in women during menstruation and high levels during ovulation.
- The liver is more active during the night than it is during the day.
- Red bone marrow produces more blood cells during the night.
- Most digestive enzymes are secreted during the day.
- Bile secretions peak at midday.
- The large bowel is most active and efficient during the early morning hours.
- Different types of cells have different life spans and are turned over at specific intervals.
- The happiness-producing brain hormone *serotonin* is produced in response to natural daylight.
- The sleep-inducing hormone *melatonin* is secreted in response to the darkness of night.

It is estimated that over 1,000 of these biological rhythms operate in and control the human body.

The Human Body Clock

Each biological timer dictates a specific rhythm or cyclic behavior to a group of cells, an organ or an endocrine gland. The various individual timers or body clocks are intrinsically linked to a common master clock. The master clock coordinates the individual clocks with one another and makes certain that every activity in the body is carried out according to its master plan. This master plan consists of nothing but the body's constant effort to maintain perfect equilibrium or balance.

The body's master clock is controlled by nature's most influential cycle, known as the *circadian rhythm*. The circadian rhythm prompts us to become active in the morning and to wind down in the evening. The sun is the main giver of life on the planet. Both organic and inorganic life forms require sunlight or sun energy for their existence, and so do all human beings. The movements of the Earth on its axis and around the sun create the precise cycles of day and night, as well as the seasonal changes. These rhythmic, repetitive patterns of the forces in nature, in turn, program our DNA to conduct all physical activities with perfect precision and ideal, accurate timing.

All external events occurring in the natural world are linked with similar events inside the body. A sunrise in nature, for example, triggers a 'sunrise' in your body. It wakes you up and gets you going. The morning light enters your eyes as soon as you open them. First, the light is broken down into its full color spectrum (seven colors) by the lenses of your eyes. Immediately, the individual light rays travel to the body's master gland, the hypothalamus. The hypothalamus, which controls the body's biological clock, then dispatches light-encoded messages to the pineal gland, which is often referred to as the 'third eye'. These messages contain specific instructions for the pineal gland to secrete hormones.

One of the pineal gland's most powerful hormones is the neurotransmitter *melatonin*. The secretion of melatonin follows a regular 24-hour rhythm. Melatonin production reaches peak levels between 1 and 3 a.m. and drops to its lowest levels at midday. The pineal gland secretes this hormone directly into the bloodstream, which makes it instantly available to all the cells in the body and tells them 'what time it is' in nature, meaning, what position the Earth is in related to the sun. It also tells a specific gene in the DNA of every single cell when it is time for it to die and be replaced by a new cell. Without the timely secretion of melatonin, the timelines of normal cell-division become extended and cancer cells develop, according to the latest cancer research (Nurses' Study 2006).

The brain synthesizes another important neurotransmitter, *serotonin*, which relates to our state of well-being. It has a powerful influence on day and night rhythms, sexual behavior, memory, appetite, impulsiveness, fear and even suicidal tendencies. Unlike melatonin, serotonin increases with the light of day - with peak secretions at midday - and also through physical exercise and the intake of sugar. It is very interesting to note that over 95 percent of this extremely important neurotransmitter is actually made in your gut, not in your brain. This gut/brain connection shows how crucial eating good food and healthy digestive functions are for the overall wellbeing of both the mind and the body, and vice versa.

The increasing and decreasing levels of melatonin and serotonin indicate to the cells whether it is dark or light outside and whether they should be more active or slow down their activities. This intricate mechanism ensures that all physical functions are synchronized with the rhythmic changes that occur in the natural environment. This is known as 'entrainment'. The health of each cell in the body depends, therefore, on the degree to which we allow the body to be in synchrony and harmony with the cycles of day and night.

Any deviation from the circadian rhythm causes abnormal secretions of the hormones melatonin and serotonin. This hormonal imbalance, in turn, leads to erratic biological rhythms, which can subsequently disrupt the harmonious functioning of the entire organism, including the digestion of food, cell metabolism and overall hormonal balance. Suddenly, we may feel 'out of sync' or shaky and become susceptible to developing an illness, which could include a simple head cold, headache, depression or even a cancerous tumor. The pineal gland controls reproduction, sleep and motor activity, blood pressure, the immune system; the pituitary and thyroid glands, cellular growth, body temperature, and many other vital functions. All of these depend on the regular melatonin cycle which, yet again, is controlled by our body's ability to be in synchrony with nature's rhythms. The amount of melatonin made available to the body in response to the darkness of the night depends on the concentration of serotonin secreted in response to the amount of natural light we are exposed to during the day. As daylight diminishes, serotonin is automatically broken down into melatonin.

If your body makes a good amount of serotonin from natural light, it will also produce sufficient amounts of melatonin during the nighttime, provided your eyes are closed. (When exposed to light, the pineal gland does not secrete melatonin in sufficient amounts.) The pineal gland starts secreting melatonin between 9.30 and 10.30 p.m. (depending on your age). Unless you use stimulants such as caffeine or food at that time, melatonin naturally induces sleepiness or drowsiness.

Melatonin may even slow the effects of aging, according to an animal study conducted by Spanish scientists associated with the Spanish Aging Research Network (RNIE). With sufficiently high levels of melatonin in the blood, the body is able to regenerate and rejuvenate itself. This sustains good health, vitality and longevity. [**Note:** Melatonin in pill form is a popular sleep aid, but it interferes with the body's own melatonin production, which dosage and timing is perfectly synchronized with the circadian rhythm.] The cycles of melatonin and serotonin totally depend on each other and are precisely controlled by our changing environment. By disregarding these rhythmic changes in nature and living against these unspoken laws, the body and mind surely move out of sync with one another. This is a leading cause of physical and mental illness.

One of the greatest secrets of good health lies in the discovery of our intimate relationship with the universe. Any sense of separateness between nature and us can only exist in the mind, not in the body. The body has formed an essential link with the external world. All its efforts are directed toward staying synchronized with our immediate and distant environment, including the moon.

Secrets of the Lunar Cycles

It is no longer just a mythological conviction that the moon exhibits a strong influence on both human beings and nature as a whole. The ebb and flow of the tides, sleep walking, and the female menstrual cycles are but a few of the countless phenomena that are stimulated and regulated by this powerful cosmic force. We are meant to use this force for our health, gardening, agriculture and almost every other area of human concern. Once you have discovered the secrets of the lunar cycles and synchronized your life and activities with them, you will greatly benefit from this newly created harmony with the natural world.

Human beings, other mammals, and most birds and insects are subjected to this mysterious force of nature. All natural processes like pregnancy, the growth of plants and their ripeness, as well as the duration of various diseases, depend on the cycles of the moon. Our ancestors were masters of 'right timing'. Their heightened sensory abilities, perceptiveness, and exact observations of the phenomena in the natural world made them aware of the following points:

- Many events in nature - the ebb and flow of the tides, birth, weather, and menstrual cycles in women - occur in direct relationship with the movements of the moon.
- Land animals and sea creatures synchronize their activities, e.g., searching for food, eating and mating with the position of the moon.
- The effectiveness and success of daily activities, such as the cutting of wood, cooking, the cutting of hair, gardening and the applying of manure in agriculture are subject to the cycles of the moon. For example, during the waning moon phase, foods cook faster and digest more quickly, and wood can be cut more easily during the waxing moon phase when moisture content is higher.

- Undergoing certain surgical operations and using medication may be successful on some days, but outright useless or harmful on others. This effect is often independent of the dosage and quality of the medication and the skills of the attending physician.
- Plants, vegetables and healing herbs are exposed to different kinds of energy on certain days and contain considerably more active ingredients at certain times than at other times. Herbs and vegetables are therefore more potent when picked during the full moon period. The waxing of the moon increases the sap flow in the plants, filling them with more nutrients, vitality and energy.

At the end of the 19th century, mankind at large was introduced to the clock as a means to know the time. The knowledge of the natural cycles of day and night and the changes in the positions of the moon and stars were gradually discarded as 'no longer important' to modern man. The clock had 'successfully' replaced the profound knowledge that most people once possessed about these natural cosmic events and their effects on all life forms on Earth. The ancient wisdom that had upheld natural ways of living throughout the centuries and had been passed on from generation to generation, quickly came to be regarded merely as superstitious belief. Today, however, a sudden and renewed interest in discovering our relationship to the lunar cycles has resurfaced. In relation to the Earth, the moon passes through the following major phases:

New Moon
The moon revolves around the Earth almost every 28 days. While the moon is positioned between the Earth and the sun, we can no longer see it. This is called new moon. New moon can be likened to the phase of exhalation in breathing, when we eliminate toxic gases and waste products from the body. You can prevent many diseases by fasting for a day at this time because the body is more than ready to purify itself from accumulated toxins. This also makes it a good time for liver flushing.

New moon also signifies a new beginning. If you wish to give up old habits like smoking or drinking alcohol, this is the best time for it. You may try hard to change such habits at other times of the month but be disappointed about your inability to do so. The old saying "Well begun is half done" applies to new moon. A sick tree, when cut back during new moon, can regain its health and vitality. Likewise, a treatment started on new moon can lead to quick healing.

The Waxing Moon
Only a few hours after new moon, we begin to see the appearance of its crescent in the sky. The journey to full moon takes about 13 days. Whatever goodness and nourishment is given to the body during this time will be much more beneficial than at other times of the month. This also explains why fertility is much increased, and more children are conceived and born during this phase of the moon and at full moon. On the other hand, it is useful to know that when the moon increases, the body's ability to heal after an injury or an operation lessens. Tooth fillings, crowns, or bridges are less likely to last if they are given during the waxing phase of the moon. Even the washing of clothes is less successful during this phase despite using the same amounts of detergents.

Full Moon
After having completed half its journey around the Earth, the moon is full, i.e. visible to us at night, and sometimes even during parts of the day. This is the time when the moon exhibits a strong influence on all planetary life forms. Sleepwalking, excessive bleeding of wounds, greater potency of herbs collected during full moon night, an increase in the number of accidents and violent crime, and a higher

birth rate, are all effects of increased lunar influence. Cutting trees during full moon can destroy them. Since the body has a tendency to hold back fluids during full moon, it is also best to avoid doing liver flushes or other cleanses at that time. Also avoid having operations, including dental work, on full moon, as you may suffer complications or infections.

The Waning Moon

During the following 13 days, the moon is gradually overshadowed again. Ancient civilizations knew that this is a good time to have an operation (if needed), as the healing capacity of the body is at its most powerful. If possible, book your visit to the dentist during this phase, or on new moon. Pulling a tooth should only be performed during the waning moon or new moon. In addition, at this time, physical activity requires less energy and meets with greater success. The digestive system also works more efficiently, even to the point that eating a little more than usual will not cause weight gain.

Man's Biological Routine

Ayurveda, which literally means 'The Science of Life' claims: "The microcosm is as is the macrocosm." Likewise, our body is the mirror of the universe. At every moment, the body undergoes profound changes by adjusting to the continually changing environment and recurring cyclic patterns. Ayurveda has a unique understanding of these cycles. It knows of three principal forces, or energies, each of which emits a powerful influence on the body and mind for a period of four hours, twice in a 24-hour day. These forces of nature, which conduct all the complex activities in the human body, as well as those that sustain the universe, are known as the three doshas: Vata, Pitta and Kapha. Let us now take a closer look at what happens in our body during a 24-hour cycle. (See **illustration 13.**)

The First Kapha Cycle

The first cycle begins with the 'birth' of a new day. Let us assume that sunrise occurs at 6:00 a.m.. Around 4:30-5:00 a.m., nature starts to awaken. It becomes increasingly active as the sun rises to higher positions. Ayurveda calls the period between 6:00 a.m. and 10:00 a.m. 'Kapha time' which means that your body is still a bit slow. This allows the body to gather strength and stamina. Whether or not you wake with an alarm clock, at around 6:00 a.m. the kidney glands secrete the stress hormones *cortisol* and *adrenaline* to get your body going; this is similar to a battery starting an engine. At this time the sex hormones in the body also reach their peak levels. And, provided your eyes actually see the natural light of day, the brain increases its production of the powerful hormone *serotonin,* which helps you to generate enough happiness and enthusiasm to experience a stress-free, joyful day. Since Kapha is composed of the heavier elements of earth and water, we exhibit more of the qualities of 'earthiness' and 'liquidity' (such as feeling grounded and easygoing) in our mind and body during the early morning hours than, for example, during the afternoon.

The First Pitta Cycle

At 10:00 a.m., the heat of the sun begins to increase considerably due to its higher position. The distribution of sun energy reaches peak levels at noon. Between 10:00 a.m. and noon, we are at our most alert and cognitive best. The Pitta period lasts from 10:00 a.m. until 2:00 p.m. At noontime, AGNI, the digestive fire, is most efficient i.e. the digestive juices (bile, hydrochloric acid, enzymes, and other digestive substances) are most plentiful and concentrated. The Pitta cycle follows the serotonin cycle, which is not surprising since most serotonin is secreted in the digestive system at noontime. Strong serotonin secretion equals strong AGNI. Low AGNI, on the other hand, goes with poor appetite, a lack of stamina, and depression. Eating only a light meal when the body has prepared itself to digest the largest meal of the day is like filling a car with 4 gallons of gas for a journey that requires a full tank. The body won't receive enough fuel (nutrients) to run the numerous, complex activities that are needed to keep you healthy and energized. For this reason, Ayurveda advises you to eat your main meal of the day between 12:00 p.m. and 1:00 p.m. **Note:** Those who don't have the liberty of going home to cook a main meal for themselves at this time, may be able to prepare a salad and vegetable dish cooked with rice or other grains in the morning. Food flasks keep the food warm for many hours. Eating at different times during the week versus the weekend, however, is even worse than eating the main meals in the evening. It is important to keep a regular eating schedule to avoid confusing the body's hormonal and digestive secretions.

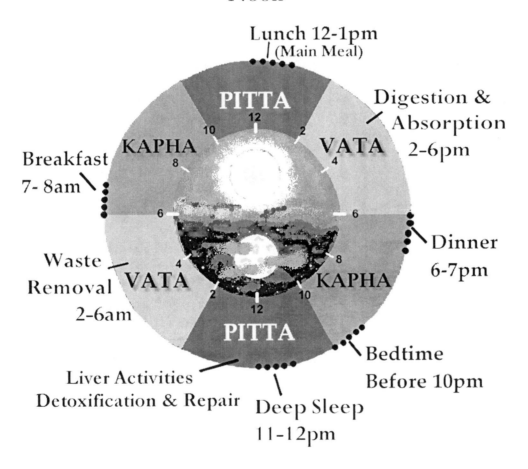

Illustration 13: The Biological Clock

Ideal Daily Routine:
1. Rise between 6:00 a.m. and 7:00 a.m.
2. Eat a light breakfast (optional) between 7:00 a.m. and 8:00 a.m.
3. Eat the main meal of the day between 12:00 a.m. and 1:00 p.m.
4. Eat a light evening meal between 6:00 p.m. and 7:00 p.m.

5. Go to sleep before 10:00 p.m.

Provided the food is wholesome and nourishing, the digestive process will provide you with most of the energy and vitality you need for the next 24 hours. If you feel tired and sleepy after the meal, this indicates that your AGNI is too weak to digest the food properly. Instead of being energized and revitalized from eating your meal, the body has to tap into its energy reserves to process the food. Consequently, there remains only a little energy for other forms of physical or mental activity. Overall, sleepiness after a meal may be due to one or more of the following reasons:

- Your meal is too heavy or consists of ill-combined food items, such as fruits with cereals, animal proteins with starches (see chapter 6 for details).
- You are not getting enough sleep during the night.
- You are eating your lunch meal much later than one o'clock.
- You are not secreting enough bile (Pitta) to keep your digestion strong (due to gallstones).

The First Vata Cycle

Vata or 'movement' controls the hours between 2:00 p.m. and 6:00 p.m. Vata conducts the physical transport of food through the intestinal tract and is responsible for absorbing the nutrients as well as taking them to the trillions of cells in the body. Vata can only perform well and on time if Pitta (bile and other digestive juices) is allowed to act on the food early enough. If you eat your lunch, for example, as late as 2:00 or 3:00 p.m., Pitta becomes disturbed. Poor secretions of bile and other digestive juices lead to poor absorption - one of the main causes for nutritional deficiencies.

The Vata period in the afternoon is conducive to more efficient mental performance and study than during other times. This is due to increased nerve and nerve cell activity. Thus, the Vata period works well for absorbing and retaining information. Studies conducted at the University of Wales showed that students who attended afternoon or early-evening classes performed better on exams than those who attended morning classes.

It may also be useful to know that going to the dentist in the afternoon is less painful than in the morning because of better neural performance and less sensitivity. Existing problems of poor intestinal absorption and unbalanced metabolism, on the other hand, become more pronounced at this time. The Vata imbalance may show up as increased irritability, nervousness, flatulence, gas, and cravings for sugary foods or other stimulants such as tea, coffee, caffeinated soft drinks, chocolate or cigarettes. Most alcoholics will start looking for their first drink of the day during the end of the Vata period. Cravings, especially during the afternoon, indicate that the body suffers from digestive problems and malnourishment, possibly caused by not eating the main meal of the day around noontime.

The Second Kapha Cycle

Sunlight energy drops considerably after 6:00 p.m., and so does Vata activity. This also marks the beginning of the evening Kapha phase, which slows down digestion, metabolism and other physiological activities. Those who are in tune with their body's cycles feel inclined to take it easy when Kapha qualities begin to dominate.

The digestive fire AGNI, which closely follows the moving positions of the sun, sharply declines with the onset of darkness. For this reason, Ayurveda recommends that you eat only a *light* evening meal, preferably around 6:00 p.m. This still gives you enough time to digest your food before bedtime. Research has found that the most important digestive enzymes are no longer produced after 8:00 p.m. A late evening meal (after 7:00 p.m.) will, therefore, not be digested properly and will decompose while it is still in the stomach. Everyone knows the feeling of having a 'rock' in the stomach or the pain of acid shooting up into the throat - both of these unpleasant sensations are signs of indigestion.

During the Kapha period (6:00-10:00 p.m.) the body and mind adopt more heavy and slow qualities. This is conducive to falling asleep. In fact, is highly beneficial to go to bed and sleep before Kapha's influence actually stops (at 10:00 p.m.). Most people feel sleepy or drowsy between 9:00 and 10:00 p.m. These feelings result from the secretion of a natural tranquillizer that the brain makes when it wants you to go to sleep. According to researchers from Harvard Medical School, during sleep most brain cells are 'turned off' by a chemical signal sent out by a group of cells located in the hypothalamus, which is often called the 'brain's brain'. This 'turning off the lights' allows us go to sleep.

It seems that melatonin has a considerable influence over sleep induction, too, since the more we secrete of it during the evening hours, the sleepier we become. Those individuals who no longer feel sleepy around 9.30-10:00 p.m. suffer from a disturbed melatonin cycle.

Around 9:00 p.m., the body's level of immunity begins to decrease, as indicated by a sudden drop in *endorphins* and *corticosteroids* - the body's weapons against inflammation. During the Kapha period, the body tries to save as much energy and as many physical resources as possible, for a very good reason, as explained next.

The Second Pitta Cycle

The body "tempts" you to go to sleep before Pitta resumes its second round in the 24 hour period. Pitta's influence begins at 10:00 p.m. and lasts until 2:00 a.m. During this time, the Pitta-energy is mostly used for cleansing, rebuilding and rejuvenating the body. The liver - a typical Pitta organ - receives most of the body's energy at this time and conducts an astonishing range of activities, totaling over 500 different functions. These include the supply of vital nutrients and energy to all parts of the body, the breaking down of noxious substances and the cleansing of the blood. In addition, the liver cells produce bile at this time, which is needed to digest food, particularly fats, the following day. One of the most important of the liver's functions is to synthesize proteins, which serve as the main building blocks of cells, hormones and blood constituents. Because the liver is such an active organ, it uses a considerable amount of energy. This organ's high metabolic rate produces a great deal of heat, making the liver the main heat-producing organ in the body. However, if you keep disregarding the body's biological rhythms and remain awake during this cycle, much less energy is available to carry out the liver's important activities, and eventually decreased liver function, intrahepatic stones, and diminished health are the result.

WHY PROPER SLEEP IS SO IMPORTANT FOR YOU!

The liver requires all the energy it can get to meet all these and many other responsibilities. This can only happen sufficiently, though, if you sleep during the Pitta nighttime. If you use up the liver's nighttime energy by forcing it to digest food or by engaging in mental or physical activities, this vital organ is left with too little energy to do its extremely crucial work. Most of the available Pitta-energy should be directed to the liver and also, to a certain extent, to the kidneys. This helps the kidneys to filter the blood plasma, to keep body fluids balanced and to maintain normal blood pressure.

Although the brain makes up merely one fiftieth of the body's mass, it generally contains more than one quarter of the body's entire blood content. However, during the Pitta period at night, most of the blood located at the back of the brain moves into the liver for storage and purification. If you are mentally or physically active at this time, the liver does not receive enough blood to function properly. It also cannot cleanse the blood sufficiently. This results in the accumulation of toxic materials in the liver and bloodstream. If toxins keep circulating in the blood, they will settle in the interstitial fluid (connective tissues) of the organs and systems, thereby raising acidity and causing them damage. This includes the liver. High blood toxicity can lead to the secretion of stress hormones, brain fog and injured capillaries, arteries and heart muscles. Most heart diseases are the result of a poorly performing liver that is unable to remove all toxic, noxious substances from the blood on a daily basis. If we don't give the liver the energy it needs to conduct its most basic activities, we sow the seeds of illness throughout the body.

Sleep may be divided into two major portions - before midnight and after midnight. Among adults, the most important processes of purification and renewal occur during the two hours of sleep before midnight. This period includes deep sleep, often referred to as 'Beauty Sleep'. Deep sleep lasts for about an hour from 11:00 p.m. until midnight. During this period, you enter a dreamless state where oxygen consumption in the body drops by about eight percent. This results in profound physical rest and relaxation. The physiological rest, which you gain during this hour of dreamless sleep, is at least three times deeper than what you get during the sleep after midnight, when oxygen consumption in the body rises again by 5-6 percent.

Growth factors, commonly known as growth hormones, are secreted profusely during this hour of deep sleep. These powerful hormones are responsible for cellular growth, repair and rejuvenation. People age faster if they don't produce enough growth hormones. The latest 'fashion' in the beauty market is to consume synthetic growth hormones which create 'fantastic' rejuvenating results but can also have devastating side effects including heart disease and cancer. On the other hand, if the body makes these hormones at the right time and in the correct amounts, as happens during deep sleep, they can keep the body vital and youthful at every age.

Deep sleep never occurs after midnight, and it comes only if you go to sleep at least two hours before midnight. If you miss out on deep sleep regularly, your body and mind become overtired. This triggers abnormal stress responses in the form of constant secretions of stress hormones such as *adrenaline*, *cortisol* or *cholesterol*. (Yes, cholesterol is a stress hormone that rises with stress!) To keep these artificially derived energy bursts going, at least for a while, you may be tempted to take such stimulants as cigarettes, coffee, tea, candy, caffeinated soft drinks or alcohol. When the body's energy reserves are depleted, though, chronic fatigue results, and stimulants will no longer work.

Fatigue is a major causal or contributing factor to today's health problems. When you feel tired, it is not just your mind that is tired. In fact, when fatigued, all the cells that make up your heart, lungs, digestive organs, kidneys and every organ and system of the body suffer from low energy and are unable to function properly. When you are tired, your brain no longer receives adequate amounts of water, glucose, oxygen and amino acids - its most essential nutrients. The short supply of brain nutrients can lead to innumerable problems in a person's mind, body and behavior, including more fatigue. When you drive a car during the night, for example, your body has to keep fighting the 'sleepy' hormone melatonin, which naturally tries to keep your body at its lowest level of performance and activity. According to research in the field of *chronobiology*, attention span after midnight drops considerably. This dramatically raises your risk for making mistakes and having an accident. Most highway road accidents occur during the nighttime, and accidents in factories are 20 percent more likely to occur on the night shift.

Doctors at the University of California in San Diego, have found that losing a few hours of sleep not only makes you feel tired the following day but can also affect the immune system, possibly impairing the body's ability to fight infection. Since immunity diminishes as tiredness increases, your body is unable to defend itself against bacteria, microbes and viruses. It also cannot cope efficiently with the buildup of harmful substances in the body.

Frequent tiredness and low energy precedes any type of chronic disease and most acute illnesses, including cancer, heart disease, multiple sclerosis, chronic fatigue syndrome, AIDS, the common cold and the flu. Studies have found a direct relationship between sleep and health conditions. Insufficient sleep even affects growth hormone secretion that is linked to obesity. As the amount of hormone secretion decreases, the chance for weight gain increases. In other words, the less quality sleep you get, the more fat you become. Furthermore, blood pressure usually falls during the sleep cycle. However, interrupted sleep can adversely affect this normal decline, leading to hypertension and cardiovascular problems. Finally, insufficient sleep impairs the body's ability to use insulin, leading to the onset of diabetes.

The Dark Side of Light in the Night - Cancer Growth

As indicated before, one of the most important findings ever discovered with regard to cancer is that low levels of melatonin in the blood drastically increase the risk of cancer. According to the Nurses' Study (reported Jan. 2006), which is the most comprehensive and longest-lasting cancer study in the world, low blood melatonin in registered nurses was found to be responsible for a 50 times higher risk of developing cancer. Nurses suffer from disrupted sleep cycles due to the nature of their work. Melatonin controls the gene responsible for keeping the life cycles of cells in the body in check. In other words, the less melatonin you make during the night, the more likely it is that cells will live beyond their natural life cycle and thus become cancerous.

The first indications of the damaging effects of light on melatonin secretions during the night were observed in rodents. "At least in rats, a little light throughout the night can have a dramatic impact on cancer," observes David E. Blask of the Mary Imogene Bassett Research Institute in Cooperstown, N.Y. By exposing rats to constant light, which causes a near-total suppression of melatonin, Blask showed that tumors can grow especially rapidly. Even small amounts of light can interfere with the body's natural biological rhythms. Blask's team reported that tumors grew almost twice as fast in animals exposed to just the crack of light coming under the room's door as they did in animals getting a night of total darkness.

Blask has performed cancer research for over 30 years and specifically studied melatonin for the last 20 years. The discoveries that melatonin inhibits cancer growth and that light inhibits melatonin production are monumental with regard to cancer treatment and cancer prevention. According to Blask, melatonin is a fundamental signal that relays rhythmic information about environmental cycles of light and darkness to all the cells in the body, including cancer cells.

He discovered that increased dietary intake of linoleic acid (a common polyunsaturated fatty acid) stimulates cancer growth rates because cancer cells take up and metabolize linoleic acid. During darkness, high levels of melatonin released by the pineal gland block the ability of tumors to take up linoleic acid and convert it to 13-HODE (a molecule called 13-hydroxyoctadecadienoic acid). While exposed to light, however, melatonin levels are extremely low, and tumors are no longer protected by melatonin from the tumor-stimulating action of linoleic acid. In other words, exposure to artificial light when it is naturally dark scrambles the molecular clocks in our brains. Light presented during the night will immediately turn off melatonin production and thus support tumor growth.

Organizations that contributed to Blask's research are members of the Basset Research Institute Laboratory of Chrono-Neuroendocrinology, the Thomas Jefferson University Medical School, the University Of Connecticut School Of Medicine, and the Northwestern University School Of Medicine. Funding for the research came from the Stephan C. Clark Foundation, the National Cancer Institute, the Laura Evans Memorial Breast Cancer Fund of the Edwin W. Pauley Foundation, the National Institute of Environmental Health Sciences and the Louis Busch-Hager Cancer Center Research Fund. Support from these organizations indicates somewhat of a shift in policy on cancer research.

More health conditions related to sleep deprivation

At one time or another almost 50% of the population of the U.S. is estimated to have suffered from the ill-effects of sleep deprivation. Lack of sleep is responsible for:

- at least 20% of motor vehicle accidents and thousands of fatalities each year
- an endless cycle of stress
- countless failed relationships and domestic violence
- poor work performance and limited earning potential
- billions of dollars in lost income due to disability and time off from work
- substance abuse
- depression, anxiety, aggression and poor judgment
- poor performance in school and on exams

An ever-increasing number of children are also victims of sleep deprivation and its consequences. The critical role of sleep and the negative impact of sleep disturbances in child development have been repeatedly demonstrated. According to published research, psychopathology in children could result from or be exacerbated by insufficient sleep and consequent fatigue and sleepiness. There exists a particularly strong relationship between sleep problems and neuropsychological functioning in children. Sleep disruptions have often been implicated in attention deficit hyperactivity disorder (ADHD) in children, because sleep deprivation and the resultant sleepiness could lead to ADHD-like symptoms. There are clear indications that learning and attention skills could be significantly compromised by insufficient sleep or by sleep disruption. This in no way is limited to children only.

Most tiredness results from missing out on the two hours of sleep before midnight, the hour of deep sleep before midnight being the most important hour of sleep. Any treatment of disease that does not include natural 'deep sleep therapy' cannot lead to lasting success, since the body's healing system itself, the immune system, depends on proper, healthy sleeping cycles to be vital and efficient.

Pitta, which controls AGNI, the digestive fire, also becomes disturbed when you regularly eat your evening meals late (after 6:30 or 7:00 p.m.) or have snacks during Pitta (night) time. By aggravating Pitta during the night, you will also disturb Pitta functions during and after lunchtime, which causes disturbances in the liver, spleen, gallbladder, stomach and pancreas.

Can't fall asleep or wake up frequently? Besides a deranged body clock (disturbed hormonal cycles caused by irregular lifestyle), the most common cause of sleep disturbance is the circulation of toxins in the blood. Most toxins result from not digesting food properly, from eating heavy meals in the evening and from eating too close to bedtime. These toxins may pass through the brain barrier just like alcohol does and enter the brain, potentially damaging brain cells. To prevent brain damage and keep the toxins diluted, the brain must hold on to as much blood as possible. To do this, it must prevent you from falling asleep or wake you up when the toxins become too concentrated (usually during the second Vata cycle). As always, you can count on the wisdom of the body. **Note:** Women at ages 40-55 may experience sleep disturbances more or less frequently when they go through the hormonal changes associated with menopause, regardless whether these include hot flashes or other symptoms.

The Second Vata Cycle

The time from 2:00 a.m. to 6:00 a.m. is controlled by Vata. Its early morning cycle is responsible for moving the body's waste products from the liver, the cells, the intestines and all other areas of the body toward the organs and systems of detoxification and elimination. Accordingly, the lymphatic system neutralizes harmful microbes, metabolic wastes, cellular debris, worn-out cells and cells damaged by disease. The rectum solidifies fecal matter and prompts the emptying of the bowel. The kidneys pass urine to the bladder, which causes urination. The skin also receives waste products that begin to surface at this time. Hence, the importance of washing or showering in the morning. The entire body is geared toward the excretion of useless waste material. About 70 percent of the body's waste is eliminated through the lungs, 20 percent through the skin, 7 percent through urine, and 3 percent through feces. Regular and complete waste excretion from these organs is vital for the smooth and balanced functioning of all the cells in the body. Any long-term congestion in the colon, liver and kidneys turns the body into a sewer reservoir.

At the end of the Pitta period, which marks the beginning of Vata time, the body temperature begins to drop and reaches its lowest point at about 4:00 a.m. (the peak of Vata time). After that, it gradually rises again. Toward the end of Vata time, when nature begins to become more active, both body temperature and stress hormone levels (such as adrenaline and cortisol) will be sufficiently high to jumpstart the day with a thorough cleanout. To support complete and efficient waste removal, though, the body needs to be awake and in a vertical position. Gravity plays an important role in the body's circulatory and eliminative functions. Therefore, Ayurveda recommends that we get up preferably before sunrise or at dawn, but not after sunrise. Since the times of sunrise vary from season to season and from country to country, Vata also undergoes certain fluctuations. Still, 6:00 a.m. is generally the recommended time to rise for most people **Note:** young children, teenagers and even adolescents whose natural melatonin cycle begins earlier in the night than that of adults, require at least one or two hours of extra sleep in the evening.

The use of an alarm clock to wake up in the morning abruptly stops the gradual phasing out of the various, sequentially-occurring sleep patterns and may cause irritability, headaches and nervousness throughout the day. You may feel as if you haven't really woken up yet. The easiest way to control your waking time is to adjust your bedtime in the evening. For example, if you generally need 8 hours of sleep to feel refreshed and rested in the morning, you would greatly benefit from going to sleep around 10:00 p.m. If you need more hours to feel refreshed, then go to bed even earlier. Should you truly require only 7 hours of sleep (although most adults need about 8 hours) then go to bed at 10:00 p.m. and get up at 5 a.m., an even better time for Vata to be effective. The bowel movement is the strongest type of movement in the body and requires a large portion of the body's energy. To support the body in this effort, we need to be up and about bright and early. Going to sleep early in the night and rising early in the morning is one of the most important health recommendations you can receive. You would be wise to apply it in your life.

Risks Of Deviating From Nature's Routine

Deviating from any of the natural biological rhythms on a regular basis may disrupt the balance of your body and mind. For example, let us presume that you sleep until 8:00 a.m., which is 2 hours into the Kapha period (slow activity). This means that the eliminative functions/movements of Vata are not able to complete the removal of waste during Vata's final phase at around 6:00 a.m. However, since Vata's influence is still very strong at this time, its movement becomes restricted and reversed, similar to the course of a river that is held up by the wall of a dam. Hence, part of the waste is forced back into the body instead of being excreted. This situation also applies to the urinary system. Some portion of the urine backs up and returns to the kidneys, which upsets fluid balance in the body and may lead to swelling of the face, eyes and abdomen. In addition, waste materials that the skin tries to eliminate are reabsorbed and begin to enter the lymph and bloodstream. As fecal matter starts backing up in the colon, congestion occurs throughout the gastrointestinal tract. Lymph ducts become obstructed, leading to edema in the intestines and other parts of the body. Such lymphatic swellings can be felt, for example, as hard lumps above or around the belly button area. These knots, which can become as big as a fist, are sensitive to the touch (detectable when lying on the back). Most edema occurs in the cisterna chyli vessels.

The occurrence of lymph congestion greatly stresses the heart and undermines its effort to maintain proper circulation. The misdirected Vata pressure may reach all the way to the respiratory system, mouth, teeth, sinuses, ears, eyes and brain, leaving toxic deposits in these areas. Among other symptoms, this can cause heaviness, dullness and swelling of the eyes and face. A round face (moon face) is a telltale sign of long-term intestinal congestion. These symptoms involve fluids such as mucus and lymph, which makes them Kapha-related issues. Since there are considerably more fluids in the body during the Kapha period to gather and build strength and prepare for the digestive process (6:00 a.m. to 10:00 a.m.), it stands to reason that we should avoid anything that could have congesting effects at this time. Ayurveda points out that sleeping during the Kapha period in the morning can cause severe congestion, leading to respiratory and circulatory problems. Both of these are Kapha disorders. Sleeping during the Kapha period can also result in dullness of mind, general heaviness and lethargy, which may last for many hours. Not being exposed to sunlight during the morning hours also keeps serotonin secretions low. This may cause a lack of happiness and enthusiasm, with the end result being chronic depression. The desire to sleep on and not wanting to get up in the morning are the first signs of depression.

A recent German study confirmed that rising late in the morning might even be a major risk factor for heart attacks. It has been known for quite some time that more people die from heart attacks at 9 o'clock on Monday mornings than at any other time and day of the week. The study found that most of the attack victims got up around 7:30 a.m., which is Ayurveda's 'danger time'. If oversleeping becomes habitual, the body cannot efficiently remove waste via the lungs and other organs of elimination, leading to congestion and exhaustion of the heart.

Remember a weekend when you slept late and woke up late. Did you feel poorly, as if you were drugged? Perhaps you were even sluggish enough to spoil the rest of the day. This is because the liver was unable to remove toxins from the blood during the night, and your condition was further aggravated by sluggish circulation during the Kapha time.

Another side effect that arises from sleeping into the Kapha period is that AGNI gets subdued, causing digestive problems. AGNI naturally increases with rising serotonin levels in the morning. For this reason, it is best to see the light of the sun as soon as it rises. This had been the custom in every part of the world before electricity was implemented and clocks were invented. Since serotonin is closely linked to happiness, and happiness is the most essential prerequisite of good health, it is obvious that exposure to natural light from dawn to dusk is one of the most important health-promoting factors.

Benjamin Franklin aptly summarizes the reason why all ancient cultures in the world have always adhered to the circadian rhythms: "Early to bed and early to rise makes a man healthy, wealthy and wise." Even the Bible in the first chapter of Genesis mentions "and the evening and the morning were the first day." It other words, the next day is determined by the evening before it. I might add to that, "Early lunch and early dinner will almost certainly make you a winner." Simply by adjusting your daily routine to the timing of natural law, you will establish the most essential preconditions for healing, health and happiness to occur in your life. Since the cycles of Vata, Pitta and Kapha are fixed by the circadian rhythms, you cannot create your own individual rhythms without finding yourself in a struggle against the powerful currents of natural law. The degree of your deviation from nature's rhythms will reflect the degree of struggle in your body, that is, the discomfort or disease you must deal with in your body and mind. Disease is a measure to motivate a person to once again, or for the first time, follow these powerful and beneficial laws of nature.

You may have experienced the phenomenon of *jet lag* when you traveled to faraway places that are located in different time zones. Sunrise and sunset occurred at different times and upset your biological clock for several days before the cells and organs of your body were able to adjust themselves to the new day and night cycles in that country. Before being your old self again, you might have felt hungry in the middle of the night, tired in the morning, and totally awake in the early morning hours.

There is one basic rule that applies to the experience of jet lag: For every hour of time difference, you require one day to adjust your biological rhythms to the circadian rhythm in the particular part of the world to which you travel. After a maximum of ten days (for a 10-hour time difference), the cellular functions in your body will return to normal, provided you adhere to the natural cycles of day and night prevalent at the new location.

Many people in the developed world suffer from the side effects of an "artificial" jet lag in their lives on a daily basis. They allow other factors such as working conditions, television or social commitments to dictate to them when they should eat, sleep and wake up, thus disrupting the body's intimate connection with nature's rhythms. This in itself may be one of the most energy-depleting influences of our time. I strongly recommend to every person who suffers from any health issue to start living in harmony with all the natural rhythms of the body, to whatever extent possible. This will greatly aid the healing process and prevent illness from arising in the future. Being in tune with the natural rhythms of life is one of the best insurance policies for healthy people to remain healthy. All it requires is that you listen to and act upon the constant messages your body is sending you.

Listen To Your Body, And It Will Keep You Healthy!

Like a switched-on radio receiver, your body continuously receives a vast amount of data and information from the external world. The earth, stars, sun and all life forms constantly emit radiation, which your body registers and processes to ensure balanced functioning and a harmonious relationship with the environment. Everything radiates a form of energy, including light, warmth, air, earth-electrical fields, microwaves, magnetic fields, radioactivity and the like. In response to all these visible and invisible influences, your body produces concrete messages, which try to let you know and feel what to do at any given moment. Sleep, hunger, thirst and any other natural urges or occurrences in your body indicate that your 'radio' is switched on, and you are 'in tune' with the natural world. All of us are constantly challenged to listen to and act on the messages we receive.

When we are no longer in tune with the outer forces, such as the cycles of the sun and moon, we begin to feel out of balance and perhaps fall ill. This means we need to take more self-responsibility, which requires a commitment to self, self-appreciation and self-love. These are the qualities that an illness can help reinforce in us. Most serious diseases result from a poor self-image or feelings of not being worthy. As with all negative things, there is a positive reason behind disease, that is, to heal us and make us whole again - not just physically, but also mentally and spiritually. Instead of merely trying to get rid of the symptoms of a disease, we may instead learn something precious about ourselves and the way we live our lives. Usually, by dealing with the origin(s) of disease, we accept and appreciate ourselves more than before.

It is much more convenient to blame a virus for the cold you catch than to acknowledge that irregular sleeping habits or eating a lot of junk food and the reasons behind this lifestyle and behavior may have something to do with it. To repeat, everything negative has an equally positive opposite hidden within it. Given the circumstances that you have created for yourself, it actually is not a stroke of bad luck or a form of punishment that makes you fall ill. All forms of ill health serve as opportunities to learn more about yourself, your body, your past actions, and the way you choose to live your life right now. Illness can lead you to a heightened state of awareness if you start seeing it as a challenge to move forward in your life rather than as being only a nuisance.

It requires an open mind and heart to be able to listen to and follow the rules that nature has laid out for the smooth and effortless functioning of the body. To insist that everything needs to be explained scientifically before it is valid and worthy of consideration is not only impractical, but also shows a lack of self-confidence and a poor sense of judgment. Waiting for the scientific proof is but an excuse for not trusting one's intuition and natural instinct. The messages that we all receive from nature are direct and need no intellectual interpretation. In fact, trying to figure out everything, to know it intellectually, tends to steer you away from the ability to listen to the inner wisdom bestowed on you by nature itself. The wisdom of how to live a healthy, happy life is intrinsic to the body, mind and spirit of every person.

The Body's Many Messages

For example, you don't really need to understand the exact mechanisms behind the hunger signal that the body gives you when it needs food. All you need to do is to eat and experience how the hunger subsides. By habitually ignoring the natural urge to eat, your stomach, pancreas and small intestines may become 'upset' and start adjusting to your new rule of living by keeping their production of digestive juices low, so as not to waste the body's precious energy and resources. As a result, when you suddenly eat a substantial, normal meal, you are likely to suffer indigestion.

On the other hand, if your stomach tells you that you are not hungry, that you don't require any food at the moment, but you still eat out of politeness, curiosity, boredom or temptation, the digestive system's vote for abstinence is overruled. Because the body is not prepared to digest food at this time, it cannot do so. This is another cause of indigestion.

If you feel the natural urge to have a bowel movement, the body sends you in the direction of a toilet. But by disregarding this signal because it comes at an inconvenient time, your body has no other choice but to hold on to the waste. Eventually, the urge to defecate subsides, and more and more water is withdrawn from the feces until it is too dry and hard to prompt a bowel movement. This condition is known as constipation. Destructive bacteria begin to break down some of the waste, leading to toxic gases and other noxious substances. This may cause blood poisoning and other disturbances in the digestive system.

When your body feels tired and sleepy you have the natural urge to lie down and sleep. However, a cup of coffee or a cigarette will provide you with enough adrenaline to keep you awake. If you ignore the body's sleep signals as a matter of routine, the oversecretion of adrenaline and other stress hormones may end up making you hyperactive and unable to relax or sleep properly.

Ignoring the natural messages of the body lies at the basis of most illnesses today. To add to the already existing confusion about health matters, books, radio, television and especially magazines bombard you with an overwhelming amount of advice and information on the latest slimming diets, routines and lifestyle programs that are supposed to be 'so good for you'. For example, not so long ago we were told that potatoes and pasta were among the most fattening foods. Shortly thereafter, nutritionists considered them good for slimming, and the latest low carb craze dismisses them as junk food. Torn between various health doctrines, we look for perfect answers to our problems. In the end, when your body is exhausted because of trying to adjust to one diet after another, you may begin to realize that your body's requirements are totally unique and that they undergo constant changes, often from one day to the next.

If you are a sensitive person, you must have noticed that on certain days of the month or at different times of the day, you are able to digest a particular food item more easily. The same food can make you feel vital and energetic on one day and cause you an upset stomach, bloating or cramping on another day. You may find that the same pasta dish may leave your stomach quickly after one meal, whereas two weeks later, the same dish will sit there like a rock, make you feel congested and even add weight to your body. Apart from the daily and seasonal cycles of change, the answer to this mysterious behavior of the body lies, among other reasons, in the continuous movement of the planets and their various positions.

Good Health Requires Natural Instinct

In 1984, Nobel laureate Carlo Rubbia proved that the human body is composed mostly of energy and of very little matter. To be exact, for each particle of matter, there are 974,600,000 units of energy (photons). In other words, only one billionth of your body consists of matter and the rest is vibrational energy. All matter that comprises your physical body, the chair you are sitting on and the planet you are living on, behaves essentially in a quantum-mechanical way. Since all external influences, such as solar storms, climate changes and the moon's passage through a particular zodiac, represent different energy states, they can instantly trigger corresponding activities, responses and transformations within your body. As a result of receiving these outer stimulations, your body sends subtle signals or intuitive messages to tell you that its requirements for such necessities as food, water, rest, exercise, warmth and coolness have changed. However, this requires sensitivity and wakefulness on your part. These will be absent if you habitually suppress your body's natural urges (hunger, thirst, defecation, urination, sleep, etc.), overload your digestive system with food and waste, and even make yourself emotionally dependent on other people's advice, however useful it may appear to be.

Any good system of health care can be recognized by one attribute: It teaches you how to listen to your body and how to become self-dependent in knowing what is useful for you at every moment in time. In any case, let experience guide you in finding out what works for you and what doesn't. A theory alone does not make you healthy. As you begin to listen to your body's subtle messages, you will find that its behavior, activities, natural urges and symptoms of disease are far from being random or coincidental.

Health trouble begins when we doubt our body's ability to make the right choices, and this is exactly what we have learned to do, almost right from the beginning of life. Many of our natural instincts were discouraged or subdued by man-made rules, beliefs, manipulation and advertising. They dictate to us our lifestyle, eating habits and times of eating, sleeping and elimination of wastes (see details in chapter 6).

If we keep ignoring the body's basic instincts, the mind begins to look for substitutes, which causes (legitimate) cravings for or addictions to foods, beverages, stimulants, sex, etc. By giving a little extra attention to your body, it will soon tell you the difference between a balanced and an unbalanced influence or message. If, for example, your stomach is still full and yet you want to eat something, you will find that it is not your stomach that wants more food. Food cravings tell you that your body is no longer able to digest and assimilate foods properly and is actually malnourished. This cellular famine is responsible for the food cravings. If your stomach is empty and you feel hungry, ask your stomach what it really would like to eat. The body's nutritional and emotional requirements shift from day to day in direct response to changes occurring in the near and far environment. A set dietary plan would, therefore, fail to meet the body's specific daily needs, while also blocking and distorting the messages it is trying to convey to you.

The body's natural instincts follow certain principal forces that are common to every part of physical creation. The unique representation of these forces in your body ultimately determines your natural inclinations and instincts. It is responsible for the specific characteristics of your body type. To restore your body's natural instincts, which is essential for regaining lasting health and vitality, you may first need to discover your personal body type.

Learning To Be Healthy
What Is My Body type?

One very important step in the pursuit of good health is, first, to find out what body type you are and, second, to discover what you can do to help your body recover its natural state of balance and vitality. Ayurveda recognizes that every person has a unique psycho-physiological body type that responds to foods, medicine, climate, seasons, stress, colors, smells, and other stimuli in a unique and specific way. No two people can exactly be the same because the three bodily humors, or doshas - Vata, Pitta and Kapha - are each represented in varied degrees in every person living on the planet. Along with the genetic makeup, this creates the individualistic qualities of looks and behavior and different instinctive choices concerning the types of foods, colors, climate and environment that each person prefers. So before we can restore balance in the body and mind, we may need to find out who we are in a psycho-physiological sense.

When we identify ourselves as Vata, Pitta, or Kapha body types (**Illustration 14**), we should keep in mind that no one constitution is better than another. The three doshas are composed of the great elements of nature, *earth, water, fire, air* and *space*. These five elements are *proto-elements*, which means that they are energies vibrating at different frequencies. For example, the photons (particles of light) that are constantly generated in the air that surrounds you have a different characteristic pattern of energy than the energy that is created by the particles sitting in a piece of clay or the water that flows in a stream. All existing matter, no matter how dense, is but a process of a constant intermingling of these five elements or vibrational energies. In the body, these elemental energies are grouped together and represented as the three *doshas,* thereby forming an inseparable link with the environment. The forces of nature work inside and outside, and the more we recognize and realize their great powers within us, the more we tend to harmonize with the outer world. Good health is the spontaneous result of harmony between the natural world and us.

Vata, Pitta, and Kapha are the main principal forces in control of all life in the universe. At present, they are greatly disturbed and cause havoc and turbulence, both within us and in our environment. By restoring balance among the three *doshas* in our body, we automatically pacify the great elements that constitute our world. This is very necessary now, since we also need to create a more healthy environment in order to become and stay healthy.

When Vata goes out of balance in nature, it causes earthquakes, droughts, hurricanes, and tornadoes. Disturbed Pitta generates heat waves and great destruction through fires. Irritated Kapha leads to excessive cold, rain and flooding. In the body, an unbalanced Vata dosha causes gas, pressure, pain, dryness, shaking and nervousness. If Pitta dosha is disturbed, the body overheats, acidifies or suffers from inflammatory diseases. An imbalanced Kapha dosha leads to congestion in the stomach, chest and sinuses, as well as water retention and weight gain, not unlike similar phenomena in the environment. As you begin to create balance in your internal spaces, the external ones will also begin to shine more brightly and become vital and fresh. Knowledge of your constitutional makeup will help you build a harmonious link with the constitution of your environment and derive all the benefits that nature can provide you with on your journey to living a healthy, fruitful and fulfilling life.

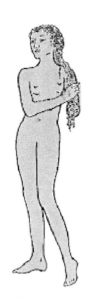 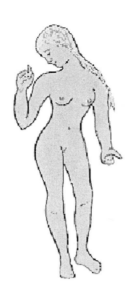 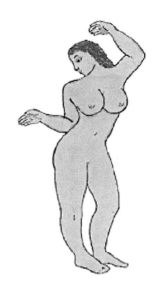

Vata Type   **Pitta Type**   **Kapha Type**

Illustration 14: The three main body types

The human constitution is composed of all three doshas or dynamic forces of nature. Human consciousness chooses a unique combination of the three doshas to carry out and fulfill its unique purpose in life. Working together in harmony, the doshas allow the individual to grow mentally, physically and spiritually to the highest degree possible. Knowledge of the three doshas and their respective concentrations in the body can hence be very beneficial for self-improvement of your body, mind and spirit.

There are ten basic body types. Ayurveda defines them as *single-dosha* types, *dual-dosha* types, and *sama-dosha* types. Sama-dosha is the rarest of all body types and manifests only when all three doshas are present in equal proportions. Single-dosha types are also relatively rare, as only a few people are influenced by one dosha alone. The most common types are the dual-doshas. Each dual-dosha can contain various proportions of the two components. Thus, a Vata-Pitta type exhibits more air energy, whereas a Pitta-Vata type has more fire energy in him. A Kapha-Pitta type is dominated by water energy, with fire energy being the subordinate force. A Vata-Kapha type is mostly controlled by air energy, with water and earth energies being secondary. And a Kapha-Vata type exhibits more water and earth principles, with Vata's air energy as the subordinate force.

THE TEN BODY TYPES

Single-dosha types:
Vata   Air/Space
Pitta   Fire/Water
Kapha   Water/Earth

Sama-dosha type
Vata-Pitta-Kapha   all elements equally present

Dual-dosha types:

Vata-Pitta   1. Air/Space   2. Fire/water
Pitta-Vata   1. Fire/Water   2. Air/Space

Pitta-Kapha   1. Fire/Water   2. Water/Earth
Kapha Pitta   1. Water/Earth   2. Fire/Water

Kapha-Vata   1. Water/Earth   2. Air/Space
Vata-Kapha   1. Air/Space   2. Water/Earth

The following questionnaire will give you an idea of your particular traits and characteristics and the possible imbalances in mind and body toward which you may tend. From there onward, you will be able to understand why each one of us has special needs and requirements and what we can do to meet all of them. Begin by answering all the questions for all three doshas. After that, add up the numbers for each section, and then study the characteristics of the body type that scored the most points. Keep in mind that your current diet, lifestyle, and physical problems may somewhat influence your evaluation. So to give you more accurate results when answering the questions, take into account the habits, characteristics and health issues that may have developed over the past 10-20 years. Because your habits may change, you may want to repeat this assessment after six months of implementing the Ayurvedic program. The results of your next evaluation will be more in line with your true constitution.

BODY TYPE QUIZ

The Vata Type

⇒ I am generally a very active person, and my body movements are quick.
⇒ My memory retention is quite poor.
⇒ I am very quick to learn new things.
⇒ I am naturally enthusiastic, vibrant and vivacious.
⇒ I am very tall (or very short), very thin and I have difficulty putting on weight.
⇒ My joints protrude, and the tendons and veins in my hands and forearms are clearly visible.
⇒ My hair is generally dry, wiry, thin and dull.
⇒ I tend to be indecisive and hesitant when it comes to making choices.
⇒ I get constipated easily and cannot tolerate gas-forming foods such as beans.
⇒ I worry a lot, even when there is no reason.
⇒ Under stress, I am nervous, agitated, restless or paranoid.
⇒ I tend to have cold hands and cold feet, even in the summertime.
⇒ I love hot weather and sunbathing.
⇒ My skin is generally dry, dark, cold, leathery and rough.
⇒ My eyes are narrow, small and dull and tend to be dry and itchy.
⇒ My sleep is often disturbed and interrupted, and I have difficulty falling asleep.
⇒ I speak quickly, and others may call me talkative.
⇒ If left on my own, I tend to skip meals and to sleep at irregular times.

⇒ Being in the midst of nature makes me calm, happy and relaxed.
⇒ I make a good counselor or teacher.

*Vata score*_____

The Pitta Type

⇒ I am generally a very efficient, precise and organized person.
⇒ I tend to perspire profusely and, sometimes, have a strong, unpleasant body odor.
⇒ I prefer cool foods and beverages; heat irritates me.
⇒ I may retain water and have a puffy face or swollen eyes.
⇒ I am quick to lose my temper and can be irritable, cynical and sharp.
⇒ I can get angry very easily but calm down again quickly.
⇒ I have a strong appetite, and I often eat more than I need.
⇒ I feel uncomfortable when I skip a meal or if it is delayed.
⇒ I have very regular bowel movements, and it is more likely for me to have loose stools than to be constipated.
⇒ Impatience is one of my greatest weaknesses.
⇒ My body is medium built, athletically toned and of medium height.
⇒ My skin is yellowish/reddish, and is prone to freckles, moles, rashes, pimples and sunburn.
⇒ I generally cannot tolerate foods that are hot and spicy, but under stress I crave them, as well as other intoxicating foods and beverages.
⇒ I am susceptible to early graying and baldness; my hair is thin, fine and straight, and is red, blond or sandy colored.
⇒ My eyes are almond shaped, green, light brown or hazel. My sclera (white of the eye) are sometimes yellow and/or bloodshot.
⇒ I am very competitive, success-oriented and somewhat forceful.
⇒ I sleep for about six to eight hours, and my dreams can be violent.
⇒ Under stress, I tend toward ulcers, insomnia, diarrhea and weight loss.
⇒ I tend to be critical of others and myself.
⇒ I believe myself to be endowed with intelligence, charisma, reliability and even brilliance. I feel very comfortable in the role of leadership, and I think I am quite good at it.

*Pitta score*_____

The Kapha Type

⇒ My body build is large, compact and wide. My thighs, arms, buttocks, chest and hips are big.
⇒ I prefer doing things slowly and methodically.
⇒ Although I have a soft, gentle and mellifluous voice, it is often congested with mucus.
⇒ Friends refer to me as calm, placid, easygoing or even 'laid-back'.
⇒ My sleep is deep, uninterrupted and profound, and I need to sleep eight to twelve hours to feel comfortable throughout the next day.
⇒ My skin is thick, oily, soft, smooth, clear, gleaming, cool; it has a somewhat pale complexion.

⇒ I feel better when I skip a meal occasionally.

⇒ I love hot weather and sunny days. Cold, damp weather bothers me.

⇒ My eyes are round, large and clear with thick eyelashes. Friends say they are sensual pools of black or blue.

⇒ I walk slowly, with a measured gait.

⇒ I am a sweet-natured, affectionate and forgiving person.

⇒ My hair is abundant, thick, blond or black and curly.

⇒ I am physically strong, have good stamina, long endurance and a steady level of energy.

⇒ When I am under stress, I tend to overeat, oversleep, feel groggy upon awakening and am slow to get going in the morning.

⇒ My digestion and metabolism seem to be slow, and I tend to feel heavy after eating.

⇒ I have a tendency toward mucus aggravation, phlegm, chronic congestion, asthma and sinus problems.

⇒ I do not learn as quickly and as easily as some people, but whatever I have learned and understood is retained in my memory for a long time.

⇒ When I feel unhappy or stressed, I become narrow-minded, stubborn, neglectful, possessive or attached.

⇒ I would love to do nothing and be lazy, but I am hard-working.

⇒ I hold on to many things, including money, relationships and body weight.

Kapha score _____

After adding up the numbers for all the applicable attributes in each section, compare the total scores for Vata, Pitta and Kapha. If, for example, your totals are Vata 15, Pitta 12, and Kapha 4, then your body type is <u>Vata</u>-Pitta (Vata-dominating.) Should Vata be 3, Pitta be 4, and Kapha be 11, then you can consider yourself a Kapha type. It may be that your score for Vata turns out to be 10, for Pitta 19, and for Kapha 10; in this case, your second dosha is not yet clear. Treat yourself as a Pitta type, and take the test again six months from now; you will then find that either Vata or Kapha has taken a clearer position, due to the removal of impurities from the body. In the rare case that your scores are something like, Vata 13, Pitta 14 and Kapha 14, then your body type is SAMA.

Initially, it may not be easy to determine one's exact body type. It took me many years of training to determine a person's body type and to separate it from the imbalances he may have had. For example, a person may predominantly be Vata, but have a Pitta imbalance, such as a skin problem (like acne, rashes or reddening of the skin). He may therefore have, perhaps, 12 points for Vata, 11 for Pitta and a few for Kapha. This may be confusing, and he may not be able sort it out for himself without the help of an Ayurvedic practitioner.

Basically, in such a case, Vata goes out of balance first (through constipation caused by irregular eating/sleeping habits, dry foods, or poor bile secretions), which then leads to toxins entering the blood and lymph. This overtaxes the liver and kidneys. Subsequently, intestinal toxins can no longer be removed by these organs and are eliminated through the skin, leading to such skin conditions as blemishes, pimples or acne. Thus, the Vata problem leads to a Pitta condition.

Once the organs are cleansed and the constipation issue is resolved, the skin problems clear up, and the Pitta score goes down. In this case, the person may now have 12 for Vata and only 7 or so for Pitta, which makes him predominantly a Vata type (with Pitta or Kapha coming second).

SAMA dosha applies only to people who have almost the same scores for each dosha, and also have no health complaints whatsoever. As I explained earlier, this is very rare. Most people have some imbalances, which can distort their true body type. In most cases, the confusion clears up as they cleanse their organs and eat a more balanced diet.

It is good to know that no one particular body type is more advantageous than another. A SAMA or Kapha type may have a stronger constitution, which seems to be more favorable, but he doesn't usually realize when he steps over the line. When out of balance, he is slower to restore his health. By contrast, those with a weaker constitution, like the Vata type, are prevented from making too many mistakes because aches, pains and other forms of discomfort won't let them.

The emphasis lies on making each body type perfectly balanced and bringing out all its inherent strength and healthy characteristics. The different percentages and associations of Vata, Pitta and Kapha in each person are responsible for structuring a unique individual. To give you an idea of the main characteristics of a Vata, Pitta or Kapha-dominated body type, see the corresponding lists below. Try to remember, though, that you are always a combination of all three doshas.

CHARACTERISTICS OF THE BODY TYPES
The Vata Type

- Light, thin physique, narrow body frame; bent or irregularly shaped nose
- Moves and performs activity quickly
- Tendency toward dry, rough, cold, and dark skin
- Aversion to cold weather
- Irregular hunger and digestion
- Light, interrupted sleep, insomnia
- Enthusiasm, vivaciousness, imagination, perceptiveness, spiritually inclined
- Excitability, changing moods, unpredictable
- Quick to grasp information, but also quick to forget
- Tendency toward worry, anxiety, restlessness
- Tendency toward bloating and constipation
- Tires easily, tendency to overexertion and hyperactivity
- Mental and physical energy comes in bursts
- Low tolerance to pain, noise, bright light

The basic theme of the Vata-type is 'changeableness'. Since Vata is composed of the elements of air and space, movement and changeability are natural characteristics of this body type. Vatas dislike any form of the status quo. They love excitement and constant change, but if that is not available to them, they create an irregular lifestyle. For example, they may choose to have different bedtimes each day or to skip meals. Their unpredictable nature makes them among the least stereotyped people.

Vata types often feel isolated and awkward when they have to stand up to the earthy Kapha type or the intense Pitta type. However, their 'airy' flair, mobility and vivacious nature particularly inspires Pittas and Kaphas, who lack these qualities. Vatas look elegant when they are dressed up. Clothing fills their need for insulation and confidence; their dry, lean and almost 'hungry' look is ideal for modeling, a reason why most high-fashion models are Vatas. Physically, Vatas are the thinnest of all the body types; their shoulders and hips are usually narrow and often rounded. Some Vatas are chronically 'underweight', and despite eating large amounts of food, they rarely put on any weight. Other Vata types are thin throughout their youth and become overweight in middle age.

Among all the body types, Vatas are the most likely to have physical irregularities. Some Vata types have hands or feet that are too large for their petite body, or they may be too small. Their teeth may be crooked, protruding or undersized. Vatas may be well shaped, but under stress and when constipated, they are prone to develop spinal deformities (scoliosis) or other skeletal problems. Some Vatas are born with very light bones, others with very heavy but elongated bones. You can recognize a Vata by his visible joints, tendons and veins. This is due to low fat content under their skin. Another typical indication of a Vata physiology is the audible cracking of joints.

A balanced Vata type is enthusiastic, energetic and uplifting in spirit. Her generally clear mind and exalted sense of awareness makes her the best candidate for spiritual development. Vatas are ruled by their heightened sense of touch and hearing. They feel and hear the world more than they see it, a reason why they need frequent cuddling and words of encouragement. Sex in itself is not so important to Vatas, but the feeling of being loved and cared for is. They have no difficulties in going for long periods of time without sex, but once they have found a partner who truly accepts and loves them for who they are, they are very fulfilling sexual partners. Vata types need matured Kapha-Pitta or Pitta-Kapha types to give their best in a relationship.

Since Vata is the principal force of movement in the body, it regulates bowel activities, absorption of food, breathing, speaking, nerve impulses, and the transport of blood and lymph. It is also in charge of the movement of the muscles and the body as a whole. Vata is very pronounced in the nervous system. Therefore, Vata imbalances are likely to show up as nervous disorders, including tremors, spasms, seizures, anxiety, depression and clinical mental disorders. Once Vata has returned to balance, such disorders, which otherwise may defy conventional treatment, often disappear spontaneously.

Vatas who are out of balance tend to worry a lot, even when there is really nothing to worry about. This may end up as insomnia, as well as constant restlessness and fearfulness. Fear, which is the Vata type's most typical emotion, affects his digestion and, particularly, the elimination of bodily waste. Vata's main seat is in the colon. When disturbed in the colon, it causes constipation and gas which, in turn, lead to increased restlessness and nervousness. Also, when Vata is deranged, the stomach and intestines may cramp due to trapped air putting strong pressure on the gastrointestinal and abdominal structures. Irregular menstrual cycles, PMT and menstrual cramps are also more often found among Vata types than other body types.

Vatas easily get unbalanced when they don't get enough rest and sleep, and particularly, when they miss out on the two hours of sleep before midnight. By pushing themselves too hard and engaging in an irregular lifestyle, they easily overexert themselves. This may lead to chronic fatigue and any of the above mental or physical problems. The main key to balancing Vata is 'regularity'.

The following factors are the most irritating for the Vata type:

- Excessive exercise and physical strain
- Sleep deprivation (especially the lack of before-midnight sleep)
- Falling
- Irregular mealtimes
- Sitting for many hours
- Tuberculosis
- Suppression of natural urges
- Cold climate
- Cold foods and beverages
- Stimulants of any kind
- Excessive noise
- Fear and grief
- Fasting
- Pungent, astringent and bitter foods
- Late autumn and winter

The Pitta Type

- Medium build, well-shaped, athletically toned
- Medium strength and endurance
- Sharp hunger and thirst, strong digestion
- Tendency toward anger and irritability when under stress
- Can be arrogant, self-centered
- Adaptable, intelligent, bright
- Tendency toward reddish skin and hair, moles, freckles, skin problems
- If out of balance, prematurely bald and/or grey
- Pointed, reddish nose
- Piercing, sometimes bloodshot eyes
- Aversion to sun, hot weather
- Prefers cool foods and beverages
- Enterprising character, likes challenges, good organizer
- Sharp intellect
- Good, precise, articulate speaker
- Can't skip meals; otherwise irritable
- Medium memory
- Successful leader

The theme that describes the Pitta type best is '**intense**'. He is mostly dominated by the fire element and its various qualities. Fire represents the dynamic force of nature and is responsible for all transformational processes in the body and mind. The mental body (non-physical), which is comprised of thoughts, feelings and emotions, is a function of Pitta. The Pitta energies are located in the central region of the body, which is the area generally referred to as the solar plexus. The solar plexus acts like a 'switchboard' for both psychological and physiological activities. The 'gut feeling' that we sometimes have about a certain person or situation is locked into the Pitta force. It gives us the natural instinct to search for pure foods, clean air, fresh water, stimulating friendships, supportive emotional relationships and the like, so that we are able to remain in physical, mental and emotional balance.

Pitta dosha also helps us to be moderate in eating, drinking, sexual activity, and in meeting our other needs. This instinctive quality is highly developed in the balanced Pitta type, which makes him a symbol of '*Sattva*', that is, one who has purity of mind. A disturbance of Pitta, however, results in a loss of discrimination as to what is useful and suitable and what is not. It is likely to lead to an excessive use of stimulants such as alcohol, tobacco and drugs, as well as a lust for power and influence. Any of these alters the proper proportion of bile constituents in the liver's bile ducts and thereby generates intrahepatic stones. Pitta also means bile. Upsetting Pitta dosha in the above way leads to the bilious personality for which this body type is known.

We all need Pitta energy to translate our ideas into concrete realities. Since this energy is most profusely available in the Pitta type, he exhibits a very dynamic, ambitious and, perhaps, even aggressive personality. Pittas get things done. Their great vision and foresight is due to the fire element that gives them a clear inner and outer vision. However, if a Pitta person abuses his power and upsets his balance, he is the first to develop eye problems and difficulties with his inner vision, too.

Pitta dosha, being situated in the most central part of the body, keeps Vata and Kapha in check. This also is represented in the Pitta's personality; he is one who always wants to be in control in every situation. When his Pitta dosha is balanced, he is indeed the most successful of all body types. His one-pointed focus and brilliance nearly always find a solution to every problem, and he excels at almost anything. His real expertise lies in the mental field, where he exerts his true power and skills. He makes an eloquent and articulate speaker and a good leader of society.

Because of Pitta's strategic position in the body, Pitta types are excellent at playing central roles in life. The solar plexus is related to sun energy, which controls all life on the planet. Pittas are aware of their solar plexus power and are, therefore, naturally self-confident. If they are able to transmute the excesses, indulgence and arrogance, which they may have acquired in their life, they are likely to have access to the most profound knowledge of Self. Pittas are also very good at passing on what they have learned through their often amazing insights and experiences.

The situation changes, though, when the Pitta energies move outside the solar plexus into other parts of the body. The Pitta type suddenly becomes fiery, jealous, cynical, angry and egotistical. He rapidly begins to lose control, like a forest fire that is quickly spread by strong winds. If his sense of 'I-ness' becomes exaggerated, he may try to subdue his Vata and Kapha counterparts, especially in the area of sexuality. Pitta's overwhelming passion for always wanting to be a winner in every area of life may leave very little room for a wholesome sexual interplay. He may not have the necessary patience and humility that is required during the most intimate moments of sharing and equality. The unbalanced Pitta type also tries to use every means to avoid admitting defeat. The most suitable partners for Pittas are the strong Kapha types, or otherwise, the Kapha-Vata or Vata-Kapha types. Having two Pitta types, for example, partnering up may not be such a good idea, though.

In physical terms, the dispersion of excessive Pitta energy can lead to heartburn, stomach ulcers, burning sensation in the intestines, diarrhea, and hemorrhoids. This type of destructive Pitta energy may also affect his skin, which becomes prone to rashes, pimples, inflammation and acne. The skin, particularly on the face and chest, may easily redden and become hot. Rosacea is not uncommon among Pittas. Hot flushes and profuse perspiration of the upper half of the body are also a typical sign of Pitta imbalance. Unbalanced Pitta women frequently experience such symptoms while going through menopause.

The Pitta's eyes can easily become bloodshot and blurry and are often oversensitive to sunlight. This sensitivity to sunlight and watering eyes are the main reasons why Pittas, whose doshas are out of balance, insist on wearing sunglasses. Their natural internal heat makes them the worst candidates for sunbathing. They prefer cool and shady places, and they love taking cold showers when outside temperatures begin to rise. If they don't follow their natural instincts regarding exposure to sun and heat, they quickly burn their skin and become prone to heat exhaustion.

Physically, Pittas are well proportioned, athletically built and of medium size. The same applies to their face. Their eyes are of medium size with a sometimes penetrating glance. You can easily recognize a Caucasian Pitta type from far away, as he is likely to have red, blond or sandy-colored hair. He is also the first among the body types to have grey hair or to go bald. Pittas rarely feel cold, even during the winter. When the sun comes out, they are the first to complain that it is too warm. Their fair, warm and soft skin is most likely marked by freckles and moles or skin blemishes. (Note: Some of these Pitta characteristics do not apply to races with dark hair and dark skin).

Pitta types have only medium physical energy, which prevents them from overexercising or going beyond their limits. Their stamina is moderate, but their digestive energy is abundant. However, overeating on a regular basis can lead to sudden intestinal problems. For this reason, they greatly benefit from moderate food intake and a balanced lifestyle. Eating more than what equals two cupped hands full at the biggest meal of the day (taken ideally at midday) gets them into intestinal trouble. Impure foods, polluted water and air, alcohol, coffee, cigarettes, soft drinks and other unhealthful substances are particularly upsetting to Pitta types and often cause very uncomfortable cleansing reactions, such as skin eruptions, stomach problems or emotional distress. Pittas are also negatively affected by wearing clothing that is made from synthetic materials.

Pitta's main warning signal that he is out of balance is anger, which may fuel his fire energy to the extent that his body becomes toxic and diseased. The main key to balancing Pitta is 'moderation'.

The following factors are the most irritating for the Pitta type:

- Anger
- Insufficient sleep
- Strong sunshine
- Fasting
- Sesame seeds and sesame products
- Wine and other alcoholic beverages
- Coffee and other stimulants

- Vinegar
- Impure foods
- Unripe fruits
- Linseed
- Yogurt
- Pungent (spicy), salty and sour foods
- Late summer and autumn

The Kapha Type

- Compact, strong and heavier build
- Well developed and lubricated joints
- Great physical strength and endurance
- Hair may be black, blond, dark brown, thick, wavy, oily
- Stable and reliable personality
- Steady energy; slow and graceful in action
- Tranquil, relaxed personality, slow to anger
- Cool, smooth, pale, often oily skin
- Hidden veins and tendons
- Slow to grasp new information, slow to forget
- Heavy, prolonged sleep
- Tendency to excessive weight, obesity
- Slow digestion, mild hunger
- Excessive need for sleep
- Calm, affectionate, complacent, tolerant, forgiving, nurturing, maternal
- Tendency to be possessive, stubborn, attached, narrow-minded.

The Kapha type is controlled by the elements of earth and water, which makes him the most grounded and stable of all the body types. One word that describes him most aptly is 'slow'. The force of Kapha pervades the food element, and in the body, it is mainly located in the upper thoracic cavity. Both stomach and lungs are central areas of Kapha activity. Proper lubrication of the mucus lining and joints plays a major role in keeping his body strong and resistant to disease.

Since Kapha types imbibe the material elements of earth and water, they are the most attuned to the pace of earthly survival. It is, therefore, not at all surprising that they have the longest life spans of all three types. In a way, they represent Mother Earth and her qualities of nurturing, vitality and stability. Kaphas, who represent the *food force*, are the complete opposites of Vatas, who represent the *mobile force*. Pitta is the *dynamic force* between them. A Kapha person is affectionate, sensual, calm and forgiving. He makes an excellent parent because he is naturally tolerant and does not become irritable even when there is a lot of noise or turbulence around him. Kapha types exist mainly on the physical and astral planes. They feel more at home on planet Earth than Vatas or Pittas do, since the earth and water elements are most concentrated in their bodies. Their dominating senses are smell and taste, which makes food one of their favorite things. This naturally makes them good cooks, a characteristic that is rarely found among Vatas.

Physically, Kaphas have great strength and stamina. Most weight lifters are Kaphas who can access and utilize vast energy reserves. Their bones and joints are heavy and well-built, but they are hidden under a protective fatty skin. They have the wide hips and broad shoulders that are often found among rugby players and heavyweight boxers. Their compact and heavy bodies thrive on athletic performance and physical activities. They are very willing to perform strenuous physical labor because they feel so much more alive afterward.

Too much sitting or sleeping, on the other hand, can make Kaphas lethargic and lazy, which slows their already low metabolic rate. A sedentary lifestyle predisposes them to putting on weight very easily; this may sometimes even happen by merely looking at food. They tend to deal with unresolved emotional issues through eating because this activity gives them the most pleasure. In this sense, food is their temporary way out of an unpleasant situation. Unbalanced Kaphas can be recognized by their excessive weight. They often become obese if 'things don't move' in their lives. They form a thick, protective layer of fat underneath their skin when they feel hurt and insecure.

Kaphas have the biggest eyes of all the body types. Their dark or blue irises stand in clear contrast to their milky white sclera, which makes them very attractive. A typical Kapha trait is their skin, which is silky smooth, soft, cool, thick, and pale, without a sign of freckles or moles. Even at an advanced age, their skin tends to be clear and without wrinkles. Its natural oiliness gives the skin a shiny glow.

Kapha types do everything slowly, including eating, walking and talking. They are slow to anger and slow to react. Calm and self-contained, they love peaceful environments. They are the most relaxed and the most romantic of all body types; a romantic dinner for two is one of the most exciting things for them. Kaphas tend to flirt innocently with everyone and to rely on bodily feelings, which makes them ideal lovers. They rarely feel obstructed in their flow of sexual energy, and they have plenty of it. Kapha types make wonderful partners for all body types, especially for those who have vital sexual prowess and a need for many offspring. Kaphas find fulfillment in caring for a family.

When Kapha types are unable to deal with inner conflicts, they tend to keep them inside the body, unlike Vata types who spurt out whatever they think and feel. Such stored unrest and antagonism can disturb the Kapha's basic metabolism and cause congestion, stagnation, and a heavy form of depression. Depression and melancholia are the vibrations that transform the Kapha's most precious assets into very destructive forces. Most cancers are caused by an imbalance of Kapha dosha, and Kapha types are the most likely to develop Kapha imbalances; hence they are more prone to develop cancers than other body types.

Because Kapha dosha controls the moist tissues of the body, the mucus lining is the first area to show signs of imbalance. Unbalanced Kaphas frequently complain of chest colds, wet coughs, asthma, sinus congestion, allergies, and painful joints, especially during the late winter and in the spring (Kapha season).

Another indication of an unbalanced Kapha type is his tendency to hold on to possessions, positions at work, money, food, energy and relationships. He would prefer everything to remain as it is. To keep it that way, he tries very hard to please everyone except himself, which again makes him a possible candidate for cancer. (Also see "Cancer - Who Makes It?" in Chapter 9)

Even though it is not necessarily a part of their nature, Kapha types benefit greatly from excitement in their lives. Status quo situations turn the Kapha's stability into inertia, which is their greatest enemy. Kaphas thrive physically, emotionally and spiritually if their focus is on having enough stimulation in their life. Engaging in activities such as exercising, going out, traveling, singing, dancing and playing musical instruments 'keeps them alive'. They need to progress in life to feel good. By contrast, watching television makes them passive and depressed. Also, lack of exercise, cold and heavy food, overeating, and receptive work (passive versus active) slow them right down. Kaphas need to be active and only recognize their great assets of inner security and steadiness when they are in action. This keeps them youthful and healthy. The main key to balancing Kapha is, therefore, **stimulation**.

The following factors are the most irritating for the Kapha type:

- Sleeping during the daytime
- Heavy food
- Sweet, sour and salty food
- Milk and dairy products
- Cold and dampness

- Spring and early summer
- Sugar and sweets
- Laziness
- Lack of exercise and physical activity
- Too much sleep

CHAPTER 6

The Simple Approach That Allows You to Maintain Peak Health *Effortlessly*

This chapter is dedicated to the main procedures, methods and insights that you can use to actually create a life of balance. Once balance has been achieved, good health results quite spontaneously. This principle of natural law applies to every living being and to nature as a whole. Yet creating balance is not something you will need to do just once in your life, rather it is an ongoing process that allows your body and mind to function in perfect coordination and harmony with each other and the natural environment. A life of balance will equip you with the ability to joyfully and passionately meet the constantly increasing challenges of our time, endowed with the tools of physical and mental strength, creativity and wisdom.

The factors that could possibly disrupt your health have increased tremendously within the relatively short period of the past several decades. Not so long ago, it was comparatively easy to live in harmony with the laws of nature and the environment. Now you have to be very alert not to get caught up in the destructive effects of man's creations. Many big city children grow up with the notion that food means highly processes junk; drinking water is not necessary, but soft drinks are; and that nature is merely something to watch on *The Discovery Channel*, an American cable television station.

The costs of forsaking a life of balance are astronomical. Many people recognize that our modern way of life, with its ever-increasing comforts and material acquisitions along with the demands to acquire and maintain them, doesn't allow for a healthful way of life. As a nation, the United States has become dependent upon a health care system that makes us sicker and which has become unaffordable for most, while pushing the country to the brink of financial ruin. Although we spend more on health care than do most developing countries taken together, 65 percent of the population is unhealthy and suffers from one health problem or another.

Never before have we had such a strong need to live a balanced life, but relatively few manage to do so. Yet balance or good health of mind, body and spirit is an option most of us can choose to create by following the simple, but powerful recommendations given in this chapter. A good number of guidelines presented here are derived from the ancient medical science of Ayurveda and my 35 years of experience in the field of complementary medicine. I have updated and improved them as a result of regular feedback that has been provided to me by thousands of patients who have applied these principles in their daily lives.

Guidelines for Daily Routine and Diet

Regularity
▶ Follow the rhythms of nature and your body as described in Chapter 5. This ensures that your body and mind can function with ease and optimal energy. This also creates the precondition for healing.

Regular rest and sleep: Optimal bedtime is between 9:00 and 10:00 p.m.
▶ Don't worry if you have difficulty falling asleep; just lie with your eyes closed and relax. You will still get 90 percent of the benefit of sleep. This program can help eliminate the causes of sleep disturbance.

Regular exercise and physical activity
▶ Morning and /or evening walk.
▶ Surya Namaskara or 'sun salutation' - the most ancient, complete and simple exercise program **(illustration 15)**.
▶ Body squatting forms a very important, natural part of life among all tribal people. Benefits include:
  - Improved respiration of almost all cells in your body. The squat incorporates the use of almost all the muscles in your body.
  - Increased Chi or life force through important meridians (which control most psycho-physiological functions in the body).
  - Improved pumping of fluids, aiding in the removal of waste and the delivery of nutrients to the cells in all bodily tissues.
  - Beneficial physiological stress to your hormonal system.
  - The squat movement encourages easier passage of feces through the colon and more regular bowel movements.

Start off with just a few squats, and increase the number by 1-5 each day. When you are capable of performing 100 squats in a row, you body will start relying on Chi (life force) for its energy requirements instead of using up its physical energy resources.
▶ Choose any other form of physical exercise that suits your body type. (See the section on *Exercise According to the Doshas*.)
▶ Whenever you exercise, try inhaling through your nose while keeping your mouth closed to avoid harmful 'adrenaline breathing'. Mouth breathing can lead to rapid depletion of one's energy reserves and trigger the release of stress hormones. You may exhale through your mouth if necessary. Some aerobic exercises are fine as long as you maintain nose breathing versus mouth breathing. (See more details on exercise in the section *'Exercise Yourself to Health'*.)
▶ Exercise only up to 50 percent of your capacity. Don't allow yourself to become tired. For example, if you can swim for 30 minutes before feeling tired, swim only for 15 minutes. In time, your capacity for more exercise will increase. Overexercising, such as in endurance training, weakens the immune system, heart and lungs and floods the blood with harmful, acidic chemicals.
▶ Expose your body to fresh air at least once or twice every day for a minimum of half an hour to ensure proper circulation and an adequate oxygen supply to its trillions of cells.
▶ Regular practice of Yoga, Tai Chi, Chi Kung, Pilates or similar fitness programs is highly recommended for maintaining energy and flexibility. The Five Tibetan Rites as described in the book *Ancient Secret of the Fountain of Youth* by Peter Kelder is one of the most excellent and simple exercise routines you can follow.

► Pranayama: Five-minute breathing exercises to increase Prana or Chi (life force energy), as explained below. These are best done before meditation and before eating.

► Meditation according to your choice: I recommend the 'Technique of Conscious Breathing', as described in my book *It's Time to Come Alive* and summarized in 'Conscious Breathing Meditation' below.

Regular Mealtimes

► Lunch should make up the main meal of the day. Eat at around 12:00 – 12:30 p.m. (The best time to eat is when the sun is in its highest position.)

► The evening meal should be light, since digestive power is low in the evening. There are very few digestive secretions after 8:00 p.m. A heavy meal taken in the evening remains mostly undigested.

► Eat dinner between 6:00 and 7:00 p.m., so that the main digestion is completed before bedtime and does not interfere with your sleep.

► Eat your meals at about the same times every day so that the digestive system can always perform at its best. Eating at different times each day makes it difficult for the body to produce the right amount of digestive juices required for each meal.

► Eat according to your hunger level. If you are not hungry, don't eat. Wait until your natural appetite (digestive power) has returned. **Note**: Food cravings have nothing to do with hunger and should be treated like an addiction. (See Chapter 7, 'Employing Nature's Healing Powers'.)

► Drink about 6-8 glasses of water each day. Pure, fresh water is best. Filtered water from a public water supply is fine. Make it a daily habit to drink one glass of water about ½ hour before each meal and one glass of water 2-2 ½ hours after each meal. This improves digestion and keeps the blood thin. (For exact directions see the section Drinking Water - The Greatest Therapy of All'.) Avoid drinking liquids with meals, since this dilutes digestive juices and interferes with stomach secretions.

► Sit down when you eat, even if it is for a small snack. The digestive system is better able to secrete balanced amounts of digestive juices when you are eating in the seated position.

► Eat in a settled environment without radio, television or reading. Any distraction from eating impairs the enjoyment of the food and the body's ability to supply the appropriate enzymes for digestion.

► Sit quietly for at least 5 minutes after the meal so that the food has a chance to settle in your stomach before you get up from the table. Lying on your left side for a few minutes and then going for a 10 to 15-minute walk afterward also greatly aids digestion.

Morning

Bowel Movement:

► For optimum health, the bowel movement should occur regularly in the morning after rising, ideally at the end of the Vata period (at around 6:00 a.m.) while Vata is still strong enough to eliminate waste materials from the system. Give yourself that extra time, but do not force a bowel movement. Also, never suppress natural urges, as this may lead to great disturbance of Vata in the body and even cause internal injuries and, possibly, hemorrhoids.

► Every morning after rising, drink one glass of warm water. This will help to end the 'drought' of the night and increase the regularity of the bowel movement. A little while later, drink a second glass of warm water, but add a teaspoon of honey and the juice from one or two slices of fresh lemon. This helps remove AMA and harmful bacteria from the gastrointestinal tract, and assists the intestines in eliminating any accumulated waste material. Wait for at least 30 minutes before eating breakfast.

Regular Dry Brushing and Oil Massage:

▶ Quickly brush your whole body with a dry body brush made of natural bristles or a good natural loofah. This will improve circulation, strengthen and rejuvenate the skin, and help with lymph drainage. The brushing of the skin also opens the pores and increases the effectiveness of the oil massage, if applied afterward. Start with the extremities, and always brush in the direction of the heart.

▶ Abyanga or oil massage: Massage yourself with either sesame oil or coconut, sunflower or olive oil (all expeller or cold-pressed and unrefined, available from natural health food stores). Abyanga helps draw out toxins and improves circulation. Conclude the massage with a warm bath or shower. (See directions for oil massage below) Sesame oil, in particular, quickly penetrates all the layers of the skin, binds to and removes toxins of various kinds (including harmful fatty acids) and helps rid the blood vessels of plaque and cellular debris. This supports the body in preventing and reversing the hardening of the arteries. Abyanga also stimulates growth hormone production and improves immunity because nearly one third of the immune system is located in the skin. Do the massage as often as is convenient for you. Some do it daily. (See more details about Abyanga below.)

Breakfast

▶ If you are not hungry, skip breakfast. (Kapha types rarely need breakfast.)
▶ If you are hungry, eat a light breakfast. Food choices may consist of nutritious wholesome foods, such as oatmeal (porridge) or any other hot cereal. (but check for a wheat or gluten allergy) Eat your cereal with expeller-pressed coconut oil or unsalted butter; unrefined sea salt; rice, hemp, oat or almond milk; and perhaps a little maple syrup, stevia, agave syrup, raw honey or xylitol sugar for sweetening. This makes a nourishing breakfast. Wetabix or toasted whole-wheat bread (finely ground) with butter, is a good choice, too. Other hot cereals include cream of buckwheat, cream of rice, millet, grits, quinoa and other such grains. By soaking oats or other grains overnight and adding 1 tbsp. or more of wheat germ (available from most grocery stores), the grains are being predigested. This may increase digestibility from 30 percent to about 90 percent.
Note: Soy milk should be avoided due to its natural food toxins (enzyme inhibitors), possible gene-manipulation, and its potentially harmful effects on hormonal balance. (Soy mimics estrogens in the body and thus increases the risk of breast cancer.) If in doubt, use the muscle testing procedure of Chapter 1. Also, do not add fruit to your cereals, as this leads to fermentation and toxicity, which will be explained further below.
▶ Avoid animal proteins such as cheese, meat, ham or eggs as well as sour foods, including yogurt and citrus fruit. All of these quickly subdue AGNI, which is naturally low in the morning. A breakfast consisting of only fruit (other than citrus) is fine.

Lunch Meal

▶ Make lunch the main meal of the day.
▶ Avoid drinking beverages with the meal since this dilutes the concentrated digestive juices and become a cause of indigestion and weight gain. Sipping a small cup of hot water during the meal, however, can help to increase the digestive power. To maintain thinness of blood and normal secretions of bile, it is best to drink a glass of water about ½ hour before lunch and again 2-2½ hours after lunch.

► If salad is part of your meal, eat it at the beginning, before eating any cooked food. Since raw foods require different digestive enzymes than those needed for digesting cooked foods, eating these food items separately, i.e. one after the other, makes it easier on the digestive system. Eating raw food items after having eaten cooked foods will leave them mostly undigested and subject to fermentation. Avoid cooked foods items in your salad, especially protein foods. (More information on this follows.) During cold days and in the winter, you may naturally desire to eat salads less often; this is due to their strong cooling effects on the body.

Note: Make certain that you use a full-fat salad dressing, such as extra virgin olive oil[12] and lemon juice for your salad. A team of researchers at Iowa State University conducted a study that showed that the salad's nutrients are only digested and absorbed properly when consumed with a full-fat salad dressing versus a reduced or no-fat product.

Evening Meal

► In the evening, Ayurveda recommends that you avoid eating meat, pork, poultry, fish, ham, eggs, nuts or any other concentrated form of protein because AGNI is too low at that time to handle protein foods. Even during the day these require 4-7 hours of digestion in the stomach. Be aware that production of digestive enzymes stops at around 8:00 p.m., and heavy food items ingested in the evening will linger in the stomach until the early morning hours. At that time, the stomach may discharge the now mostly undigested food into the small intestine, prompting destructive bacteria to decompose it.

► Yogurt, cheese, fruits and salads should also be avoided in the evening. These foods have a naturally high bacteria content. When exposed to the warm and moist environment of the stomach and small intestine during the night, they end up causing indigestion and fermentation (along with plenty of low-grade alcohol).

► Oily, fried and deep-fried foods, as well as root vegetables such as potatoes (with the exception of cooked carrots, beets, or white radishes), are also very difficult to digest at night. Coconut oil and unsalted butter or ghee are fine to use.

► An example for a light dinner is freshly prepared vegetable soup, perhaps blended, served with whole wheat pita or spelt bread, whole wheat toast or rye crackers with unsalted butter, ghee or coconut oil. Another option is cooked vegetables with rice or other light cooked grain foods. The soup/vegetables may be seasoned with spices and herbs, vegetable bullion, unrefined sea salt, as well as butter, ghee or coconut oil added during or after cooking - about one teaspoon of butter, ghee or coconut oil per person (avoid other oils in the evening since they are more difficult to digest.

---

[12] A recent study in Italy found only 40% of olive oil brands were actually 'pure' olive oil. The same is true for olive oil sold in the U.K. In 1995, the Food and Drug Administration (FDA) testing olive oils for purity found that only 4 per cent of the 73 brands of olive oils tested proved to be pure olive oil. Most olive oil products were adulterated with vegetable oils, such as canola, corn, cottonseed and soy oils, which have been shown to cause, not prevent heart disease. Some 'olive oils' contained only 10 percent olive oil. Buy your olive oils preferabgly at whole food stores. The cheaper the oils are, the more likely they are not pure. **Avoid the Following brands:** Andy's Pure Olive Oil (Italy), Bertolli (Italy), Castel Tiziano (Italy), Cirio (Italy), Cornelia (Italy), Italico (Italy) Ligaro (Italy), Olivio (Greece), Petrou Bros. Olive Oil (California), Primi (Italy), Regale (Italy), Ricetta Antica (Italy), Rubino (Italy), San Paolo (Italy) Sasso (Italy), Terra Mia (Italy).

General Guidelines

▶ It is best to avoid heavy, oily and fried food; aged cheeses; yogurt; onion and garlic, especially uncooked; highly processed and refined foods; fizzy drinks, alcohol, coffee, regular tea; artificial sweeteners; and commercial sugar.

▶ Try to include one or two pieces of fresh fruit per day in your diet. If you use fruit juice, make sure it is freshly prepared and not older than one hour (best diluted with water). Packaged fruit juices are pasteurized, which makes them acid-forming, deprives them of natural enzymes, and depletes the body of important minerals and vitamins. Many brands contain artificial sweeteners, which dehydrate the body and may damage the brain, nervous system and immune system. It is preferable to eat one kind of fruit at a time.

Fruit or fruit juices should always be taken on an empty stomach. Since fruit leaves the stomach within 20-40 minutes without requiring any stomach action, it is important not to eat them with other foods; doing so leads to fermentation, bloating, and even diarrhea. The best times to eat fruit are midmorning and midafternoon, or for breakfast with nothing else.

For optimal digestion, fruit should preferably be consumed when it is in season. When picked too early, they have not reached their natural ripening stage and lack most vitamins and important sugars. They may also irritate the intestinal walls due to their high concentration of antibodies (acting as antigens in the body) and enzyme inhibitors (highly toxic). Once fully sun-ripened, the fruits' toxins become neutralized. If you find that you have trouble digesting fruit, the reason could most often be that the fruit has been harvested too early.

Since they have a cooling influence, you may want to eat fruits more often during the summer months. They are less suitable during the cold season when we need more warming foods.

The best types of fruit are the ones that grow naturally in your environment. To properly digest fruit from another country, we require different digestive enzymes. We can only produce these enzymes if we have lived there for some time and our bodies have adapted to that new environment.

▶ You may eat soaked dried fruit such as sultanas, figs, dates or prunes, either for breakfast (without other foods) or as a snack like other fruit. 'Muscle test' which ones are the most suitable for you! Dried fruits contain enzyme inhibitors, which can make them gas-forming and constipating. Soaking them overnight or for at least a few hours breaks down these natural chemicals and makes them more easily digestible.

▶ Eat 8-12 almonds on a daily basis. This provides vital nutrients to the cells of the body, and particularly to the eyes and bones. Remove the skin by placing the almonds in boiled water for 15-20 minutes. The skins will easily slip off. Soaking them overnight increases their digestibility.

Note: The skin contains harmful acids used to protect the nut from insect attack and fungus. These acids may cause some irritation, or even allergies, in some sensitive individuals.

▶ It is best to avoid leftover foods, with the exception of rice and beans, which you may keep for a day or two and then reheat. Research has shown there are more destructive bacteria in Grandma's reheated soup than on a month-old kitchen sink sponge. With regard to vegetables, the active life force (Prana or Chi energy) and important enzymes and vitamins dissipate after one hour of cooking them. Frozen food is void of the life force, and thus has diminished nutrient-absorption. Fruit should be eaten only fresh. Microwaves used to cook food cause total disintegration of the food's molecular structure and destroy its life force. Without its life force, food cannot be digested and assimilated properly[13].

▶ For deep tissue-cleansing, drink hot (ionized) water frequently: Boil water for 15-20 minutes. Keep it in a thermos flask. Every half hour, take 1-2 sips or more according to your thirst. To have a cleansing effect, the water must be boiled this long and be taken as hot as you would take tea. You may put a small piece of fresh ginger in the flask to improve taste. By boiling the water continuously for at least 15 minutes, large numbers of negatively charged oxygen ions are generated. When ingested by taking frequent sips of this water throughout the day, these negatively charged ions systematically begin to cleanse the tissues of the body and help rid them of positively charged ions - those associated with high acidity and toxins. If you have excessive body weight, this cleansing method can help you shed many pounds of body-waste without any major undesirable side effects. (See more details in Chapter 7) It can be used for any health issue related to congestion in any part of the body.

▶ Avoid ice-cold foods or beverages as they can 'extinguish' AGNI, the digestive fire, for many hours. They may also damage the nerve endings of the stomach. A hand, held in icy water, becomes numb. Similarly, cold drinks or food items cause the stomach cells to contract and prevent them from secreting the required amounts of digestive juices. They also make the stomach insensitive to potentially harmful foods or beverages, and effectively disrupt its communication and potential warning signals to the brain. In addition, digestive enzymes require a very specific temperature to operate optimally. By cooling down the enzymes' environment, their digestive and anti-cancer properties begin to diminish, too, predisposing a person to excessive weight gain and even cancer. Also, the sudden cold influence, as caused, for example, by ice cream or iced beverages, forces the body to increase its internal heat generation in order to compensate for the harmful drop in temperature. This response wastes the body's energy reserves and may make it feel even hotter and thirstier than before, particularly during the summer period. Foods and beverages that are of room temperature or warm are the most suitable and natural ones for the human body.

▶ Use the spices appropriate for your body type generously. You will find them listed in the Ayurvedic food charts below. Spices not only enhance the flavor of food, but also contain vital nutrients and aromas that help with the digestion and metabolism of food. People who suffer from low metabolism (mainly Kapha types) can speed up their metabolic rate by as much as 30 percent by using warming or heating spices in their food. Chili peppers or chili-containing spice mixes should be avoided, though, as they affect the chest and cause mucus irritation in the stomach and intestines. If you like food to be hot and spicy, cayenne pepper is the best option.

▶ If available, drink 2 to 4 ounces of freshly prepared carrot juice before lunch. Note: Pitta types should do the muscle test for carrot juice before attempting this regimen, since carrots can increase Pitta.

▶ For one day per week or month, you may want try taking only a liquid diet (soups, freshly made juices, water, herbal teas, ionized water, etc.). Then gradually build up to a normal diet again. This may greatly relieve the digestive system of its daily workload and improve its ability to remove any accumulated toxic waste. Women benefit greatly if they have a 'liquid day' about one or two days before the onset of menstruation: this can help to make the menstrual period more comfortable and effective.

Drinking Water - The Greatest Therapy of All

Dehydration is perhaps the most common, yet largely unrecognized problem prevalent in modern societies today. Alcohol, coffee, tea and soft drinks have become the primary choice for satisfying thirst, especially among the younger generations. The principal effect of these beverages, however, is to remove water - the most important and precious resource in the body - from the blood, cells and organs. Drinking enough fresh water is an essential prerequisite for avoiding disease and slowing the aging process. Anyone who is healthy and wants to stay that way needs to drink about 6-8 eight-ounce glasses of fresh water each day. This will ensure that the 60-100 trillion cells in the body receive their daily-needed ration of water in order to maintain efficient digestion, metabolism and waste removal. Children may need to drink 4-6 glasses of water per day, depending on how physically active they are.

Suggestions:

⇒ Start the day by drinking one glass of warm water to end the 'drought' of the night and remove accumulated wastes from the excretory organs. As previously mentioned, this can be followed by a glass of warm water with lemon and honey.

⇒ About half an hour before each meal, drink one glass of water. Doing this will keep your blood thin and thereby enable it to take up nutrients and distribute them to the cells. The water also helps increase the secretion of digestive juices and prevents bile from becoming too viscous. Drinking a lot of water or other beverages *with* your meal, however, dilutes the digestive juices. This should be avoided because it undermines the digestive process.

⇒ Following a meal, the blood uses up a considerable amount of water to distribute nutrients to the cells and can, therefore, become water deficient quite quickly. Drinking another glass of water approximately 2 ½ hours after each meal restores the blood's water requirements.

These simple guidelines can help prevent the most serious major diseases that are prevalent in modern societies today. Drinking sufficient amounts of water at the right times can and should be part of every other therapy used in the treatment of disease.

A note of caution: Any attempt to restore the proper state of hydration of the body should be made gradually. otherwise this may cause serious harm. A dehydrated person, that is, someone who has not taken the minimum required amount of water for several weeks, months or years, and/or has depleted the cells of excessive amounts of water by consuming caffeine or sugar-containing foods or beverages for a considerable length of time, is susceptible to becoming ill. During dehydration, the body's cells are no longer able to function efficiently. To protect themselves against further loss of water, they make their membranes less penetrable to water diffusion by pulling in extra amounts of fats, including *cholesterol*. This survival mechanism, however, also prevents metabolic waste from leaving the cells, causing them to suffocate in their own waste. Some of the cells, in order to survive in this toxic environment, may eventually need to undergo genetic mutation and become cancerous.

During the state of dehydration, the kidneys hold on to water and so does the rest of the body. At this point many people start craving and overeating salt or salty foods because the body needs more salt to hold on to the little water it has left. This, however, causes the kidneys to contract and filter even less water than before. Urine becomes more and more concentrated and scarce. In this condition of extreme dehydration, it would be unwise to suddenly start drinking even the recommended 6-8 glasses per day of water. Since the cells have created a barrier in order to save water, they are in no position to absorb a quantity of water to which they have become unaccustomed, all at once. The water would simply stagnate outside the cells and lead to water retention and weight gain. Given these circumstances, the kidneys are not able to filter much of it, and urine will remain scarce. Any sudden intake of large amounts of water can indeed cause severe lymph congestion, swelling, and in some cases, even death. The effect would be water intoxication, a potentially fatal disturbance in brain function that results when the normal balance of electrolytes in the body is pushed outside of safe limits by a very rapid intake of water. The transition from a state of severe dehydration to improved hydration should be very gradual and is best monitored by a health practitioner who knows the basics of water metabolism.

Guidelines for Gradual Rehydration

Add *only* about one glass of water per day to the amount of water you usually drink and check whether urination increases. If it does, drink another 1-2 glasses per day. If not, reduce the additional amount to a third or half glass of water per day. It is of principal importance that your kidneys begin to filter more water when you drink more water. You don't want to create a 'dam' in your kidneys, which could end up flooding even your lungs. In time, the kidneys will recognize that water is no longer a scarcity in the body and will make the necessary adjustments to increase urination. At the same time, the body will naturally decrease its salt production and salt retention. When this occurs, the urge to eat a lot of salt or salty foods will also lessen. This response is caused by the water's own natural diuretic effects.

If you are on diuretic drugs, it is important for you to know that water is a much more efficient diuretic than any drug can possibly be, and it has no harmful side effects. Diuretic drugs should be decreased gradually and under the supervision of a health practitioner.

Once the kidneys have no more difficulties with eliminating urine, you can increase your water intake to the natural minimum daily requirement of 6-8 glasses per day. This will drastically reduce the health risks imposed by an illness. To undo years of dehydration and to be completely hydrated again, however, may take up to a year, and sometimes even longer.

A note of caution: When the body is dehydrated, it tries to retain its salt in order to hold on to water. Once urination increases following improved hydration, these salts are gradually passed out with the urine. If the hydration attempts are implemented too quickly, those areas with the most salt retention may develop lymph edema. Any emerging puffiness of or around the eyes or swelling of the ankles indicates that the hydration process should be done more gradually. As the swellings decrease, you may resume drinking normal quantities of water. With increased water intake, your body will also be able to remove any excessive salt. However, you do not want to become salt-deficient. You should, therefore, be certain to include some unrefined salt[13] as an important part of your diet. If don't use your muscles enough and they start to cramp, particularly during the night, your body is most likely not getting enough salt (or it is getting the wrong type of salt, which is commercially produced table salt).

Both water and salt are absolutely essential for keeping the water metabolism balanced and for generating enough hydroelectric energy to maintain cellular activities. Drinking water is the most important therapy of all therapies because absolutely nothing in the body does not depend on it. Drinking water and cutting out any energy-depleting (overstimulating) influences should be the very first treatment in the case of an illness, before attempting to do anything else. In most cases, the problem will disappear naturally when the body is properly hydrated and allowed to rest.

---

13 Regular, refined table salt (sodium chloride) is a major cause of heart, lymph, and kidney problems and should be avoided. See also the section on the great benefits of unrefined salt in Chapter 7.

Exercise Yourself to Health

The Purpose of Exercising

Under normal circumstances, exercising one's body would not be necessary. Man, like every other animal, was meant to live in nature, have plenty of fresh air, and be involved in enough physical activity to keep the body fit and vital. Technological and economic advancements, however, have led to an increasingly sedentary lifestyle, which requires physical exercise to keep our bodies healthy and strong.

The purpose of physical exercise is not just to prove to ourselves that we are able to defy the aging process, look good, or prevent a heart attack. Exercise also enhances our capacity to digest food and eliminate physical and emotional impurities. Furthermore, it increases firmness and suppleness, as well as our ability to deal with stressful situations. The lymphatic system, especially, which drains toxic and noxious substances from the connective tissues of the organs and muscles, depends on the daily movement of all the parts of the body. Unlike the blood, which has a heart to circulate it around the body, the lymph fluid has no such direct pumping device to do the same. The lymphatic system heavily relies on the breathing mechanism and how well we use it. When the muscle responsible for the breathing action of the lungs (diaphragm) extends into the abdomen, it exerts great pressure on the intestinal lymph vessels, thereby squeezing their contents. This forces the lymph to move through the lymph ducts, such as the thoracic duct. Thus, each inhalation and exhalation acts as an indirect pump for the lymphatic system. Shallow breathing that results from a sedentary lifestyle (and intestinal congestion) has a detrimental effect on proper lymph drainage. Exercise can greatly improve lymphatic functions and thereby prevent a multitude of diseases.

Physical exercise is a great immune-stimulant if done in moderation, and it also improves neuromuscular integration in all age groups. Its effect of boosting self-confidence and self-esteem stems, to some extent, from the improved oxygen supply to the cells and the resulting well-being in all parts of the body and mind. Exercise is an excellent means of increasing happiness in life, especially if it involves challenges that require creativity.

The conventional approach to exercise promotes the belief that a good workout takes you to the limits of your endurance, leaving you exhausted and tired. This is not true. Exercise that exhausts your body is an indirect act of violence that the body perceives as a kind of punishment for not performing well enough. The pain that shows in people's faces when they struggle through a tough workout program is an indication that the body is suffering from overexertion. This sort of exercise defeats its purpose. Any form of strong physical exertion upsets Vata and causes the secretion of abnormal amounts of stress hormones such as adrenaline; this leaves the body restless and shaky. The body, thus depleted of energy, is unable to do the repair work that arises from the demanding workout, leaving the cardiovascular system weak and vulnerable to other stress factors.

Post-exercise exhaustion is a serious cause of illness that affects many unsuspecting people who think they are doing themselves a favor by pushing their bodies to the limit. In the excitement of competitive sports, you may not be aware at first how strenuously you are exerting yourself, but once the *adrenaline rush* is over, the side effects start kicking in. Besides exhaustion and possible injury, professional athletes are more likely to suffer from a deficient immune system, which makes the body prone to infections and other ailments. For this reason, athletes consume a much larger quantity of prescribed drugs than the average person does. The thymus gland, which activates *lymphocytes* and controls energy supplies, may actually shrink in size and leave the body weak and debilitated as a direct result of over conditioning the body and stressing the mind.

Exercise According to the Doshas

Exercise is best done according to one's capacity and psycho-physiological body type. A Vata type, who has the lowest capacity for exercise, benefits mostly from such easy ways of keeping fit as walking, dancing, bicycling, taking short hikes, balancing and stretching. Vatas generally do well with Yoga, Tai Chi, and Chi Kung. Since Vata types experience energy in bursts, they should be particularly careful not to overexert themselves. When their energy suddenly drops, they can feel depleted for a long time afterward. This often results in depression.

Pitta types, being competitive by nature, are equipped with more drive and energy than Vatas. They generally are not satisfied with the more ordinary forms of working out. To achieve physical satisfaction, they need a more goal-oriented exercise program. However, they also do not have boundless energy and are better off exercising in moderation. Pittas feel challenged by hiking in the mountains, skiing, jogging, swimming, playing tennis or engaging in other sports that generate in them a sense of achievement.

In sports, you can easily recognize the unbalanced Pitta types. They are often bad losers and may get angry if they feel they are 'not good enough'. Pittas who get angry while performing should look for a less competitive exercise program to increase their level of satisfaction. Since excessive heat is a sign of unbalanced Pitta, swimming, which has a cooling influence, is one of the best forms of exercise for them. A walk in the cool forest is another excellent way to pacify an unbalanced Pitta type.

Kapha types are the ideal candidates for a good or moderately heavy workout. Weight training, running, rowing, some aerobics, long distance bicycling, dancing for a long time, playing football, basketball and tennis are all very suitable for a Kapha. The Kapha type's steady energy gives him the necessary endurance and stamina to last through long competitive games without feeling tired. Exercise will clear out any excessive Kapha congestion, remove excessive water and fat, and improve general circulation. This will leave him feeling refreshed and buoyant afterward.

Basic Guidelines for Healthy Exercise

- It is best not to exercise at more than 50 percent of your capacity, whatever that means to you. The purpose of exercising is not to prove to others how capable you are, but to derive personal benefit and satisfaction from it. If you are able to run for 30 minutes before you are tired, then make the choice to run for only 15 minutes. Getting tired during exercise defeats its very purpose. Feeling refreshed, revitalized and energetic afterward indicates that the workout has been successful. In due time, your capacity for exercise will naturally increase on its own.

- Stop exercising when you feel the need to breathe through the mouth. Once you are forced to breathe through the mouth, rather than through the nose, you have gone beyond the 50 percent threshold of your capacity for exercise at that time. This is a sign that your body has moved into the adrenaline-breathing mode, which uses up your basic energy reserves and depletes cellular oxygen. You have reached your limit when you feel your heart pounding violently, you begin to sweat profusely, or your body shakes. In that case it is good to finish off with a short period of walking and breathing normally. The basic rule is always to breathe through the nose and not through the mouth. Exercise to the point of perspiration once a day.

- You need good, strong muscles to meet the typical demands of the day, such as climbing stairs, carrying groceries, picking up young children, cleaning your home, riding horseback, swimming in a lake, going for a hike or bike ride, or performing other natural activities, without being at risk for injury. The best way to increase muscle tone and strength is to quickly raise heart and muscle activity to the point of panting, followed by a period of low activity (called 'active recovery'). One to two-minute intervals (of activity and rest) are ideal. Doing this for 10-20 minutes per day has more benefits than engaging in hours of strenuous exercise. Besides, it increases muscle tone, lung capacity and heart health. During the panting phases, the body uses up its complex sugar reserves in the muscles. For those who desire weight loss, this method causes you to lose weight after exercising, as the body tries to replenish its lost sugar reserves by breaking down fat deposits while you are resting. Weight loss achieved during strenuous endurance exercise programs, on the other hand, tends to be reversed because the body tries to quickly replenish the lost fat deposits in order to prepare itself for the next energy-depleting round of exercise. The body perceives the strenuous exercise as a threat. Vata and Pitta types are those who are affected most negatively by strenuous exercise. Pure Kapha types are the only people who can benefit from it.

- It is best to exercise during daylight hours. The best capacity for exercise is available during the Kapha period in the morning (6:00-10:00 a.m.) and at the end of the Vata period in the afternoon (5:00-6:00 p.m.). The benefits of exercise increase dramatically when it is done in sunlight. (See Chapter 8, Sunlight - Medicine of Nature)
- Ayurveda discourages exercising after sundown. Allow the body to slow down in the evening and prepare itself for a restful and rejuvenating sleep. Never exercise just before or after a meal, as this impairs AGNI, the digestive fire, and causes indigestion. However, walking for 15 minutes after meals works as a good digestive aid. Always drink water before and after exercising to prevent the blood from thickening and the cells from becoming dehydrated.

A note of caution about aerobic exercise: The medical journal, *Lancet*, reported that aerobic exercise can cause deadly arterial clogging and heart disease in those who had never before had heart trouble. According to *The American Journal of Cardiology*, jogging has similarly caused some runners to drop dead from heart attacks. Their autopsies show severe coronary artery disease. Any regular, strenuous form of exercise actually does about as much damage to your heart as continuous stress does. The heart literally comes under constant attack via the excessive exercise sessions. Marathon runners are known to lose muscle mass, both in the heart and the rest of the body. Many have dropped dead just after reaching the finishing line. Short distance sprinters, on the other hand, develop healthy muscles and strong hearts, as explained in point 3 above.

Vigorous weight training can be equally damaging. It leads to abnormally enlarged, bloated muscle fibers that actually become dysfunctional and prone to injuries. Oversized muscles constantly use up a lot of precious energy (complex sugar reserves), energy that your body requires for its more important activities. Weight training also adds excessive muscle tissue to parts of the body where it was never designed to be, thus hindering natural patterns of movement. Lifting heavy weights can also raise your blood pressure and increase the risk of strokes and aneurysms. By nature, the human body was not made to deal with the additional gravitational force imposed upon it while lifting heavy weights. Frequently stressing the joints, muscles and tendons causes them to age prematurely. Excessive weight training can cause permanent damage to the body.

Surya Namaskara (Sun Salutation)

Surya Namaskara (**illustration 15**) is one of the most ancient and integrated exercise programs around. It forms an integral part of Yoga, which benefits both the mind and the body. It is unique in the sense that it strengthens and stretches all major muscle groups, massages all the internal organs, supports lymph drainage from every part of the body, and enlivens the energy centers and acupuncture points of the body. This exercise program increases blood flow and circulation, conditions the spine, and improves flexibility of the joints. Grace, suppleness, as well as physical stability are the natural results arising from daily practice. You may not get the handle on this exercise right from the first time, but with regular practice you will be able to go through the different positions easily and naturally.

SURYANAMASKARA

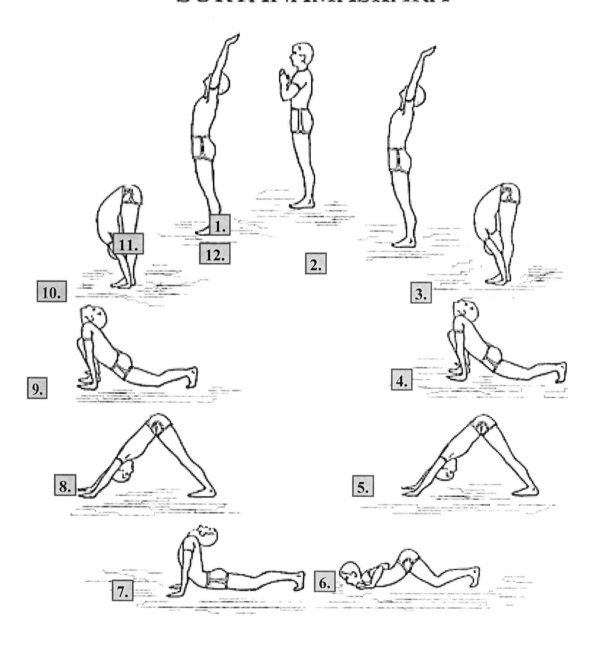

Illustration 15: Surya Namaskara

Directions: Surya Namaskara consists of two cycles of twelve postures each. During the first cycle, in positions #4 and #9, the right knee is brought forward to the chest, and during the second cycle the left knee is brought forward. Apart from this exception, all the movements are exactly the same for both cycles. The twelve postures or positions are performed one after another in fluid sequence and coordinated with one's breathing. It is important not to strain while performing this exercise because benefits can only be felt when it is done easily and effortlessly. When you feel tired, lie down and rest, and breathe freely. Begin with one or two complete cycles and see how you feel afterward. This way, the exercise will gradually increase your capacity for more. As a general guideline, men can eventually do as many as twelve complete (double) rounds, women as many as six.

You will find that after a few cycles your breathing will naturally adjust itself to the different movements. After having done this exercise for a few days, the sequence of movements will be automatic, and you will no longer need to look at the instruction pictures.

Breathing Exercises (Pranayama)

Ayurveda recommends simple breathing exercises or *Pranayama* that help to refresh energy and restore vitality to both mind and body within minutes. The word Pranayama is composed of two Sanskrit words. *Prana* means 'the life force' or 'the breath of life'. It carries vital energy from the surroundings into the body. *Yama* means exercise that increases the flow of Prana and thereby stimulates all the functions of body and mind. *Pranayama* can cause an extraordinary balance in consciousness. It has a deep cleansing effect, and it purifies the *nadis*, which are the pranic currents of energy - the pathways (meridians) for Prana also known as 'meridians' in acupuncture). The benefits of Pranayama include a reduction of stress and tension, improved respiration and circulation, as well as a heightened awareness and clarity of mind. Those suffering from respiratory ailments, headaches or migraines, and depression, may especially derive great relief from Pranayama. For maximum results, any of the following three types of Pranayama (according to body type) should be performed twice a day for five minutes each, preferably on an empty stomach in the morning and in the evening, before meditation or when under stress. There is one Pranayama that is most suitable for each of the different body types, although Vata Pranayama can be done by anyone who is suffering from any kind of affliction. Breathing should be normal and effortless. For maximum benefits, one should sit straight but comfortably, and with eyes closed.

Breathing should be coordinated with the natural movements of the body. Whenever you extend the spine or elongate the body, inhale, and when you bend or fold the body, exhale.

Vata-Pranayama

A person of Vata constitution or Vata imbalance benefits most from *alternative nostril breathing*, which brings balance on all levels of mind and body. For this exercise:
  ⇒ **Close your right nostril with the thumb of your right hand, and inhale through the left nostril.**
  ⇒ **Then close the left nostril with the middle or ring finger of the same hand, and exhale through your right nostril.**
  ⇒ **Hold your finger there and inhale. Release, and once again close the right nostril with your**

thumb, and exhale through your left nostril.

⇒ **Remain there and breathe in again.**

Repeat this sequence for five minutes. Be sure to breathe in a relaxed and natural way while sitting straight and comfortably. This Pranayama supplies a larger and equal amount of oxygen to both hemispheres of the brain, empties the lower lobes of the lungs from excessive amounts of carbon dioxide, and makes room for more oxygen to be taken to the cells, giving them an 'oxygen bath'. Vatas who feel tense, restless and stressed can quickly return to balance by practicing this Pranayama. Asthmatics also benefit from it.

Pitta-Pranayama

A person of Pitta constitution or Pitta imbalance can 'cool down' and enhance female energies in the body by performing *left nostril breathing*. The left nostril corresponds to the cooling system in the body. If it is blocked, the body overheats. For this exercise:

⇒ **Close your right nostril with the thumb of your right hand, and inhale through your left nostril.**

⇒ **Then close your left nostril with your middle or ring finger, and exhale through your right nostril.**

Repeat for five minutes, breathing normally and naturally while sitting upright and comfortably.

Kapha-Pranayama

A person of Kapha constitution can literally warm up and increase male energies in the body by performing *right nostril breathing*. The right nostril corresponds to the heating system in our body. If it is blocked, the body becomes too cold. For this exercise:

⇒ **Close your left nostril with the middle or index finger of your right hand, and inhale through your right nostril.**

⇒ **Then close the right nostril with your thumb and exhale with your left nostril.**

Repeat for five minutes, breathing effortlessly and sitting upright and comfortably.

Obese-Pranayama

A person who suffers from obesity should perform a fast Pranayama.

⇒ **Sit in a comfortable position, take a deep breath and exhale quickly and forcefully through the nose. You will naturally inhale after each exhalation.**

⇒ **Repeat for one minute; then rest for one minute.**

⇒ **Do this exercise for a total of five times, resting for one minute after each time.**

This exercise speeds up the metabolic rate and is the *equivalent of running two miles*. You will begin to feel hot and start sweating. It is important at this stage not to drink cold or chilled beverages, as they shut down AGNI and increase the buildup of fat in the body. Drink water of room temperature.

Conscious Breathing Meditation

Conscious Breathing is practiced in a comfortable sitting position (in a chair or on the floor) and with the eyes closed. It is best to sit straight to make it easier for the body to breathe without strain. For maximum results, this meditation should be practiced for about 15 minutes once a day, although twice a day in the morning and/or in the evening is preferable. Meditate before, or at least 2-3 hours after, eating food.

As you close your eyes, simply bring your attention to the end of your nose or to your chest and experience the movements of inhalation and exhalation. Breathe easily and naturally. The longer you practice, the more readily your mind will follow the rhythm of breathing and become relaxed. To go into a peaceful state, your mind does not have to stop thinking. In fact, the only mistake you can make with this practice is to try to stop thinking or to prevent thoughts from coming. If you are carried away by your thoughts, feelings or emotions, please do not do anything to stop them. Instead, simply bring your awareness back to the breathing, to your nose or chest, and if the thoughts continue to be there, that is fine. An increase in thought activity during this practice indicates that stress is being released from the nervous system. Stress release naturally results in increased physical activity. This, in turn, increases mental activity, i.e. thoughts, feelings and mental pictures.

Continue this process until you feel that about 15 minutes have passed. There is no reason to be anxious about doing this correctly. Breathing is natural, and having your attention on it is natural, too. There is nothing you can do to improve upon what nature is already doing perfectly. Do not try to breathe with greater emphasis or more deeply than you would normally do in the sitting position.

By repeatedly allowing your mind to follow the inhalation of fresh air into the body and the exhalation of used air out through your nose, your mind will become increasingly quiet and peaceful. If for a brief moment your mind becomes still altogether, you will only be aware of yourself, without a thought or feeling. For this brief moment you are Self-realized because your Self is the only thing to which it can refer. It is for this instant that your mind has given up thinking; your body follows suit by becoming very relaxed. This is the time when body and mind are perfectly coordinated, a moment of healing for both body and mind. There is nothing you can possibly do from your side, though, to produce or experience these moments. They occur when you least expect them, i.e. when you are totally relaxed about the process, with no expectations or effort.

With regular practice of conscious breathing you will find that this peaceful and relaxed state of your mind will extend in time and accompany you during mental and physical activity throughout the day. There will be a strong sense of calmness and of being centered and self-confident, even in stressful situations or amidst noise and chaos. The depth of this experience will increase to the point that your own unbounded awareness, the deepest aspect of your consciousness, will coexist with the most dynamic activity of your body and mind.

Directions:
⇒ Close your eyes and sit comfortably.
⇒ Bring your attention to the end of your nose or to your chest, and breathe consciously but naturally.
⇒ When you are aware of other thoughts, let them be there, while gradually bringing your attention back to the breathing.
⇒ After about 15 minutes open your eyes slowly.
⇒ Ideally, meditate twice a day, in the morning and evening before eating.

Abyanga - Ayurvedic Oil Massage

The main purpose of *Abyanga* or oil massage as part of the Ayurvedic daily routine is to assist in preventing the accumulation of physiological toxins (**AMA**) and to lubricate and promote flexibility of the muscles, tissues and joints. Once applied to the skin, the oil passes quickly through the various layers of the skin and the underlying connective and fat tissues. The oil combines with any toxins present there, especially those that are fat-soluble. Within several minutes of massaging the skin, the oil becomes expelled through the skin along with the toxins.

The classical texts of Ayurveda indicate that daily oil massage promotes softness and luster of the skin, as well as youthfulness. The skin is a major producer of endocrine hormones and is connected to every part of the body through thousands of cutaneous nerves. Daily oil massage can, therefore, balance the two master systems of the body - the nervous system and the endocrine system. The following are directions to assist you in learning the Ayurvedic daily do-it-yourself oil massage.

- Unless specific oil has been recommended for you, cold-pressed (also called expeller-pressed) and unrefined sesame oil (not roasted sesame oil) should be the preference. Although sesame oil is suitable for all body types (for external use), if you find it irritating to the skin, you may try olive oil or coconut oil as an alternative. To purify the massage oil, 'cure' it by heating it to about 100 degrees Celsius, the boiling point of water. Add a drop of water to the oil at the beginning, and when the water begins to splutter, you will know that the proper temperature has been reached. You may prepare the entire contents of the bottle at once or do so as needed.

- Before beginning the massage, the oil should be at or slightly above body temperature, especially during the wintertime. Start by massaging the head, if you intend to shampoo afterward. Place a small amount of oil on the fingertips and palms, and begin to massage the scalp vigorously. Since the head and feet are considered the most important parts to be emphasized during Abyanga, spend proportionally more time on the head and feet than on other body parts.

- After massaging the head, gently apply oil with your hands to your face and the outer parts of your ears.

- Massage both the front and back of the neck, and the upper part of the spine.

- You may want to apply a small amount of oil to your entire body and then continue with the massage in each area.

- Next massage your arms. The proper motion is back and forth over the long bones and with a circular motion over the joints. Also massage your hands and fingers.

- Now apply oil to the chest and abdomen. A very gentle circular motion should be used over your heart. Repeat this circular motion, following the 'bowel pattern' from the right lower part of the abdomen, moving clockwise toward the left lower part of the abdomen.

- Massage the back and spine. Some areas are more difficult to reach, so you may want to ask your partner to help you.

- Massage the legs. Like the arms, use a back and forth motion over the long bones and a circular motion over the joints.

- Lastly, massage the soles of the feet. Since all body reflex points are situated in the feet, a good amount of time should be spent on massaging the feet.

Ideally, one should spend about 5-10 minutes on the massage, possibly every morning. If there is not enough time for a full body massage, then a mini-massage of 1-2 minutes on the head and feet is preferable. After your massage, take a warm shower or bath. Use soap only on the genital area and under the arms. This will leave a thin film of oil on the skin that is very beneficial for toning the skin and keeping the body muscles warm throughout the day. If, however, you have applied too much oil, a mild soap made from natural ingredients can be used to wash it off. Sesame oil in particular has a disinfecting action, which helps to ward off harmful microbes.

Daily Oil Therapy - Oil Swishing

Oil therapy is a simple, yet astoundingly effective, method of cleansing the blood. It is helpful for numerous disorders, including blood diseases, lung and liver disorders, tooth and gum diseases, headaches, skin diseases, gastric ulcers, intestinal problems, poor appetite, heart and kidney ailments, encephalitis, nervous conditions, poor memory, female disorders, swollen face and bags under the eyes. The therapy consists simply of swishing oil in the mouth.

To apply this therapy you need expeller-pressed, unrefined sunflower, sesame or olive oil. In the morning, preferably after awakening or anytime before breakfast, put 1-2 tablespoons of oil in your mouth, but do not swallow it. Slowly swish the oil in your mouth, chew it, and draw it through your teeth for 3 to 4 minutes. This thoroughly mixes the oil with saliva and activates the released enzymes. The enzymes draw toxins out of the blood. For this reason, it is important to spit out the oil after no more than 3 to 4 minutes. You do not want any of the released toxins to be reabsorbed. You will find that the oil takes on a milky white or yellowish color as it becomes saturated with toxins and with billions of destructive bacteria.

For best results, repeat this process two more times. (If this releases too many toxins and you feel uncomfortable, do this only once.) Then rinse out your mouth with half a teaspoon of baking soda or unrefined sea salt (take either of these dissolved in a small amount of water). This solution will remove all remnants of the oil and toxins. Additionally, you may want to brush your teeth to make sure your mouth is clean. Tongue scraping is also advised.

Some of the visible effects of oil swishing include the elimination of gum bleeding and the whitening of teeth. During times of illness, this procedure can be repeated 3 times per day, but only on an empty stomach. Oil therapy greatly relieves and supports liver functions, as it takes toxins out of the blood that the liver is not able to remove or detoxify. This benefits the entire organism.

Diet According to Body Types

"No illness which can be treated by diet should be treated by any other means," said Moses Maimonides (1135-1204). The use of food as medicine is not just a treatment model that was almost common knowledge in ages past, but it is now increasingly being recognized as a matter of survival. Most chronic diseases share nutritional deficiency as the number one cause for the underlying degeneration of cells, tissues and organs. Instead of food being our best medicine, modern food production has turned our best foods into man's most harmful poisons. Many among the younger generations have almost completely lost touch with the simple truth that *they are what they eat*. Even educated doctors tell their patients that their heart attacks, cancers and arthritic pains have nothing to do with the foods they eat. Well, not too long ago, doctors told their patients that smoking was good for them. Only rarely does a doctor question his patient about his eating habits, something that should be dealt with before subjecting the diseased person to a series of tests that have no other purpose than to find a label and a corresponding drug or procedure to suppress the symptoms from which he suffers. The treatment consists of methods that make the symptom(s) disappear. If successful, the patient is considered disease-free, at least for a little while. Buying into the illusion of a cure is costly, but only to the patient. Everyone else profits from it. At $7,8 billion a year, Pfizer is now the most profitable of all Fortune 500 companies. Who wins, and who loses? Consider the following facts. In the United States:

- Adverse prescription drug reactions are responsible for the death of 105,000 people each year.
- 95 percent of all drug reactions are not properly identified or reported by doctors, hence their true

risks and potentially deadly consequences are not known.

- Doctors not only treat the symptoms of disease but also the side effects these treatments produce. These side effects are now considered new diseases that require further treatment. Hence there has been a massive escalation of illness in the U.S., at a cost of at least $2 trillion each year.
- Doctors' sloppy handwriting on prescriptions kills 7,000 patients each year.
- 1.5 million people are injured each year because of preventable medication errors.
- Every year 7.5 million Americans undergo unnecessary medical and surgical procedures.
- The number one food item consumed is sugar, in the form of corn syrup. This has generated an epidemic of obesity, diabetes, cancer and heart disease. This epidemic is not being treated at the causal level. **Note:** Since the fructose in corn syrup does neither stimulate insulin secretion nor reduce the hunger hormone *ghrelin*, you will continue to feel hungry while the body converts the fructose into fat. The resulting obesity increases the risk of diabetes and other diseases.

Since you obviously cannot expect to receive much help from those who only know how to treat the effects of illness and not its causes, you may need to take your health into you own hands. Foods have an almost immediate effect on the body. In fact, it is known that the body's biochemistry changes within several minutes of eating a meal. You can easily verify the powerful influence that food has on your body through muscle testing. (See Chapter 1 for details.) If you eat something that is outright harmful to you, your stomach will signal indigestion. Some foods can be even more damaging than just causing heartburn. Research has shown that eating meat in the evening can trigger a heart attack in the morning.

To make it easier for you to figure out which diet and lifestyle are the most beneficial for you, determine which body type you are. As discussed earlier, different people digest and utilize the same food in a different way. If a Vata and a Pitta type go to a restaurant and order the same meal, one of them may feel invigorated afterward and the other one dull and heavy. If Vata and Pitta are about equal, go by the imbalances you experience. For example, if you suffer from regular skin eruptions, internal heat or constant perspiration (Pitta imbalances), choose foods from the Pitta food list. If you are prone to constipation, dry skin or headaches (Vata imbalances), choose foods from the Vata food list. Likewise, if you feel cold and suffer from an oily skin or nose and sinus congestion, follow the Kapha diet plan.

The following food charts provide you with specific lists of foods that are most suitable for each of the three main body types and imbalances. In an ideal situation, you would not require any lists to know which foods are good for you because your natural instinct would make that decision for you. But most people's doshas were thrown off balance with their first taste of manufactured baby formula and whatever manmade foods became their source of nourishment after that. Once a dosha is out of balance in your body, you tend to yearn for exactly those kinds of foods that maintain that imbalance. When the body is congested, the natural urges and signals of the body are also subdued, and cravings result. For example, an unbalanced Pitta type may crave spicy, sour and salty foods, and an unbalanced Kapha type chooses to eat cake, candy and oily foods. Healthy Pittas and Kaphas would have a natural aversion to those foods. Our natural instincts also fail us when we orient our tastes toward nutritional information, time schedules, and the promises of advertisements.

Since the three forces of nature (doshas) are represented in our body in a unique and individual way, each one of us has different requirements for the various nutrients contained in food. Our body is only able to utilize the nutrients of those foods that are suitable for our body type, just as certain feeds are only suitable for certain animals and not for others. Try giving a rabbit olive oil to eat, and it will get sick in no time. Give the oil to a rat, and it will have no problem digesting it.

Now, first determine your body type or dominating dosha by reading the sections below and, perhaps, filling out the body type questionnaire at the end of Chapter 5. Then look at the charts and choose the foods that balance that dosha. For example, if you have scored Vata 6, Pitta 15, and Kapha 8 in the Body Type Quiz, refer to the section 'Pitta Pacifying Diet' found in this chapter.

In order to know yourself better, familiarize yourself with the food charts that are applicable to your body type, and choose to eat more of those foods that are on the 'favor' list while avoiding those that are on the 'avoid' list. Those items in the 'reduce' category should be eaten in moderation, i.e. only occasionally and in small amounts.

You don't need to become overly fixated about sticking to the food lists, especially if you are not just one clear body type. However, these lists can be very helpful in your quest for discovering the most ideal foods for you to return to a balanced state of body and mind. If you feel attracted to a particular food that is not on your list, double check by doing the muscle test, and you will have a better sense of whether your body can benefit from it or not. Both the food lists and the muscle test may help you to get to know yourself better and to restore your natural instincts. If you are an experienced dowser, you can also use dowsing tools to confirm the correctness of your choice of foods. If in doubt about what body type you are, you may even use these methods to determine your exact body type. If most items on the Vata favor list, for example, test positive for you, you are most likely a Vata type. If you suffer from chronic constipation, and/or had such a tendency when you were a child, you are most likely a Vata type. Pitta types are rarely constipated but have a greater tendency toward loose stools and frequent bowel moments.

Children usually share the same body types as their parents. For example, Pitta parents tend to give birth to Pitta children who often have red hair, fair skin and freckles (if Caucasian white). In this situation, the whole family can basically eat the same foods. If one parent, though, is a Vata type and the other parent is a Kapha type, the children may not have such a clear body type configuration. In that case, addressing each family member's dietary needs can be somewhat challenging. However, if healthy foods are offered to the children right from the beginning, they will soon let you know which foods are best for them.

VATA PACIFYING DIET

Favor: Warm foods and beverages; moderately heavy; added *ghee*, butter, oil; mostly high fluid-containing and nourishing foods; foods that have the sweet, sour and salty tastes.

The Vata type - influenced mainly by the elements of air and space - is naturally sensitive to foods that are light, dry and cold. Vata types lack the qualities of *heavy, oily* and *hot* that, when taken in the form of food and beverages, keep them balanced. In addition, foods that contain the dominant tastes of *sweet, sour* and *salty* pacify Vata, whereas those that are *pungent* as in spicy foods, *bitter* as in bitter greens, and *astringent* as in regular black tea or beans, greatly upset it. A meal consisting of a lettuce salad, hot vegetable curry with steamed potatoes, kidney beans and ice cream can derange Vata for many days, whereas a meal consisting of an avocado with lemon and salt, stir fried asparagus, and Basmati rice with butter and almonds can keep the Vata type balanced and strong.

Vata dosha is cold, dry, and light by nature, which are the qualities dominant in autumn and early winter. Especially during that time of year, Vata needs to be soothed and nourished by soft and warming foods such as hearty stews and soups, long-cooked vegetable casseroles, freshly prepared bread, puddings and hot cereals. Butter, oils and cream, too, keep Vata in check. Since sensitivity is one of his characteristics, the Vata type becomes upset when there is too much noise and disturbance around meal times.

Vata types are the most likely to need a more nourishing breakfast. Hot cereals such as oatmeal/porridge cooked with almond milk or oat milk soothe Vata, and so does cream of rice or cream of wheat. Vatas, however, get agitated and nervous by caffeine-containing beverages such as coffee or tea, due to their bitter and astringent tastes and stimulating effects.

Vata types tend to suffer from constipation with dry and hard stools if they have too much rice, pasta or wheat products. Yet when eaten with plenty of well-cooked, juicy vegetables, these foods are Vata pacifying, too. Potatoes in any form are likely to cause Vata problems since they have a drying and dehydrating effect. Popcorn is another typical Vata-raising food. Vata's main rule regarding starch-containing foods, often referred to as carbohydrates, is to add copious amounts of fats; otherwise, they tend to pass too quickly through the small intestine and end up being fermented by bacteria in the large intestine. This causes the typical gas and bloating about which Vatas so frequently complain.

Vatas also benefit from spices that are mild, soothing, sweet and heavy, as listed below. Since their digestive fire (ANGI) tends to fluctuate and be irregular, ginger, cardamom, fennel and cinnamon can stimulate the appetite and improve digestion. These also help to reduce gas, a problem that Vatas are particularly prone to develop.

The Vata type is the only body type that requires more salt in his body and can greatly benefit from adding it to his food, although it is always better to do so during the cooking process. Care is to be taken, however, when the salt is eaten in a dry form, such as on salted crackers or crisps. Processed, commercial salt aggravates Vata, whereas unrefined salt calms it. (Also see Chapter 7)

It is better for the Vata type to choose unprocessed foods such as unsalted nuts, which are sweet, heavy and oily, all qualities that pacify Vata. Be aware that nuts and seeds are very concentrated and rich foods, which means they should be consumed only in small quantities. Vatas can digest them more easily when they are ground or made into butters. Be careful, however, with commercial nut butters. They become rancid within a few days of being ground, even if kept in the refrigerator. Nut butters are notorious for causing food poisoning and inflammation in the gastrointestinal tract. It is best to make nut butter fresh and keep it for no longer than 2-3 days. One of the best nuts for pacifying Vata is almonds (8-10 a day) without the skin. Soaking nuts and seeds overnight greatly enhances their digestibility.

Ripe and sweet fruits are also very beneficial to the Vata, provided they are eaten on an empty stomach and not in the evening. Vata types should avoid fruits that have an astringent taste, as in unripe bananas or persimmons, whereas the sour taste of grapefruit helps to pacify Vata.

The drying, cooling and light elements of air and space/ether are the most dominating elements in the Vata type. Therefore, when he is in a balanced state, Vata shows a natural aversion to the following air/space foods:

AIR/SPACE FOODS
(To be reduced or avoided)

- All cabbage families
- All dry, rough, and stale foods
- Bitter vegetables
- Hollow vegetable with tiny seeds (except peppers)

- Greens and lettuce
- Most nightshade fruits and vegetables
- Most dry and compact legumes

Vata Food Chart

FRUITS
Favor

Apricots	Coconut	Lemons
Avocado	Dates, fresh	Mango
Bananas	Figs, fresh	Stewed fruits
Berries	Grapefruit	Soaked dried
Cherries	Grapes	fruits
Oranges	Pineapple	Melons (sweet)
Papaya	Plums	Tangerines
Peaches	Rhubarb	

Reduce

Apples	Dried Fruits, cooked	Pomegranate
Cranberries	Pears	Quince

Avoid

Persimmon	Prunes	Watermelon

Note: all fruits should be ripe and sweet. They should be consumed on an empty stomach. Apples and pears should be cooked.

VEGETABLES
Favor

Artichokes	Leeks, cooked	Summer squash
Asparagus	Okra, with fat	(yellow crookneck,
Beetroot	Pumpkin, orange and	zucchini)
Carrots	white	Watercress
Celery(cooked)	Radishes, cooked	Winter squash
Cucumber, seedless	Sweet potatoes, with fat	(acorn, buttercup,
Green beans		butternut)

Reduce

Broccoli	Lettuce	Plantain
Collards	Mustard greens	Radishes
Corn, fresh	Onion, cooked	Spinach
Jerusalem artichoke	Parsnips	Turnip greens

Avoid

Bell peppers	Eggplant	Potatoes, white
Brussels sprouts	Endive	Swiss chard

Cabbage	Kohlrabi	Sprouts
Cauliflower	Mushrooms	Tomatoes
Celery, raw	Onion, raw Peas	

Note: The *Reduce* and *Avoid* items, with the exception of cabbage, potatoes and sprouts, are acceptable if cooked well, and with oil and Vata spices added. Raw vegetables should be avoided altogether.

GRAINS
Favor

Basmati rice, white	Whole rice, well cooked,	Wheat cereal, not dry
Oats, cooked	Chia Seeds (super grain)	Wild rice

Reduce

Amaranth	Whole Wheat Pasta	Unbleached white flour,
Barley	Quinoa	Whole wheat flour
Bulgur	Rice flour	
Couscous	Udon noodles	

Avoid

Buckwheat	Millet	Rye
Corn	Oats, dry	
Cereals, dried	White flour pasta	

LEGUMES, BEANS, PEAS
Favor

Aduki beans	Pink lentils	Toor dhal
Mung beans (split or whole)	Tofu, fermented and cooked*	

*Soy milk and commercially produced tofu contain at least two highly toxic enzyme inhibitors. They can increase the risk of cancer and other illnesses. (See more information in *A Note on Legumes and their Digestibility* below) Japanese tofu is properly fermented through a process that takes several years and renders these poisons harmless. Also see chapter 13, *A Warning Note about Soy Products.*

Reduce

Black chickpeas	Urad dhal
Muth beans	

Black beans	Kidney beans	Soybeans
Black-eyes beans/peas	Lima beans	Split peas
Chick peas	Navy beans	White beans
Lentils, brown	Pinto beans	

DAIRY
Favor

Buttermilk, home-made	Cow's milk, certified raw	Ghee
Cottage cheese, homemade	Unsalted butter	Yoghurt, home-made

Caution: With the exception of ghee and butter, use these foods very sparingly. If they cause mucus, coating on the tongue or congested nose/sinuses, discontinue them immediately and avoid them altogether. Dairy products can lead to serious lymphatic congestion and thickening of the blood vessel walls. (See more details in the section *Milk Controversy* in Chapter 14)

Reduce

Cheeses, hard and soft	Goat's milk	Sour cream

Avoid

All commercially produced dairy products, including low fat milk and ice cream, with the exception of unsalted butter and cream

NUTS AND SEEDS
Favor

Almonds	Pecans	Sesame seeds, roasted
Brazil nuts	Pine nuts	Sunflower seeds
Cashews	Pistachios	Walnuts
Chestnuts	Pumpkin seeds	

Note: peanuts should be avoided.

SWEETENERS
Favor

Brown rice syrup	Rock sugar	Unrefined sugar
Date syrup	Stevia	cane
Honey, raw	Sugar cane juice	products
Palm sugar		Xylitol

Reduce		
Barley malt	Maple syrup	Molasses

Avoid		
Honey, heated or cooked White sugar	Sugar substitutes (Aspartame, Saccharin,	Sweet 'N Low, NutraSweet, etc.)

Note: If Candida is an issue in your body, avoid all sweeteners except stevia and small amounts of xylitol.

Oils/Fats

Favor		
Almond Unsalted Butter	*Ghee* Sesame	Sunflower

Reduce		
Coconut Mustard	Olive Safflower	Walnut

Avoid		
Animal fats, except butter and *ghee* Corn	Canola Mixed vegetable oils Light fat products	Synthetically Derived fats

Note: All refined and heat-pressed oils are harmful to your health!

HERBS. SPICES. CONDIMENTS
Favor

Allspice	Cumin	Paprika
Almond extract	Dill, leaves or seed	Peppermint
Anise	Fennel	Rosemary
Asafetida	Gomasio	Sage
Basil	Ginger, dried or fresh	Rock salt
Bay leaf	Lemon juice	Unrefined Sea
Black cumin	Licorice root	Salt
Black pepper	Mace	Savory
Carraway	Marjoram	Spearmint
Chutney, coconut or	Mango powder	Tamarind
mango	Mustard seeds, black and	Tarragon
Cardamon	yellow	Thyme
Cinnamon	Nutmeg	Vanilla
Cloves	Olives, black or green	
Cilantro	Oregano	

Cayenne	Fenugreek	Parsley
Chili peppers	Garlic, cooked	Saffron
Coriander seed	Horseradish	Turmeric
Curry, leaves and powder	Mint	

Note: You may use these spices in moderation, but avoid raw garlic and all very bitter and astringent tasting spices and herbs.

BREWS, BEVERAGES, TEAS
All are acceptable except for:

Alcohol	Cranberry juice	Blackberry tea
Apple juice	Pear juice	Burdock tea
Caffeinated beverages	Prune juice	Dandelion tea
Carbonated beverages	Pungent beverages	Power Drinks
Cold beverages	Tomato juice	

PITTA PACIFYING DIET

Favor: Cool or warm foods and beverages; moderately heavy; less added butter and fats except for *ghee* and *coconut oil*; foods that are of sweet, bitter and astringent tastes.

The Pitta type is naturally equipped with a strong digestive power that allows him to choose from a larger variety of foods than suitable for the other body types. His main adversary, however, is overeating. As long as he does not abuse his strong digestive power, it is hard to throw him off balance. When suffering from digestive trouble, just eating lesser amounts of food can restore his physical balance.

The dominating elements in the Pitta type are fire and water. Therefore, pungent and sour foods (both have heating properties) as well as salty food (containing commercially produced salt) upset Pitta and should be used sparingly. The sodium chloride in common table salts causes water retention, malabsorption of nutrients, and blood pressure problems. If used in moderation, unrefined sea and rock salt, on the other hand, have beneficial effects even for the Pitta type. The dominating presence of the fire element makes the Pitta type prefer cooling, refreshing foods and beverages, especially during the hot summer season.

Unlike the Vata type who benefits from oily, sour, salty and heating foods, the Pitta type is greatly disturbed by them. (**Note:** if you are a Vata/Pitta type and not sure which one of the two doshas is the dominant one in your body, apply the muscle test for a couple of major food items from the Pitta list and see whether the results match your body type score). Pitta types benefit more from bitter and astringent tastes, both of which are contained in lettuces, herbs and green leafy vegetables. Legumes are mainly astringent and are generally liked by all Pitta types. Foods that have cold, heavy, and dry qualities are generally more suitable for the Pitta type. Mint, for example, has cooling properties whereas honey is heating. Wheat is both cooling and heavy compared to the light and heating properties of buckwheat or millet. Potatoes or cauliflower are very dry in comparison to the oiliness of eggs or peanuts. The Pitta's strong AGNI has no problem digesting the more dry, cold and heavy foods, and they are, therefore, not gas-forming for him. Grain foods, on the other hand, cause him trouble if they are left whole. Brown rice and heavy whole-wheat breads can upset Pitta dosha, so does brown unrefined cane sugar. The Pitta type is the only one that can get away with eating white sugar from time to time. Maple and carob syrups are also more easily digested by the Pitta type, unless he eats these in large amounts (which unbalanced Pittas tend to do).

The fats that are contained in meat, eggs, pork, etc., strongly irritate Pitta types. Fried and oily foods, too, upset a Pitta's stomach, causing heartburn and even ulcers. He also has great difficulties digesting meat and fish proteins. These foods tend to heat up his body and cause circulatory problems. Most of the Pitta types who eat meat or other animal foods on a regular basis develop a pouch around the stomach, hold on to excessive lymph fluid and suffer from coronary heart disease. Their skin, especially around the face, neck and upper chest may redden. Pitta types thrive on a purely vegetarian diet, but fall ill if they don't. Their digestive system is not equipped with the specific enzyme systems needed to successfully handle flesh or other concentrated protein foods, such as cheese. Carbohydrates such as vegetables, grains, pulses, fruits and salads, and some nuts and seeds greatly satisfy a Pitta's stomach.

A steak can make a balanced Pitta bad-tempered and aggressive. So can alcohol, tobacco and coffee. These items are far too acidic-forming for the already sour-taste-dominated Pitta type. Mint, fennel, and Liquorice teas are all pacifying Pitta, whereas regular tea aggravates it. The liver breaks down regular tea into large amounts of uric acid, which tends to cause sluggishness and thickening of the blood. Eventually, it can cause gout or other painful conditions. Fresh, cool water is the best beverage for this body type.

Pittas are better off staying away from Indian or Mexican restaurants whereas Chinese and Japanese foods suit them better, as long as they stick to the vegetarian food selections. Salty snacks, like crisps, can also upset their sensitive stomach lining. Pitta types thrive on fresh and unprocessed foods, preferably organically grown. The remnants of pesticides or other impurities contained in foods are more likely to be felt by the Pitta type, and can even cause 'food' allergies. In many cases, it is not the food the Pitta type reacts to, but the chemical poisons and additives they contain. **Note:** To test for food allergies, take your pulse; then place a small piece of the food under your tongue and take your pulse again; if it is higher than before you may be allergic to that particular food. *Ghee (clarified butter)* is one of the main foods to pacify irritated Pitta and can be used for cooking, and on breads. It pacifies imbalances resulting from excessive secretions of bile and stomach acid.

Pitta types should be particularly careful not to eat unripe and prematurely picked fruits, as they tend to ferment in the intestines and cause loose stools or diarrhea. Unripe fruits are packed with toxic antibodies which the Pitta's immune system will quickly try to purge from the intestines.

Since the heating properties of the fire element are dominating in the Pitta type, in a balanced state he has a natural aversion to 'fire foods', which can be summarized as follows:

FIRE FOODS
(To be reduced or avoided)

- Acidic foods and medicines
- Meat and its products
- Fish
- 'Heating' grains
- Vinegar
- Pickles

- Hot spices
- Most nuts
- Salt and salty foods
- Sour/pungent fruits and vegetables
- Oily foods
- Red-color foods

Pitta Food Chart

FRUITS
Favor

Apples	Mangoes	Plums, sweet
Coconut	Melons	Pomegranate
Dates, fresh	Oranges, sweet	Prunes, soaked
Figs, fresh	Pears	Raisins, soaked
Grapes, dark	Pineapple, sweet	Watermelon

Reduce

Apricots	Kiwi, sweet	Quince, sweet
Avocado	Lemons	Strawberries,
Dried fruits, sweet	Limes	sweet

Avoid

Bananas	Grapefruit	Oranges, sour
Berries	Grapes, green	Peaches
Cherries	Papaya	Pineapples, sour
Persimmon	Plums, sour	Rhubarb

Note: Pitta types are very sensitive to unripe, sour and chemically-treated fruits, which can cause fermentation-related diarrhea and gas.

VEGETABLES
Favor

Artichokes	Dandelion greens	Potatoes, white
Asparagus	Endive	Pumpkin, white
Bitter and sweet	Green beans	Sprouts
vegetables	Jerusalem artichoke	Sweet peppers
Broccoli	Leafy green	Winter squash
Brussels Sprouts	vegetables	(acorn, buttercup,
Cabbage	Lettuce	butternut,
Cauliflower	Mushrooms	spaghetti)
Chicory	Okra	Watercress
Collards	Parsnips	Zucchini
Cucumber	Peas	

Reduce

Bamboo shoots	Kohlrabi	Pumpkin, orange

Carrots, cooked	Leeks, cooked	Spinach
Celery	Mustard greens	Tomatoes, in
Corn, fresh	Parsley	salad
		Turnip greens

Red Beets	Leeks, raw	Swiss chard
Beet greens	Horseradish	Tomatoes, cooked
Carrots, raw	Hot chili peppers	Tomato sauces,
Eggplant	Onions, raw and cooked	Ketchup
Horseradish	Radishes	Turnips

GRAINS
Favor

Barley	Oats, cooked	Chia Seeds (super
Basmati rice, white	Pasta	grain)
		Wheat
		Wheat germ

Reduce

Barley flour	Couscous, all types	Wheat bran
Bulgur	Unbleached white flour	Whole wheat flour
Pasta, whole wheat		

Avoid

Amaranth	Millet	Pasta in excess
Buckwheat	Oats, dry	Rye
Brown rice	Quinoa	
Corn	Rice in excess	

LEGUMES, BEANS, PEAS
Favor

Aduki beans	Lima beans	Split peas, all
Black beans	Mung beans, split or	kinds
Black-eyes beans	whole	Urad dhal
Chickpeas	Navy beans	
	Pinto beans	

Note: Consume not more than 1-2 times a week, and avoid brown and pink lentils, as well soy beans, soy milk and tofu. Soy milk and commercially produced tofu contain at least two highly toxic enzyme inhibitors. They can increase the risk of cancer and other illnesses. (See more information in *A Note on Legumes and their Digestibility below*. Japanese tofu is properly fermented through a process that takes several years and renders these poisons harmless.)

DAIRY		
Favor		

Butter, unsalted	Cottage cheese	*Ghee*
Milk, certified raw (from non-grain fed cows		

Reduce		

Lassi, sweet	Yoghurt, home-made	Cream cheese

Caution: With the exception of ghee and butter, use dairy foods very sparingly. If they cause mucus, coating on tongue, or congested nose/sinuses, discontinue immediately and avoid them altogether. Dairy products can lead to serious lymphatic congestion and thickening of the blood vessel walls, (See more details in section *Milk Controversy* of Chapter 14).

Avoid		

Buttermilk	Commercial dairy products, Goat's cheese	Ice cream
Cheeses, hard		Sour cream

NUTS AND SEEDS		
Favor		

Almonds (8-10 a day)	Pumpkin seeds, raw or roasted	Water chest nuts, cooked
Coconut	Sunflower seeds, raw or roasted	
Poppy seeds		

Reduce		

Walnuts	Pecans	

Avoid		

All other nuts and seeds

OILS/FATS
Favor

Coconut	Sunflower	Unsalted butter
Ghee		

Reduce

Avocado	Olive	Safflower

Avoid

Almond	Corn	Vegetable, mixed
Animal fats, except butter	Mustard	Canola
Apricot	Sesame, dark, roasted	

Note: All refined and heat-pressed oils are harmful to your health!

SWEETENERS
Favor

Barley malt	Rock sugar	White sugar, in
Date syrup	Stevia	moderation
Maple syrup	Xylitol	Palm sugar

Note: With the exception of xylitol and stevia, eating sweeteners in large amounts or regularly can lead to blood sugar problems and high acidity in the body (candidiasis).

Avoid

Brown, unrefined cane sugar	Honey (except small amounts,	All Sugar substitutes (artificial)
Brown rice syrup	1-2 tsps per day)	
	Molasses	

HERBS, SPICES, CONDIMENTS
Favor

Black cumin	Coriander	Peppermint
Cilantro (green coriander)	Curry leaves	Rose water
Coconut, grated or roasted	Dill leaves	Saffron
Coconut milk/cream	Fennel	Spearmint
	Mint	Turmeric
		Wintergreen

Almond extract	Cloves	Orange peel
Basil, fresh	Dill seed	Parsley
Black mustard seeds	Ginger	Salt
Black pepper	Lemon juice	Tamarind
Caraway	Mace	Vanilla
Cardamom	Nutmeg	
Cinnamon	Olives, black	

Avoid

Allspice	Garlic	Rosemary
Asafetida (hing)	Gomasio	Sage
Barbecue sauce	Horseradish	Salt, iodized
Basil, dried	Mango powder	Salty foods
Anise	Mustard	Soy Sauce
Asafetida (hing)	Marjoram	Thyme
Bay leaves	Mayonnaise	Pickles
Catsup	Onion, raw	Vinegar
Cayenne	Oregano	Yellow mustard
Fenugreek	Paprika	Seeds
Food additives, chemicals,		Preservatives

Brews, Beverages, Teas
All are OK except:

Alcohol	Clove tea	Power drinks
Milk shake	Bottled, boxed juices	Protein drinks
Caffeinated beverages	Cranberry juice	Papaya juice
(coffee, tea)	Ginger tea	Sour fruit juices
Carbonated beverages	Ginseng tea	Tomato juice
Chocolate beverages	Grapefruit juice	Sage tea

KAPHA PACIFYING DIET

Favor: Warm foods; light and dry in texture; cooked without much water; only small amounts of butter, oil and sugar; foods of pungent, bitter and astringent tastes; foods and beverages that have a naturally stimulating effect.

The Kapha type imbibes profuse amounts of the water and earth elements. This makes him naturally strong, heavy and stable. The qualities present in the air energies, however, are not well represented in his body, which makes him naturally want foods that can give him the drive, movement and agility he requires to maintain physical and mental balance. The Kapha dosha has the exact opposite properties of the Vata dosha, which prompts him to eat mostly Vata-increasing foods. These are the dry, light and heating foods. Honey, beans and barley, for example, are foods that have a drying effect and are, therefore, able to remove excessive fluids from the Kapha's body. Potatoes, too, produce a similar benefit in this body type.

An ideal food for the Kapha type is the astringent legumes that help to purge his intestinal tract from excessive mucus. Combined with heat-producing spices, they stimulate his digestion and help with the removal of stagnant waste material. Many vegetarian Mexican and Indian dishes are good for the Kapha type. Since his sense of smell is highly developed, the exotic smells of herbs and spices satisfy him. His often sluggish and slow metabolism can benefit greatly from an eye-watering spicy meal. A spicy and bitter appetizer such as romaine lettuce with added pepper can kindle his AGNI, so can chewing on a piece of fresh ginger. Kaphas don't need or even want much of a salad dressing that is sour and oily.

Generally, Kapha types should ensure that there are enough pungent, bitter and astringent tastes present in each meal. Spices such as cumin, fenugreek and turmeric are both astringent and bitter. Green leafy vegetables, including kale and spinach, that are cooked with plenty of spices also help to pacify Kapha, but care should be taken not to add too much water during cooking.

During the summer, the Kapha's body is warm enough to eat fruits, salads and some raw vegetables. These foods, however, can greatly upset his balance in the winter, when his body requires mainly cooked foods with hot spices. Cayenne pepper is especially beneficial for him, since it breaks down excessive mucus. Chili pepper, however, can sometimes cause congestion in his lungs. Other peppers are usually well tolerated by him. Cooling foods such as dairy products like milk shakes, ice cream, cream and butter, and sugary sweets like cake and cookies make the Kapha's system cold, cause mucus discharge and lead to heaviness, lethargy and depression. Besides their dulling effect on the Kapha type, these foods also increase his body weight, whereas the heating influence of pungent, bitter and astringent foods keeps his weight in check.

Fats and oils are far too heavy for the Kapha type and should be used sparingly. Kaphas not only secrete fats in their external skin, which makes their skin smooth and silky, but also through their internal skin - the gastrointestinal lining. In other words, they are oily inside and out. Unlike the Vata type who must add fats to their food in order to digest it, the Kapha type supplies his own fats; hence, the reduced need to add them to food. However, expeller-pressed corn, sunflower or safflower oil are more digestible for him, since they possess heating qualities. (Use in small quantities only.) Ghee is an acceptable choice, too, when used in cooking.

Deep-fried foods quickly subdue the Kapha's AGNI, which is the lowest among all the body types.

Salt or salty foods quickly imbalance the Kapha type because they tend to cause him to retain water. Many Kaphas suffer from swollen feet and arms because of too much salt consumption, especially if it is refined, processed salt.

Since the balanced Kapha type is mainly influenced by the elements of Earth and Water, he has a natural aversion to Earth/Water foods, which are listed below:

EARTH/WATER FOODS
(To be avoided or reduced)

- Salty tasting foods
- Sweet, juicy fruits
- Sweets and sweet tasting foods
- Sweet, watery vegetables

- Cool, milky foods
- Oily foods
- Sticky and cold foods

Kapha Food Chart

FRUITS
Favor

Apples	Dried fruits	Pomegranate
Apricots	Figs, dried	Quince
Berries	Peaches	Prunes
Cranberries	Pears	Raisins
Cherries	Persimmon	

Reduce

Grapes	Limes	Strawberries
Kiwi	Mango	Tangerine
Lemons	Oranges	Tamarind

Avoid

Avocado	Grapefruit	Rhubarb
Bananas	Papaya	Watermelon
Coconut	Pineapple	Melons
Figs, fresh	Plums	

VEGETABLES
Favor

Asparagus	Broccoli	Carrots
Beets	Brussels sprouts	Cauliflower
Bell peppers	Cabbage	Celery
Corn, fresh	Endive	Green beans
Eggplant	Garlic	Jerusalem
Leafy green vegetables	Onions	artichoke
Leeks	Parsley	Sprouts
Lettuce	Peas	Turnips
Mushrooms	Potatoes, white	Turnip greens
Mustard greens	Radishes	Watercress
Okra	Spinach	

Reduce

Artichoke	Plantain	Zucchini
Parsnips	Summer Squash	

Avoid

Cucumber	Sweet potatoes	Winter squash
Pumpkin, all kinds	Tomatoes	(acorn, buttercup, butternut)

GRAINS
Favor

Barley	Corn	Rye
Buckwheat	Millet	

Reduce

Amaranth	Cornmeal	Pasta, rye
Basmati rice, white (small amount)	Millet cereals	Quinoa
	Oats, dry	Rye cereals
Barley cereals	Oat bran	Rye flakes
Couscous	Chia seeds (super grain)	

Avoid

Brown rice	Steamed grains	Wheat
Oats, cooked	Rice flour	Whole wheat flour

LEGUMES, BEANS, PEAS
Favor

Aduki Beans	Lentils, pink	Pinto beans
Black beans	Lima beans	Split peas
Chickpeas	Navy beans	

Reduce

Black-eyes beans	Urad dhal
Mung beans	White beans

Avoid

Kidney beans	Soybeans
Lentils, brown	Tofu

DAIRY
Favor

Caution: With the exception of small amounts ghee and butter, use dairy foods very sparingly. If they cause mucus, coating on tongue, or congested nose/sinuses, discontinue immediately and avoid them altogether. Dairy products can lead to serious lymphatic congestion and thickening of blood vessel walls. (See more details in section *Milk Controversy* of Chapter 14)

Ghee	Butter	Ice cream
Goat's cheese, unsalted	Buttermilk	Sour cream
Goat's milk	Cheese	Yoghurt
Lassi, spiced and with	Cow's milk	
Honey	Dairy products	

NUTS AND SEEDS
Reduce

Coconut	Pumpkin seeds, roasted	Sunflower seeds,
Poppy seeds	Sesame seeds	roasted

Avoid

All nuts

OILS/FATS
Reduce

Almond	Safflower	Sunflower
Corn	Ghee	
Mustard	Unsalted butter	

Note: These oil/fats are OK in small amounts

Avoid

Apricot	Coconut	Sesame
Avocado	Olive	Soy

SWEETENERS
Favor

Honey, raw and unheated (but not more than one tablespoon a day) and stevia

Reduce

Maple Syrup	Dates syrup
Brown rice syrup	Barley malt

Avoid

Brown cane sugar	Honey, cooked	Sugar cane juice
Fructose	Molasses	All Sugar
Glucose	Palm sugar	substitutes
		White sugar

HERBS, SPICES, CONDIMENTS
Favor

All are good for Kapha types except mango powder, miso, olives, salt, tamari, vinegar

BREWS, BEVERAGES, TEAS
Favor

Aloe Vera juice	Carob beverages	Pear juice
Apple juice	Carrot juice	Pineapple juice
Apricot juice	Cherry juice	Pomegranate juice
Berry juice	Mixed vegetable juice	Prune juice

Note: all fruit juices should be freshly pressed, diluted with water, and taken on an empty stomach. Use only in moderation, since too much fruit sugar can upset Kapha dosha.

Reduce

Almond drink	Grape juice	Lassi
Almond milk	Mango juice	
Caffeinated beverages	Vegetable broth, salted	

Avoid

Alcohol	Cold beverages	Orange juice
Banana shake	Grapefruit juice	Papaya juice
Carbonated beverages	Lemonade	Sour beverages
Chocolate beverages	Licorice tea	Tomato juice
Coconut milk	Milk shakes	Sports drinks

Important for all body types

In the above food charts I have omitted beef, pork, poultry, fish, eggs and similar foods because they can create major imbalances in all three body types. (See the section on vegetarianism later in this chapter) When heated, their proteins coagulate, which makes them even more harmful for the body. All cadaver foods are deprived of their life force. The body is not able to bring them back to life. It has to mobilize extra energy to get rid of these foods. This strongly stimulating effect, which always engages an immune response, may give you the false impression that these foods make you stronger. The overall, long-term effect is physical, mental and emotional deterioration. Ayurveda claims that these foods reduce *Ojas* in the body, which is the chemical equivalent of bliss. Bliss results when the body and mind vibrate at a high frequency.

The following foods have similar detrimental effects: Heavy, deep-fried and oily foods, hard cheeses, leftover and processed foods, refined and genetically altered foods, as well as excessively sour and salty-tasting foods. Also, overeating any food prevents the body from producing *Ojas*, and leads to gastrointestinal disturbances.

Ghee - Its Value and Preparation

Ghee is clarified butter. Although it is prepared completely from butter, its properties, according to Ayurveda, are very different from butter itself. Once of the most obvious differences is that all of the milk protein has been removed. Ghee is pure fat with none of the impurities that may be found in butter. Unlike butter, ghee contains no bacteria and it is not prone to turning rancid, even after storing it for several months outside the refrigerator.

In many cases, ghee is recommended in the diet. Ghee is particularly useful for the Pitta constitution; it helps to digest and absorb food better and makes food tastier, although not everyone will agree. Its benefit lies in the fact that it stimulates AGNI without upsetting Pitta dosha. Also Vata and even Kapha types benefit from ghee. Unless you have access to an Indian health food store that sells ghee, you will have to prepare it yourself, using the following recipe:

How to Prepare Ghee
1.   Place any amount of unsalted butter in a deep porcelain, Pyrex or stainless steel pan over medium-low heat. (Be sure that the butter does not scorch while melting) Allow complete melting to occur, and then reduce the heat to low.
2.   During the next 30-40 minutes, the water in the butter will boil away. (Approximately 20 percent of butter is composed of water) Milk solids will appear on the surface of the liquid and at the bottom of the pan.
3.   Be alert to remove the liquid from the heat as the milk solids turn golden brown on the bottom of the pan. Otherwise, the ghee may burn. At this point, you may notice that the ghee smells like popcorn, and you can see tiny bubbles in the ghee rising from the bottom.
4.   Strain the ghee while still hot or warm, pouring it through a cotton cloth into a stainless steel or heavy glass container. At this point it is very hot, so you should always be cautious. Another way of doing this is to let the ghee cool down, and then strain it by pouring it through a cotton cloth or handkerchief directly into clean glass jars or bowls.
5.   Ghee can be stored at room temperature for several weeks, and it keeps indefinitely when kept in the refrigerator. Put a teaspoonful (per person) into food or on food after cooking it. Ghee can be used in the same way as cooking oil, in place of butter, or as a digestive aid dripped over food.

Note: Caution should always be observed when handling hot liquids. Ghee should never be left unattended during the heating process.

If ghee is not available, other good alternatives are coconut oil, olive oil and butter (Check the body type list to see which is most suitable for you.)

A Summary of General Principles Regarding Diet

- A half teaspoon of grated ginger taken with a pinch of salt is an excellent appetizer and kindles AGNI, the digestive fire. Splashing cool water over your face, neck, and hands before meals also stimulates AGNI.
- Eat in a settled environment and quiet atmosphere, with a settled mind. Your company and environment should be pleasant. Do not work, listen to music, read or watch TV during meals.
- Always sit down to eat. Eat at roughly the same times each day.
- Eat neither too quickly nor too slowly (about 20 minutes) and without interruption.
- Eat to about ¾ of your stomach capacity at your biggest meal; this equals the amount of your

cupped hands full. Ideally, one third of the meal should consist of liquid food of a soupy consistency. Stop eating when you notice a small burp coming from your stomach.

- Avoid eating a meal or snack before the previous meal has been digested, unless it is a piece of fruit. Allow approximately 3 to 6 hours between meals, depending upon the types of food consumed.

- If you desire to drink anything with your meals, it is best to sip a little hot or warm water. Also avoid drinking large quantities of liquids right before and within the first 2 hours after meals.

- Drinking excessive amounts of water (3-4 liters a day) may produce obesity, kidney disorders and mineral/vitamin deficiencies, whereas drinking too little water causes dehydration. To meet the minimum requirements for water, drink 6-8 glasses of water (at room temperature or warm) each day. You may need to increase the amount during hot, dry weather, when exercising or during stressful times in your life. If the color of your urine is dark yellow, drink more water; if colorless, drink less.

- Consuming cold foods, such as ice cream, and drinking iced beverages may reduce your resistance to disease, impair AGNI and cause mucus congestion.

- The diet should be balanced by including all six tastes - sweet, sour, salty, pungent (spices), bitter and astringent - in at least one meal per day. However, check the previous section concerning specific taste requirements and physiological needs or imbalances for your particular body type.

- It is best not to heat or cook with honey; heat destroys it and makes it toxic.

- Never eat just before going to bed. To avoid developing sleeping disorders, there should be at least three hours between eating and sleeping. If your bedtime is 10:00 p.m., eat no later than 6:00 p.m.

- Chew your food thoroughly - the digestive process starts in the mouth.

- Ayurveda does not favor the intake of too much raw food like raw vegetables, uncooked oat flakes, uncooked grains, etc. Fruits are an exception as they are already 'cooked' or ripened by the sun. (See also the section in Chapter 14, *Raw Versus Cooked Foods*) The Pitta type is the only one among the body types who is able to digest more raw foods.

- It is best not to eat when the mind is dominated by strong emotions such as anger, worry or sorrow. Wait until it has become more settled, since the digestive system does not work under stress.

- Sleeping after meals causes sluggishness and increases Kapha and body weight. However, it is good to rest for about 10 minutes after meals and, if possible, to go for a 10 to 15 minute walk.

- Food should always be delicious and pleasing to the senses and should be prepared by a happy cook.

Sequence of Dishes - The Ideal Lunch Recipe

1. Before you eat, be certain that your stomach is empty and that you actually feel hungry. If you feel you need to kindle your digestive fire, AGNI, take ¼ to ½ teaspoon of grated ginger with a pinch of salt before eating. Spraying or sprinkling your face, neck and hands with a little cold water before your meal also increases AGNI.

2. Liquid foods, such as soup, should be eaten toward the beginning of the meal, unless your meal includes a fresh, raw salad. In this case, eat the salad first, followed by the soup. Raw foods can only be digested at the beginning of a meal, not once you have eaten cooked food.

3. Normally, the stomach processes and removes liquids before it can attempt the digestion of the

more solid and concentrated food items. Therefore, drinking a lot of liquid with your meals will greatly hinder digestion and also dilute the concentrated digestive juices, rendering them less effective.

4. It is helpful to realize that the stomach does not operate like a washing machine, but stores the ingested foods in layers, one on top of the other. To avoid digestive problems and flatulence, I recommend the following sequence of dishes. The foods listed are examples only. Ideally, you would choose those foods that are listed in your body type food chart:

Stage A

A salad made with raw food items that may include such ingredients as lettuce, endive, avocado, cucumber, carrot, tomato, celery, bell pepper, jicama, sprouts, cilantro, basil, mint, parsley, young white radish, roasted or raw pumpkin seeds and sunflower seeds. Ideally, there should be no more than 4-5 main ingredients in a salad. Recommended dressings include lemon juice or Balsamic vinegar with sunflower, sesame or olive oil for Vata types, almond or rice milk with sunflower or olive oil and a very small amount of lemon juice for Pitta types, or a little sunflower oil with herbs and spices and a very small amount of lemon juice for Kapha types. Vatas and Kaphas are better off eating small portions of salad, whereas Pittas may eat a larger amount.

Note: Avoid adding any cooked items, such as beans or chicken, to the salad, even if they are cold. Nuts are better added to stages B or C, if desired.

Stage B

Cooked vegetables such as asparagus, cabbage, broccoli, carrots, cauliflower, okra, summer or winter squash, Swiss chard, green beans, peas, sugar snap peas, mushrooms, or other wholesome fresh vegetables. To make the vegetables more digestible and delicious-tasting, add spices and herbs such as turmeric, coriander, cumin, cardamom, fennel, basil, oregano and thyme. (See your food chart for those best for you) Add about 1-2 teaspoons of fat per serving such as coconut oil, olive oil, butter, or another oil that is compatible with your body type. Adding some unrefined salt and perhaps a small piece of vegetable bouillon, coconut milk, or other natural condiment will further enhance the flavor of the vegetables. Perhaps the easiest, most efficient and healthy method of cooking involves the use of *Waterless Stainless Steel Cookware.* (See details in section 9 of Chapter 7)

Note: Vegetables should be cooked until exactly tender, not too little, and not too much. Both overcooked and semi-cooked vegetables may generate toxins, bloating and dullness.

Stage C

Grain foods such as basmati rice, bulgur wheat, oats, barley, buckwheat, Kasha, millet, whole wheat couscous, quinoa, amaranth, Chia, whole wheat pasta, or other grains. Proper digestion of grain foods requires fat (oil, butter or ghee). You may add spices, herbs and salt and/or vegetable bouillon. Stage B and C foods may be cooked together in one pan.

Stage D

Beans, including mung beans (dhals), lentils, chickpeas, kidney beans, fresh lima beans and others. Add fat or oil, spices, herbs, salt, and/or other condiments. Do not eat stage D foods more often than 1-2 times per week.

Important for non vegetarians: Stages C and D should be omitted if you include animal protein in your meal. Animal protein and starch foods, such as meat and potatoes, or fish and rice, cannot be digested properly when eaten at the same meal. Meat, for example, requires acid secretions, whereas potatoes require alkaline secretions to digest them. When eaten in one meal, these secretions neutralize one another, and the food remains mostly undigested. Acid reflux disease and putrefaction may result.

The amount of stage A and D food eaten should small, while the stage B and C quantities should be more substantial. If desired, food items from stages B, C and D may be eaten together. The total amount of food at lunchtime should not exceed two cupped hands full.

Lunch does not always have to consist of all four stages. In fact, it is easier on the digestive system to have only 3-5 main types of food in one meal, such as a raw salad, vegetables and rice.

You should also, try to avoid eating two concentrated food items in one meal, such as rice with potatoes, rice with bread, beans with cheese, pasta with cheese, or chicken with bread or another starchy food. Eating beans with rice, or barley with almonds, however, is a compatible combination.

Lunch should always include a substantial serving of cooked vegetables to support proper bowel activities.

A Note on the Digestibility of Legumes, Grains and Seeds

Due to the large quantity of enzyme inhibitors and antinutritional compounds - antigrowth factors - in legumes, grains and seeds, there is a limit to how many of them humans and animals can eat without suffering gas-related digestive problems. The normal cooking time of half an hour to several hours for most beans does not entirely destroy these toxic compounds. Soaking legumes, grains and seeds in water overnight or at least for several hours, ideally with some sodium bicarbonate, greatly helps digestibility, according to research in India.

The substances in beans that cause gas are mainly the indigestible carbohydrates *raffinose*, *stachyose and verbascose*. These provide substrate for intestinal micro flora to produce flatus.

Many of the legumes' enzyme-inhibitors, which protect the plants against insect attacks or fungal infestation, cannot be destroyed by the heat generated during cooking. The protein *alpha-amylase* inhibitors, for example, may represent as much as 1 percent of wheat flour and, because of their heat resistance, persist through bread-baking. Consequently, they are typically found in large amounts in the center of loaves. For that reason, when people eat a lot of the inner parts of bread, instead of the crusty parts, they tend to develop flatulence.

The problem with the legume soybean is even more pronounced than that found with other legumes or grains. With regard to soy products' production, there needs to be a balance between the amount of heat necessary to destroy the enzyme inhibitors while still preserving some nutritional properties of the soy. That balance is impossible to achieve. Most commercially available edible-grade soybean products retain 5 to 20 percent of the enzyme inhibitor activity (for trypsin) originally present in the raw soybeans from which they were prepared. In addition, most of their nutrients are destroyed. Recently, the parents of twins were imprisoned for committing involuntary manslaughter of their babies. They fed the twins soy milk, which starved them to death. Soy products (unless properly fermented for several years) have a toxic effect on the body, and should not be consumed on a regular basis, if at all. Likewise, eating other legumes more often than 1-2 times per week can impair immune functions and cause GI-tract disturbances.

Yellow mung beans (dhal), if soaked overnight or at least 30-60 minutes prior to cooking for 15 minutes, contain the least amount of these compounds and are relatively easy to digest. However, once again, the rule of thumb is not to eat them more often than 1-2 times per week.

Ideal Daily Routine - Dinacharya

The following outline summarizes an ideal daily routine, which can help anyone to restore his health or prevent illness from arising. Many people find that they can stick to some of the points but not to all of them. This is fine. Begin implementing those first that seem to be the easiest for you. As they become a natural part of your way of life, you may discover that you can implement more and more of them into your daily routine. The most important points appear in bold letters.

Morning:

- **Arise early in the morning (before sunrise)**
- **Clean teeth, scrape and clean tongue**
- **Drink a glass of warm water**
- **Drink another glass of warm water with lemon and honey**
- **Evacuate bowels and bladder**
- Dry brush the body
- Apply oil massage to head, body and soles of feet
- While massaging, swish 1-2 tablespoons of cold-pressed sunflower or sesame oil in your mouth for 3-4 minutes, and then spit it into the toilet
- **Warm bath or shower, ideally followed by a brief cold shower**
- Yoga Asanas (postures) and Pranayama (breathing exercise). If you wish to do vigorous exercise that causes you to perspire, do this after evacuating your bowels and bladder, and before dry brushing or the oil massage
- Meditation
- **Light breakfast before 8:00 a.m. (optional for Kapha types)**
- Work or study

Afternoon:

- **Lunch at 12-1:00 p.m.: Substantial meal according to body type and season**
- Brief rest after lunch, ideally followed by a walk of 10-15 minutes
- Work or study
- Yoga Asanas and Pranayama (optional)
- Meditation (optional)

Evening:
- **Dinner: Light meal according to body type, between 6:00 p.m.-7:00 p.m.**
- Brief walk for 10-15 minutes
- Pleasant relaxing activity such as listening to music
- **Early to bed (before 10:00 p.m.)**

Note: Exercise should be done on a daily basis, away from meals (up to 1/2 hour before or 2-3 hours after meals) and according to body type. The best time for exercise is in the morning during the Kapha period or else during the late afternoon.

Vegetarian Diet - One Solution to Many Health Problems

Vegetarians Live Longer and Healthier Lives

It is not necessary to be a vegetarian to enjoy the benefits of an Ayurvedic diet and lifestyle. However, a balanced vegetarian diet is often considered necessary, particularly when the body is afflicted with disease. Vegetarians have believed all along that living on a purely vegetarian diet can improve health and one's quality of life. More recently, medical research has found that a properly balanced vegetarian diet may, in fact, be the healthiest diet. This was demonstrated by the over 11,000 volunteers who participated in the *Oxford Vegetarian Study*. For a period of 15 years, researchers analyzed the effects a vegetarian diet had on longevity, heart disease, cancer and various other diseases.

The results of the study stunned the vegetarian community as much as it did the meat-producing industry: "Meat eaters are twice as likely to die from heart disease, have a 60 percent greater risk of dying from cancer and a 30 percent higher risk of death from other causes." In addition, the incidence of obesity, which is a major risk factor for many diseases, including gallbladder disease, hypertension and adult onset diabetes, is much lower in those following a vegetarian diet. According to a Johns Hopkins University research report on 20 different published studies and national surveys about weight and eating behavior, Americans across all age groups, genders and races are getting fatter. If the trend continues, 75 percent of U.S. adults will be overweight by the year 2015. It is now almost considered the norm to be overweight or obese. Already more than 80 percent of African-American women over the age of 40 are overweight, with 50 percent falling into the obese category. This puts them at great risk for heart disease, diabetes and various cancers. A balanced vegetarian diet may be the answer to the current obesity pandemic in the United States and many other countries.

Those who include less meat in their diet also have fewer problems with *cholesterol*. The American National Institute of Health, in a study of 50,000 vegetarians, found that the vegetarians live longer and also have an impressively lower incidence of heart disease and a significantly lower rate of cancer than meat-eating Americans.

What we eat is very important for our health. According to the *American Cancer Society*, up to 35 percent of the 900,000 new cases of cancer each year in the United States could be prevented by following proper dietary recommendation. Researcher Rollo Russell writes in his *Notes on the Causation of Cancer:* "I have found of twenty-five nations eating flesh largely, nineteen had a high cancer rate and only one had a low rate, and that of thirty-five nations eating little or no flesh, none of these had a high rate."

Could cancer lose its grip on modern societies if they turned to a balanced vegetarian diet? The answer is 'yes' according to two major reports, one by the World Cancer Research Fund and the other by the Committee on the Medical Aspects of Food and Nutrition Policy in the United Kingdom. The reports conclude that a diet rich in plant foods and the maintenance of a healthy body weight could annually prevent four million cases of cancer worldwide. Both reports stress the need for increasing the daily intake of plant fiber, fruits and vegetables and reducing red and processed meat consumption to less than 80-90 g.

If you are currently eating meat on a regular basis and wish to change over to a vegetarian diet, unless you suffer from a major cardiovascular illness, *do not* give up all flesh foods at once! The digestive system cannot adjust to a substantially different diet from one day to the next. Start by reducing the number of meals that include meats such as beef, pork, veal and lamb and substituting poultry and fish during these meals. In time, you will find that you are able to consume less poultry and fish also, without creating strain on the physiology due to too rapid an adjustment.

Note: Although the uric acid content of fish, turkey and chicken is less than in red meat and, therefore, not quite as taxing to the kidneys and tissues of the body, the degree of injury that is sustained to the blood vessels and intestinal tract from eating these coagulated proteins is no less than it is with the consumption of meat. (More details on this subject follow)

Death in the Meat

Research has shown that *all* meat eaters have worms and a high incidence of parasites in their intestines. This is hardly surprising given the fact that dead flesh (cadaver) is a favorite target for microorganisms of all sorts. A 1996 study by the United States Department of Agriculture (USDA) showed that nearly 80 percent of ground beef is contaminated with disease-causing microbes. The primary source of these bugs is feces. A study conducted by the University of Arizona found there are more fecal bacteria in the average kitchen sink than in the average toilet bowl. This would make eating your food on the toilet seat safer than eating it in the kitchen. The source of this biohazard at home is the meat you buy at the typical grocery store.

The germs and parasites found in meat weaken the immune system and are the source of many diseases. In fact, most food poisonings today are related to meat-eating. During a mass outbreak near Glasgow, 16 out of over 200 infected people died from the consequences of eating E. coli contaminated meat. Frequent outbreaks are reported in Scotland and many other parts of the world. More than half a million Americans, most of them children, have been sickened by mutant fecal bacteria (E. coli) in meat. These germs are the leading cause of kidney failure among children in the United States. This fact alone should prompt every responsible parent to prevent their children from eating flesh foods.

Not all parasites act so swiftly as E. coli though. Most of them have long-term effects that are noticed only after many years of eating meat. The government and the food industry are trying to divert attention from the escalating problem of meat contamination by telling the consumer it is his own fault that these incidents happen. It is very obvious that they want to avoid hefty lawsuits, and bad-mouthing of the meat industry. They insist that dangerous bacterial outbreaks occur because the consumer does not cook the family's meat long enough. It is now considered a crime to serve a rare hamburger. Even if you have not committed this 'crime', any infection will be attributed to not washing your hands every time you touch a raw chicken or to letting the chicken touch your kitchen counter or any other food. The meat itself, they claim, is totally safe and meets the standard safety requirements imposed by the government; of course, this holds true only as long as you keep disinfecting your hands and your kitchen countertop. It evades all good reasoning to propose such a 'solution' to the 76 million cases of meat-borne illnesses a year, except to safeguard the vested interests of the government and the meat industry. If a particular imported food produced in China is found to be contaminated, even if it hasn't actually killed anyone, it is immediately taken off the shelves of grocery stores. Yet, with all the research proving that meat-consumption harms and kills millions of people each year, meat continues to be sold in all grocery stores.

The new mutant bugs found in today's meat are extremely deadly. For you to come down with *Salmonella* poisoning, you have to consume at least a million of these germs. But to become infected with one of the new mutant bugs, you need to ingest a measly five of them. In other words, a tiny particle of uncooked hamburger, making it from a kitchen utensil to your plate, is enough to kill you. Scientists have now identified more than a dozen food-borne pathogens with such deadly effects. The

Center for Disease Control admits that we don't even know the bugs behind most food-related illnesses and deaths.

Much of the germ-infestation of meat is caused by feeding farm animals foods that are unnatural to them. Cattle are now fed corn, which they are unable to digest, but it makes them fat very quickly. Cattle feed also contains chicken feces. The millions of pounds of chicken litter (feces, feathers and all) scraped off the floors of chicken houses are recycled as cattle feed. The cattle industry considers this 'good protein'. The other ingredients of cattle feed consist of ground-up parts of animals, such as deceased chickens, pigs and horses. According to the industry, giving the cattle natural, healthy feeds would be far too costly and so unnecessary. Who really cares what the meat is made of, as long as it looks like meat?

Combined with hefty doses of growth hormones, a diet of corn and special feeds shortens the duration of fattening up a steer for market from a normal time period of 4-5 years to a mere 16 months. Of course, the unnatural diet makes the cows sick. Like their human consumers, they suffer from heartburn, liver disease, ulcers, diarrhea, pneumonia and other infections. To keep the cattle alive until the deadline for slaughter at the 'ripe old age' of 16 months, the cows need to be fed enormous doses of antibiotics. In the meantime, the microbes that respond to the massive biochemical assault of antibiotics, find ways to become immune to these drugs by mutating into resistant new strains.

Those unfortunate cows that don't drop dead prematurely due to all the poisons fed to them during their short earthly existence, experience an undignified and gruesome end of life in the slaughterhouse or meat-packing plant. From there, the diseased, germ-infested meat ends up in your local grocery store, and a little later, on your dinner plate, if you so dare.

Is Meat Natural For Humans?

Vegetarians have long been warned that they are not getting enough of the essential proteins humans are supposed to eat on a daily basis. It is well known that the eight amino acids making up these proteins can be found in a simple meal of rice and beans or in one serving of the supergrain 'Chia', available through web sites such as www.chiaforhealth.com. Rice contains the amino acids that are missing in beans, and beans contain the amino acids missing in rice; Chia has all 16 amino acids and more of them than are contained in meat. Although many more meat-free foods contain these proteins than there are types of meat, meat as a source of protein is still considered to be the better option. The fact that eating *too much* protein is linked to many more serious health problems than eating too *little* protein is only rarely, if at all, considered in the protein discussion.

Typical disorders caused by the overconsumption of protein are osteoporosis, heart disease, rheumatoid arthritis and cancer. By contrast, those who never eat animal protein as contained in meat, poultry, fish, eggs and dairy products, have very low rates of these diseases and don't suffer from protein deficiency either, provided they eat adequate amounts of fruits, vegetables, grains, legumes and a few nuts and seeds. No scientific evidence exists that indicates a protein deficiency in people who never eat animal protein, such as me and billions of others. By contrast, our modern societies consume at least 50 percent more protein than they actually need. We may not be suffering from a lack of protein at all, regardless whether this relates to essential or nonessential amino acids, but from an overconsumption of protein. By filling up the connective tissues of our body with unused protein, we turn the body into an overflowing pool of harmful acids and waste, thereby laying a fertile ground for disease, including arteriosclerosis and bacterial or viral infections. To consider meat a natural food for humans is, therefore, more than farfetched, especially when it is known to kill so many people.

At the root of the problem lies man's inability to properly break down meat protein into amino acids. Chunks of undigested meat pass into the intestinal tract and, along with them, parasites. Most of these parasites, also known as intestinal flukes, can neither be destroyed by the heat applied during cooking nor by human stomach acid. Carnivorous animals, on the other hand, kill these parasites instantly while the meat is passing through their stomach. This is because their stomachs produce twenty times more hydrochloric acid than ours do. This massive amount of acid helps the animal break down the meat proteins into their essential components. If a healthy young man eats a piece of meat, he may be able to digest 25 percent of it. By contrast, carnivorous animals can digest almost the whole thing, including bones and fibrous tissue. Parasites and other bugs cannot survive this acid 'assault'.

The main digestive work in carnivorous animals takes place in the stomach and not in the small intestine. Meat stays in their relatively short intestinal tract for only a little while. Our small intestine, which is about 5-6 meters long (16-20 feet), processes most natural foods within several hours. Meat, however, may stay in the small intestine for as long as 20-48 hours, by which time much of it is putrefied or decomposed. The rotting process results in the generation of the meat poisons cadaverine, putrescine, amines and other highly toxic substances. These poisons begin to act as pathogens (causal factors of disease) in the body. Many of them end up in the lymphatic system, causing lymph congestion as well as fluid and fat buildup, first in the mid-section of the body, and eventually throughout the body. Since the remnants of undigested meat can accumulate and be kept in the large intestinal walls of humans for 20-30 years or longer, it is not surprising that colon cancer is highly prevalent among meat-eaters but virtually non-existent among carnivorous animals and vegetarians. Colon cancer, in most cases, is just another name for constant poisoning through putrefying meat. While being digested, meat is known to generate *steroid metabolites* possessing *carcinogenic* (cancer-producing) properties. In other words, even if you were able to digest meat properly or ate 'healthy' meat from free-range and non-grain-fed cattle, you would still increase your risk of colon cancer.

The kidneys, which extract waste products from the blood, also suffer from the overload of meat poisons, consisting mostly of nitrogenous wastes. Even moderate meat-eaters demand three times more work from their kidneys than vegetarians do. Young people generally may still be able to cope with this form of stress, but as they grow older, the risk of kidney damage increases greatly.

After many years of regular meat consumption, the body may suddenly succumb to the flood of poisonous substances emanating from undigested meat. A research study conducted in Germany showed that middle-aged people who consumed meat in the evening were more prone to suffer a heart attack the next morning than those who didn't. Too many proteins entering the blood can thicken it and drastically cut oxygen supplies to the heart and other vital organs, such as the brain.

Animal cells, unlike plant cells that have a rigid cell wall and a simple circulatory system, die very rapidly once they are cut off from their blood supply. When the animal dies, its cell proteins begin to thicken and harden (coagulation), and destructive enzymes immediately begin to break down the cells. This, in turn, results in the formation of a degenerative substance called *ptomaine,* which is a known cause of many diseases. Cellular destruction occurs in the cells of all types of dead animal flesh, as well as chicken and fish. All meat products have already been poisoned with decomposed and putrefied protein. A dead animal, bird or fish is no longer 'fresh'. Regardless of what you do with it, you cannot bring it back to life or turn it into living food for your body. Putrefaction and bacterial growth start immediately after death and are very advanced by the time the meat is several days or weeks old, as is the case by the time it is offered for sale in most grocery stores or meat markets.

Whether it is E. coli, other bacteria, or enzymes acting on the dead ingested protein, they effectively send the body's immune system on a 'mission of war', hence, the stimulating effect of meat. Depending on one's physical resources and immune capacity, the body may eventually get overwhelmed by the influx of virulent poisons and destructive germs and begin to signal 'dis-ease'. Those with the weakest immune system are usually the first to suffer from meat poisoning.

Yes, food can actually turn into deadly poison and kill someone! The kinds of poisons resulting from the putrefaction (decomposition) of meat or fish in the body are some of the most powerful found in the natural world. Many of the hundreds of thousands of fragile, elderly people lying in hospitals today will die unnecessarily simply because they are given meat or fish to eat - an impossible feat for the digestive system to handle after surgery, a heart attack or during treatment for a chronic illness. Often constipated, these patients do not succumb to their illness; rather, they die from rotting flesh sitting in their gastrointestinal tract and releasing cadaverine, putrescine, amines and parasites into their digestive system.

Man's entire anatomy (jaw, teeth, digestive system, hands and feet), not unlike that of a gorilla or orangutan, shows that he must have evolved for millions of years living on fruits, grains, vegetables, nuts and seeds. Before the last sudden pole shift and ice age, no humans inhabited the cold regions of the world. They all lived in the warm, tropical places where plant foods were plentiful and accessible. But suddenly, without warning, the formerly tropical areas of Siberia and the Arctic region experienced a massive drop in temperature. Animals froze to death within a moment while still chewing on tropical fruit. Such animals were recently found fully intact with the fruit still in their mouth, thousands of years later. The deep freeze occurred so quickly that they didn't even have the chance to swallow the fruit they were eating. Those humans and animals that happened to live in other tropical areas of the world experienced more moderate climate shifts and thus survived the sudden start of the ice age. However, they had to learn to live with the seasons as we know them today. During the cold seasons, they had no other option but to kill animals for food. This is when hunting and meat-eating became a necessity. Yet this has nothing to do with the original constitutional design of the human body. Furthermore, meat-eating is not somehow programmed into certain blood types, as the promoters of the blood type diet would have us believe.

Non-carnivorous animals, including the human animal, have long bowels, designed for the slow digestion of nutrient-rich vegetables and fruits. Our dental structure is only conducive to the cutting of fruits and vegetables with incisors (think of how useful they are when you eat an apple) and to the grinding/chewing of nuts, grains and seeds with the help of molars. Our short, dull canines have no real capacity for slashing or tearing meat. We have, indeed, nothing in our anatomy that compares with the sharp claws of a tiger or an eagle. The human hand with its opposable thumb is better suited for harvesting fruits and vegetables than to killing prey. Had it been in our nature to eat flesh, we, too would have been equipped with the same or similar hunting faculties as carnivorous animals.

Misleading Theories

Unfortunately, mainstream medical and nutritional science base their theories not so much on the basic processes that occur in the body, but rather on the contents of food. This can be very misleading, to say the least. We are being told, for example, that when we lack calcium we should drink milk because it contains a lot of calcium. We are not being told, however, that in order to digest and metabolize milk calcium, we must first dispose of the phosphorus contained in milk. To process and remove the phosphorus, though, we require calcium. Since there is more phosphorus in milk than there is calcium, the bones, teeth and muscles have to supply the extra calcium. This fact alone makes milk a major calcium-depleting food. Loss of calcium can cause osteoporosis and such diseases as Crohn's and Irritable Bowel Syndrome, diabetes, heart disease, respiratory ailments and cancer.

The above principle can be applied to almost everything else we believe is so good for us. Giving vitamins to people with vitamin deficiencies can make their bodies even more deficient. (More details follow in Chapter 14) Those lacking in Omega-3 fats don't necessarily gain them by eating these fats in the form of fish oils, fish or linseeds. People whose digestive functions have been impaired do not suddenly make better use of certain foods or nutrients simply because they begin to eat more of them.

Just because fish has good things in it does not mean that the body can actually absorb and make use of them. (One must, of course, ignore the mercury or other metals they absorb from the sea, lakes and rivers, or the antibiotics, coloring agents and other food additives that farmed fish are fed.) Fish has to be rich in nutrients otherwise we wouldn't have whales, dolphins and bears, or any life at all on this planet. This doesn't mean, though, that everything nutritious that exists in nature should also appear on our dinner plate.

As previously explained, once a fish or an animal has been killed, the oxygen supply to the cells is cut off. This immediately starts the process of cell-destruction through intracellular enzymes. Unless you eat the fish or chicken right away after it dies, and yes, raw, most of what you will get is degenerated and putrefied protein. Unless treated with carcinogenic coloring agents, a piece of meat will start to look greenish/gray in a matter of hours. To make matters worse, the baking, roasting or frying of meat, fish, eggs and poultry applies enough heat to cause any proteins that may still be intact to coagulate. Think of a raw egg that has been boiled or fried. The liquid egg quickly becomes hard and stiff. The protein molecules lose their three-dimensional structure and are destroyed as they are exposed to the heat.

The body cannot utilize coagulated protein for cell-building. Rather, it is treated as a pathogen or disease-causing agent by the body. As a result, these now toxic foods may, at best, stimulate the immune system in the small intestine and initially induce a strong eliminative response in the large intestine. The immune response makes you feel energized, and you may think it is because of eating the animal foods, but this is far from the truth. Deceiving as it may be, with each immune response, the body actually becomes weaker; more liver bile ducts get clogged with stones and the cardiovascular system becomes increasingly congested as more and more proteins are deposited in the blood vessel walls (See also chapter 9, The Secrets of Heart Disease.) These are the most common causes of chronic illness.

Eating meat also stimulates the body's growth hormones and male hormones, which can lead to the overgrowth of tissues. Many young men today are extra large, very tall, and have bulging muscles, something you rarely see in most regions of Asia, South America and Africa, where meat is scarce and plant foods plentiful. Having an oversized, bulky body is a great disadvantage, for it can predispose one to diabetes, heart disease and other physical as well as mental problems later in life. Besides, a lot of energy is lost in maintaining large muscles, which can reduce one's lifespan considerably.

As is the case with the strongest animals in the world, e.g. the elephant, water buffalo, giraffe, horse, cow, gorilla and orangutan, humans don't need to eat protein in order to produce and make it available to the cells in the body. A healthy newborn baby triples its size and the number of protein-packed cells within its first 16 months, without ever eating any protein foods at all. You might object here by saying: "But isn't mother's milk filled with protein?" Not by a long shot! Human breast milk contains only a trace of protein, namely 1.1 – 1.6 grams per 100 grams of milk. Most of the healthy children in the world don't receive any food other than mother's milk during their first year. With breast milk containing, let's say, 1.4 percent protein, this is by far not enough to account for a baby's 15 pound weight increase within the first year.

By design, humans and most other non-carnivorous animals don't depend on eating protein foods to make or maintain their muscles, cells and organs. Actually, all of us derive the most essential nutrients we need from the air we breathe, right from the first breath we take. Everyone knows that in order to live we need oxygen molecules from the air, but very few of us know that we also need and make use of the nitrogen, carbon and hydrogen molecules with which the air is saturated. These four molecules are the ingredients that make up every amino acid in the body and anywhere else on the planet. Our DNA and the liver are perfectly able to synthesize these molecules into amino acids and complete proteins. The brain produces billions of neuropeptides (peptides consist of amino acids) each day. The trillions of enzymes the body makes are also made of proteins. Similarly, most hormones in the body are made of pure protein.

A protein deficiency occurs only in people whose liver, respiratory and immune functions are seriously impaired, or who eat too much protein. This is because excess proteins that accumulate in the basal membranes of the blood capillaries actually inhibit protein supplies from reaching the cells. Personally, I have not eaten any concentrated protein foods, e.g. fish, meat, chicken, cheese, milk or eggs, during my 35 years of adulthood, and my body has hardly aged during all those years (being 54 years old at the time of writing this). On the other hand, I have seen thousands of people who have aged prematurely or suffered debilitating illnesses because of eating too much protein. At no other time in human history has humankind consumed so much meat and other concentrated protein foods as today.

The Pitta body type is especially susceptible to becoming poisoned by protein foods, such as meat, fish and cheese. Their ability to digest these foods is very limited. Naturally, the body doesn't want to digest something it doesn't need and cannot make use of. Using this example, I recommend you to be extremely cautious about taking the advice of any person or institution that persists in handing out general food guidelines without regard to a person's individual body type and physical condition, if applicable.

It is also worth noting that carnivorous animals have an unlimited capacity to handle saturated fats and *cholesterol*. Dogs, for example, who received one half pound of butterfat with their daily ration of meat for two years, showed no signs of damage to their arteries or change of their serum cholesterol. By contrast, the purely vegetation-eating rabbits quickly developed arteriosclerosis when fed meat or as little as 2 grams of cholesterol daily. Humans, too, have a very limited capacity to digest and process meat proteins and meat fats. If you placed a hungry child into a cage with a chunk of meat on one side and an apple on the other, which of the two do you believe the infant would choose to eat? That's correct, it would choose the apple! Place a lion cub in the same cage, and you will see the cub heading straight toward the meat. If we only listened to our basic instincts, and not to the food industry's advertising slogans, we would discover that meat was never meant for humans.

Meat - A Major Cause of Disease and Aging

Populations that eat meat regularly have the shortest life spans and the highest incidence of degenerative diseases. According to published reports of national health statistics from around the world, one out of two people in the industrialized world will die from heart disease or a related blood vessel disease. In other words, heart disease is the leading killer disease in the world, with cancer following closely behind. As long ago as June 1961, the American Medical Association reported that a vegetarian diet could prevent 90 percent of our thromboembolic diseases[14] and 97 percent of our coronary occlusions. This means that by adopting a vegetarian diet, we would be able to eradicate heart disease almost completely. Compared with meat-eating, smoking seems only a minor risk factor for heart disease! It is disconcerting that this important research has long been forgotten and is basically ignored today.

---

[14] A condition in which a blood vessel is obstructed by an embolus carried in the bloodstream from the site of formation

Heart disease is virtually unheard of in societies where meat consumption is low, and the majority of the population eats mostly traditional foods. A group of Harvard doctors and research scientists examined 400 people in a remote mountain village in Ecuador and were surprised to find that except for two men, none of the people above 75, including all the centenarians and a 121-year-old man, showed any signs of heart disease. All the villagers turned out to be complete vegetarians. Examinations of similar age groups in the United States would typically reveal a 95 percent incidence of heart disease.

Cancer, the second most common killer disease, now closely rivaling heart disease, may largely be caused by meat-eating, too. Modern cancer research claims to have found specific protein compounds responsible for certain types of cancers. This, in itself, may be a very important finding, but it is even more important to discover where these proteins come from. Putrefying meat is one answer, and the decaying protein of dead human cells is another. Meat consumption slows or hinders the complete removal of dead cells in the body by congesting the lymphatic system (which removes dead cells) and by using up the body's resources of energy, enzymes, minerals and vitamins (needed to break down dead cells and dispose of them safely). Both undigested meat proteins and decaying cell protein can, therefore, damage human cells and impair their genetic programs.

Another reason why meat-eaters have more cancers than vegetarians may be the fact that they ingest large quantities of sodium nitrates, which are carcinogenic preservatives that are used to make meat look 'fresh'. But meat is no longer fresh after the animal has died. As already mentioned, if left untreated animal flesh begins to turn a sickly grayish-green color within several days. Since nobody would buy meat in that condition, the meat industry uses these toxic nitrates to make it look red and palatable. In reality, though, it is already decomposed and highly toxic.

The most appalling news from cancer research, however, is that secondary *amines*, prevalent in beer, wine, tea and tobacco, react with chemical preservatives in meat to form *nitrosamines*. The American Food and Drug Administration (FDA) has labeled *nitrosamines* as "one of the most formidable and versatile groups of *carcinogens* yet discovered." In other words, if you are a smoker or if you drink beer, wine, or tea *and* eat meat, you produce one of the most deadly toxins that can be found anywhere. As it turns out, most meat-eaters also drink wine or beer, and many of them smoke, too. When fed to test animals, *nitrosamines* produced malignant tumors in *one hundred percent* of the animals; the cancers appeared everywhere, including the lungs, pancreas, stomach, adrenals, intestines and the brain.

A meat-eater's immune system also has to combat many other cancer-producing agents. Farm animals are regularly injected with hormones to stimulate growth, are fed appetite stimulants to 'force' them to eat non-stop, and are given antibiotics, sedatives and chemical feed mixtures. Over 2,500 drugs are routinely given to animals to fatten them and to keep them alive. Most of these harmful chemicals are still in the animals at the time of their death. Many other drugs are added after the animal has been slaughtered. These drugs will still be present in the meat when it is eaten, but the law does not require a listing of the cocktail of drugs that have been added. Hence, you have no way of knowing what kind of drug interactions and allergic reactions you could become a victim of by eating a juicy steak at your favorite restaurant. It is difficult to imagine how many people today become sick for no apparent reason, due to being drugged with poisonous medicines contained in the meat they eat. Sadly, when they go to see their doctor, they are most likely given even more drugs to combat those they have already unwittingly ingested.

One of the chemicals added to animal feed in the United States is the growth hormone *diethylstilbestrol* (DES). The FDA estimates that the use of this chemical earns meat producers in the United States $500 million annually. DES is highly carcinogenic and has been banned as a serious health hazard in thirty-two countries. According to another report by the FDA, the antibiotics *penicillin* and *tetracycline* alone save the meat industry $1.9 billion a year. Yet these drugs may be breeding deadly antibiotic-resistant organisms in the consumer's body.

Animal protein foods are nearly always propagated as being the safest choices for people with Type 2 diabetes and also for those who want to avoid developing this condition. Nothing could be further from the truth. Most people believe that high blood sugar comes from eating too much sugar or refined carbohydrates. They are correct. It has recently been proven that women who drink one regular soda such as Coke or Pepsi per day have an 83 percent chance of developing diabetes. (One can of soda contains about 12 teaspoons of sugar or the equivalent amount of high fructose corn syrup, amounting to 200 calories.) However, sugar pales as a cause for diabetes when compared with meat.

If you eat concentrated protein foods such as meat or chicken, your body requires much insulin to synthesize proteins from the amino acids derived from these foods. According to research, the stimulation of protein synthesis is a classic action of insulin. Loss of the stimulatory effect of insulin on protein synthesis would reduce growth and result in weight loss, which are hallmarks of . To make certain that the amino acids derived from the protein meal are synthesized into proteins, the pancreas has to secrete insulin. In other words, the more protein you eat, the more insulin your body needs to make, thus increasing the chances of insulin resistance and Type 2 diabetes.

Accordingly, eating a normal-sized steak forces your pancreas to secrete more insulin than it would need to produce in response to eating 12 times the amount of sugar contained in one can of soda. In addition to that, if you also eat potatoes, a sweet desert, and drink a soda along with your meal, like most Americans do, you can expect to further increase insulin resistance. Currently, diabetes is the fastest growing epidemic in America, and it is easy to see why. (More on diabetes in Chapter 11)

The effect of insulin on protein metabolism is complex, and it involves changes in both the synthesis and degradation of protein. If protein intake is excessive, insulin secretions increase to help with its degradation. Protein synthesis and the control of carbohydrate and fat metabolism have now been linked in unexpected ways, and many of the same signaling systems utilized by insulin to control glucose metabolism, for example, have been found to be involved in the control of protein synthesis as well. The bottom line is that excessive intake of protein is a direct cause of insulin resistance and may lead to the onset of Type 2 diabetes.

Other very harmful effects that may occur as a result of eating meat are generated indirectly by the tragic conditions to which farm animals are exposed during their short lives. Most animals never see the light of day. They spend their entire lives in cramped and cruel surroundings, merely to die a brutal death. High rise chicken farms breed animals that have never been exposed to fresh air or allowed to take as much as one step. This not only greatly upsets their body chemistry but also causes malformations and the growth of malignant tumors. These sick animals are slaughtered and sold to unsuspecting customers. In the United States, chicken with *airsacculitis* (a pneumonia-like disease), which causes pus-laden mucus to collect in the lungs, are permitted to be sold. Other examples of common diseases include eye cancer and abscessed livers among cows. Carcasses contaminated with rodent feces, cockroaches, and rust are routinely found in meat-packing companies, but meat inspectors are very lax about enforcing regulations because this would effectively close down the whole industry.

Modern research on diseases such as cancer and diabetes is mostly focused on how to combat the *effects* of an unbalanced lifestyle and unhealthy eating habits. Billions of dollars are spent on discovering everything about the symptoms of these diseases, with little or no attention being paid to their underlying causes. By contrast, some people have adopted vegetarianism as a way of life and subsequently have significantly lower disease rates, especially of cancer, diabetes and heart disease. Vegetarians do not claim to understand the mechanisms of or treatments for these diseases, yet through the elimination of meat from they diets, they have attained a significant degree of success in preventing and conquering these illnesses.

Benefits of a Vegetarian Diet

A major study conducted in California revealed that the cancer rate among Mormons, who are known to eat very little meat, was 50 percent lower than that of the normal population. Researchers in an even more comprehensive, carefully controlled study compared 50,000 vegetarians of the religious group, *Seventh Day Adventists*, with the same number of non-vegetarians of the same age and gender. This study, known as the *Oxford Vegetarian Study*, produced similar results. The members of the vegetarian group had an astonishingly low rate of cancer of all types, their life expectancy was notably longer, and they suffered significantly less from cardiovascular disease than those in the control group.

Overall, life expectancy ranking of the United States compared with the rest of the world dropped from position 19 in 1999 to position 42 in 2007. The stark increase of obesity and related vascular diseases can be blamed for this trend. And both these chronic conditions are largely caused by the consumption of animal protein.

From a historical perspective, the 'forced' vegetarianism of the Danes due to the allied blockage of Denmark during World War I, led to a 17 percent reduction of mortality rates in the first year of meat rationing. Norway experienced a similar positive side effect from meat-rationing during the years of World War II (1940-1945). There was an immediate drop in national mortality rates from circulatory diseases during the period of meat shortage. Mortality rates returned to pre-war levels when the population fully resumed meat consumption.

Studies from the University of Belgium that tested endurance, strength and the rate of recovery from physical exhaustion in vegetarians clearly showed that vegetarians had far superior scores in all three categories. A study at Yale University proved that vegetarians have nearly twice the stamina of meat eaters. Other findings confirmed that during endurance tests, the vegetarians were able to perform two to three times longer than the meat eaters before reaching a point of complete exhaustion. They also needed only one-fifth the time to recover from fatigue after each test than did their meat-eating counterparts.

The common belief that eating meat makes you strong is unfounded and misleading. The super-strong elephant, gorilla, rhinoceros and horse all sustain their great physical strength and stamina by eating only vegetation. Based on present evidence, there is nothing to suggest that meat is beneficial to our health. The fact that populations like the Eskimos (Inuits) can survive on a meat diet without suffering heart disease is known. However, the Eskimo's average life span is still not more than 40 years. An important observation has been made relative to the rapid shortening of the average lifetime by Dr. V. E. Levine and Professor C. W. Bauer, of Creighton University, Nebraska, who reported on October 26, 1934: "Due to susceptibility to tuberculosis and other diseases the average life span of the Eskimo of Alaska is only 20 years and their race is doomed to extinction within a few generations unless modern medical science comes to their aid." The *Masai* tribes of East Africa live on mostly cows' blood and milk, and meat. Their average life span is 60. A typical 45-year-old man looks about 20 to 30 years older. During my many visits to Masai villages in East Africa between 1983 and 2006, I observed that those Masai tribes who have adapted to grow and include fresh vegetables in their diet, look much healthier and don't age as quickly.

Another major benefit of the vegetarian diet is that, statistically, vegetarians are thinner and healthier. On the average, vegetarians weigh about 20 pounds less than their meat-eating counterparts. According to the U.S. Worldwatch Institute, 1.1 billion people worldwide are underweight, and another 1.1 billion are overweight. In the U.S., 23 percent of adults are obese and 60 percent are overweight. But obesity besets poor countries, too, from Brazil to China. The traditionally 'lean' and mostly vegetarian populations in the world are now quickly following in the footsteps of the typically non-vegetarian populations. Eating meat is becoming increasingly synonymous with a higher standard of living. The country/subcontinent of India, for example, which traditionally has been vegetarian for thousands of years, is rapidly adopting carnivorous eating habits, much to the benefit of that country's cardiologists and oncologists. (Ayurveda, the traditional medicine of India, was largely responsible for keeping the Indian population vegetarian.)

Harvard research has shown that a vegetarian diet also reduces colds and allergies. Children especially benefit greatly from meat abstinence. Studies show that vegetarian children have better teeth and are afflicted with fewer children's diseases than non-vegetarian children. They are also less prone to obesity, high cholesterol, diabetes and heart disease.

Food For Thought

According to Harvard nutritionist Jean Mayer, we would have enough food for the entire developing world if we ate half as much meat. Reducing meat production by merely 10 percent could release enough grain and other natural foods to feed 60 million people! Albert Einstein had this to say about vegetarianism: "Nothing will benefit human health and increase the chance for survival on Earth as much as the evolution to a vegetarian diet." He predicted that producing and eating so much meat would literally kill us and our environment. Leo Tolstoy stated, "Vegetarianism is the taproot of humanitarianism."

The world's output of meat increased fivefold in the second half of the 20th century. Given the current trend, by 2050, the increases in meat production will have reached a point where we could feed 4 billion extra people with the plant food that is now being used to raise cattle. Only 10 percent of the protein and calories we feed to our livestock are recovered in the meat we eat. In the case of the United States, for the 20 million tons of humanly edible and nutritious protein that is fed to livestock yearly (apart from the waste products and drugs), only about 2 million tons of meat protein are obtained; and out of that amount, less than 27 percent can be utilized by the human body. If you are concerned about the world's survival, consider the following statistics:

- One acre of grain produces 5 times more protein than an acre of pasture set aside for meat production. An acre of beans or peas produces 10 times more protein and an acre of spinach 28 times more protein. Almost all land can be used for growing some crop or another.
- One portion of meat contains only 20 grams of protein, whereas a typical 100-gram portion of beans yields 35 grams of protein. The meat, however, costs about 20 times more than the beans do. Being a vegetarian saves not only lives, but also money.
- The food energy supplied by meat production uses 10 times more fossil fuel than the food energy supplied by plant production. Given the current shortage of fossil fuels on the planet, meat production may soon become unaffordable.
- The world's livestock now produces at least 10 percent of all the greenhouse gases. In other words, emissions from livestock have become a significant source of atmospheric methane. As of 1990, domestic animals currently account for about 15 percent of the annual *anthropogenic methane* emissions, and the number has been steadily increasing ever since.
- 85 percent of the topsoil lost in the USA each year is directly associated with the raising of livestock. In this way, 4 million acres of cropland is destroyed every year. In the same way, precious rain forests have had to give way to satisfy the demand for more meat in the world.

- To grow one pound of wheat requires only 60 pounds of water, whereas the production of one pound of meat requires a staggering 50,000 pounds of water. To produce one pound of chicken, 1,800 pounds of water are needed. Large chicken slaughtering plants, in fact, expend up to 100 million gallons of water daily, enough to supply a city of 25,000 people!
- According to research published in *Chemical & Engineering News*, Vol. 85, No. 15, April 9, 2007: 34-35, *roxarsone*, an arsenic-based additive used in most chicken feed, could pose health risks to humans. Roxasone is used to promote growth, kill parasites and improve the color of chicken meat. Under certain conditions, which can occur within live chickens or on farm land, this compound converts into more toxic forms of inorganic arsenic. This form of arsenic has been linked to bladder, lung, skin, kidney and colon cancers, and low-level exposure can lead to partial paralysis and diabetes. Of course, arsenic is also a deadly poison. Over 70 percent of the 9 billion broiler chickens produced annually in the United States are fed roxarsone.

The meat production process is so wasteful and costly that, in order to survive, the meat industry needs hundreds of millions of dollars in tax subsidies every year. You never pay only for the meat you eat; the subsidies come out of your pocket. In 1977, the governments of Western Europe spent almost half a billion dollars purchasing farmers' overproduction of meat and additional millions to store it. This trend has not been different in the United States and is worsening each year. All this is precious money lost, thereby heavily burdening every national economy. In this sense, meat consumption is directly impoverishing the wealthy nations. Any wars fought in the future will revolve about energy, food and water, all three of which are heavily wasted through meat production. The worldwide increase of meat consumption is driving the world closer and closer to the brink of international conflict.

But Fish Is Really Good for You, Isn't It?

Not quite so. Besides the above reasons for avoiding dead and coagulated protein foods, tests on both wild and farm-raised fish have revealed that their levels of toxic chemicals and metals are endangering the lives of pregnant mothers, developing fetuses and young children. Does this mean it is acceptable for adults to eat fish? Scientists now say that salmon, for example - long considered to be one of the safest of all fish - should be eaten only once per month. We are exposed to numerous other sources of indoor and outdoor pollution almost all the time, not to mention the chemicals contained in most foods today. Our immune system simply cannot afford such high concentrations of toxins as found in fish without developing a toxemia situation.

Specifically, tests on farmed salmon uncovered high levels of toxins linked to cancer and birth defects. These findings recently triggered a 'scare-mongering' row as other experts insisted salmon was safe to eat regularly - and important for a healthy diet. A study released in the journal, *Environmental Science & Technology*, found much higher levels of some chemicals in farmed salmon compared with wild salmon. The study, which is being considered the most thorough analysis of farmed and wild salmon to date, found in most cases that consuming more than one serving of farmed salmon per month could pose unacceptable cancer risks. These standards for determining safe fish consumption levels are according to United States Environmental Protection Agency (EPA). Farmed salmon were found to have up to 10 times higher levels of PCBs and dioxins than wild salmon. Farmed salmon are frequently fed antibiotics, which contribute to the growth of drug-resistant bacteria. In addition, chemicals are often added to their food to color their flesh pink to resemble their wild cousins. Otherwise, they would remain an unappetizing grayish-brown color.

Sales have increased up to 15 percent a year as more people eat oily fish to prevent heart attacks, or so they are made to believe. But when samples from around the world - some from stores in London and

Edinburgh - were analyzed, it was discovered that levels of 14 'organochlorine' toxins, the most hazardous of which include *PCBs*, *dioxins*, *dieldrin* and *toxaphene*, were significantly higher in European and North American farm-raised salmon than in fish caught in the wild. According to U.S. and Canadian scientists and reported by the journal *Science*, fishmeal was traced as the source of most of these poisons. New research shows dioxins to cause breast cancer.

Not just that poisons in fish can cause cancer, they also can cause diabetes. Korean researchers have recently found evidence that people who consume fish containing high levels of persistent organic pesticides (POPs) are more prone to developing insulin resistance, a precursor to diabetes. POPs are synthetic chemicals that accumulate in the fatty tissue of animals.

While farm-raised catfish, trout, haddock, salmon, flounder and other fish are unsuitable for consumption due to the toxic additives in fishmeal, deep ocean fish are even more harmful than farmed fish due to their excessively high levels of mercury.

Even if fish consumption were shown to prevent heart attacks (for which there is no proof), would it be justified and wise to propagate it as being a healthy food when it is known to cause other chronic or fatal diseases? Eating food that saves one person but kills another is much like gambling with one's life. You can never really know whether you will win or lose. As always, the final judge is you, the consumer. If in doubt, I suggest that you use Kinesiology muscle testing to determine whether fish is or is not conducive to your health and well-being. Vegetarian foods such as nuts, seeds, chia, avocado, beans, vegetables, have superior health benefits to fish, which is still a cadaver food. Cadavers, especially when their proteins are destroyed (coagulated) through heat, do very little to provide nourishment for the body.

Mercury gets into water primarily through solid-waste incinerators, mines and power plants. Algae typically absorb the mercury and tiny zooplankton animals eat the algae. In turn, small fish eat the zooplankton, and from there the mercury moves up through the aquatic food chain, with the large, deep-ocean fish at the top of the chain carrying the highest mercury concentration. Even waterways that are far away from any ocean, such as the Elkhorn River in Nebraska or the Colorado River in the Western part of the United States, are known to have mercury-contaminated fish. The Environmental Working Group (EWG) issued the following list of high-mercury fish:

1. Swordfish
2. Tuna
3. King mackerel
4. Halibut
5. Sea bass
6. Tilefish
7. Pike
8. Walleye
9. Largemouth bass
10. White croaker
11. Marlin
12. Shark
13. Gulf coast oysters

There are other environmental concerns related to fish farming. For example, presently, over 85 open net cage fish farms operate in the coastal waters of British Columbia, producing waste that is equivalent in volume to the raw sewage released from a city of 500,000 inhabitants. This excessively 'wasteful' usage of precious water resources for few or no health benefits is yet another example of how misinformation and vested interest groups control the eating and living habits of the masses today.

A Note on the Blood Type Diet

Eat Right for Your Type by Peter J. D'Adamo has become widely known as the blood type diet. Since I am constantly asked to give my input on this dieting system, I have decided to add my comments here.

I agree with and respect quite a few of D'Adamo's insights and perspectives but have major reservations about others. The book suggests that you use your blood type to determine which foods you should be eating. According to the theory, when you eat foods that 'agree' with your blood type, you reduce the risk of cancer, heart disease, diabetes, infections and liver disease. Type A people supposedly had ancestors that were farmers. If you are of this type, you should be a vegetarian and avoid meat and dairy products. According to the author, people with Type B blood had ancestors that were nomads; therefore they should eat red meat and fish. Those with Type O blood had ancestors that were hunters and gatherers; this means they should eat lots of animal protein and few carbohydrates. Finally, those with Type AB blood, had mixed ancestry, and are supposed to eat a combination of the Type A and B diet. Does this mean, for example, that all nomads used to have the blood type 0, and all farmers used to have type A blood? What about people who didn't farm and who didn't move from place to place?

Unfortunately, these theories are not supported by scientific literature, traditional knowledge and records of the world's oldest medical systems, such as Chinese Medicine and Ayurveda. D'Adamo's discoveries have not been confirmed anywhere else. There is little or no distinction made between individuals who have lived in the Andes, the tropical rain forests, or plains of Africa for hundreds of thousands of years. The Indian subcontinent thrived and flourished for thousands of years on a vegetarian diet, and so has most of the world's population. And where does ancestry begin anyway? Two thousand years ago, 100 centuries ago, or 60 million years ago? How far do we go in the bloodline of our ancestors to determine our dietary needs? When the last Ice Age began, many vegetarians living in formerly tropical lands were suddenly forced to eat animals in order to survive. Some ate a mixed diet, because of more moderate climates. Others in the all-year-round tropical places of the Earth continued with vegetarian foods until quite recently. The proposed theory is highly inconclusive about all of these facts.

When I went on the high protein diet (very similar to the type O diet plan) at age five, I felt great for about 18 months, as do so many others who go on the popular Atkins diet. Then I started developing stones in my liver, a dangerous arrhythmia and juvenile rheumatoid arthritis, among other diseases. I had no idea that these ailments were due to protein poisoning. Ten years later I switched to a balanced vegan diet, and most of my illnesses went away within a matter of weeks. However, I still had to live with the many stones that had been produced in my liver and gallbladder as a result of what is known today as the O-type blood diet. Forty gallbladder attacks later, I did a series of liver and gallbladder flushes, which cleaned out these vital organs. Finally, I was free of any illness or discomfort.

You won't notice the effects of a high protein diet until the blood vessel walls are well-thickened with excessive protein. Eating lots of animal protein triggers a powerful immune response in order to get rid of the foreign DNA and the dead, coagulated and damaged protein of meat, fish, eggs, poultry and dairy products. This immune response involves a powerful release of energy, thereby cleaning out impurities, improving skin functions and making you feel more grounded. However, as soon as the immune system is exhausted by the constant excessive activity, which took a mere 18 months in my case, the situation begins to backfire and the body becomes increasingly congested.

The blood type diet theory is flawed in the sense that it does not recognize the basic body type requirements generated by the three forces/humors of nature (Vata, Pitta and Kapha) that control the physicality of matter and the body of humans and animals. Only a fraction of the body's energy requirements are met through food, and there are many more influences on the body than one's blood type. The 6,000-year old medical system of Ayurveda accounts for most of these influences. One's constitutional body type is not as simply and easily determined as one's blood type. The theory of blood type foods is really based on guesswork, not on science or time-tested traditional knowledge as found in Ayurveda, Chinese Medicine, Greek medicine or ancient Egyptian medicine.

If concentrated protein foods were a necessary part of the human diet, as the blood type diet advocates for the O-type, for example, why does nature not reflect that need when it formulates human milk in a mother's breast? Its protein content is a mere trace amount of 1.1-1.6 percent, provided to a baby at the time of its biggest growth spurt. Wouldn't O-type babies die if they lived on so little protein for up to 18 months, since most babies in the natural world only get mother's milk as food? On the contrary, the babies actually develop perfect organs and systems, and are emotionally the most content. If nature's most perfect food doesn't give you much protein at the time when you are growing more rapidly than at any other time in your life, why would you need to eat concentrated proteins, such as meat, when you are older and no longer growing?

If you are on the blood type diet and decide to continue following it, I recommend that you be vigilant about how your body feels. If you start feeling a dull sensation in your gallbladder or pain in your joints, muscles or head, or if you develop mucus and sinus problems, a coated tongue or other signs of congestion, you may need to reconsider your dietary regimen.

"The time will come when men such as I will look on the murder of animals as they now look on the murder of men." ~ *Leonardo da Vinci*

CHAPTER 7

Over 100 Secrets for
Igniting Nature's Healing Power Inside You

*"The art of healing comes from nature and not from the physician.
Therefore, the physician must start from nature with an open mind."*
~ Paracelsus

The Liver and Gallbladder Flush

Cleansing the liver and gallbladder of gallstones is one of the most important and powerful approaches you can take to improve your health. The liver flush requires six days of preparation, followed by 16 to 20 hours of actual cleansing. To remove gallstones you need the following items:

Apple juice	Six 32 oz. containers
Epsom salts* (or magnesium citrate)	Four tablespoons dissolved in three 8-oz. glasses of water**
Extra virgin olive oil, cold-pressed	One-half glass (4 oz.)
Either fresh grapefruit (pink is best), or fresh lemon and orange combined***	Enough to squeeze ¾ glass (6 oz.) of juice
Two pint jars, one with a lid	

Note: * Look for Epsom salts (magnesium sulfate), usually found in the laxatives section or drugstores. In German-speaking countries it is known as "Bittersalz." For those in the U.S., check out any drugstores or natural food stores. Some packaging labels describe it as a natural laxative. If it is not available, use magnesium citrate.

** I have chosen 'glass' instead of 'cup' as a measuring unit to avoid confusion about the meaning of 'cup' on different continents.

*** If you cannot tolerate grapefruit juice or if it tends to make you nauseated, you may use equal amounts of freshly squeezed lemon and orange juice instead. The effect is the same with either choice.

Preparation

➤ **Drink 1 container (32 oz.) of packaged or freshly prepared apple juice (or see other options below) per day for a period of six days:** (You may drink more than that if it feels comfortable to do so.) The *malic acid* in the apple juice softens the gallstones and makes their passage through the bile ducts smooth and easy. The apple juice has a strong cleansing effect. Some sensitive people may experience bloating and, occasionally, diarrhea during the first few days. Much of the diarrhea is actually stagnant bile, released by the liver and gallbladder (indicated by a brownish yellow color). The fermenting effect of the juice helps widen the bile ducts. If this becomes somewhat uncomfortable, you can dilute the apple juice with any amount of water, or use other options described later. Drink the apple juice slowly throughout the day, between meals (avoid drinking the juice during, just before, and in the first two hours after meals, and in the evening). This is in addition to your normal water intake of six to eight glasses. *Note:* Preferably, use organic apple juice, although for the purpose of the flush, any good brand of commercial apple juice, apple concentrate, or apple cider works just as well. It may be useful to rinse your mouth out with baking soda and/or brush your teeth several times per day to prevent the acid from damaging your teeth. (In case you are intolerant of apple juice or allergic to it, see the other options explained in *Having Difficulties with the Cleanse* at the end of this chapter)

➢ **Dietary recommendations:** During the entire week of preparation and cleansing, avoid foods or beverages that are cold or chilled; they chill the liver and, thereby, reduce the effectiveness of the cleanse. All foods or beverages should be warm or at least room temperature. To help the liver prepare for the main part of the cleanse, try to avoid foods from animal sources, dairy products, and fried food items. Otherwise, eat normal meals, but avoid overeating.

➢ **The best times for cleansing:** The main and final part of the liver flush is best done over a weekend, when you are not under any pressure and have enough time to rest. Although the liver flush is effective at any time of the month, it should preferably coincide with a day between the full moon and new moon. Try to avoid doing the actual flush on full moon day (the body tends to hold more fluids in the brain and tissues on this day than on others). The day of the new moon is the most conducive for cleansing and healing[15].

➢ **If you take any medication:** While on the liver flush regimen, avoid taking any medication, vitamins, or supplements that are not absolutely necessary. It is important not to give the liver any extra work that could interfere with its cleansing efforts.

➢ **Make sure that you cleanse your colon before and after you do a liver flush:** Having regular bowel movements is not necessarily an indication that your bowel is unobstructed. Colon cleansing, done either a few days before or, ideally, on the sixth day of preparation, helps to avoid or minimize any discomfort or nausea that may arise during the actual liver flush. It prevents back-flushing of the oil mixture or waste products from the intestinal tract into the stomach. It also assists the body in swiftly eliminating the gallstones. Professional colonic irrigation (colon hydrotherapy) is the fastest and easiest method to prepare the colon for the liver flush. Colema-board or home-kit colonic irrigation are the second most preferable methods (see details in the next section on Intestinal Cleansing).

➢ **What you need to do on the sixth day of drinking apple juice:** Drink all the 32 ounces of apple juice in the morning. You may start drinking the juice soon after awakening. If you feel hungry in the morning, eat a light breakfast, such as a hot cereal - oatmeal would be an ideal choice. Avoid sugar or other sweeteners, spices, milk, butter, oils, yogurt, cheese, ham, eggs, nuts, pastries, cold cereals, and the like. Fruit or fruit juices are fine. For lunch eat plain cooked or steamed vegetables with white rice (preferably basmati rice) and flavor it with a little unrefined sea or rock salt. To repeat, *do not eat any protein foods, butter, or oil,* or you might feel ill during the actual flush. *Do not eat or drink anything (except water) after 1:30 p.m.,* otherwise you may have difficulties passing stones! Follow the exact schedule below.

---

[15] For a detailed explanation about lunar influences on the body, see Chapter 5.

The Actual Flush
Evening

6:00 p.m.: Add *four* tablespoons of Epsom salts (magnesium sulfate) to a total of 24 ounces (three 8-oz. glasses) of filtered water in a jar. This makes four 6-oz servings. Drink your first portion (¾ glass) now. You may take a few sips of water afterward to neutralize the bitter taste in your mouth, or may add a little lemon juice to improve the taste. Some people drink it with a large plastic straw to bypass the taste buds on the tongue. Closing the nostrils while drinking it works well for most people. It is also helpful to brush your teeth afterward or rinse out the mouth with baking soda. One of the main actions of Epsom salt is to dilate (widen) the bile ducts, making it easy for the stones to pass. Moreover, the salts clear out waste that may obstruct the release of the stones. (If you are allergic to Epsom salts or are just not able to get them down, you may instead use the second best choice - magnesium citrate - at the same dosage) Set out the citrus fruit you will be using later, so that it can warm to room temperature.

8:00 p.m.: Drink your second serving (¾ glass) of Epsom salts.

9:30 p.m.: If you have not had a bowel movement until now and have not done a colon cleanse within the past 24 hours, take a water enema; this will trigger a series of bowel movements.

9:45 p.m.: Thoroughly wash the grapefruits (or lemons and oranges). Squeeze them by hand and remove the pulp. You will need ¾ glass of juice. Pour the juice and ½ glass of olive oil into the pint jar. Close the jar tightly and shake hard, about 20 times or until the solution becomes watery. Ideally, you should drink this mixture at 10:00 p.m., but if you feel you still need to visit the toilet a few more times, you may delay this step for up to 10 minutes.

10:00 p.m.: Stand next to your bed (do not sit down) and drink the concoction, if possible, without interruption. Some people prefer to drink it through a large plastic straw. Drinking it while keeping the nostrils closed seems to work best. If necessary, use a little honey between sips, which helps the mixture go down more smoothly. Most people, though, have no problem drinking in one go. Do not take more than five minutes for this (only elderly or weak people may take longer).

PLEASE LIE DOWN IMMEDIATELY!

This is essential for helping to release the gallstones! Turn off the lights and lie flat on your back with one or two pillows propping your head up. Your head should be higher than your abdomen. If this is uncomfortable, lie on your right side with your knees pulled toward your head. **Lie perfectly still for at least 20 minutes, and try not to speak!** Put your attention on your liver. Some people find it beneficial to place a castor oil pack over the liver area.

You may feel the stones traveling along the bile ducts like marbles. There won't be any spasms or pain because the magnesium in the Epsom salts keeps the bile duct valves wide open and relaxed, and the bile that is excreted along with the stones keeps the bile ducts well lubricated. (This is very different than in the case of a gallstone attack where magnesium and bile are not present.) Go to sleep if you can.

If at any time during the night you feel the urge to have a bowel movement, do so. Check if there are already small gallstones (pea-green or tan-colored ones) floating in the toilet. You may feel nauseated during the night and/or in the early morning hours. This is mostly due to a strong, sudden outpouring of gallstones and toxins from the liver and gallbladder, pushing the oil mixture back into the stomach. The nausea will pass as the morning progresses.

The Following Morning

6:00–6:30 a.m.: Upon awakening, but not before 6:00 a.m., drink your third ¾ glass of Epsom salts (if you feel very thirsty, drink a glass of warm water before taking the salts). Rest, read, or meditate. If you are sleepy, you may go back to bed, although it is best if the body stays in an upright position. Most people feel fine and prefer to do some light exercises, such as yoga.

8:00–8:30 a.m.: Drink your fourth and last ¾ glass of Epsom salts.

10:00–10:30 a.m.: You may drink freshly pressed fruit juice at this time. One half-hour later, you may eat one or two pieces of fresh fruit. One hour later you may eat regular (but light) food. By the evening or the next morning you should be back to normal and feel the first signs of improvement. Continue to eat light meals during the following two to three days. Remember, your liver and gallbladder have undergone major 'surgery', albeit without the harmful side effects or the expense.

Note: Drink water whenever you are thirsty, except right after drinking the Epsom salts and for the first two hours after drinking the oil mixture.

The Results You Can Expect

During the morning and, perhaps, afternoon hours following the liver flush, you will have a number of watery bowel movements. These initially consist of gallstones mixed with food residue, and then just stones mixed with water. Most of the gallstones are pea-green and float in the toilet because they contain bile compounds (**Illustration 16a**). The stones will be in different shades of green and may be bright-colored and shiny like gemstones. Only bile from the liver can cause this green color.

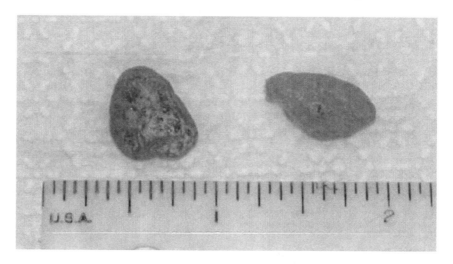

Illustration 16a: Green-colored gallstones

Gallstones can come in many sizes, colors, and shapes. The light-colored stones are the most recent. Dark-green stones are the oldest. Some are pea-sized or smaller, and others are as big as 1 inch in diameter. There may be dozens and, sometimes, even hundreds of stones (of different sizes and colors) coming out at once (see **Illustration 16b**).

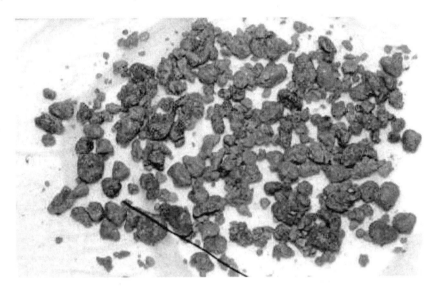

Illustration 16b: Mixed types of gallstones

Also, watch for tan-colored and white stones. Some of the larger tan or white stones may sink to the bottom with the stool. These are calcified gallstones that have been released from the gallbladder. They contain heavier toxic substances, with only small amounts of cholesterol (**Illustration 16c**). All the green and yellowish stones are as soft as putty, thanks to the action of the apple juice.

You may also find a layer of white or tan-colored chaff, or "foam," floating in the toilet. The foam consists of millions of tiny white, sharp-edged cholesterol crystals, which can easily rupture small bile ducts. They are equally important to release.

Try to make a rough estimate of how many stones you have eliminated. To permanently cure bursitis, back pain, allergies, or other health problems, and to prevent diseases from arising, you need to remove **all** the stones. This may require at least 8 to 12 flushes, which can be performed at three-week or monthly intervals. *(Do not flush more frequently than that!)* The three-week break between flushes may include the six-day preparation for the next liver flush, but most ideally, it should start after the three weeks have passed. If you cannot flush this often, you may take more time between flushes.

The important thing to remember is that once you have started cleansing the liver, you should keep cleansing it until no more stones come out during two consecutive flushes. Leaving the liver half clean for a long period of time (three or more months) may cause greater discomfort than not cleansing it at all. The liver, as a whole, will begin to function more efficiently soon after the first flush, and you may notice sudden improvements, sometimes within several hours. Pains will lessen, energy will increase, and clarity of mind will improve considerably.

However, within a few days, stones from the rear of the liver will have traveled 'forward' toward the two main bile ducts (hepatic ducts) in the liver, which may cause some or all of the previous symptoms of discomfort to return. In fact, you might feel disappointed because the recovery seems so short-lived. Yet all of this merely indicates that some stones were left behind, ready to be removed with the next round of cleansing. Nevertheless, the liver's self-repair and cleansing responses will have increased significantly, adding a great deal of effectiveness to this extremely important organ of the body.

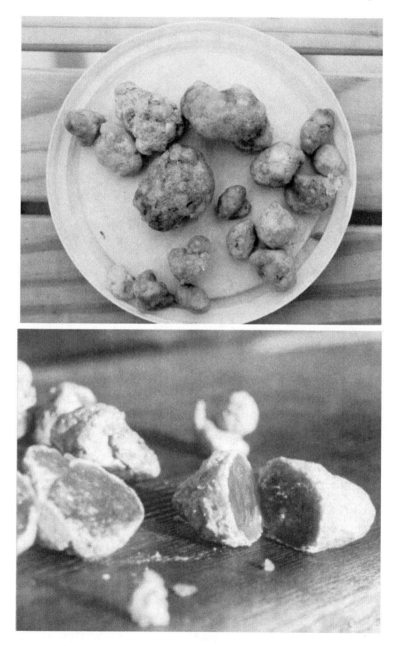

Illustrations 16c: Calcified and semicalcified gallstones (cut in halves)

As long as there are still a few small stones traveling from some of the thousands of small bile ducts to any of the hundreds of larger bile ducts, they may combine to form larger stones and produce previously experienced symptoms, such as backache, headache, earache, digestive trouble, bloating, irritability, anger, and so forth, although these may be less severe than they were before.

If two consecutive new cleanses no longer produce any stones, which may happen after 6 to 8 flushes (in severe cases it may take 10 to 12 or more), your liver can be considered 'stone-free'. Nevertheless, it is recommended that you repeat the liver flush every six to eight months. Each flush will give a further boost to the liver and take care of any toxins or new stones that may have accumulated in the meantime.

Caution: Never cleanse when you are suffering an acute illness, even if it is just a simple cold. If you suffer from a chronic illness, however, cleansing your liver may be the best thing you can do for yourself. However, don't attempt the flush if you are using prescribed medications, such as antibiotics, steroids, painkillers, statins or others suppressive drugs. The liver cannot both break down/release these drugs and suppress this activity (which drugs do) at the same time. It is best to wait with liver flushing until drug intake has been discontinued for at least 10 days.

Important! Please read carefully:

The liver flush is one of the most invaluable and effective methods to regain your health. There are no risks involved if you follow all the directions to the letter. Please take the next cautionary note very seriously. There are many people who have used a liver flush recipe that they received from friends or through the Internet, and they suffered unnecessary complications. They did not have complete knowledge of the procedure and the way it works, believing that just expelling the stones from the liver and gallbladder was sufficient.

It is likely that, on their way out, some gallstones will be caught in the colon. They can quickly be removed through colonic irrigation. This should ideally be done on the second or third day after the liver flush. If gallstones remain in the colon, they can cause irritation, infection, headaches, abdominal discomfort, thyroid problems, and so on. These stones can eventually become a source of toxemia in the body. If colonics are not available where you live, you can take a coffee enema followed by a water enema, or else, do two or three consecutive water enemas. Still, this may not guarantee that all the remaining stones will be removed. There is no real substitute for colonic irrigation when it comes to liver flushing. Doing a Colema Board® enema, though, is the closest you can attain to a professional colonic. If you settle for anything less than a colonic irrigation or Colema enema, mix one level teaspoon of Epsom salts with one glass of warm water and drink it first thing in the morning on the day of any other chosen colon cleanse following the liver flush. (To acquire a Colema Board®, see *Product Information* at the end of the book.)

On the importance of colon and kidney cleansing: Although the liver flush on its own can produce truly amazing results, it should ideally be done *following* a colon and kidney cleanse. Cleansing the colon (see also section on *Preparation*) ensures that the expelled gallstones are easily removed from the large intestine. Cleansing the kidneys makes certain that toxins coming out of the liver during the liver flush do not put any burden on these vital organs of elimination. However, if you have never had kidney trouble, kidney stones, or a bladder infection, you may go ahead with the *colon cleanse - liver flush - colon cleanse sequence*. Nevertheless, make certain that you cleanse the kidneys at a later stage. You should do a kidney cleanse after every three to four liver flushes and after your liver has been completely cleaned out (for details, see *The Kidney Cleanse* later in this chapter). In addition, you may drink a cup of kidney tea (see 'Kidney Cleanse' recipe) for two to three days after each liver flush. Follow the same directions given for the preparation of the main kidney cleanse. The kidney and liver flushes can be combined (overlap), but be sure to avoid drinking the kidney tea on the day of the actual liver flush.

People whose colon is severely congested, or who have a history of constipation, should consider doing at least two or three colon cleanses before their first liver flush. Moreover, to reemphasize, it is very important that you cleanse your colon within three days of completing each liver flush. Removing gallstones from the liver and gallbladder may leave some of the stones and other toxic residues in the colon. To prevent possible toxemia problems resulting from trapped stones in the colon, it is essential to clear them out.

A note on drinking water during the cleanse

To reiterate, you may drink water at any time during the liver cleanse, except right after and before taking Epsom salts (allow about 20 minutes). Also, avoid drinking water from 9:30 p.m. until 2 a.m. (if you happen to wake up). Apart from that, you can drink water whenever you are thirsty.

Having Difficulties with the Flush?

Intolerance to Apple Juice

If you cannot tolerate apple juice (or apples) for some reason, you may substitute the following herbs: *gold coin grass* and *bupleurum.* The herbs are made into a tincture and sold as *Gold Coin Grass* (GCG), 8.5 oz. (See *Product Information* at the end of the book)

Malic acid in apple juice does exceptionally well at dissolving some of the stagnant bile and making the stones softer. (See details on *malic acid* below) Cranberry juice also contains malic acid and can be used instead of apple juice. (See below)

The aforementioned herbs are also effective in softening gallstones and, therefore, can be used as a preparatory step for the liver flush, although it may take a little longer than with using apple or cranberry juice. The proper dosage for the tincture is 1 tablespoonful once daily on an empty stomach, about 30 minutes before breakfast. Keep this regimen for eight to nine days before the day of the liver flush.

Intolerance to Epsom Salts

If you are allergic to Epsom salts or just cannot tolerate them, you may use magnesium citrate instead (although it is not quite as effective as Epsom salts). Magnesium citrate is readily available at most drugstores.

Intolerance to Olive Oil

If you are allergic to olive oil or cannot tolerate it, you may use clear macadamia oil, expeller-pressed or cold-pressed grape seed oil, sunflower oil, or other expeller-pressed oils instead. Don't use canola, soy oil, or similar processed oils. Please note that extra virgin olive oil still appears to be the most effective oil for liver cleansing.

You Suffer from Gallbladder Disease or Don't Have a Gallbladder

If you suffer from gallbladder disease or your gallbladder has already been removed, you may need to take cranberry juice or gold coin grass for two to three weeks (approximately a 1-bottle supply) before liver cleansing. For details, see the previous and following sections.

As a general recommendation, you may also need to consider taking a bile supplement. Most bile supplements contain ox bile. Without a gallbladder, you may never again obtain the right amount of bile needed for the proper digestion of food. If you develop symptoms of diarrhea, lower the dosage or discontinue it. Consult with your health practitioner about which product may be the most suitable for you.

Those Who Should Not Use Apple Juice

Some people may have difficulty drinking apple juice in the large quantities required for the liver flush. These include those who suffer from diabetes, hypoglycemia, and yeast infection (Candida), cancer, and stomach ulcers.

In any cases of this kind, you may replace apple juice with *malic acid* in powdered form. Try to avoid malic acid capsules, especially if they contain other ingredients. It is best if the malic acid is properly dissolved before ingesting it. The preparation period is the same as for the apple juice regimen, except that ½ to 1 teaspoon of malic acid, taken with 32 ounces of room-temperature water (or more if it tastes too acidic for you), substitute for the 32 ounces of apple juice per day. Drink this solution in small amounts throughout the day. Food-grade malic acid powder (not mixed with magnesium or other ingredients) is very inexpensive and can be purchased over the Internet or from some natural health food stores. All wineries use malic acid to produce wine. (See *Product Information* at the end of the book)

Cranberry juice also contains much malic acid and can be used for the preparation period (4 ounces of juice mixed with 4 ounces water, four times per day for six days). It can also be combined with apple juice. There is added benefit if some cranberry juice is used each day for two or three weeks before liver cleansing.

Another alternative is gold coin grass. Use the same directions as given for those who are intolerant to apple juice. You may try malic acid or cranberry juice during one flush and gold coin grass during the next, to see which works best for you.

A fourth alternative is apple cider vinegar: mix 1 to 2 tablespoons in a glass of water and drink four servings per day, for six days.

Headache or Nausea During the Days Following Liver Flushing

In most cases of headache or nausea in the days after a liver flush, it occurs when the directions have not been followed carefully. (See above section) However, on some rare occasions, gallstones may continue to pass out of the liver after completing a liver flush. Some toxins released by these stones can enter the circulatory system and cause discomfort. In such a case, it may be helpful to drink about 4 ounces of apple juice for seven consecutive days, or for as long as the discomfort lasts, following the liver flush. It is best to drink the apple juice at least ½ hour before breakfast. In addition, a repeat colon cleanse may be necessary to clear out any of the late-coming stones. The tissue-cleansing method (ionized water), as mentioned in chapter 5, also helps to remove the circulating toxins. If you place a small piece of fresh ginger into the thermos flask, drinking this water will quickly stop the nausea. Drinking two to three cups of chamomile tea per day also helps to calm the digestive tract and the nervous system. Chamomile is also a good 'stone-breaker' of calcified stones.

Feeling Sick During the Flush

If you have properly followed all the directions given in the outlined procedure, but still feel sick sometime during the actual liver flush, please do not feel alarmed that something is wrong. Although it occurs rarely, a person may vomit or feel nauseated during the night. This happens when the gallbladder ejects bile and gallstones with such force that bile forces the oil back into the stomach. When the oil, combined with some bile, returns to the stomach, you are likely to feel sick. In such an instance, you may be able to feel the expulsion of stones. It will not be a sharp pain, just a mild contraction.

During one of my 12 liver flushes, I spent a miserable night. But, despite throwing up most of the oil mixture, this flush was just as successful as all the others I had done. By the time I vomited, the oil had already done its job; that is, it prompted the release of gallstones. If this happens to you, remember that this is only one night of discomfort. Recovery from conventional gallbladder surgery may take many weeks or months. Surgery may also lead to major pain and suffering in the years to come.

Instant relief: There is a good remedy, though, that can stop nausea within seconds. Take one tablet of hydrochloric acid (HCL) or two tablespoons of aloe vera juice. This closes the sphincter of the esophagus, thus preventing the oil mixture from moving up into the esophagus and making you feel sick.

The Liver Flush Did Not Deliver the Expected Results

In some cases, albeit very rarely, the liver flush does not produce the results you expect. The following are the two main reasons, and their remedies, for such difficulties:

1. It is likely that severe congestion in your liver's bile ducts, due to extremely dense structures of stones, has prevented the apple juice from softening them sufficiently during the first cleansing attempt. In some individuals, it may take as many as two or three liver flushes before the stones start coming out.

Chanca piedra, also known as 'stone-breaker', can help prepare your liver and gallbladder for a more efficient release of stones, especially if you have calcified stones in the gallbladder. Take 20 drops of chanca piedra extract (see *Product Information* at the end of the book) in a glass of water, three times daily for at least two to three weeks before your next flush. Enteric peppermint oil, taken in capsule form, is also very useful in dissolving calcified gallstones or reducing their size. It may not be easy to find it in pure form, though. It is often mixed with other ingredients, which can reduce its effectiveness.

Drinking two to three cups of chamomile tea per day also helps to dissolve calcified stones.

Another useful method to help support the liver and gallbladder during the flush, and to encourage the release of more stones, is to soak a piece of flannel with heated apple cider vinegar and apply it to the liver/gallbladder area during the 20 to 30-minute period of lying still. Some people have found increased benefits from doing this using warm castor oil instead.

The herbs *Chinese gentian* and *bupleurum,* help to break up some of the congestion and can, thereby, prepare your liver for a more successful flush. These herbs are prepared as a tincture. They are more commonly known as Chinese Bitters. (See *Product Information* at the end of the book) The proper dosage for this tincture is ½ to 1 teaspoonful once daily on an empty stomach, about 30 minutes before breakfast. This regimen should be followed for three weeks before drinking the apple juice (or using the other alternatives discussed in the previous section). Any unpleasant cleansing reactions usually disappear after three to six days; they can be minimized by following the tissue-cleansing method of using hot, ionized water and by keeping the colon clean with capsules of OxyFlush™, Oxy-Powder®, Colosan, a Colema, or an enema (see Chapter 5).

Another method is to drink three tablespoons of undiluted, unsweetened lemon juice, 15 to 30 minutes before breakfast daily for one week. This stimulates the gallbladder and makes it ready for a more successful liver flush.

2. You may not have followed the directions properly. Leaving out any one item from the procedure, or altering the dosages or timing of the steps laid out, may prevent you from obtaining the full results. In quite a few people, the liver flush does not work at all unless the large intestine has been cleansed first. The backup of waste and gases cuts down adequate bile secretion and prevents the oil mixture from moving easily through the GI tract. In people who are severely constipated, the gallbladder may barely open up during the liver flush. The best time for a colonic irrigation or an alternative colon cleansing method is the day of the actual liver flush.

Intestinal Cleansing - For Prevention and Cure

Your body's health and vitality largely depend on the effortless and complete elimination of waste products from the intestinal tract. Most physical problems are caused and exacerbated by a buildup of waste material that may at first accumulate in the intestines and then spread to other parts of the body such as the liver, kidneys, heart, lungs, face, and skin.

Accumulated or trapped waste material in the large intestine may consist of impacted feces, hardened mucus, dead cellular tissue, gallstones that were released from the gallbladder, dead and living bacteria, parasites, worms, metals and other noxious substances. It undermines the colon's important role in absorbing essential minerals and some bacteria-produced vitamins, including the all-important vitamin B12. Parts of the waste matter may enter the lymph and blood systems, which can make you feel tired, sluggish or ill.

Colon-related complaints include constipation, diarrhea, bloating, headaches, dizziness, nausea, sinusitis, eye and ear disorders, backaches, bad breath, body odor, sciatica, skin blemishes and diseases, abdominal gas, low energy, disorders of the nervous system, etc. A clean colon is a prerequisite for the balanced functioning of the rest of the body. Cleansing of the large intestine should, therefore, be part of every healing therapy.

Keep Your Intestines Clean!

A weak, irritated and congested large intestine is a breeding place for destructive bacteria which have no other purpose than to break down potentially hazardous waste material. As an unavoidable side effect of their truly life-saving activities, these microorganisms produce toxic, poisonous substances. Some of the toxins produced by the bacteria enter the blood, which delivers them straight to the liver. Constant exposure of liver cells to these toxins greatly dampens their performance, causes bile stones and reduces bile secretion, all of which leads to further disruption of digestive functions. Eventually, the toxins can no longer be removed from the blood by the liver, and they end up accumulating in the tissues of organs and systems in the body. Those toxins that enter the lymphatic system, end up causing lymph congestion, fluid retention, bloating and weight gain.

When you eat highly processed foods that have been stripped of most of their nutrients, natural fiber and life force, your colon has great difficulty in moving the food mass or chyme along. Processed foods tend to make for a dry, hard or sticky chyme that does not pass easily through the intestinal tract. The muscles wrapped around the colon can easily squeeze and push a more fibrous, bulky chyme along, but they struggle with fiberless, gooey, sticky chyme. When chyme sits too long in the colon, it becomes harder and drier each day. If that were the only thing that happened - chyme turning into hard, dry feces

- you would only need to worry about constipation, from which millions of Americans suffer. But there is more. After the chyme/feces gets plastered onto the walls of the colon, it begins to do several things, including:

- Ferment, rot and harden, thereby becoming a breeding ground for parasites and pathogens (disease-causing agents), and a storehouse for toxic chemicals that can pollute the blood and lymph and slowly poison the body.
- Form a barrier that prevents the colon from interacting with and absorbing nutrients from food chyme.
- Restrict movement of the colon walls, making it difficult for the colon to rhythmically contract (peristalsis) in order to speed the chyme along its way. How well could you do your job if you were covered with thick sludge?

The following are some of the symptoms manifesting as a result of colon dysfunction:

- Lower-back pain
- Neck and shoulder pain
- Skin problems
- Brain fog (difficulty concentrating)
- Fatigue
- Sluggishness
- Colds and flu
- Cold hands and feet
- Constipation or diarrhea
- Digestive problems

- Flatulence/gas
- Bloating
- Crohn's disease
- Ulcerative colitis
- Colitis/Irritable Bowel Syndrome (IBS)
- Diverticulitis/Diverticulosis
- Leaky Gut Syndrome
- Pain in lower stomach

The large intestine absorbs minerals and water. When the membrane of the large intestine is impacted with plaque, it cannot properly assimilate and absorb minerals and certain vitamins. Accordingly, no matter how many supplements you take, your body will begin to suffer from nutrient deficiencies. Most diseases are, in fact, deficiency disorders. They arise when certain parts of the body suffer malnourishment; particularly minerals (see also *Take Ionic Minerals* in this chapter). The main cause of malnourishment is intestinal congestion. I recommend several possible methods to aid intestinal cleansing; they are *Colonic Irrigation*, *Magnesium Oxides* and *Enema* treatments. I understand that not everyone has access to a colon hydrotherapist, so I have included some other options.

Colonic Irrigation

We all know how important it is to clean the outside of the body. However, few people realize that the same applies to the inside of the body. Historic writings dating back to the ancient Egyptians show that cleaning the inside of the body with water was considered to be the fastest and most effective way to lower a fever, alleviate abdominal pain and help ease any discomfort or ailment. The ancients knew that most diseases were merely manifestations of one single condition, the condition of autointoxication. Autointoxication results from being poisoned by one's own wastes. Incomplete elimination of waste matter from the intestines turns the body into a cesspool of toxins.

Although prescribing colonic irrigation used to be standard medical procedure in every good hospital until the 1920s, doctors now consider it unnecessary, ineffective or even harmful; not that they ever tried one for themselves or their patients. In Russia however, colonic irrigation remains standard procedure in all hospitals and clinics for all patients, regardless of what types of ailment they suffer from. Patients undergo the colon cleansing treatment upon entering the hospital. Russian physicians believe that a toxic, congested body does not properly respond to their treatment programs. Some Israeli hospitals don't even treat patients until they had a colon cleanse.

Colonic irrigation, also called colon hydrotherapy or colonic, is perhaps one of the most effective colon cleaning therapies. Within a short passage of time a colonic can eliminate large amounts of trapped waste that may have taken many years to accumulate. During a 40-50 minute session of colonic irrigation, a total of two to six liters of distilled or purified water is used to gently flush the colon. Through gentle abdominal massage old deposits of mucoid fecal matter (waste mixed and hardened by old mucus) are loosened and subsequently flushed out by the water.

A colonic removes not only harmful, toxic waste, but it also tones, hydrates and rejuvenates the colon muscles. The repeated uptake and release of water improves the colon's peristaltic action and reduces the transit time of fecal matter. In addition, colonic irrigation helps restore the colon's natural shape, and stimulates the reflex points that connect the colon with all the parts of the body. This form of colon cleansing can detach old crusted layers of waste from the colon walls, which permits better water absorption and hydration of the colon and the body as a whole. However, it may take a minimum of two to three colonic sessions for these latter benefits to take effect.

Colonic irrigation can also help with emotional problems. It is no coincidence that the transverse colon passes right through the solar plexus, which is the body's emotional center. Most of our unresolved or 'undigested' emotional issues are stored in the solar plexus and result in the tightening of the colon muscle. This may slow bowel movement and cause constipation. Colonics can help clear the physical obstruction and release the tension that causes the emotional repression in the first place.

Colonics have a truly relieving effect. During a colonic, you may feel a slight discomfort or chills from time to time when larger quantities of toxic waste detach themselves from the intestinal walls and move towards the rectum. However, the feeling of lightness, cleanness, and clarity of mind soon afterwards make up for that.

Colonic irrigation is a very safe and hygienic system of cleansing the colon. Rubber tubing carries water into the colon and waste out of the colon. The released waste material can be seen floating through a tube, showing the type and quantity of waste eliminated. Although some critics claim that there are risks involved in this procedure, in the many years I have worked with colonics, I have never seen any justification for these claims. Not having a colonic from time to time, on the other hand, can be very risky, given today's high incidence of irritable bowel syndrome and colon cancer.

Colonic cleansing is best done when the stomach is empty. It is beneficial to drink one to two glasses of water afterwards and eat a piece of fruit or have some freshly prepared fruit juice ½ hour later. The first one or two meals after the treatment should be light and not contain food items such as meat, eggs, cheese, fried food, etc.

Some people have expressed their concern about losing friendly, probiotic bacteria in the colon as a result of a colonic. It is actually much easier for the friendly colon bacteria to repopulate in a clean environment than in one filled with putrefied and fermented waste matter. Once the colon is properly cleansed, it takes less than 36 hours to restore normal bacteria populations. If you still feel concerned about this, you may use soil-based microbes, such as *Nature's Biotics* (upwardquest.com), or similar products. Be certain that whatever product you use contains live, not dead, bacteria. Personally, I am not an advocate for probiotics because I have not seen any convincing benefits, despite the convincing theory behind their use.

After a colonic, the bowel movement will become naturally restored within about two days. If it takes longer than that, it indicates that the colon has accumulated unduly large amounts of waste over a period of many years. To soften up and flush out all the waste may require a series of colonics and, of course, liver flushes and a balanced diet and lifestyle.

Once the colon has been thoroughly cleansed through colonics, nutritional improvements, exercise, liver and kidney cleanses, and any other health programs will become many times more effective. Since an estimated 70-80 percent of the immune tissue resides in the intestines, cleansing the colon from immune-suppressive toxic waste, in addition to removing gallstones from the liver and gallbladder, can make a crucial difference in the treatment of cancer, heart disease, arthritis, AIDS and other illnesses.

Colema Board®

If no colon therapist is available in your area, you may greatly benefit from using a *Colema Board®* (see illustration 17, and *Product Information*) as a second best choice. The Colema treatment is based on the same principle as colon-hydrotherapy, although it may not be as effective and thorough. The advantage is that the Colema Board® allows you to clean your whole colon in the comfort of your own home. The Colema colon cleanse is a do-it-yourself treatment that is easy to learn and perform.

Another similar method, the "Home-kit Colonic Irrigation," (see *Product Information*) is perhaps not as easy to perform as a Colema treatment, but it is the closest you can get to a professional colonic irrigation. However, most people find the Colema Board® to be more user friendly, and I tend to agree.

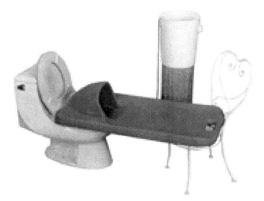

Illustration 17: Colema Board

Colosan Treatment

Colosan (formerly known as *ColoZone*) is a proprietary blend of various oxides of magnesium designed to gently release oxygen in the digestive tract for cleansing. Please note that there are other brands of magnesium oxides available that have similar effects, including Oxy-Powder®, Homozon and Oxy-Cleanse®, and Aerobic Mag 07. Some are easier to take than others, but they all work pretty much the same. The preferred method of use is in capsule form.

In my practice I have found Colosan (or similar) to be a very useful product to counteract the following problems:

- Build-up of undigested material in the intestines and colon

- Impeded assimilation of nutrients
- Presence of pathogens and parasites that breed in the putrefaction of the digestive tract
- Detoxification or healing crisis associated with many health regimens
- Insufficient oxygen to maintain homeostasis

The main actions of Colosan:
- It releases oxygen in the intestines and colon to help speed the elimination of wastes.
- It provides needed oxygen for proper digestion and cleanses digestive membranes to allow improved uptake of nutrients.
- It eliminates the unwanted buildup of toxins, creating a clean and healthful environment where there is no room or 'food' for disease-causing microbes.

How does Colosan Work?
The various oxides of magnesium contained in Colosan involve the bonding of oxygen and ozone to magnesium. This alkaline compound requires an extremely low pH in order to liberate its oxygen. For this reason, the hydrochloric acid in the stomach is commonly assisted with the juice of a lemon or apple cider vinegar. The average size tablespoon of approximately 7-10 g of pure magnesium oxide would produce a total volume of 3.85 cubic meters of oxygen. In the use of Colosan, one teaspoon would provide approximately 7.5 liters of available oxygen. This oxygen is made bio-available to the stomach which is 40 percent more efficient at assimilating oxygen than are the lungs. It also assists in oxidizing the undigested putrefaction that is known to be impacting the intestines and the colon. The average person has six to twelve pounds of putrefaction rotting away in their gut, breeding pathogens and creating a welcome home for parasites, germs, bacteria and viruses.

Digestion is known to be a process of oxidation. By introducing oxygen into the intestines and the colon, one can assist the process of assimilating nutrients, as well as oxidizing the undigested material. It is common for Colosan to turn undigested material into CO_2 and water. For this reason, Colosan is a cathartic. It is not unusual to have very liquid stools during the use of Colosan; this is a sign that the product is working. If the stools are not liquid during the first one to two treatments, it shows that most of the magnesium is absorbed straight away, indicating a mineral deficiency. After a few treatments, the situation returns to normal and stools become liquid and more frequent following each dose of Colosan. Many people use Colosan once or twice weekly as a maintenance product for staying clean and maintaining regularity.

The most common health problem besides irregular bowel movement that Colosan has shown great benefit for is Candida (also see chapter 10). Colosan provides an aerobic environment in the intestines and colon. Therefore, it is beneficial to the 'friendly' bacteria, which are desirable and inhibitory toward toxin-producing, undesirable bacteria. In other words, this product helps beneficial intestinal flora to flourish.

Colosan can be used to prevent any type of healing crisis or detox reaction that you might have when you follow a certain cleansing protocol. Anyone versed in natural therapies is usually familiar with these occurrences. These undesirable experiences stem from attempting to clean out the body before the organs of elimination have been cleansed. This results in backing up of toxic waste. The body frequently attempts to rid itself of these wastes through the skin. The back-flushed waste can result in feelings of nausea, headaches, tiredness, ear and eye trouble, aching joints or pain in the neck and shoulders. This influx of toxicity may also affect the liver and kidneys.

By cleaning out the organs of elimination through the use of Colosan you can avoid detox reactions associated with the use of herbal cleansing programs or other regimens that are administered for this purpose. Colosan is available from 'The Family News' in the United States (see *Product Information* at the end of the book) and many online health stores.

Note: The products Oxy-Powder®, Oxy-Cleanse®, or similar, have about the same beneficial effects as Colosan, and may be used instead. Prices for each product vary.

The Salt Water Flush

If you wish to cleanse the intestinal tract just for one day, you may take an oral salt-water enema upon arising. To do this cleanse, add 2 level teaspoons of non-iodized, unrefined, unprocessed sea salt to a quart (32 ounces) of lukewarm water. Shake well and drink the entire quart. You get used to the taste as you continue drinking it. **Important note**: Make sure you use only non-iodized, unprocessed sea salt; regular or iodized sea or table salt will make you feel sick and have harmful side effects.

If you cannot find natural sea salt at your local health food store, you can order it through the Internet. An equally good product is mineral or rock salt, which has a grayish-white color. You can perform this cleanse when you feel congested from having eaten something you know is causing you harm. However, do not follow this procedure more often than once per week. An added benefit here is that there are usually no cramps or discomfort accompanying the salt-water cleanse. However, this cleanse doesn't work for everyone. Those with very congested colons may not find much relief, and those sensitive to water retention may find that their hands and feet become tight and hold on to water.

Epsom Salts

Another method of intestinal cleansing uses Epsom salts. Epsom salts not only cleanse the colon, but also the small intestine. This may become necessary if you have major difficulties absorbing food, repeated kidney/bladder congestion, severe constipation, or are simply unable to have a colonic or Colema. For one week, mix one teaspoon of Epsom salts (magnesium sulfate) with one glass of warm water and drink first thing in the morning. This oral enema flushes your entire digestive tract and colon, from top to bottom, usually within an hour, prompting you to eliminate several times. It clears out plaque and debris from the walls, along with parasites that may have been living there. Anticipate the stools to be watery for as long as there is intestinal waste to be disposed of. Stools adopt a more normal shape and consistency once the entire intestinal tract is clean.

This treatment can be done twice a year. In the beginning, and whenever the intestines release some major pockets of waste and toxins, you can expect gas, bloating and even some cramping. Your tongue may become covered white and be thicker than normal. This indicates increased intestinal cleansing. If you are allergic to Epsom salts or just cannot tolerate this product, you may use Magnesium Citrate, Colosan, Oxy-Powder® or similar methods of cleansing instead.

Some practitioners have raised the concern that Epsom salts may be harmful to the kidneys and affect blood pressure. In 35 years of working with Epsom salts, I have not seen such side effects, but only benefits. However, Epsom salts, unlike magnesium oxides, have laxative properties, which means they should not be overused. If you are taking prescribed drugs, although there are only relatively few known reactions to medication, it is best to use other methods of intestinal cleansing. Do not use magnesium sulfate as a laxative if you have stomach (abdominal) pain, nausea, or vomiting, unless directed by a doctor.

Castor oil

Castor oil is a traditionally used, excellent remedy to clear waste material from the intestines. It is less irritating than Epsom salts and has no side effects other than normal cleansing reactions. Take one to three teaspoons of castor oil in 1/3 glass of warm water on an empty stomach in the morning or before going to sleep at night (depending on which works better for you). It is a very beneficial treatment for stubborn cases of constipation. It can also be given to children (in smaller dosages). While castor oil is not recommended to replace Epsom salts or magnesium citrate during the liver cleanse, in case of an allergy to the above, castor oil may be used as a substitute.

Four Major Rectal Enema Treatments

Enema treatments involve introduction of liquids into the rectum for the purpose of cleansing and nourishment (see **illustration 18**). Since the colon is the seat of Vata, an enema has an immediate effect on all the functions of Vata. It alleviates constipation, distension, chronic fever, the common cold, headache, sexual disorders, kidney stones, pain in the heart area, vomiting, low backache, stiffness and pain in neck and shoulders, nervous disorders, hyperacidity and tiredness. Disorders such as arthritis, rheumatism, sciatica and gout also greatly benefit from an enema.

Please note: A colonic or Colema treatment would still be a better choice for balancing disturbed Vata functions. For liver flushes, colonics or Colemas are preferable. If not available, two to three back-to-back water enemas can be used instead.

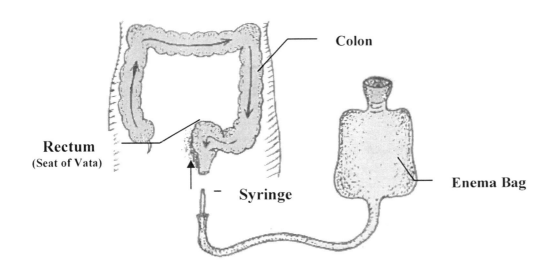

Illustration 18: Enema treatment

Since the disturbance of Vata dosha is responsible for the retention of feces, urine, bile, and other excreta, by pacifying it through an enema, most of the eliminative functions in the body are improved. Besides the colon, Vata also controls lung functions and the bones. All chronic colon disorders are likely to manifest as lung and bone disorders as well. Although less effective than colonic irrigation, which irrigates the entire colon, enemas can offer quick relief when the rectum is congested with fecal matter.

The first three types of enemas can be used to balance Vata and the fourth can improve digestion and liver functions.

1. Oil enema: Half a cup of warm sesame oil for above problems and chronic constipation once or twice a week. Perform the enema while lying on your back with your legs elevated. Hold the oil in your intestine as long as possible, ideally for 30 minutes or longer; turning to your right side may help make this easier. **Note:** Those with diabetes, obesity, indigestion, low AGNI, and enlarged spleen should avoid oil enemas and opt for the second type enema.

2. Decoction or water enema: Up to half a liter (16 ounces) of Lapacho, Comfrey or Chaparral tea, or one liter of plain water, at room temperature. These types of enema are indicated for acute constipation and above problems, but should not be taken more often than once or twice a week. **Note:** Avoid if you suffer from debility, hemorrhoids, inflammation of anus, diarrhea, or if pregnant. If you are diabetic, consult your physician. The effects increase if an enema type 2 is followed by an enema type 1. Patients who are lying in bed and are constipated can take enemas type 1 and 2 alternately.

3. Coffee enema: The main purpose of the coffee enema is that of lowering serum (blood) toxins. The coffee stimulates the visceral nervous system, promoting peristalsis and the transit of toxic bile from the duodenum out the rectum. This enema is indicated when you feel very sluggish and tired, particularly when you have pain in your middle/upper back, which are all indications of a toxic liver. The effect is often immediate. Place three heaped tablespoons of ground organic coffee (not instant coffee) into 16 ounces (two glasses) of boiling water. Boil for three minutes and let simmer (on a low flame) for 15 minutes. Filter through a coffee filter or cotton cloth. Make sure that no coffee substance is left at the bottom. Let it cool to body temperature and perform the enema while lying on your back with your legs elevated. Ideally, retain the coffee solution for 15 minutes, then release; turning to your right side may help make this easier. This enema can be taken if time or circumstances (such as feeling ill) don't permit a person to do the liver cleanse. When seriously ill with cancer, liver or heart disease, it can be taken more frequently, as often as every other day.

4. Urine Enema: If you suffer from persistent skin conditions, such as acne, a series of urine enemas can help you restore skin health within a matter of a few weeks. Collect your urine starting in the morning (use mid-stream only) until you have a jar of one to two liters. Administer the enemas in the late afternoon before eating. You may want to add a little amount of hot water to the urine to warm it up. Once you remove the nozzle, you may lie on your back, gently lift your knees up towards your chin, and if possible, move into the yoga posture "shoulder stand" for one minute. Continue lying on your back with your knees up for five more minutes and then gently roll over to your right side for about 10 minutes. The most important thing with regard to this enema is to keep the urine in the colon for as long as possible. If you feel strong discomfort, though, release it. While you are in the process of releasing the urine and waste, you may gently massage the abdomen with or without oil (ideally sesame or coconut oil) in a clockwise direction. For serious illnesses, use the following protocol for about five weeks:

1st week – one enema per day, late afternoon
2nd week – one enema every 2nd day, late afternoon
3rd week – one enema every 3rd day, late afternoon
4th week – one enema every 3rd day, late afternoon
5th week – one enema every 3rd day, late afternoon

Since urine contains the perfect mix of vitamins, hormones, minerals, antibodies, etc., doing urine enemas so frequently does not deplete the colon of these nutrient components. In fact, urine enemas can greatly increase colon health and help restore intestinal flora. Candida sufferers, especially benefit from urine enemas.

A Note on Auto Urine Therapy (AUT):

Auto-urine therapy is an age-old practice of India and China and is gaining popularity worldwide, but mainly in Europe. It has shown success in the treatments of a wide array of disorders, including multiple sclerosis, colitis, lupus, rheumatoid arthritis, cancer, hepatitis, pancreatic insufficiency, psoriasis, eczema, diabetes and herpes. For three million Chinese, drinking their own urine is an accepted health practice. Former Prime Minister of India Morarji Desai, who lived up to the age of 99, has been the most well known proponent of this therapy. In Germany, a former president's wife openly admitted drinking her own urine on national television.

AUT entails using your own urine internally or externally as a way to treat or prevent illness. Most people are under the wrong impression that urine is a toxic waste product that could harm us if we were to ingest it. Toxic or otherwise harmful substances are removed from the body through the liver, intestines, lungs, and skin. The main role of the kidneys is to maintain proper fluid balance in the body and ensure that the blood always contains a balanced amount of minerals, salt, hormones and enzymes. Urine is sterile after secretion and has an antiseptic effect. Many who were shipwrecked or were lost in the desert survived by drinking their own urine. Urine contains everything that a person needs to survive, including water, minerals and vitamins.

Dr B.V. Khare, an allopathic doctor and Mumbai-based follower of AUT, says: "The Italian surgeon Stanislau R. Burzynski, now settled in America, separated antineoplaston from human urine and showed remarkable results in the treatment of cancer. Another substance found in large quantities in the urine is called dehydroepiandrosterone (DHEA). It is a hormone related to testosterone. This, as research showed, has anti-cancer, anti-obesity and anti-aging properties. It has also been found that urea when recycled by ingesting, is converted into essential amino acids." All in all, urine contains 15 known ingredients that work synergistically to keep the body cancer-free. Among them are the anti-cancer drugs interferon, and interleukins 1 & 2, urea, uric acid, 3 methylglyoxal, DHEA, H-11, directin, antineoplaston,

The most common method of AUT is to consume your morning urine (mid-stream part) completely and without dilution. It can also be used to gargle or swished through teeth for gum protection. As described above, urine can also be administered to the body through enemas. When applied to wounds and broken bones, urine helps prevent scarring and swelling. It draws toxins out of areas of inflammation and permits the healing to occur faster than it normally would.

Important note for those doing liver and gallbladder flushes: If for some reason you cannot have a colonic irrigation or Colema treatment before and after liver flushes, taking two to three back-to-back water enemas may be your next best option. Begin the second or third enema only after you have released the previous one. You need to make certain that the water reaches into the ascending colon.

You can massage your abdomen to help bring the water to this part of the colon. Enema kits are available at most pharmacies.

The Kidney Cleanse

You may also need to cleanse the kidneys, if the presence of gallstones in the liver, or other causes, have led to the development of stones in the kidneys or the urinary bladder. The kidneys are very delicate, blood-filtering organs that easily get congested as a result of poor digestion, stress and an irregular lifestyle. The main causes of congestion in the kidneys are kidney stones. Most kidney stones/crystals/sand, however, are too small to be recognized through modern diagnostic instruments, such as X-rays.

The following herbs, when taken daily for a period of 20-30 days, can help dissolve and eliminate all the various types of kidney stones, including uric acid stones, oxalic acid stones, phosphate stones and amino acid stones. If you have a history of kidney stones and want to completely clean out your kidneys, you may need to repeat this cleanse several times, at intervals of six to eight weeks.

Ingredients:

- Marjoram (1oz)
- Cat's Claw (1oz)
- Comfrey Root (1oz)
- Fennel Seed (2oz)
- Chicory Herb (2oz)

- Uva Ursi (2oz)
- Hydrangea Root (2oz)
- Gravel Root (2oz)
- Marshmallow Root (2oz)
- Golden Rod Herb (2oz)

Note: If you need to know the Latin names for the above herbs, see Product Information at the end of the book.

Directions:

Take 1 oz. each of the first three herbs and 2 oz. each of the rest of the herbs and thoroughly mix them together. Keep them in an airtight container. Before bedtime, soak two to three heaping tablespoons of the mixture in two cups of water, cover it and leave covered overnight. The next morning bring the concoction to a boil; let it simmer for a few minutes and strain. If you forget to prepare the tea in the evening, in the morning bring it to a boil and let it sit or lightly simmer 10-15 minutes before straining.

Drink a few sips at a time in six to eight portions throughout the day. This tea does not have to be taken warm or hot, but do not refrigerate it. Do not add sugar or sweeteners. Leave at least one hour after eating before taking your next sips.

Repeat this procedure for 20-30 days. If you experience discomfort or stiffness in the lower-back area it is because of salt crystals from kidney stones passing through the ureter ducts of the urinary system. Any strong smell and darkening of the urine at the beginning of or during the cleanse indicates a major release of toxins from the kidneys. Usually, the release is gradual and does not significantly change the color or texture of the urine. Important: During the cleanse, support the kidneys by drinking extra amounts of water, a minimum of six and a maximum of eight glasses per day.

During the cleanse, avoid consuming animal products, dairy foods, tea, coffee, alcohol, carbonated beverages, chocolate and any other foods or beverages that contain preservatives, artificial sweeteners, coloring agents, etc. While cleansing the kidneys, harsh substances such as chemicals may not only interfere with the cleanse, but may also injure the kidneys.

In addition to drinking this kidney tea each day, you may chew a small piece of rind from an organic lemon on the left side of your mouth and a small piece of carrot on the right side of your mouth 30-40 times each. This stimulates the kidney functions and triggers the release of specific enzymes that help with the breakdown of certain acidic deposits in the kidneys. Make certain that there about half an hour in between chewing 'cycles'. Although this is not an essential part of the cleanse, it can enhance its effectiveness.

Sipping Hot Ionized Water

The sipping of hot ionized water has a profound cleansing effect on all the tissues of the body. It helps reduce overall toxicity, improves circulatory functions, and balances bile. When you boil water for 15 to 20 minutes, it becomes thinner (its molecule clusters are reduced from the normal number of about 10,000 to one or two clusters), and it is charged and saturated with negative oxygen ions (hydroxide, OH^-). When you take frequent sips of this water throughout the day, it begins to systematically cleanse the tissues of the body and help rid them of certain positively charged ions (those associated with harmful acids and toxins).

Most toxins and waste materials carry a positive charge and, thus, naturally tend to attach themselves to the body, which is negatively charged overall. As the negative oxygen ions enter the body with the ingested water, they are attracted to the positively charged toxic material. This neutralizes waste and toxins, turning them into fluid matter that the body can remove easily. For the first couple of days or even weeks of cleansing your body tissues in this way, your tongue may take on a white or yellow coating, an indication that the body is clearing out a lot of toxic waste. If you have excessive body weight, this cleansing method can help you shed many pounds of body waste in a short period of time, without the side effects that normally accompany sudden weight loss.

Directions: Boil water for 15 to 20 minutes and pour it into a thermos. Stainless steel thermoses are fine. The thermos keeps the water hot and ionized throughout the day. Take one or two sips every half hour all day long, and drink it as hot as you would sip tea. You may use this method anytime you do not feel well, have the need for decongesting, wish to keep the blood thin, or simply want to feel more energetic and clear. Some people drink ionized water for a certain duration, such as three to four weeks; others do it ongoing.

The oxygen ions are generated through the bubbling effect of boiling water, similar to water falling on the ground in a waterfall or breaking against the seashore. In the thermos, the water will stay ionized for up to 12 hours or for as long as it remains hot. The total amount of water you need to boil to give you enough hot, ionized water for one day would be about 20 to 24 ounces. This specially prepared water should not substitute for normal drinking water. It doesn't hydrate the cells like normal water does; the body uses it to only cleanse the tissues.

Clearing Allergies

In the United States, food allergies claim the lives of 100 to 200 people and send another 30,000 to the emergency room each year. In addition, millions of people suffer from allergies or sensitivity to chemicals added to common foods, including artificial colors or preservatives. There are many environmental contaminants contained in food packaging materials such as plastic bottles or plastic wraps, not to mention the exhaust fumes, pesticides, paint or carpet vapors and other environmental chemicals so many of us are exposed to every day. It would be harmful for the body if it did not react at all against the massive onslaught of poisons it has to deal with.

In many cases, growing up in an overly sterile environment may cause the immune systems to overreact when they get in contact with harmless substances. Food processing, genetically engineered foods, or the age when solid foods are first given to infants, may also be contributing factors to the escalation of allergies. Among the most common foods to cause allergic reactions are milk, eggs, peanuts, tree nuts (like cashews), fish, shellfish, soy and wheat (gluten). These foods account for about 90 percent of all allergy reactions in the United States. However, in the above examples, with the exception of tree nuts and wheat, it is actually normal for the body to try to defend itself against these potentially damaging foods. They were never meant for human consumption, but for animal consumption. The very toxic enzyme inhibitors in soy, for example, prevent the digestion of soy proteins, which makes it very difficult for the human body not to react. The same applies to peanuts, and even to other nuts and legumes, unless they are soaked overnight before consumption. Creating shortcuts in the baking process of wheat products such as adding yeast, which prevents the destruction of harmful antibodies, or adding extra gluten, has made many people sensitive to wheat.

Keeping a food diary helps you sort out the allergy triggers. To test for food allergies, take your pulse for one minute; then place a small piece of the food under your tongue and take your pulse again; if the count is higher than before you may be allergic to that particular food.

Although the liver cleanse helps remove the main physical cause of allergies in the body, you may need other methods to 'persuade' the cells of the immune system to stop producing antibodies against antigens present, for example, in dust, pollen, duck feathers, cat hair, or such foods as milk, wheat, oranges, tomatoes, etc. In fact, allergic reactions, which might have had their root cause in a congested liver and impaired digestive system and have not disappeared, may be responsible for causing gallstones again. *Bio-resonance Therapy* is one method to deal with any remaining antibody complexes in the blood responsible for allergic reactions.

It is known in the circles of natural health practitioners that almost every person suffering from a chronic disease, illness, or long-term complaint has one or several allergies. An allergy results when repeated exposure of the body to a normally harmless substance or antigen stimulates the immune system to produce antibodies. In whichever part of the body the defense reaction is most pronounced, that's where the symptoms of disruption and discomfort will occur more intensely. If it happens to occur in the nose, sinus cavities or chest area, you may suffer from severe mucus congestion and breathing difficulties. Likewise, a similar immune response in the ovaries can cause ovarian cysts; in the prostate gland, it may lead to prostate enlargement. In some instances, the reaction may trigger anaphylactic shock, nausea, skin rashes, breathing difficulties, fainting, diarrhea, and death. There may be many more diseases linked to allergic reactions than are currently known.

Research in the field of *Radionics* has shown that there are four main allergies which cover most other possible allergies. These take account of the body's reactions to *duck feathers, milk, wheat, and mint*. Accordingly, if you happen to be allergic to duck feathers you may also be allergic to a number of allergens that belong in the category of duck feathers, such as certain fruits, vegetables, dust particles, metals, pollutants, etc. There may, in fact, be hundreds of such substances. By annulling your body's allergic response to duck feathers through *Bio-resonance Therapy*, all these other allergies linked to duck feathers are likely to disappear as well. Similarly, when a wheat allergy has been cleared up, the body's immune system will stop to react to all the antigens that fall in the wheat category. The same principle applies to the groups pertaining to the milk and mint allergies.

Most people with health problems have at least one major allergy, which may, for example, be against wheat and its subordinates. Almost everyone who has tooth fillings made with mercury-containing amalgam is allergic to milk, as well as to its products and subordinates. Research has shown that all AIDS patients, who have been tested for all the four allergy categories, are allergic to each one of them. Cancer patients have allergies to at least three groups.

Bio-resonance therapists who test not only the entire physical body as a whole for existing allergies, but each energy center (chakra) separately, seem to have the best results. Subsequent tests show no further allergies against anything; that is, provided that a balanced diet and lifestyle remain or become an integral part of daily life. Recent research conducted in Germany on the value of *Bio-resonance Therapy* in the treatment of the severest forms of allergy showed that out of 200 tested patients, 83 percent were completely cured of all allergies and 11 percent had improved significantly. Although *Bio-resonance Therapy* may be effective even without cleansing of the liver, the benefits are much more pronounced if it is applied after the liver has been cleansed. The success of this treatment is determined by exposing oneself to the former antigens such as orange juice, flower pollen, or gluten that is contained in wheat.

In my experience, my method of Sacred Santémony (see end of book or my website for details) has shown the most powerful and immediate effects for common allergies or chemical sensitivities. I was able to remove gluten allergies and even chemical allergies in a large number of people who had them for decades within a matter of half an hour or less. In some cases, a repeat session was necessary to solidify the results. Also, the *Emotional Freedom Technique* (EFT), available for download from the Internet, has helped people clear up allergies. Most allergies actually have an emotional component to them, which makes them resistant to standard medical treatment.

Replacing Metal Tooth Fillings And Removing Toxic Metals/Chemicals from the Body

Metal Fillings - A Ticking Time Bomb?

Metal dental ware is a constant source of poisoning and allergic reaction in the body (especially to milk and its products). All metal corrodes in time, especially in the mouth where there is a high concentration of air and moisture. Among other harmful metals, amalgam fillings contain the extremely toxic mercury. Mercury makes up 50 percent of the filling! Their vapors are being released into the lungs through inhalation and enter the digestive system while eating and drinking. When they enter the blood and lymph, they can cause considerable damage in the body, including the nervous system. Recently, researchers produced a special video that showed constant mercury vapor escaping from the mouths of people with metal fillings in their teeth. That's not very nice, if you are into kissing.

In Germany, a federal law passed in the mid-nineties prohibits dentists to give mercury fillings to their patients. For the same reason, most North-European countries have limited the use of amalgam, and Sweden, Spain, Austria, and Denmark, among others, also banned this product in the year 2000. The amalgam compounds are so toxic that dentists are instructed not to touch amalgam with bare hands and store excess amalgam in tightly sealed containers. If it is so dangerous to touch amalgam, it certainly is dangerous to keep it in the mouth 24 hours a day, year after year, or get it injected in the blood with the flu vaccine!

The World Health Organization (WHO) issued a report showing that mercury absorbed from amalgam fillings is up to ten times higher than mercury absorbed from environmental and dietary sources. It is noteworthy to point out that patients with Multiple Sclerosis (MS) and Alzheimer's disease have up to ten times the normal mercury levels in their brains. Post-mortem studies show that the mercury level in some organs is directly proportional to the number of amalgam fillings in a diseased person.

The most vulnerable of all to mercury poisoning seems to be the developing fetus in pregnant women. A fetus accumulates more mercury than even the mother does, and in amounts directly proportional to the number of her amalgam fillings. [For the same reason, pregnant women should avoid tuna, salmon and other mercury-containing fish.]

The gradual, continuous release of mercury and other toxic metals into the body by metal fillings affects particularly the liver, kidneys, lungs and brain. Cadmium, for example, which is used to produce the pink color in dentures, is five times as toxic as lead. It does not take much of this metal to raise the blood pressure to abnormal levels. Yet how many people are aware that they are developing a heart condition as a result of the dental fillings in their mouth?

Thallium, which is also found in mercury amalgam fillings, causes leg pain and paraplegia. It affects the nervous system, skin, and cardiovascular system. All wheelchair patients who have been tested for metal poisoning tested positive for thallium. Many people, who were in a wheelchair several years after they received metal fillings, completely recovered once all metal had been removed from the mouth. Thallium is lethal at a dose of 0.5-1.0 gram.

Other metals contained in dental fillings are known for their cancer-producing (carcinogenic) effects. These include nickel, which is used in gold crowns, braces and children's crowns. Also chromium is extremely carcinogenic. All metals corrode, (including gold, silver and platinum) and the body absorbs it. Women with breast cancer have accumulated large amounts of dissolved metals in their breasts. When the mouth is cleared of all metals, they will also leave the breasts and the metal-caused cysts will shrink and disappear by themselves. Yeast infections often improve quickly after removal of metal fillings. Some people report complete relief of prostate problems as well as nose and sinus congestion.

Porcelain can be toxic, too. It is made of aluminum oxide, with other metals added. The body's immune system naturally responds to the presence of toxic metals in the body and eventually develops allergic reactions which may show up as a sinus condition, ringing in the ears, enlarged neck and glands, bloating, enlarged spleen, arthritic symptoms, headaches and migraine, eye diseases, and more serious complications such as paralysis or heart attacks.

Composites

Although metal toxicity may not be the only cause for these conditions, replacing all metal fillings with *composites* certainly assists your immune system in its effort to protect your body against disease. A composite filling is one that is primarily non-metallic. There are a large variety of materials used in composite fillings, but some metals may be present. Ordinary composites are not suitable for large cavities. Whenever used for large cavities, they tend to last no more than five or six years. *Indirect composites*, on the other hand, can be placed in large cavities. They can even be used in place of gold crowns. They look like a real tooth and last as long as gold. If selected properly, indirect composites are quite non-allergenic and non-toxic. They are fairly new and can be as expensive as gold fillings, but they can save you a lot of trouble and money in the long-term. Since many dentists don't know how to place them properly, you may need to do a bit of research to find an experienced mercury-free dentist who also works with indirect composites. The fillings should be replaced cautiously and gradually, one or two (if small ones) at a time. It is best not to replace metal fillings more often than once every two months.

Preventing Heavy Metal Toxicity

If you decide to replace your amalgam fillings, make certain that your dentist provides for protection (through a special plastic device) against the inhalation and absorption of the generated amalgam dust. Otherwise, you may end up suffering severe migraine attacks, memory loss, weakening of eyesight, etc. Before attempting to have any larger fillings removed you may need to take selenium (if possible in ionic form) for one to two months. Eat more foods that contain Vitamin C, such as the supergrain Chia, or red-colored fruits and vegetables, for about ten days. Use cilantro leaves and green leafy vegetables in every main meal to help clear mercury and other metal deposits from the body. Drinking several cups of Pau d'Arco (Lapacho) tea per day, or taking four capsules of its extract three times daily for two weeks may greatly assist you in the detoxification of the blood, liver and kidneys (see section 7 for details on this powerful immune balancer). The kidney cleanse is also very beneficial in preventing injuries from any released metals. The native American tea formula, Ojibwa tea (see section 8), is also excellent for metal removal. It contains large amounts of vitamins.

Metallic Clay - And How To Remove Noxious Metals, Chemicals and Radiation

A safe and direct way to remove noxious chemicals, toxic metals radioactive isotopes (generated by x-ray equipment and other sources) from the body is to take several baths with metallic clay - ideally, using clay bath kits (http://www.magneticclay.com or http://www.magneticclaybaths.com, 800-257-3315) or any other unpolluted bentonite clay. *Calcium Bentonite Clay,* such as Pascalite clay (www.relfe.com) is particularly useful for radiation removal. While lying in the bathtub, apply some wetted clay to the whole head and make a facemask with it. One pound per bath is sufficient. Soak in the water for about half an hour. Let the bathwater stand for a few hours, or overnight, and then drain off the water, but keep the settled clay in the bathtub. Check for black, gold, silver-colored sediments in the clay (metals). Remove the clay.

If a full bath is impractical, take a number of foot baths instead. Soak your feet in bentonite clay for 20-30 minutes in the evenings, let the water sit over night the next day and view at the results the following morning. Like with the full bath, you may find that at the bottom there are with flecks of gold, silver or stuff that looks like black sand. **Note:** although part of the black sand consists of metals, it may partially be due to impurities in the clay.

A note on tooth extractions: In case a tooth needs to be extracted, be aware that tooth extractions can cause lasting illness if the 'cavitations' are not cleaned properly. When a tooth is extracted, dead tissue can be left behind and attract infectious bacteria. This has been known to cause serious lasting fatigue. Cleaning out such cavitations can improve your well-being dramatically.

A note on root canals: Root canals can become a source of sickness in the body. During a root canal operation, the center of the tooth including the nerve is drilled out, leaving behind what is really a dead tooth. The dead tooth may become subject to attack by bacteria that try to eat it away (which is their job). The tooth may become infected, but since there is no nerve left there will also be no pain. Even such minor infections can progressively weaken the immune system and undermine the most basic functions in the body. Pulling a root canal filled tooth is a bit complicated, besides being more expensive, since the tooth will have to be replaced with some kind of bridge. But the alternative (leaving it as is) may end up causing you more harm.

Heal Your Gums and Teeth

A 1980 survey by the U.S. Department of Health and Human Services concluded that only 5 percent of dentists' time is spent in attempting to treat gum disease (gingivitis and periodontitis) and yet the majority of all teeth that are pulled (or fall out) are lost due totally to gum disease! This has not changed since then but has actually become worse. A study conducted by dental authorities in North Carolina states that gum disease in America is "rampant". And it continues to escalate at epidemic proportions.

The diagnosis of the gum disease and its predictable solution is based on over 30 years of study, research, and private practice, of Dr. Robert O. Nara. Dr. Nara is the founder of Oramedics International, the world's only group dedicated to helping people avoid tooth and gum disease rather than treating the results of the disease process with needles, knives, drugs, drilling, pulling and false teeth! Dr. Nara's solution is simple and effective, and it makes sense.

He says that American forefathers used brine to preserve their food and kill bacteria. The same germ-removing action of salt water can be harnessed to keep the gums free of infection. Millions of people have used warm salt water rinses to cure oral abscesses, gum boils, etc. Apparently, the warm salt water helps to draw excessive toxic fluid out of the gum tissue, thereby reducing swelling, alleviating pain, and killing harmful bacteria. This allows the gums to heal and keep the teeth healthy, too. If used in an irrigating device, the warm salt water reaches all gum line crevices and periodontal pockets, which is important for complete reversal of gum disease and tooth decay. Dr. Nara says brushing and flossing are not sufficient to stop gum disease, that's why so many people who followed their dentists' standard advice still wound up with gum disease (infection).

Most people believe that gum disease is caused by plaque. Research studies by Socransky at Forsyth Dental School in Boston, and by Loesche at the University of Michigan showed that the plaque theory does not hold. The presence of up to five different types of destructive bacteria in gum diseases actually shows that plaque and tartar are not primary causal factors, but effects. Healthy gums attract only good bacteria, such as gram-positive *faculative rods* and *cocci* - predominately *Actinomyces* species and *streptococci*. Sick gums attract gram-negative *anaerobic rods* - primarily *Bacteroids* and *Fusobacteria.*

Rinsing or irrigating the mouth with salt water several times a day is usually enough to prevent and reverse gum disease. For situations of advanced gum disease, however, Dr. Nara recommends you also use *Sanguinaria*, a herbal extract, which has been used as a mouth rinse for centuries by native cultures.

Gum disease indicates the presence of large amounts of toxins in the body, especially in the alimentary canal which begins in the mouth and ends in the anus. In addition to the above rinsing procedures, it is also important to address the underlying causes i.e. poor diet, dehydration, irregular lifestyle, congested liver and intestinal tract, and emotional stress.

This is what Jim Humble, the inventor of *Miracle Mineral Supplement* (MMS), said dealing with his own gum issues: "All of my life I have had trouble with my teeth. Most of my teeth were missing and I wore dentures. My gums were quite soft and my teeth were somewhat loose in the gums. They often got sore and at that particular time they started to hurt and I thought I would have to have one or two pulled. Then I finally decided that I should brush my teeth with the MMS…again I was amazed. All of the infection and soreness disappeared in hours. Within a week my gums had hardened up.

Jim recommends the following procedure for abscessed teeth, infected gums, and pyorrhea: "Use six drops in a glass, add ½ teaspoon of vinegar or lemon, or lime, wait three minutes and add ¼ glass of water. Use this solution to brush the teeth. Use a new solution every morning. Do not leave this solution in the mouth for longer than 60 seconds. Expect the pain of an abscessed tooth to be overcome by the immune system in about four hours. Expect all infection and all pyorrhea to be gone in one week. Expect all loose teeth to be rock solid in two weeks. Expect a completely healthy mouth in less than three weeks. Keep in mind that the MMS solution is the most powerful health solution ever developed and it will indeed do exactly what is described here." For more information about MMS, see *Some Of Nature's Greatest Healing Secrets* in this chapter.

Soladey's Dental Solution

I personally use a *Soladey* toothbrush to clean my teeth. Soladey has a patented design that is scientifically and clinically proven to significantly eliminate plaque more effectively than your regular toothbrush, without the use of toothpaste or dental floss. Soladey features a Titanium Oxide (TIO_2) metal rod, which is sensitive to light. It creates a natural ionic chemical reaction that separates the plaque from your teeth enamel and removes tobacco, coffee and other stains using the natural attraction of ions. You might have heard of a room ionizer that also produces ions. Plaque has particles with a positive charge - positive ions, and when the Titanium Rod reacts with light, it creates negative ions that attract the positive ions, like a magnet. The plaque just disintegrates and falls off your teeth washing away when your rinse. Other stains are sucked right out of your teeth using this process.

There have been four clinical trials at four different dental universities in Canada and Japan, and they all found that the people who used Soladey had significantly less plaque on their teeth as compared to the people who used the ordinary brush. The research also showed an improvement in gingivitis. So Soladey works to protect your gums - as well as reducing plaque.

The scientific principals behind Soladey have been around since the 1970s and Soladey has now been sold in Japan for a few years - where it sells two million brush units and five million replacement heads every year. Clinical studies on the effectiveness of Soladey technology to remove dental plaque have been conducted at Osaka Dental University, Nippon Dental University, Nihon University and the University of Saskatchewan in Canada. All institutions certify that Soladey was more effective in the removal of plaque and whitening of dental enamel than any regular bristle toothbrush on the market today. (See *Product Information* or visit www.ener-chi.com/soladey.htm)

Find a dentist who practices toxic-free dentistry at http://www.hugnet.com/
Essential dental health information at: http://mizar5.com/omedia2.htm

How To Give Up Smoking And Other Addictions

Addiction - An Unconscious Signal of Not Being in Control

If you are substance-addicted, this may be accompanied or caused by the inability to fulfill one or more of your deepest desires. Although unconscious of it, you may have this idea that there is a power beyond your control that stops you from achieving your dreams, big or small. You may even admit self-defeat by maintaining the belief that it is just too difficult for you to give up old habits like smoking, drinking alcohol or eating addictive foods.

Many smokers argue that they cannot quit smoking if they constantly see other people smoking. Others do not want to face the possibly unbearable withdrawal symptoms that often accompany a sudden abstinence from smoking. Quite a lot of people managed to quit smoking, but when they suddenly put on a lot of weight, they resumed the habit.

Most smokers who wish to end their addiction feel that they don't have enough willpower to stop smoking. Why are we giving a small cigarette such great power that it is able to rule over our freedom to make conscious choices in our life? Smoking, like any other addictive habit, is merely a symptom of an underlying void or deficiency of some sort. What is really missing in our lives that we continue to desire substitutes? This question is impossible to answer in this context due to a vast number of possible answers, many of which may only be known by the addict himself. But the need to smoke can become very useful in as much as it can reveal and actually overcome this inner lack, whatever it may be.

Instead of criticizing or judging yourself for giving your power to a habit that has the potential to make you ill or kill you, you can learn a great deal from it and make yourself feel complete again. Because you may not be able to understand the underlying message that smoking entails, you tend to resign yourself to the expectation that quitting the habit is a difficult and frustrating task. Yet smoking can make you aware that you are no longer completely in control of your life, and even offer you a way to reclaim that control.

The excuse that "I cannot give up smoking because..." is an unconscious recognition that I am a victim of some kind, and that I am suffering from low self-worth. There is a part of me that I consider weak and inadequate. A part of me is not alive and well. The act of smoking makes me admit in a way that my desire for a cigarette is greater than my desire to stay healthy or, in other words, to love myself. It is very difficult to give up smoking or other addictions for as long as I preserve this underlying weakness, projected by such exclamations as "I can't give it up" or "I go crazy if I don't have my cigarettes".

Learning to Recover Your Free Will

Similar to using a thorn to pull out another thorn, learning to give up the habit of smoking may be one of the most effective ways to uproot any underlying incompetence and dependency in your life. By suppressing or fighting the habitual desire to smoke, you merely feed it with more of your own energies. This all but increases the addiction. Desires want to be fulfilled, or at least we should be able to decide whether we want to fulfill them or not. The addiction to smoking, which reflects a lack in inner competence and completeness, can actually become a very effective method to fill you up again and regain conscious control over your life. What does that mean, you'll ask. Smoking is not the problem you need to combat. Just seeing smoking as an addiction that may have horrible consequences is a depressing notion, and fighting it doesn't raise your self-esteem. Even if you succeed in quitting this habit, you still haven't regained your inner sense of freedom and are likely to develop an addiction to something else, like eating sweets, drinking alcohol or having sex. Instead of waging a war against your anxiety or poor self-confidence, all you need to do is increase that sense of inner freedom to make your own choices in life.

If understood and dealt with properly, smoking can be one of the most important things that has ever happened to you. It can lead you to adopt an entirely new way of thinking, thus reshaping your destiny. If you are a smoker and wish to give up the habit, you first need to understand that your addiction is not an accidental mistake you made during one of your lower moments in life. You have created this habit not to suffer because of it, but to learn from it. It is likely to stay with you or change into another addictive habit until that day when you will have acquired the ability to refer all power of fulfilling your desires back to yourself. Giving up smoking is not about quitting one addictive habit just to adopt another one; it is about recovering your sense of free will.

To use one's willpower to fight an undesirable habit is defeating its purpose and likely to backfire because fighting something is based on the premise that you are being attacked or in some sort of danger. With what we know today about the powerful mind/body connection, the fear that underlies the fight against an addiction is enough to keep the cells of the body jittery, anxious and dysfunctional. They can never find the peace, balance, and energy they need in order to be 'happy' cells for as long as the fear of not being in control prevails in the awareness of their master. The enzyme-based messages that cells are sending to the brain and heart are simple cries for help. The host interprets these signals, though, as depression and nervousness. To 'overcome' the discomfort, at least for a few moments, the host feels compelled to grab the next cigarette or look for another drink. Each time the discomfort reemerges, he or she feels defeated and weakened, and so the addiction carries on.

True willpower, however, is about learning how to make conscious choices. Addictions stick like glue to everyone who wishes to overcome them. They are the 'ghosts of memory' who live in our subconscious and pop up every time the addictive substance is in sight or is imagined. The subsequent urge is not under conscious control, hence the feeling of 'dying' for a cigarette, a cup of coffee, or a bar of chocolate. It is important, though, to realize that **you always have a choice**. This is all you need to learn when it comes to overcoming an addiction.

You cannot successfully exorcise the ghost of memory by throwing away your cigarettes, avoiding your smoking friends, or living in a smoke-free environment. Society has condemned the act of smoking so much that many smokers already feel deprived of that sense of personal freedom they need to feel in order to make their own choices in life. If you are a sensitive person, be aware that a nagging spouse, a doctor, and the warning written on cigarette packs that smoking is harmful to your health may make you feel ridden with guilt. When all of this external pressure succeeds in making you give up smoking, you will continue to feel deprived of your free will and, therefore, look for other more socially acceptable forms of addiction.

Making Smoking a Conscious Choice

We all remember our childhood days when our parents told us not to eat chocolate before lunch or would not allow us to watch television when we wanted. The subconscious mind reacts negatively when it is deprived of its ability to make choices or when it feels forced to do something against its will. Disappointments resulting from not being able to fulfill one's desires can add up and lead to an inner emptiness that wants to be filled. Smoking is simply a subconscious rebellion against the external manipulation of our freedom to choose what we want, and it appears to fill that uncomfortable space within, at least for a little while. However, this inner lack can only subside permanently when we have regained the freedom to make our own choices. You must know that you are free to smoke whenever you like and as often you like. If you have a cigarette and a match to light it, you will certainly find a way to smoke it, too.

The unconscious association of smoking, with all the other 'don'ts' in your past, will be negated by accepting your desire to smoke. I had my first cigarette when I entered high school at age ten. I felt like a criminal because the law said I was only allowed to smoke when I was sixteen years old. My parents were certainly strictly against smoking. Years of hiding my 'secret' from my parents and my teachers left me with no other choice but to continue smoking until I felt I *had* a choice. When I finally got the legal permission to smoke, I lost interest and chose to quit. I was able to give up the habit at once, without any withdrawal symptoms.

The first and most important step to quit smoking is to give yourself permission to smoke. Guilt from the act of smoking will only prevent you from gaining satisfaction and urge you to have another cigarette that may 'at last' give you what you have been looking for. But you are not really looking for the short sensation of satisfaction that smoking provides but for the lost freedom to make your own choices in life. By trying to avoid lighting up, you also deprive yourself of this potential satisfaction. The resistance to smoking creates powerful psychosomatic side effects. These are known as withdrawal symptoms. Symptoms may include depression, lack of interest in life, sleeplessness, anger, nausea, ravenous hunger, obesity, cardiovascular disease, lack of concentration, and shaking. However, these symptoms can only manifest if you believe that you have been deprived of your freedom to smoke.

Choosing To Smoke Less, But...

Don't fight your desire to smoke. Contrary to general belief, to give up smoking you *do not* need to abolish your desire to smoke. **You will start giving up the habit automatically once you choose not to follow your desire to smoke each and every time you have it** (the desire to smoke). This will take the fuel out of your subconscious, rebellious mind and stop you short of becoming a victim of external forces, situations or people. A master of yourself, you can choose to smoke or choose not to smoke. Keep your cigarettes with you as long as you feel you want to have this choice. It may even be a good idea to encourage your desire to smoke by keeping your cigarette pack in front of you, smelling it from time to time. Watch other people around you light up and inhale, imagining that you inhale deeply too. Do not count the days that pass without you smoking and do not look ahead in time either. You neither need to prove to yourself nor to anyone else that you can beat this addiction. In fact, you don't want to beat it all. You want to benefit from it. You are neither a better person if you quit, nor are you a worse person if you don't. You are free to stop smoking today and begin again tomorrow. You will always have this choice, and you will always be only a puff away from being a smoker, just like the rest of us.

The choice of using and training your free will has to be made in the ever-present moment, right now, and has to be done anew repeatedly many times each day. The longer the periods of time during which you actualize your choice not to smoke, the more quickly diminishes your urge to smoke, becoming less intense each day. Whenever the desire to smoke returns, which is possible because the ghost of memory doesn't just leave your subconscious overnight, you are once again compelled to make a new choice. This time, however, your conscious mind finds it much easier to stick with its previous successful choice because of the newly improved self-confidence and self-esteem. Setbacks don't exist in this program; only exercising your freedom of choice does. One way or the other, you are in charge.

The conscious retraining of your mind will benefit your entire life. It will restore your power of using your free will and remove the 'victim' within you. Because you have been told so many times in your life that *you cannot do this* or *cannot do that*, you began to use this belief dogma to accept your addiction as being too difficult to quit. By reclaiming your power of making conscious choices you will be able to break the self-fulfilling 'I can't' pattern in your life for good. This will become a great asset in every part of your life.

Ending the Addiction

Before you decide to stop smoking (or any other addiction), make sure that you are aware of the following points:

- Make ending your addiction a priority in your life.
- Don't try to make too many other changes in your life at the same time.
- Don't reward yourself for ending the habit; quitting is enough of a reward.
- It is good not to tell anyone about your intention to stop smoking because this only undermines your freedom to choose to smoke.
- Carry your cigarettes or tobacco with you, so you can choose to smoke whenever you decide to. Also, people will assume you are still smoking; this way you don't have to prove to anyone that you are capable of quitting the habit.

- Unless for health reasons, don't try to avoid places where other people smoke; you want to remain in charge under all circumstances.
- Realize that unless you are traveling on an airplane or a bus you are always free to smoke whenever you wish to, even if you have to do it out in the cold air.
- Avoid substituting things like tea, coffee, chocolate, chewing gum, more exercise, drinking mineral water, etc. for cigarettes, as they won't satisfy your desire to smoke in the long run.
- Choose a starting time of your program to stop smoking that does not coincide with an emotional upheaval or stressful situation. It is best to link the starting date with a positive event in your life. New moon day is one of the best days to start quitting.
- Think about all the benefits that will come to you when you stop smoking, i.e., better health, less mucus discharge from the lungs, cleaner breath, saving money, etc.
- Acknowledge your desire to smoke when it comes up by saying to yourself: "I really have the desire to smoke now and I feel free to do so, but right now I decide not to smoke." When the desire to smoke returns in an hour or so, you may choose to fulfill it this time. This will teach you to consciously accept your desire to smoke, but not always fulfill it. By choosing not to smoke each time the desire emerges, you train your mind to make conscious choices.
- Often, your desire to smoke is coupled with clues like drinking a cup of coffee, the ringing of the telephone, waiting for a bus or a taxi, or switching on the television set. Your addiction is a 'program' that you have written in your subconscious mind and associated with such clues. As the clues occur, your desire to smoke pops up, too. The next time you want to smoke when the telephone rings, while you drink a cup of coffee, or after you switch on the TV, make the conscious choice to wait for a few minutes until you have the time or opportunity to smoke consciously. Another suggestion is to smoke somewhere in the house or garden where you usually don't smoke. This will sever the ties to your subconscious and make your decision whether to smoke or not a more conscious one.
- Allow your desire to smoke to become quite strong before you actually reach for the cigarette; in other words, you will still have the freedom to smoke but postpone your decision for a while until you really feel the discomfort. Notice where in your body you feel tense, irritable or nervous. It is important to feel how strong your desire to smoke becomes before you light up. Most smokers give into the slightest urge to smoke and do not even notice when they light up. You want to break the pattern of doing things unconsciously.
- To make it easier to quit smoking (or any other addiction), drink half a glass (or more) of water (at room temperature) before you choose to smoke a cigarette every time you have the urge to smoke. Physically speaking, the urge to smoke is directly linked to toxins that were deposited in the connective tissues of the body and are now entering the blood, increasing blood thickness. The thickening of blood generally causes irritation, nervousness and anxiety, even panic. Instead of pushing the toxins back into the connective tissues (as they will surely reemerge) drinking a glass of water will make your blood thinner, which will help to remove the toxins from the body. Thus, the urge to smoke lessens each time you do this and eventually disappears altogether.
- Finally, your addiction to smoking is not something terrible that you need to get rid of. It is rather an opportunity to train yourself to become the master of your destiny. In this sense, your addiction can become one of the very best teachers you have ever had.

Summary of the Technique to Stop Smoking:

1. Whenever you feel the urge to smoke, repeat to yourself: **"I want to smoke now."** This will bring your desire to smoke from your subconscious into your conscious mind and allow you enough time to make the conscious choice of whether to smoke or not to smoke. Drinking half a glass of water also brings the desire into your conscious mind.

2. Then say to yourself: **"I have the free choice to smoke now."** If you do not remind yourself of your inherent freedom of making choices, your subconscious, addicted mind may believe that you can't smoke anymore and may go into a state of rebellion. This may cause withdrawal symptoms.

3. If you feel a desperate need to smoke, acknowledge your desire by saying: **"I choose to begin smoking again."** Before you reach for a cigarette check whether this is what you really want. Or you may repeat to yourself: **"For the moment I accept that I want to smoke, but I choose not to at this time."** Think about how you would feel if you stopped smoking altogether.

Follow this simple sequence every time you have the desire to smoke. The technique is fool proof because you cannot go wrong, whatever the outcome. Whether you decide to continue smoking or not, you have begun to become 'aware' and exercised your free will - a prerequisite to consciously taking charge of your life. The majority of people who follow this simple program give up smoking within one week, others take a little longer. How long it takes to quit is not important. What is important, though, is that you experience a major positive shift in your thinking and in your attitude towards yourself and others.

All the research studies which show that smoking is a hazard to your health have missed the point. Instead of condemning people who smoke, we should show them ways to learn from this addictive habit as we can learn from any other problem in life.

This technique works equally well for any other addiction, including coffee, alcohol, drugs, sleeping pills, sugar, salt, sex, and even work. I suggest that you read this section as often as it takes to familiarize yourself with the major points, or at least once a week.

<u>Some Of Nature's Greatest Healing Secrets</u>

Amazing Food Cures

Hippocrates was the first physician in the Western Hemisphere to state that food is man's best medicine. It is very obvious that if food can nourish and create healthy, strong bodies, it must also be able to heal them if they are ill. Research on naturally grown foods is the least biased and most authentic of all because there is no drug company or manipulative food industry that could take advantage of these findings and market something that is already freely available to everyone.

I have listed just a few examples out of hundreds of foods which all have some amazing healing properties. It can be said that by not eating enough foods made by Mother Nature, a person is most likely to fall ill sooner or later. On the other hand, eating from her table, you may never become ill in the first place. But if you are ill now, in your search for a real cure to your ailment, you may discover that food is still the best medicine you can buy.

When you consider using foods as medicine, please refer to your body type charts to check whether these foods are actually beneficial for you. Although the foods listed below may have great potential healing properties, if your body is not designed to utilize them (for example, Vata types don't do well with broccoli), or is otherwise unable to digest them properly, they may not do you any good regardless of what nutrients they contain.

Broccoli's Anti-Cancer Properties

Small quantities of fresh broccoli sprouts contain as much cancer protection as larger amounts of the mature vegetable sold in food markets, according to researchers at Johns Hopkins University. You would have to eat about two pounds of mature broccoli a week in order to reduce, say, your risk of colon cancer, by about 50 percent. Although this is certainly possible, just 5 grams (0.17 ounces) of broccoli sprouts contain concentrations of the compound *glucoraphanin* equal to that found in 150 grams (5.2 ounces) of mature broccoli. The active compound is a precursor to *sulforaphane*, proven in animal studies to boost cell enzymes that protect against molecular damage from cancer-causing chemicals.

Like other cruciferous vegetables, broccoli speeds up removal of estrogen from the body, helping suppress breast cancer. It has also anti-viral, anti-ulcer activity. In addition, broccoli is a super source of chromium that helps regulate insulin and blood sugar.

Note for the Vata type: You may still benefit somewhat from broccoli and other cruciferous vegetables if you cook them with a good amount of oil or butter.

Cabbage - The Romans' Cancer Cure

Cabbage was revered in ancient Rome as a cancer cure. Today, we know its cancer-curing effects are from its numerous anti-cancer and antioxidant compounds. Cabbage speeds up estrogen metabolism, which is thought to help block breast cancer and suppress growth of polyps, a prelude to colon cancer. According to research, eating cabbage more than once a week cut men's colon cancer odds by as much as 66 percent.

As little as two daily tablespoons of cooked cabbage protected subjects against stomach cancer. Cabbage also contains powerful anti-ulcer compounds; its juice has shown to help heal ulcers in humans. It even has anti-bacterial and anti-viral properties. Red cabbage has twice the fiber as white cabbage. It is known for its balancing effects on blood cholesterol. Cauliflower and Brussels sprouts have similar benefits.

Bok choy, which is brimming with minerals, has been found to lower high blood pressure by 30 points or more. No need for expensive prescription drugs that ruin your liver, kidneys and digestive systems.

Cauliflower Helps With Breast Cancer

Cauliflower is a cruciferous family member that contains many of the same cancer-fighting, hormone-regulating compounds as its cousins, broccoli and cabbage. Cauliflower is one of the least popular vegetables, but this doesn't make it less important. Researchers have found it helps women to break down estrogen and produce estrogen-byproducts in a safe way, slashing breast cancer risk by 40 percent. It also helps ward off colon cancers.

The Great Carrot Phenomenon

Carrots are a rich source of beta carotene, a powerful anti-cancer, artery-protecting, immune-boosting and infection-fighting antioxidant. Recent research has shown that a single carrot a day slashed stroke rates in women by 68 percent! No drug can even get close to that. Even beta carotene supplements had no benefits at all, according to a recent study (2007). If you are or were a smoker, the beta-carotene in one medium carrot cuts your lung cancer risk in half.

Your eyes will be grateful for that carrot per day as well. It has been shown that high doses of beta carotene, as found in carrots, substantially reduces odds of degenerative eye diseases (cataracts and macular degeneration). It also helps with chest pain (angina). The high soluble fiber in carrots balances blood cholesterol and promotes regularity. Cooking has shown to make it easier for the body to absorb the beta-carotene.

Celery - Better Than Viagra

Celery has long been known to be one of the best foods to keep your blood pressure normal. It dilates blood vessels like most potent drugs, but without the harmful side effects. Who would have thought, though, that this common food could turn out to be far more effective than Viagra or any other sex-enhancing drug ever produced? According to an exhaustive study of purported aphrodisiac foods, celery is the 'sexiest' substance on earth. This unlikely-sounding candidate combines ideal amounts of vitamin E, magnesium, niacin, potassium and zinc - all required for optimum sex.

And it gets even better. Celery contains *arginine*, a natural amino acid that expands blood vessels much like Viagra. Yet, unlike Viagra, arginine also increases blood flow to the clitoris and makes female genitals more responsive.

Furthermore, the actual aroma of celery contains two steroids called *androsterone* and *androstenol*. The research showed that the subtle odor of these two chemicals travels through the nose and attracts the opposite sex.

Celery has other benefits, too. It contains an ingredient *acetylenics*, which has been shown to stop the growth of cancer cells. Celery is an excellent source of organic sodium, which gives it a slightly salty taste. Along with potassium, sodium helps to maintain the body's electrolyte balance. Sodium is also necessary for hydrochloric acid production in the stomach and is involved in many glandular secretions. Celery is also an excellent source of vitamin C, a vitamin that helps to support the immune system.

Celery is a natural diuretic, and thus useful in circulatory disorders, such as high blood pressure and lymphatic congestion. Chinese physicians have long used celery to dependably reduce blood pressure. Now scientists have discovered exactly why it works so well. Celery contains unique oil which relaxes the muscles that regulate blood pressure, improving flow, and lowering pressure. Just a few stalks every other day (or some celery juice, perhaps, combined with carrot juice) do the trick.

Avocado - The Delicious Super Fruit

Avocado is a very dense fruit, packed with nutrients. It is especially rich in vitamin A. It also contains plenty of B vitamins, especially niacin, folic acid, calcium, iron, 9 essential amino acids, and a mountain of potassium.

The avocado has shown to benefit circulation, lower cholesterol, and dilate blood vessels. It's true, avocados are high in fat - one reason they've earned the nickname 'butter pear'. But it's primary fat, monounsaturated oleic acid (also concentrated in olive oil), acts as an antioxidant to block LDL cholesterol. A 1996 study by researchers at the Instituto Mexicano del Seguro Social in Mexico looked at the health benefits of daily avocado consumption. The 45 subjects who ate avocados every day for just one week experienced an average of 17 percent drop in total blood cholesterol. Their cholesterol ratio also changed in a healthy way: Their LDL (low-density lipoprotein) and triglycerides dropped significantly while their HDL (high-density lipoprotein) levels climbed.

Avocados are also rich in *beta-sitosterol,* which was shown to reduce cholesterol in 16 human studies. Beta-sitosterol is a widely prescribed anti-cholesterol drug that interferes with cholesterol absorption, but has serious side effects. Avocados have four times the amount found in oranges that had previously been cited as the richest fruit source of beta-sitosterol.

Avocado has also been found to have three times the amount of *glutathione* than in any other fruit. Glutathione is a powerful antioxidant shown to block thirty different carcinogens and proliferation of the AIDS virus in test tube experiments. Studies have revealed a strong correlation between increased glutathione intake (from food) and decreased risk of oral and pharyngeal cancer.

I have been eating avocado in my daily lunch salad (avoid eating it in the evening) for over 20 years and found it to be one of the most nutritious foods around.

Mashing an avocado and rubbing it into your hair for five minutes after washing will add luster to your hair; rinse afterwards. In South Africa, an avocado mask made of mashed avocados, honey, and lime juice is applied to the face as a moisturizing treatment to counteract the drying effects of the hot sun.

Blueberries and Cranberries Protect Kidneys, Heart, Eyes, Skin

Urinary tract infections (UTI's) are triggered by bacteria, primarily E. coli, adhering to the walls of the bladder or kidney. Many scientific studies have found that blueberries and cranberries are beneficial in fighting UTIs by blocking or prohibiting the growth of bacteria. Cranberry juice has traditionally been known to clear up a bladder infection or urinary tract infection within one to two days. Take two to three ounces of juice three to four times per day, about ½ hour before meals and just before going to sleep.

Research shows that blueberries contain high concentrations of antioxidant compounds with medicinally beneficial properties. Blueberry's reported medicinal benefits include preventing urinary tract infections, stimulating anti-cancer activity, reducing heart disease risk, strengthening collagen, regulating blood sugar, improving night vision, reducing replication of the HIV virus, and treating diarrhea.

Cranberries are rich in bioflavonoids and natural vitamin C which stimulate the immune system and ward off infection. Just eating cranberries during the wintertime can prevent colds and the flu. In addition, cranberries can reduce the occurrence of kidney stones. They can also help dilate the bronchial tubes during an asthma attack. They are even beneficial for acne sufferers. Cranberries prevent acne-causing bacteria from entering the skin, so breakouts are less frequent and less severe.

The malic acid contained in cranberries helps soften stones in the bile ducts of the liver, and thus may be helpful in the preparatory phase of the liver cleanse. It is best to use a pure form of organic, concentrate which can be diluted at the ratio of one part juice to four parts water.

The Healing Power in Green Beans

Also known as snap beans, green beans are loaded with nutrients of significant medicinal value. They are an excellent source of vitamin K (154.9 percent of the daily value in one cup). Vitamin K is essential for maintaining strong bones.

Greens beans are also a rich source of the equally important vitamin A (notably through their concentration of carotenoids, including beta-carotene). And, as you may know, when you chew on green beans they contain loads of useful fiber, which helps prevent colon cancer. In addition, green beans are packed with vitamin C, riboflavin, potassium, iron, manganese, folate, magnesium, and thiamin. Plus, they are a good source of thiamin, phosphorous, calcium, niacin, vitamin B6, copper, protein and zinc.

For arteriosclerosis, diabetic heart disease (diabetis-caused heart disease), and stroke, few foods compare to green beans in their number of helpful nutrients. Magnesium and potassium work together to help decrease high blood pressure, while folate and vitamin B6 help convert the potentially dangerous protein molecule *homocysteine* into other, benign molecules. Homocysteine can directly damage blood vessel walls if not promptly converted; high levels are associated with a significantly increased risk of heart attack and stroke.

The iron content in green beans is twice as high as in spinach. This useful plant iron comes in ionic, organic form, unlike the toxic rust (iron oxide) contained in food supplements and breakfast cereals. Iron is an integral component of hemoglobin, which transports oxygen from the lungs to all body cells, and is also part of key enzyme systems for energy production and metabolism. To properly utilize iron for hemoglobin synthesis the body requires copper, which is also amply present in green beans.

The vitamins C, A, and Zinc present in green beans help to maintain optimal immune function and acne-free skin. Last but not least, green beans help maintain your memory with thiamin (Vitamin B1).

The many nutrients in green beans can help to prevent a number of different conditions, including Alzheimer's, arteriosclerosis, diabetic heart disease, colon cancer, asthma, arthritis, acne, ear infections, and even colds and flu.

Note: Green beans contain a measurable amount of oxalates. So if you suffer from oxalic acid stones in the kidneys, make certain to cleanse your kidneys before eating green beans on a regular basis.

The Bone-Building Power of Brussels Sprouts

By age 70, one of every two women in the United States will likely suffer a painful fracture due to weak bones. Hip fractures are often fatal. But, a recent woman's study shows that by eating a 3-ounce serving of Brussels sprouts several times a week, women can slash the risk of a hip fracture by 30 percent. In addition, phytochemicals found in Brussels sprouts enhance the activity of the body's natural defense systems to protect against disease, including cancer. Scientists have found that *sulforaphane*, a potent phytonutrient found in Brussels sprouts and other *brassica* vegetables, boosts the body's detoxification enzymes.

Brussels sprouts are a good source of fiber and folate and an excellent source of vitamin C. Vitamin C supports immune function and the manufacture of collagen, a protein that forms the basic substance of body structures including the skin, connective tissue, cartilage, and tendons. In addition, a cup of Brussels sprouts contains a whopping 1122 IU of vitamin A, plus 669 IU of beta-carotene, both of which are important for defending the body against infection and promoting supple, glowing skin.

Artichoke—For Good Digestion

The artichoke (*Cynara scolymus*) has been known for centuries for its beneficial effects on digestion. Its most noted effect is increased bile production. Because the body uses cholesterol to make bile acids, increasing bile acid production may balance blood cholesterol. Increasing bile acid secretions also aids digestion - one reason why artichokes have traditionally been used for indigestion. Its leaves contain phytonutrients with numerous health-enhancing effects.

Kale

This nutritious vegetable comes in quite a few variations and colors - green and purple being the most common. It is part of a typical traditional diet in parts of Africa where people live very long and healthy lives.

Kale is a rich source of various anti-cancer compounds. Being a member of the cruciferous family, it is endowed with anti-cancer indoles that help regulate estrogen and fight off colon cancer. It contains more beta carotene than spinach and twice as much lutein, the most of any vegetable tested. Kale is also high in the antioxidant Vitamin C. Collard Greens and other green leafy vegetables share similar benefits.

Nuts

All nuts have anti-cancer and heart-protective properties. Almonds and walnuts particularly help balance cholesterol levels. Both contain high concentrations of antioxidant oleic acid and mono-unsaturated fat, similar to that in olive oil, known to protect arteries from damage. Almonds, however, seem to be the most valuable of the two. A total of six studies showed the resounding results of the almond's ability to lower total and LDL cholesterol and reduce the risk of heart disease by 10 percent. All it takes is to eat one small handful of almonds (1 ounce) a day. It is best to remove the skin by putting the almonds into boiled water for a few minutes. Soaking the almonds overnight makes them more digestible.

Nuts generally are high in antioxidant vitamin E, shown to protect against chest pain and artery damage. Brazil nuts are extremely rich in selenium, an antioxidant also linked to lower rates of heart disease and cancer. Walnuts contain ellagic acid, an antioxidant and cancer-inhibitor, and are high in omega-3 type oil.

Nuts are also good regulators of insulin and blood sugar, preventing steep rises. This makes them appropriate foods for those with glucose intolerance and diabetes. It is interesting to note that nuts have been found lacking in the diets of those who later develop Parkinson's disease.

Beware of allergies and rancid nuts: Nuts, particularly peanuts (which are actually legumes), are a prime cause of acute allergic reactions in susceptible individuals. Avoid nuts that are broken, for they become rancid easily. Nut butters are also notorious for causing adverse reactions in the digestive system. When ground and, thereby, exposed to oxygen, they easily oxidize, i.e., become rancid. Rancid fats are very toxic and a major cause of illness. They can even cause irritable bowel syndrome and Crohn's disease. Eat only fresh nuts, or if you prepare fresh nut butter, make sure to consume it in no less than two to three days. Avoid eating nuts that come mixed up with dried fruits or in commercially produced breakfast cereals (the nuts are pre-rancid or rancid, and the dried fruits contain fungi).

Note: All nuts and seeds (and also grains) should ideally be soaked overnight, after which they can be heat-dried in the oven for 6-12 hours, and stored in a dry container. Soaking removes phytic acid, which can combine with important minerals in the intestinal tract and block their absorption, and thereby cause serious mineral deficiencies. Soaking also neutralizes toxic enzyme inhibitors that prevent digestion of proteins.

Chia - Ancient Supergrain

Chia - a white variety of the 'Salvia Hispanica L' plant - possesses an astonishing assortment of oils, vitamins and minerals. This ancient supergrain was part of a 6-month study, headed by famed scientist and pioneer of the functional foods movement, Dr. Vladimir Vuksan - one of the developers of the revolutionary glycemic index at the University of Toronto. For the research, Vuksan used a brand of chia called *Salba®*.

The following are a few of the many superior nutritional properties Dr Vuksan discovered. An amount of 3 ½ ounces of Chia has:

- the highest known whole food source of omega-3s found in nature (it contains as much omega-3 as 28 ounces of Atlantic salmon);
- more calcium than three cups of whole milk ;
- higher, and more bioavailable protein content than soy, and more vegetable protein content than1½ cups of kidney beans;
- highest natural fiber content of any food - more fiber than 1 ¼ cups of all-bran cereal;
- the iron equivalent of 3 cups of raw spinach;
- the potassium content of 1 1/2 bananas;
- as much vitamin C as 7 oranges;
- an antioxidant capacity 3 times the strength of blueberries with Myrecetin counts 270 times the strength of red wine.

Chia is safe for diabetics and those suffering from Celiac disease or gluten allergy.

Dr. Vuksan and his colleagues concluded that chia "could be considered the world's most nutritious food crop and thus can be used as a global remedy for world hunger". In separate studies, Dr Vuksan demonstrated that chia

- reduced after-meal blood glucose and plasma insulin levels;
- lowered C-Reactive protein, a marker of inflammation, by 40 percent;
- significantly lowered the systolic and diastolic blood pressure (>10mm/5mmGH);
- decreased coagulation (blood thinning) by 30 percent;
- had no adverse effect on glycemic control or blood lipids as previously seen with high doses of omega-3 fatty acids.

There is evidence that (Salvia hispanica L), called 'chia' by the ancient Aztecs, was first used as food as early as 3500 B.C. and served as a cash crop in central Mexico between 1500 and 900 B.C. The Aztecs ate the seeds of this semitropical plant to improve their endurance. They called it their 'running food' because messengers could purportedly run all day on just a handful. They also used it as medicine. Chia can be taken in its whole form or ground when used in cooking. Chia can be added to cereal, salads, beverages, and used in baking. Refrigerate chia after grinding. It can be found by searching 'chia seeds' on the Internet. I have provided one inexpensive source for chia seeds under *Product Information.*

Fresh Corn Can Help Reverse Vision Problems

Almost every person with age-related macular degeneration, which is the leading cause of blindness, suffers from lutein-deficiency. A recent study showed that consuming 6 mg of lutein in your food per day reduces your risk of this disorder by a whopping 43 percent. Fresh corn is an excellent source of lutein.

Rice

This common food has anti-diarrheal and anti-cancer properties. Like other grains, rice contains anti-cancer protease inhibitors. Of all grains and cereals, it is the least likely to provoke bowel distress, such as intestinal gas or spastic colon. In Vata types, whole rice (brown) is excellent for constipation; it lowers cholesterol and tends to block development of kidney stones. For Pitta types, white Basmati rice is preferable (they don't do well with rough fiber and the high concentration of plant antibodies in brown rice).

Basmati rice appears to have the highest nutritious value. It is a rich source of iron, selenium, thiamine and niacin. It contains also a good amount of vegetable protein.

Coconut Oil - A Gift from the Tropics

Virgin coconut oil is rich in lauric acid, a proven antiviral and antibacterial agent. It is currently being used in treating AIDS. Monolaurin is a monoglyceride of lauric acid. Lauric acid is also found in human mother's milk, which makes coconut milk an excellent alternative to milk-formula foods. In fact, coconut milk has been used in the tropics to bring up very healthy children when breast milk was unavailable.

Delicious-tasting coconut oil is not only satisfying to your taste buds, but it also cleanses your colon by gently softening and loosening old fecal material, and helping to remove it without unpleasant side effects. It has a strongly alkalizing effect in the body, which is beneficial for every disease process. The tropical oil has a substance that has been shown to raise HDL cholesterol levels, the good kind, thereby lowering the risk of heart attack.

For those who are concerned about infestation with intestinal parasites and Candida albicans, coconut's anti-parasitic properties help purge pathogenic organisms by robbing them of their protective coating. A natural anti-yeast treatment, coconut oil has been known for many centuries to prevent yeast infections in women in the Pacific islands. During scientific tests, both capric and lauric acid (found in coconut oil in very large amounts) were found to be absolutely lethal to all major strains of Candida albicans.

Research comparing Pacific Islanders with people from several developed nations showed that their health was extremely good compared to Western standards. These Islanders had no signs of kidney disease or hypothyroidism that might influence fat levels. There was no hypercholesterolemia (high blood cholesterol). All inhabitants were lean and healthy despite a very high saturated-fat diet from coconut oil. In fact, the population as a whole had ideal weight-to-height ratios as compared to the Body Mass Index figures used by nutritionists. Digestive problems were rare. Constipation was uncommon.

They averaged two or more bowel movements a day. Atherosclerosis, heart disease, colitis, colon cancer, hemorrhoids, ulcers, diverticulitis, and appendicitis are conditions with which they were generally unfamiliar.

Coconut oil also assists with dissolving and removing toxins that are trapped in fatty deposits, thereby making fat accumulation increasingly unnecessary (accumulation of fat is a survival mechanism to keep toxins engulfed within fatty tissue). This may explain why coconut oil helps to build lean muscles. Many body builders, personal trainers, Olympic athletes, and others use it for building lean body mass.

Coconut oil is easily digested, even by weak and compromised digestive systems. It is the only oil that doesn't require bile to digest it, which makes it useful for those whose gallbladder has been removed. Coconut oil assists with most digestive disorders, such as Crohn's disease and irritable bowel syndrome. This oil does not require any enzymes or carriers to be transported across cell membranes. Once it has reached the cell interior, it is used for energy. This makes coconut a readily available energy source.

Coconut oil has also been shown to balance hypothyroidism. It is a saturated fat made up primarily of medium chain fatty acids. Also known as medium chain triglycerides (MCTs), medium chain fatty acids are known to increase metabolism, and promote weight loss, and immobilize yeast bacteria. If required, coconut oil raises basal body temperatures while increasing metabolism, which is great news for those suffering low thyroid functions, and those afflicted with Chronic Fatigue Syndrome.

Coconut oil is useful for the very young and the very old. It is one of the healthiest and safest oils. Unlike most oils, coconut oil will not oxidize upon heating. This makes coconut oil the ideal cooking oil. With the exception of Kapha types, the average adult can safely include about 3.5 tablespoons of coconut oil per day in their diet. It will not make you fat. But, start out with a low dose until you find out how the breakdown of yeast affects you. Apart from its internal benefits, when applied to the skin, coconut oil will protect from sunburn, drying, chapping and harmful germs.

A Banana a Day May Keep the Doctor Away

When you compare it to an apple, the banana has four times the protein, twice the carbohydrates, three times the phosphorus, five times the vitamin A and iron, and twice the other vitamins and minerals. It is also rich in potassium and is one of the best value foods around. Bananas contain three natural sugars - sucrose, fructose and glucose - combined with fiber. In this form a banana gives an instant, sustained and substantial boost of energy (otherwise, the sugar could be harmful). Research has shown that just two bananas can provide enough energy for a strenuous 90-minute workout. The banana has also been found helpful for a number of illnesses and conditions:

Depression: Depressed people often feel better after eating a banana. This is because bananas contain tryptophan, a type of protein that the body converts into serotonin. This powerful hormone is known to make you relax, improve your mood and generally make you feel happier.

PMS: The banana's vitamin B6 helps regulate blood glucose levels, which can positively affect your mood and calm the nervous system.

Anemia: High in organic iron (versus inorganic iron used in supplements), bananas can stimulate the production of hemoglobin in the blood and thereby improve anemia.

Blood Pressure and Brain Power: High in potassium, yet low in sodium, bananas are very effective in balancing blood pressure. This effect led the U.S. Food and Drug Administration to allow the banana industry to make official claims for the fruit's ability to reduce the risk of blood pressure and stroke.

And, for the same reasons, students were found to be more alert and to show increased academic performance when eating bananas regularly.

Constipation: High in fiber, bananas in the diet have helped restore normal bowel functions in people suffering from constipation.

Heartburn: Having a natural antacid effect, bananas have helped people suffering with heartburn. Banana neutralizes over-acidity and reduces irritation by coating the lining of the stomach.

Morning Sickness: Snacking on bananas between meals helps to keep blood sugar levels up and avoid morning sickness.

Mosquito bites: If bitten by an insect, try rubbing the affected area with the inside of a banana skin. Banana skin is known for reducing swelling and irritation.

Nerves: Bananas are high in B vitamins that help calm the nervous system.

S.A.D.: Bananas can help SAD sufferers because they contain the natural mood enhancer tryptophan.

Smoking: Bananas have also helped people trying to give up smoking. The B6, B12 and the potassium and magnesium found in them, help the body recover from the effects of nicotine withdrawal.

Stress: The banana's potassium helps normalize the heartbeat, sends oxygen to the brain and regulates the body's water balance. During stress, our metabolic rate rises; this in turn drops potassium levels. Bananas can reverse this effect of stress.

Strokes: According to research published in The New England Journal of Medicine, eating bananas as part of a regular diet can cut the risk of death by stroke by as much as 40 percent!

Please note that the above food recommendations do not apply to all body types equally. Before you start eating these foods, verify with your body type food charts whether these foods are beneficial for you or not.

SHOULD WE EAT ORGANIC FOODS?

For the reasons given below, the answer is a definite 'yes'. Whether you are able to afford to buy organic foods or even have access to such foods is a question that only you can answer. Organic foods are still very expensive when compared with pesticide-treated produce. If your budget is very limited, but you still want to feed your body the best possible food available, you may either need to grow your own fruits and vegetables or increase your spending on food.

In a report on organic foods, published in 'Coronary and Diabetic Care' in the U.K. in 2004, it was stressed that the use of pesticides in food production correlated with a significant reduction in the health benefits of foods. For example, there exists a strong connection between pesticide use and the antioxidant content of food. Crops that are visited and stressed by insects are known to produce *polyphenolic* compounds, which are naturally potent antioxidants. These compounds not only ward off insects, but also increase the nutritional value of the plants. However, when crops are treated with pesticides, they don't need the natural protection of polyphenolics, and produce less of these compounds.

Foods that contain pesticides are not only less beneficial in the nutritional sense, but also quite harmful. The U.K. report noted that pesticide use has been associated with a variety of health risks, including cancer, fetal abnormalities, chronic fatigue, and Parkinson's disease. One study showed that women with breast cancer are five to nine times more likely to have traces of pesticides in their blood than women who don't have the cancer. If you are concerned about breast cancer, you may definitely need to weigh the risks of cancer against budgetary stress.

Furthermore, organic foods are free of food additives such as MSG, hydrogenated fats, and artificial sweeteners and coloring agents, which have been associated with a risk of asthma, headaches, growth retardation, and hyperactivity in children. As the U.K. report further pointed out, these additives have been linked to the development of allergies.

Another advantage of organic food is that it is free of genetically modified (GM) organisms. The report notes that only ten studies of GM foods have been conducted so far. Among those, the ones that were completely independent of funding or input from companies with GM affiliations found evidence of harmful effects in the gut lining of humans.

Overall, organic foods have been found to be more nutritious than conventionally grown foods. In one study comparing the vitamin and mineral content of organic foods versus non-organic foods, the organics showed higher levels in all 21 of the examined nutrients. For example, the vitamin C and magnesium levels in the organic foods were 27 percent and 29 percent higher, respectively, compared to the non-organic samples. The study also showed minerals to be significantly higher in organic spinach, potatoes, cabbage, and lettuce.

So, if you have a choice, choose organic foods over chemically treated foods. This may burden your budget somewhat, but will lift the burden on your stomach.

Cinnamon - Medicine for Diabetics

Who would have thought that this culinary spice possesses numerous profound healing properties! Taking one-quarter to one-half teaspoon of cinnamon works just as well as the statin drugs in lowering cholesterol and triglycerides as well as blood glucose. Plus, you can get a pound of cinnamon for less than $5, and save yourself dreadful side effects.

According to research conducted by the U.S. Department of Agriculture, cinnamon helps to control blood sugar levels in type 2 diabetics. Ground cinnamon helps stimulate the production of glucose-burning enzymes and boosts insulin's effectiveness. In one study, cinnamon made insulin 20 times more capable of breaking down blood sugars. To benefit type 2 diabetes you will need to eat about ½ teaspoon of ground cinnamon per day. [According to other research, diabetics also benefit from ground fenugreek, turmeric, ginger, bitter melon extract, bilberry extract and gymnema sylvestre extract; the latter has been shown to heal damaged pancreas cells.] Cinnamon has also been shown to lower triglycerides and cholesterol levels, and to prevent and improve heart disease.

More recent research shows that cinnamon does more than just ward off diabetes and heart disease. It

- supports digestive function;
- constricts and tones tissues;
- relieves congestion;
- alleviates pain, inflammation, and stiffness of muscles and joints;
- eases menstrual discomfort;
- stimulates circulation;
- neutralizes destructive bacteria, including E. coli.

Cinnamon also makes you smarter. In a study testing cognitive abilities, participants were given cinnamon, both orally and nasally. The conclusion of the study was that cinnamon is effective in enhancing cognitive functions. Cinnamon also reportedly scores high as an aphrodisiac for males.

So whether you use cinnamon to improve your health, your mental capacity, your love life, or all of the above, it makes good sense to include cinnamon in your diet whenever possible. You may add it to your cereals, vegetables or favorite beverage, such as herbal tea.

Scientists have also discovered that curry powder (mainly turmeric, cumin, cardamom, coriander, ginger, red pepper, fenugreek and fennel) with cinnamon, bay leaves and cloves triples the effectiveness of insulin. What a delicious way to help diabetes and numerous other disorders!

Turmeric - A Powerful Decongestant and Anti-Cancer Drug

Turmeric, *Curcuma longa* is the bright yellow constituent of curry powder. Medicinally, it is both an *adaptogen* and a *bioprotectant*. Practitioners of Ayurvedic medicine have used turmeric for millennia. The active principles, known as 'Curcuminoids', possess anti-inflammatory properties comparable in strength to steroidal and nonsteroidal drugs. Curcuminoids are distinguished further for their antiviral, antibacterial, antifungal, antiparasitic, antimutagen, anticancer and detoxifying properties. Curcuminoids prevent the formation of free radicals while scavenging and neutralizing those already formed.

Traditionally, turmeric has been used to treat jaundice and other liver problems, promote circulation, dissolve blood clots, relieve the pain of arthritis and rheumatism, and cure diarrhea, sinus congestion, and ear infections. Today, it is also used by AIDS patients as an alternative, organic, natural herbal medicinal remedy to relieve throat and chest congestion. You can add generous amounts of turmeric to your cooked foods every day. Added to vegetables, rice, beans, soups, etc., turmeric does not just taste delicious, but is also healthy.

Turmeric can be applied externally (as a paste) to help heal hemorrhoids, wounds, cuts, and burns (but beware of its yellow-staining effect).

Curcumin, the main ingredient in turmeric, has now been shown to be a potential cancer preventive or treatment, according to a report by Johns Hopkins University. A laboratory study published in the journal, *Clinical Cancer Research* (Volume 12, page 5346), looked at the effects of curcumin on cell activity and found it interferes with neurotensin, a gastrointestinal hormone suspected of setting off the cancer process in colon cells. Apparently, University of Texas researchers treated some human colorectal cancer cells with neurotensin, with and without curcumin. They confirmed that neurotensin started a chain reaction of chemicals that can increase the growth of cancer and also the migration of cancer cells and that curcumin blocked the process. The researchers concluded that curcumin may have the potential to both treat and prevent colon cancer and other cancers.

Ginger Combats Motion Sickness and More

Conducted by Svensborg Hospital in Denmark, a seasickness trial and clinical study has shown that ginger was as effective as, or superior to, over-the-counter drugs in dealing with motion sickness. It is indeed a safer option than over-the-counter drugs, which cause drowsiness. In another clinical trial conducted by the Department of Anesthesiology at St. Bartholomew's Hospital in London, researchers were able to show that 1 gram of ginger powder was as effective, and much safer, at preventing postoperative nausea and vomiting as the tranquilizer commonly used by hospitals.

Ginger is also effective in relieving the severity of nausea and vomiting of pregnancy. Using ginger to quell morning sickness does not raise the risk of birth defects, according to a new study co-authored by Dr. Gideon Koren, director of the Motherisk Program at the Hospital for Sick Children in Toronto,

Canada. The sickness-reducing effects seem more pronounced when the ginger is taken along with some honey.

Ginger has been used in Ayurvedic medicine for the treatment of inflammation and rheumatism. Indian research showed that a highly purified and standardized ginger extract had a statistically significant effect on reducing symptoms of osteoarthritis of the knee.

Research confirms that ginger acts as an anti-thrombotic and anti-inflammatory agent in humans. It has shown to have antibiotic properties in test tubes (kills salmonella and staph bacteria), and acts as an anti-ulcer agent in animals. Also, it has anti-depressant, anti-diarrheal and strong antioxidant activity. Ginger is also high in anti-cancer activity.

Ginger has been successfully used in the treatment of vomiting, headaches, chest congestion, cholera, colds, diarrhea, stomachache, and nervous diseases.

Other research on *gingerols* demonstrated, the active components of ginger (the rhizome of Zingiber officinale, Roscoe), represent a potential new class of platelet activation inhibitors. Ginger's blood thinning effects provide great benefits for heart disease patients.

Chewing on a small piece of fresh ginger with a little honey, drinking some water with a few drops of ginger extract, or taking capsules of ginger powder are the best options of choice. To stimulate gastric juices, take some grated ginger with a pinch of unrefined sea salt before meals.

Cayenne pepper - To Protect your Heart and Stomach

According to research by Italian doctors, red pepper powder (cayenne) has been shown to reduce symptoms in more than half of patients suffering with functional dyspepsia. The subjects consumed 2.5 grams of red pepper powder each day (divided into capsules taken before each of three meals).

Many herbalists believe that Cayenne not only aids the digestive system, but also benefits the heart and circulatory system. It acts as a catalyst and increases the effectiveness of other herbs when used with them. Cayenne is very rich in vitamins A & C, has the complete B complexes, and is very high in organic calcium and potassium, which is one of the reasons it is good for the heart. Cayenne has been known to stop heart attacks within 30 seconds (a teaspoon of Cayenne extract in a glass of hot water every 15 minutes until the crisis has passed). Pitta types may not benefit as much from red pepper as Vata and Kapha types.

Cloves - Nature's Pharmacy

Cloves have warming, antibacterial and antiseptic properties. This herb relieves pain, lessens nausea and prevents or relieves vomiting. It combats and neutralizes pathogenic bacteria and prevents infection. It is often used as a topical tooth and gum painkiller. Chewing on a piece of clove after meals helps remove bad breath.

Clove has great preventative value for a number of disorders. For example, it discourages blood platelet clumping, which is associated with cardiovascular disease. This herb contains volatile, essential oils that aid digestion and relieve gas pain and distention; it promotes peristalsis. Its astringent effect helps keep hemorrhages under control.

In addition, clove encourages the loosening of phlegm from the respiratory tract. It also stimulates blood flow to the skin causing localized reddening. For those who easily get cold inside the body, this herb increases internal heat, dispels internal chill and strengthens metabolism and circulation. Clove strengthens stomach functions, and restores, nourishes, and supports the entire body; it exerts a gently strengthening effect on the body. For those afflicted with parasites, clove expels or repels intestinal worms.

One of the most promising effects of cloves is derived from its cholesterol lowering effects. Every day for about one month, let six pieces of clove soak in half a glass of water overnight, remove the cloves in the mornings with a spoon or fork, and drink this water every day for about one month. This should help restore your cholesterol levels back to what is normal for your body.

Honey - The World's Best Wound Healer?

Would you have ever guessed that this delicious food made by honeybees is actually one of mankind's oldest-known medicines? Dating as far back as 5,000 years, honey has been successfully used to treat burns, coughs and ulcers. Hippocrates, the Greek physician, also praised honey's healing powers and came up with many honey-based treatments for ailments such as skin disorders, ulcers and sores. In World War I, German physicians used a mixture of honey and cod liver oil to treat gunshot wounds. According to John Riddle, professor of ancient science at North Carolina State University, a medical text written on papyrus from 3000 years B.C. specifies the use of honey for head wounds. He says that perhaps "the honey helped prevent swelling and sealed off the wound to keep air and infection out".

Recent Research shows that honey is far superior to antiseptics and antibiotics. Israeli researchers took honey to the test. They applied the sweet, sticky food twice a day to wounds of nine infants after two weeks of intravenous antibiotic treatment and daily antiseptic cleansing failed to heal them. Following just five days of honey treatment, the babies' wounds improved significantly. After 16 more days, they were closed, clean, and sterile.

In a Yemeni study, honey was shown to have a significant advantage over antiseptics used for infected surgical wounds. Fifty women whose wounds became infected were divided into two groups. One group was treated with honey, the other with antiseptics. The patients in the honey group recovered within 7 to 11 days, whereas the antiseptic group needed 12 to 27 days.

Although modern creams and antibiotics may have healing effects, they have the disadvantage of killing tissue and causing scabs and scars. But how many of us would think of putting honey under that Band-Aid or bandage? Like in the above studies, results of a three-year clinical trial at the University Teaching Hospital in Calabar, Nigeria, showed that unprocessed honey can heal wounds when more modern dressings and antibiotic treatments fail. In 59 patients treated for wounds and external ulcers, honey was effective in all but one case. Much to the surprise of the researchers, topical applications kept sterile wounds sterile until they had time to heal, while infected wounds became sterile within a week. Astonishingly, honey was even shown to remove dead tissue from persistent wounds, helping some patients avoid skin grafts or amputations.

According to the European Journal of Medical Research, topical honey proved to have positive effects on post-operative wound infections due to gram-positive and gram-negative bacteria[16] following Caesarean sections and hysterectomies.

"Honey provides a moist healing environment, yet prevents bacterial growth even when wounds are heavily infected," notes Dr. Peter Molan of the Honey Research Unit at the University of Waikato, New Zealand. "It is a very effective means of quickly rendering heavily infected wounds sterile, without the side effects of antibiotics, and it is even effective against antibiotic-resistant strains of bacteria."

---

[16] Two types of bacteria types marked by their different cell membrane structures

The reason honey is able to stop infection may actually be quite simple. Ordinary honey ties up water so that bacteria in a wound have insufficient water to multiply. The water activity of honey inhibits bacterial growth. In addition, the pH of honey is between 3.2 and 4.5 - low enough to inhibit the growth of many common bacteria. The major antibacterial activity in honey, however, is thought to be due to hydrogen peroxide, which is produced enzymatically. The level of hydrogen peroxide produced is antibacterial, but doesn't damage the cell tissues.

In July 2007, the U.S. Food and Drug Administration - believe it or not - gave Derma Sciences, a New Jersey-based manufacturer of wound-care products, clearance to sell *Manuka* wound and burn dressings as medical devices. Now Manuka honey can officially be used in wound and burn care in the United States. Manuka honey has already been used as wound dressing for several years in Great Britain, Australia, and its native New Zealand. Canada also approved it for use as an antimicrobial dressing in early 2007. Honey used to be a standard conventional therapy in fighting infection up until the early 20th century. With the advent of penicillin, knowledge of honey's powerful healing ability began to fade from public awareness, and doctors were simply too excited over using the new miracle drug.

Compared to other types of honey, Manuka has an extra ingredient with antimicrobial qualities, called the Unique Manuka Factor (UMF), according to an article published in the Washington Post August 7, 2007. Apparently, the higher the concentration of UMF, the darker, thicker and more expensive the honey is. In this situation, it may pay off to use the most expensive honey available. However, even ordinary natural honey has amazing healing properties.

Applications:
- Apply honey to cuts, scrapes, or burns and cover with a clean bandage. Change dressings one to three times daily, as needed.
- Use honey as a first-aid dressing material where there could be time for infection to set in before medical treatment is obtained.
- For internal disinfection and as a preventative measure, every morning, drink a glass of warm water with a teaspoon of honey and a little lemon juice.
- Honey also has sleep-inducing, sedative and tranquilizing properties.
- Nursing salve: Nursing mothers, try covering cracked, sore nipples with honey-soaked gauze to prevent infection.
- For heartburn, take 1 teaspoon of raw honey mixed with 1 teaspoon of apple cider vinegar.

Note: Excessive heat (don't cook or bake with it) or prolonged exposure to light can rob honey of its antibacterial properties. Always store in a dark, cool place.

Hydrogen Peroxide for Colds and Flu

Speaking of *hydrogen peroxide*, this naturally occurring substance has great benefits for the flu and colds. It can be effective 80 percent of the time, especially if used when the symptoms first appear.

In 1928 Richard Simmons, M.D., hypothesized that colds and flu viruses enter the body through the ear canal, not through the eyes, nose or mouth, as most have believed. His findings were dismissed by the medical community. But he insisted you catch the flu or the cold via the ear canal, and he may be correct. In 1938 German researchers had great success using hydrogen peroxide for treatment of colds and the flu. However, their data has been ignored for over 60 years, perhaps because there is not much money to be made selling hydrogen peroxide.

As a general rule, keeping your fingers out of your ears will greatly reduce your chances of coming into contact with these viruses, however, since they are microscopic and can be air-borne, they may settle on or even in your ear. According to the German findings, once the germs have entered the inner-ear (middle-ear) they will start breeding. From there, they have easy access to the rest of the body, infecting it throughout (provided there is fertile ground for them to spread).

The treatment is simple, and involves administering a few drops of 3 percent Hydrogen Peroxide (H_2O_2) into each ear, although often only one ear is infected. The (H_2O_2) starts acting immediately and after two to three minutes all germs will be neutralized. There will be some bubbling noise sensation in the ears, and perhaps even mild stinging. Start with one ear by holding the head toward one side, and once the bubbling has subsided, drain onto tissue and repeat with the other ear. One or two applications are usually enough.

Hydrogen peroxide at 3 percent solution is perfectly safe for infants/children and available at any drugstore for a couple of dollars. The best way to administer it is to use a dropper. If the (H_2O_2) gets into the eyes, immediately rinse them with water.

The Miracle of Unrefined Salt

Natural sea salt contains ninety-two essential minerals, whereas refined adulterated salt (a byproduct of the chemical industry) contains only two elements, sodium (Na) and chlorine (Cl). When cells suffer from a dietary deficiency of trace elements, they lose their ability to control their ions. This has dire consequences on the human body. Even if ion equilibrium is lost for just one minute, cells in the body begin to burst. This can lead to nervous disorders, brain damage, or muscle spasms, as well as a breakdown of the cell-regenerating process.

When ingested, natural sea salt (reconstituted seawater) allows liquids to freely cross body membranes, blood vessels walls, and glomeruli (filter units) of the kidneys. Whenever the natural salt concentration rises in the blood, the salt will readily combine with the fluids in the neighboring tissues. This, in turn, will allow the cells to derive more nourishment from the enriched intracellular fluid. In addition, healthy kidneys are able to remove these natural saline fluids without a problem, which is essential for keeping the fluid concentration in the body balanced. Refined salt, however, may pose a great risk to the body. It prevents this free crossing of liquids and minerals (see the reasons for this below), thereby causing fluids to accumulate and stagnate in the joints, lymphatic ducts and lymph nodes, and kidneys. The dehydrating effect of commercial salt can lead to gallstone formation, weight increase, high blood pressure, and other health problems.

The body requires salt to properly digest carbohydrates. In the presence of natural salt, saliva and gastric secretions are able to break down the fibrous parts of carbohydrate foods. In its dissolved and ionized form, salt facilitates the digestive process and sanitizes the GI tract.

Commercially produced table salt has just the opposite effect. To make salt resist the reabsorption of moisture and, thereby, be more convenient for the consumer, salt manufacturers add chemicals such as desiccants, as well as different bleaches, to the final salt formula. After undergoing processing, the salt can no longer blend or combine with human body fluids. This invariably undermines the most basic chemical and metabolic processes in the body. Water retention and kidney and blood pressure problems are the most obvious consequences of refined salt consumption. Refined salt is still added to thousands of different manufactured foods. Some 50 percent of the American population suffers from water retention (the leading cause of weight gain and obesity). The consumption of large amounts of refined salt is much to blame for that.

Before salt was commercially produced, versus harvested naturally, it was considered the most precious commodity on earth, even more precious than gold. During the Celtic era, salt was used to treat major physical and mental disturbances, severe burns, and other ailments. Research has shown that seawater removes hydroelectrolytic imbalance, a disorder that causes a loss of the immune response, allergies, and numerous other health problems.

In recent years, salt has earned a bad reputation, and people have learned to fear it, in the same way they fear cholesterol and sunlight. Many doctors warn their patients to stay away from sodium and sodium-rich foods. However, to live a salt-free life means that you will suffer an increased risk of mineral and trace mineral deficiencies, as well as numerous related complications. Eating unrefined salt fulfills the body's need for salt without upsetting the hydroelectrolytic balance. If your diet contains a good amount of potassium in natural form, you should have no concern about being harmed by the relatively small amount of sodium in real sea salt. Foods that are particularly high in potassium are bananas, apricots, avocados, pumpkin seeds, beans, potatoes, winter squash, and many other vegetables. However, if potassium levels in the body drop below normal, sodium (even in natural salt) can become a source of imbalance.

Celtic ocean salt (grayish in color) is a good product to ingest because it is naturally extracted through sun drying. Other great salts are sold at whole food stores such as Whole Foods Market® or co-ops. Some are multicolored; others have a pink color. Himalayan salt is considered the best and most nutritious of all. The Hawaiian Black Sea salt is also excellent, and it tastes great. If taken dissolved in water or added to the water in which foods are cooking, these salts have profound, positive effects at the cellular level. Unrefined salt also helps to cleanse and detoxify the gastrointestinal tract, and it keeps harmful germs at bay.

Refined salt has virtually no benefits for the body. On the contrary, it is responsible for causing numerous health problems, including gallstones. The only salt that the body can digest, assimilate, and utilize properly is unrefined, unprocessed sea salt or rock salt. For salt to be useful to the body, it needs to penetrate foods - that is, the moisture of the fruits, vegetables, grains, and legumes must be allowed to dissolve the salt. If salt is used in its dry state, it enters the body in a non-ionized form and creates thirst (a sign of being poisoned). It causes further harm because it is not being properly assimilated and utilized.

You may dissolve a pinch of salt in a small amount of water and add that to fruit or other foods that are not usually cooked. This will aid in the digestion of those items while helping to de-acidify the body. Adding a pinch of salt to drinking water generates alkaline properties and provides you with important minerals and trace elements.

It may be worth mentioning that food should taste delicious, but not salty, in and of itself. Pitta and Kapha body types require less salt than does the Vata body type.

Important Functions of Real Salt in the Body:

- Stabilizes irregular heartbeat and regulates blood pressure - in conjunction with water
- Extracts excess acidity from the cells in the body, particularly the brain cells
- Balances sugar levels in the blood, which is particularly important for diabetics
- Is essential for the generation of hydroelectric energy in the cells of the body
- Is vital for the absorption of nutrient components through the intestinal tract
- Is needed to clear the lungs of mucus and sticky phlegm, particularly in those suffering from asthma and cystic fibrosis
- Clears up catarrh and congestion in the sinuses

- Is a strong natural antihistamine
- Can prevent muscle cramps
- Helps prevent excess saliva production; saliva that is flowing out of the mouth during sleep may indicate salt deficiency
- Makes bones firm; 27 percent of the body's salt content is located in the bones; salt deficiency and/or eating refined salt versus real salt are major causes of osteoporosis
- Regulates sleep; acts as a natural hypnotic
- Helps prevent gout and gouty arthritis
- Is vital for maintaining sexuality and libido
- Can prevent varicose veins and spider veins on the legs and thighs
- Supplies the body with over 80 essential mineral elements; refined salt, such as the common table salt, has been stripped of all but two of these elements; In addition, refined, commercial salt contains harmful additives, including aluminum silicate, a primary cause of Alzheimer's disease.

Sugars That Heal

There are a number of sugars that can actually end infections without even destroying the germs that trigger them:

1. FOS

FOS is a concentrated chain of fructooligosaccharides composed of carbohydrates found naturally in fruits, vegetables and grains. FOS has been a popular supplement in Japan for years and is becoming increasingly respected in the Western Hemisphere for its 'prebiotic' effects. Prebiotics serve as intestinal nutrients for the probiotic beneficial bacteria that naturally populate the gut, such as bifidobacteria and lactobacilli. FOS thus promotes the ability of these bacteria to support proper digestion.

Among those who may particularly benefit from FOS's healthful effects on intestinal bacteria are people who have used antibiotics (antibiotics can seriously disrupt the balance of intestinal bacteria), people who have eaten a poor diet for several months or years, visitors to foreign countries where 'travelers' diarrhea' is a risk, and those who face constant stress.

Japanese research has demonstrated that supplemental FOS is digested only to a small extent in the upper gastrointestinal tract. FOS passes virtually unchanged to the colon, where it is fermented and used as a fuel by beneficial bacteria. Both beneficial and potentially detrimental organisms inhabit our lower gastrointestinal tracts, but fortunately, many pathogenic and putrefactive bacteria cannot break the bonds that hold FOS together. According to the research, FOS can help promote up to a tenfold increase in the populations of bifidobacteria and lactobacilli. As a result, the intestinal environment becomes increasingly uninhabitable for potentially harmful bacteria such as Escherichia coli, clostridia, Veillonella and Klebsiella. As the detrimental bacteria die off, the beneficial bacteria of the colon are allowed to grow and proliferate, establishing a beneficial intestinal balance for them to exert their health-promoting effects.

In addition to aiding digestion, FOS may also benefit diabetics by preventing swings in blood sugar. By helping to eliminate or prevent the formation of toxic compounds in the intestines, blood and lymph, FOS may assist the liver in its effort to keep the body toxin-free. FOS has already been shown to support cardiovascular functions by lowering blood pressure and reducing blood fats and total cholesterol levels. FOS's naturally induced ability to increase resistance to infection may be especially helpful for people at increased risk of bacterial infections. FOS also supports the production of various vitamins and minerals. Animal studies suggest that FOS may help prevent anemia and loss of bone density by promoting absorption of iron and calcium in the intestines.

FOS is a mildly sweet, white, sugar-like powder that can be taken in tablet/capsule form (see *Product Information*). Very high dosages may cause intestinal gas in some people.

2. Xylitol Curbs Tooth Decay

Xylitol is a sugar alternative that looks and tastes like real sugar but contains less than 40 percent of the calories. Xylitol is a natural carbohydrate that is found in fibrous plants and vegetables, including birch and other hardwood trees, berries, almond hulls and corncobs. The human body produces small amounts (5-15 grams per day) during normal metabolism. It has been approved for use as a sugar substitute in over 35 countries.

Xylitol has been shown in studies to reduce plaque and cavities up to 80 percent by neutralizing plaque acids and inhibiting the growth of Streptococcus mutant, the plaque-producing bacteria most responsible for causing cavities (dental caries). Xylitol stimulates remineralization of tooth enamel. In clinical trials, Xylitol has also been known to boost the immune system, and in children, it specifically inhibits the growth of Streptococcus pneumonia bacteria, reducing ear and sinus infections by 40 percent.

In addition, Xylitol has been shown to improve breath odor, retard loss of tooth enamel, reduce infections in the mouth and nasopharynx, and relieve dry mouth. It is safe for diabetics and hypoglycemics. Xylitol does not encourage growth of yeast, including Candida albicans. In contrast to ordinary sugar, xylitol increases the absorption of B-vitamins and calcium.

Xylitol enjoys wide acceptance in Japan, Finland, and the Scandinavian countries. In the Soviet Union it has been used for decades as a sweetener by diabetics, and in Germany in solutions for intravenous feeding. Numerous clinical and field studies performed over the past 30 years have demonstrated the safety and efficacy of Xylitol as a healthy alternative to sugar and artificial sweeteners. Xylitol is recommended and used by dentists, periodontists and nearly all other medical and dental professionals worldwide.

Xylitol is added to chewing gum, gumdrops and hard candy, mints, toothpastes and mouthwashes. Recent studies at the Dental Schools of Michigan and Indiana Universities have tested the effect of xylitol/sorbitol blends in chewing gum and mints on plaque. They showed a significant decrease in plaque accumulation. In the United States, xylitol is approved as a direct food additive for use in foods for special dietary uses. It can be purchased in bulk form from health food stores and many online stores (see *Product Information*). Many people use it in their breakfast cereals and for baking.

3. D-Mannose for Bladder/Kidney Infections

D-Mannose is considered to be a simple sugar, like glucose. It is naturally found in cranberry and pineapple juice. When D-Mannose is ingested into the body, most of it is rapidly absorbed through the stomach and upper gastrointestinal tract before reaching the intestines. The result is that almost all of the sugar is emptied into the urine through the kidneys, and only a very small amount of D-Mannose is actually metabolized by the body. Although it may not be obvious at first, the fact that the body treats D-Mannose essentially as a waste product turns out to have very positive implications for people suffering form urinary disorders, such as bladder infection.

Escherichia coli (or E. coli) is the normal bacterium found in every intestinal tract as part of the natural microbe population therein. When E. coli bacteria find their way into the urinary tract, they may infect the urinary bladder. This is quite common. In fact, 80-90 percent of all bladder infections (cystitis) can be attributed to E. coli entering the urinary tract, a problem 50 times more widespread among women than among men. Provided there exists a predisposing weakness of the immune system, E. coli bacteria present in the vagina are able to migrate into the urethra and onward to the bladder, which is why many women end up with a bladder infection every time they have intercourse. Unless the immune system destroys them, *E. coli* bacteria have the ability to attach themselves like glue to the inner walls of the urinary tract and bladder.

A bladder or urinary tract infection may be indicated by incontinence, burning sensation upon urination, sensation of urgency to urinate without the ability to void completely, reddish or cloudy urine, foul smelling urine, lower abdominal pain, and frequent urination.

If left untreated, a bladder infection may lead to a kidney infection when bacteria continue to migrate up the ureters to the kidneys. In such case, there will be additional symptoms such as burning sensation during urination, frequent urination, increased urgency to urinate, lower-back pain, chills, nausea, vomiting and diarrhea.

D-Mannose has a unique chemical structure that causes it to adhere to *E. coli* bacteria even more tenaciously than *E. coli* adhere to human cells. Normal urination, therefore, with a sufficient level of D-Mannose present in the urine, becomes a simple and effective treatment for the above conditions. As remarkable as it sounds, *E. coli* cells coated by D-Mannose in the urine become unglued and get flushed right out of the body.

The first-time use of antibiotics in the treatment of bladder or kidney infection almost always leads to repeat infections. Although these deadly drugs successfully kill the unwanted microorganisms, they also destroy the beneficial flora responsible for keeping any infectious bacteria at bay. Essentially, the immune system depends on these 'friendly' microbes to protect the body against being decomposed while still living. Use of antibiotics has caused many women to end up having yeast infections, which indicates that this protective mechanism has already been broken.

D-Mannose has no anti-fungal properties. It does not kill bacteria, friendly or unfriendly. D-Mannose simply helps to remove misplaced *E. coli* from inside of the urinary tract by the natural process of urination. Apart from having no side effects and being of virtually no burden to the digestive system, it also tastes good, like sugar.

Interstitial Cystitis (IC) is a chronic bladder disorder that mimics the symptoms of an ordinary urinary tract infection (UTI). Normal therapeutic dosage is 1/2 tsp. daily for chronic sufferers of ICs and UTIs, or weekly for preventative measures (see *Product Information*).

In addition to the use of D-Mannose, UTI sufferers require thorough cleansing of the large intestine, liver bile ducts and kidneys, and an adjustment of diet and lifestyle as advocated in this book. Taking SSKI iodide may also be beneficial.

Please note that Stevia, although it is very sweet, is not a sugar, but can be used as one. It is also perfectly safe for diabetics and for people suffering from Candida issues.

Caution: Beware of an elaborate gimmick by a global, multimillion dollar marketing company that claims: "Medical research has discovered that eight **glyconutrient sugars** are needed at the cellular level for optimum immune function." The idea is to take expensive supplements that contain these eight sugars, which are supposedly missing in your diet. These special nutrients are supposed to cure the most serious diseases, including cancer, Lupus, Diabetes, and MS. The fact is that there are no 'glyconutrients' discovered by science. That term doesn't even exist in the medical literature. There are no scientific studies that appeared in medical journals (search Medline) that can back the claims made for any of their products, including Ambrotose. The only 'research' that exists is the one promoted by the company and its affiliations. As of July 2007 - Greg Abbott, the Texas Attorney General has charged Mannatech, Inc., its owner, Samuel L. Caster, and several related entities with promoting an illegal marketing scheme that encourages consumers to believe that its products are effective against many serious diseases.

The Miraculous Yucca Extract

Yucca root contains steroidal saponins, which are natural detergents found in many plants, especially certain desert plants, such as Yucca schidigera. Its extract has traditionally been used as an intestinal cleanser, which may explain the vast array of its benefits.

Yucca
- helps form a protective coating on the intestinal walls, preventing damage of the lining and toxins from seeping into the blood and lymph (leaky gut)
- helps eliminate disease-causing organisms, including viruses
- encourages growth of beneficial bacteria
- helps with lower-grade intestinal infections, while reducing inflammation and swelling
- reduces intestinal disorders including colitis, diverticulitis, constipation, intermittent diarrhea, intestinal gas
- aids digestion and absorption of fats
- decreases accumulated intestinal wastes in the colon
- breaks down and eliminates hardened intestinal mucus in the intestines
- relieves cramping and abdominal pains, often within several minutes
- reduces soreness, stiffness and swelling of joints (as found in arthritis and gout)
- relieves migraine headaches
- helps heal sores, scabs and skin rashes
- lowers elevated blood levels of cholesterol and triglycerides
- helps offset stress due to its cortisone-like action
- helps some people to stop smoking
- has been used to stop hair loss
- has benefited people suffering from Addison's disease
- helps normalize high blood pressure
- inhibits cancer cells

Dr. Bingham, in the Journal of Applied Nutrition (Vol.27, No.2 and No.3), reported that 60 percent of people who took the yucca supplements experienced diminished pain, swelling, and stiffness in their joints. Native Americans of the Southwest used yucca as shampoo, to treat wounds and sores, as well as symptoms of arthritis and rheumatism. Yucca root extract has no known unpleasant or harmful side effects. It is a rich source of vitamin A and B complex. It has a high content of calcium, potassium, phosphorus, iron, manganese and copper. It is best to buy the liquid Yucca extract, without alcohol, from 'Herb Farm' or other sources found on the Internet. Yucca capsules are being absorbed poorly by the body.

Slippery Elm Bark

Slippery elm inner bark is very rich in mucilage, a complex mixture of polysaccharides that form a soothing gelatinous fiber when water is added. Slippery elm is also considered a wholesome nutritional food, similar in texture to oatmeal and can be prepared as porridge. Consumed three times per day, unsweetened 'elm food' may be a good source of nutrients. Because it is gentle and easily digested, it is well tolerated by people with gastritis and other forms of intestinal problems. The pleasant tasting highly nutritious porridge was traditionally used as both a food and a medicine by First Nations peoples, and later by European colonists. The mucilage was traditionally used internally for soothing sore throats and tonsillitis, coughs, dryness of the lungs and digestive upsets, and externally for healing wounds and other skin inflammations. Slippery elm tree and root bark were also used as folk remedies for treating many serious degenerative diseases. The bark is particularly recommended for soothing gastric diseases. The viscous fiber has several beneficial effects on digestion.

Slippery Elm
- reduces bowel transit time
- absorbs toxins from the bowel
- increases fecal bulk and dilutes stool materials thereby reducing stool contact with the intestinal mucosa
- enhances beneficial bacteria in the gut and provides an excellent substrate for bacterial fermentation

Eliminating estrogenic anaerobes from the gut can significantly help the body to regain critical hormone balances that are required for basic health. The bark has noted anti-inflammatory activity and because the mucilage resists hydrolysis and digestion by stomachs acids and enzymes, it therefore maintains its soothing action throughout the entire digestive system. Slippery elm bark mucilage also helps to moisten the throat, nasal passages, and lungs. Slippery elm bark was also traditionally used for treating abscesses, dysentery, urinary conditions and fever. Poultices were traditionally used to support bone and joint health, reduce swollen glands and stop the spread of infections.

The bark contains a complex mixture of polysaccharides including pentoses, methyl-pentoses and hexoses that form a soothing gelatinous fiber or mucilage. The bark also contains high concentrations of anti-oxidants including beta-sitosterol, traces of beta-carotene and flavonoids including proanthocyanidins.

Porridge of the bark can be taken throughout the day, as required. It is best suited for Vata and Pitta and types, but Kapha types may also benefit. Sufficient amounts of water (1:10) should be taken at the same time (especially Vatas) to ensure maximum therapeutic benefits and to prevent impacted bowel. If these directions are followed, there are no known side effects. As with any type of fiber, it is important not to take too much all at once and overdo it. Slippery elm bark is also a main ingredient of the American Indian herbal remedy 'Ojibwa tea'. Any major herbal store, such as MountainRoseHerbs.com sells slippery elm bark in larger quantities.

Ojibwa Herb Tea - One Remedy for All Ailments?

Ojibwa Indian herb tea is a 280-year old Native American Indian root and herb tea remedy made in the 1700s by the Ojibwa Indian medicine society. Ojibwa people used it to survive a small pox genocide started by the early European settlers.

Native Americans have since used the tea formula to cure all types of cancers, Type 1 and Type 2 diabetes, liver infections and other liver/gallbladder conditions, tumors, arthritis, gout, asthma and other respiratory ailments, obesity, high blood pressure, elevated cholesterol, fibromyalgia and chronic fatigue syndrome, ulcers, irritable bowel syndrome (IBS), kidney and bladder disorders, sinus congestion, influenza (flu) and chest colds, measles, mumps, chicken pox, small pox, herpes, diarrhea, constipation, lymph edema (fluid retention), heart disease, allergies, skin disease, auto immune diseases such as Lupus, AIDS, Lyme disease, addiction to alcohol, drugs, tobacco, etc., clinical depression, and many more.

Blessed Thistle is used for digestive problems such as gas, constipation, and upset stomach. This herb is also used to treat liver and gallbladder diseases.

Burdock Root is a mild diuretic. It increases the production of both urine and sweat, potentially making it useful in treating swelling and fever. Burdock Root might play a role in preventing liver damage caused by alcohol, chemicals, or medications. The exact reason for this protective effect is not known, but it is thought to involve opposition of a chemical process called oxidation, which occurs in the body as a natural function of metabolism. Although oxidation is a natural process, that doesn't mean it isn't harmful to the body! One result of oxidation is the release of oxygen free radicals, which are chemicals that may suppress immune function. Antioxidants such as Burdock Root may protect body cells from damage caused by oxidation.

Kelp is a sea vegetable that is a concentrated source of minerals, including iodine, potassium, magnesium, calcium, and iron. Kelp, as a source of iodine, assists in making the thyroid hormones, which are necessary for maintaining normal metabolism in all cells of the body. This increases energy levels and helps make it easier to maintain a healthy body weight. Kelp is the most nutrient-dense of all the Native Ojibwa Tea ingredients - and it isn't found in the commonly sold Essica tea four-herb formulas. (Unless you suffer from hyperthyroidism, it is best to use the eight-herb formula)

Red Clover is a source of many valuable nutrients, including: calcium, chromium, magnesium, niacin, phosphorus, potassium, thiamine, and vitamin C. Red Clover is also one of the richest sources of isoflavones (water-soluble chemicals that act like estrogens and are found in many plants). The isoflavones found in Red Clover have been studied for their effectiveness in treating some forms of cancer. It is thought that the isoflavones prevent the proliferation of cancer cells and that they may even destroy cancer cells.

Sheep Sorrel is a rich source of oxalic acid, sodium, potassium, iron, manganese, phosphorous, beta carotene, and vitamin C. This native Ojibwa tea ingredient is a mild diuretic, mild antiseptic, and a mild laxative.

Slippery Elm Bark has been used as a poultice for cuts and bruises, and also for aching joints due to gout or other causes. Besides being a native tea ingredient, this herb is also used to alleviate sore throats. Slippery elm bark is found in many lozenges that claim to soothe throat irritation. Since a sore throat and a cough are often linked, slippery elm bark has also been used in cough remedies. It also regulates the elimination process of digestion, easing both constipation and diarrhea.

Turkish Rhubarb Root is a detoxifying herb and is world-famous for its healing properties. Turkish Rhubarb Root purges the body of bile, parasites, and stagnating food in the gut by stimulating the gall duct to expel toxic waste matter. It has been shown to alleviate chronic liver problems by cleansing the liver. Tjis root improves digestion and helps regulate the appetite. It has also been shown to help heal ulcers, alleviate disorders of the spleen and colon, relieve constipation, and help heal hemorrhoids and bleeding in the upper digestive tract.

Watercress is high in Vitamin C, Watercress is used as a general tonic, and its bitter taste is thought to regulate the appetite and improve digestion. It can be used to alleviate nervous conditions, constipation, and liver disorders. Watercress is a popular cough and bronchitis remedy. It contains a remarkable substance called rhein, which appears to inhibit the growth of pathogenic bacteria in the intestines. It is believed that rhein is also effective against Candida albicans (yeast infection), fever and inflammation, and pain.

Caution: As with other sources of food and remedies that contain soluble fiber, such as slippery elm bark, Ojibwa tea can interfere with the absorption of other medicines within the gut if they are taken at the same time. As such, take prescription medications at an alternate time to consuming this tea.

One company sells this tea formula under the name Essiac tea http://www.premium-essiac-tea-4less.com. Another one, NaturesAlternatives.com, sells it as "Native Essense™ Plus dry tea," available on the internet (see *Product Information*). For those who wish to purchase these herbs separately, the exact breakdown of herbs (ratio) is available at this web page: http://www.biznet1.com/p2699.htm. This site also sells the Ojibwa tea in larger quantities.

Lapacho (Pau d'Arco)

An Amazing Incan Herbal Remedy

South American physicians are using a recipe derived from the ancient civilization of the Incas to successfully treat various forms of cancer - including leukemia and other life-threatening diseases. They use the inner bark of the Lapacho Colorado Tree, or Red Lapacho - called so because of its scarlet flowers. Also known as Pau d'Arco, Ipe Roxa and Taheebo, the red Lapacho tree grows in the warmer parts of South America: Brazil, northern Argentina, Paraguay, Bolivia, etc. The tree apparently only grows where there is high ozone content in the air, with high concentrations of vital negative oxygen ions. It is virtually free of contaminants caused by pollutants such as pesticides or exhaust fumes.

The tree has vibrant, trumpet-shaped flowers—pink, purple, or yellow, depending on the species. The Lapacho tree with the purple flowers has the most potency. The unusual thing about the flowers is that they are carnivorous and eat insects, protecting the tree against pests, parasites, viral infections, and fungal growth.

The power of the tree lies in the inner bark. It can be removed without damage, dried, from which an extract is obtained. The tree renews its bark and, therefore, serves as a continuous supply source. The active ingredient is known as Lapacho. The herbal remedy is valued for its ability to strengthen and balance the body's immune system. With all the herbal cures and the treasures the Incas left us, there appears to be none as precious as Lapacho, which their descendants - the Callaway - are still using today.

Lapacho is commonly applied in the alternative treatment of cancer, AIDS, and Candida Albicans overgrowth and other fungal problems as well as many other diseases of the immune system. Moreover, Lapacho is highly valued for its ability to detoxify the body, particularly the liver, kidneys, and intestinal tract. It also helps babies cope with food allergies and intestinal cramps. Research in South America on Lapacho has shown it to help reduce counter-reactions to antibiotics and to allow other medicines to work more effectively by reducing the danger of toxic effects on the liver.

Lapacho can be used safely along with other medicines and even minimize their side effects. I personally have recommended it to thousands of people, with very good results, especially for infections. Many medical doctors and dental surgeons now routinely prescribe Lapacho to their patients for infection instead of giving them antibiotics. This herb seems to work both at the causal and symptomatic level, which may explain the absence of side effects.

Medicine of the Highest Caliber

The following is a list of ailments that South American doctors found were helped by Lapacho:

- Anemia Tonic
- Asthma Ulcers
- Arteriosclerosis
- Blood builder
- Bronchitis
- Cancer
- Cystitis
- Diabetes
- Gastritis
- Hernias
- Infectious diseases
- Leukemia
- Liver ailments
- Osteomyelitis
- Psoriasis
- Pyorrhea
- Parkinson's disease
- Ringworm
- Rheumatism
- Skin problems
- Varicose veins
- Venereal diseases
- Wounds

Further research showed that Lapacho is also helpful in colds, influenza, gonorrhea, polyps, prostate infection and enlargement, tuberculosis, growths, multiple sclerosis, typhus, dizziness, impotence, hair loss, boils, snake bites, food allergies, and chemical allergies. When applied topically, it can help against dandruff, eczema and skin cancer. Scientists believe that Lapacho may even have potential in the treatment of AIDS. *Aveloz* is a herbal remedy which when used in combination with Lapacho is capable of practically breaking down cancer cells while Lapacho itself addresses more the cause of the disease.

The fascinating revelation about the properties of Lapacho is that there has never been any record in medical research of an antibiotic chemical agent capable of destroying both bacteria and viruses. Any other known type of vegetation when exposed to water and the weather is eventually covered with spores that lead to the formation of fungus. This does not occur in the case of Lapacho, indicating an uncommon resistance. Following are the known properties of Lapacho:

- ANALGESIC - agent that diminishes pain without the loss of consciousness
- SEDATIVE - agent that alleviates nervousness, irritation and distress
- DECONGESTANT - agent that relieves congestion throughout the body
- DIURETIC - agent used to stimulate secretion and the flow of urine
- HYPOTENSIVE - powerful nervine relaxant that induces sleep when necessary
- VIRUCIDAL - agent capable of destroying a virus

The dramatic cures caused by Lapacho in Brazil were so astounding that the government of Brazil began to study and confirm its healing properties. Research at the University of Illinois, U.S.A, supports the research in Brazil, and the claim that Lapacho does indeed contain a substance to be highly effective against cancers. Dr. Teodoro Meyer of the State University of Tucuman, Argentina, was the first researcher to discover an antibiotic substance called *Zyloiden*, that he found is capable of killing viruses. *Lapachol,* the main ingredient of the herb, also was discovered to have powerful antitumoral action without toxic side effects. The antineoplastic activity was confirmed in 1968 when the use of Lapachol on rats carrying *Yashida's Sarcoma* inhibited the growth of the tumors in 84 percent of the animals treated with high doses.

Professor Accorsi of Sao Paulo University also found Lapacho to be of excellent therapeutic value in the treatment of various forms of cancer, including leukemia. A Japanese research group led by doctors from the National Cancer Center confirmed Professor Accorsi's findings. The researchers were able to extract an anti-cancer substance from Lapacho, which they found acted against leukemia and malignant tumors including those in stomach cancer.

Besides its powerful healing properties, Lapacho is a powerful tonic and blood builder that increases the hemoglobin content and the number of red corpuscles. This is not surprising because Lapacho contains easily absorbable (colloidal) iron. It also assists with the proper assimilation of nutrients and the elimination of wastes, which is essential for recovery from any illness. Lapacho seems to be capable of revitalizing the body, by creating new vital elements and normal cell growth. It permits control of 'incurable' diseases, lengthening life span and enhancing the quality of life both at the same time. Lapacho is a gift of nature to us humans and we may greatly benefit from accepting this gift.

Dosage: To strengthen the immune system, drink two to three cups each day, or take two capsules three times daily. For infection/inflammation, cancers, or other serious illnesses, double the dosage.

Beware: Not all Pau d'Arco products sold in today's grocery stores, on the internet and even in herbal stores are potent enough to have the effects mentioned. Look for the most reputable stores known for their high quality products, even if their prices are somewhat higher, than at stores that sell the common brands. However, I found that even the extracts offered at local health food stores still have some good benefits, effective enough to balance a simple infection or immune weakness. Although the tea tends to be more potent than capsules, it is less convenient.

Olive Leaf Extract

This ancient herbal remedy has very similar and equally powerful healing properties as Lapacho, so I will omit repeating them here. I will mention, though, one particular ailment for which olive leaf extract has especially astounding and fast-acting effects - *Shingles*. In most cases, five 150 mg capsules, or two 500 mg capsules a day, taken with food, helps to end this painful affliction within just three to four days. For the very elderly patients, though, it might take as long as a week or two for full recovery.

Olive leaf extract is one of the natural alternatives to pharmaceutical antibiotics. It has long been known for its antimicrobial properties, and has been officially tested as an antimicrobial agent, with sufficient power to achieve a published status in peer-review journals.

Astragalus

Astragalus membranaceus (Dong Quai in Chinese Medicine) is mostly used to strengthen immunity and assist the body with preventing colds, the flu and other illnesses. However, according to Chinese tradition, astragalus **should not** be taken during the early stage of infections. It may still ward off the flu, however, if taken just as the first signs or symptoms begin to appear. Its greatest effects are preventative.

Other ailments which Astragalus may be used to treat are: AIDS, arteriosclerosis, chemotherapy side effects, chronic active hepatitis, diabetes, genital herpes, high blood pressure, hyperthyroidism, and insomnia.

Sage Oil - A Memory Booster

In the 17th century, noted herbalist Nicholas Culpepper wrote that the herb sage could 'heal' the memory while 'warming and quickening the senses'. Sage has always had that reputation, but no one knew why. Researchers from the Medical Plant Research Centre (MPRC) at the Universities of Newcastle and North Umbria in the U.K. have possibly uncovered sage's ancient secret. An enzyme called acetyl cholinesterase (AChE) breaks down a chemical called acetylcholine that is typically deficient in Alzheimer's patients. According to a 2003 study at MPRC, sage inhibits AChE. Researchers gave 44 subjects either sage oil capsules or placebo capsules containing sunflower oil, and then conducted word recall tests. The group that received sage oil turned in significantly better test results than subjects that took the placebo.

Sage can be found in health food stores and from many Internet sites. There are no known side effects.

Guarana - An Energy Booster

There is yet another South American plant that has very unusual and beneficial health-promoting properties. The plant is known as paullinia cupana, and its seeds as *Guarana*. Like Lapacho (Pau d'Arco), Guarana can be found in most health food stores

Guarana is regarded as a natural elixir or energy booster. Often, the Amazonian Indians would eat only Guarana when they went into the jungle. They would grind the seeds, mix them with water, and drink the concoction. This alone would sustain them on their long treks. They also used Guarana to combat fever, headaches and pain.

Research has shown that Guarana gently stimulates the adrenal system to combat fatigue without producing the harmful adrenaline shots. The large amount of bulk prevents its natural caffeine from being released in bursts, as is the case with coffee or black tea. The gradual release of caffeine makes much energy available to the body without depleting the body's own energy resources. Guarana soothes the nervous system and is, therefore, useful for stress related conditions including anxiety and depression. It has become highly valued as a tonic herb, improving both concentration and physical stamina. Many professional sportsmen and gymnasts use it regularly. Recommended uses are:

- When you need an energy boost (take it instead of coffee which can exhaust the nervous system)
- As a general tonic and stress reliever
- For those who live an active lifestyle or have a demanding day ahead
- During periods of hard work, either mental or physical
- As a gentle stimulant and to remove fatigue
- When recovering from an illness or feeling weak
- To slow or reverse signs of aging
- To help relieve headaches and migraine
- As a natural diuretic, to rid the body of excess fluid
- To relieve menstrual pain[17]

---

[17] There are other herbs that have shown great benefit for relieving menstrual pain: Chinese angelica root, Szechuan lovage root, red peony root, white peony root, Chinese motherwort, and cinnamon bark. In one trial, 53 percent of the women who took these Chinese herbs had less pain, compared with 26 percent in the placebo group. The herbs were more effective than non-steroidal anti-inflammatory drugs (NSAIDs), oral contraceptive pills, acupuncture, heat compressions, placebos, or no treatment at all.

- As a non-addictive anti-depressant

Whatever brand you use, make sure it is 100 percent pure Guarana and not mixed with any other ingredients or preservatives. Beware of chewing gums or similar products that claim to contain Guarana. The large amount of chemicals and preservatives, colorings, and artificial sweeteners they contain cause considerable harm to the body, which you can confirm by doing the muscle test.

The Bloodroot Paste and Indian Herb

Both of these products can basically accomplish the same thing. When used topically, they are able to completely remove malignant and non-malignant skin cancers, moles, large freckles and other growth-type skin blemishes. When a tiny amount is applied to a mole, for example, about one week later the mole, along with its roots and toxic deposits, is discharged from the skin and falls off. Even large cancerous tumors come out in one piece, without the need for surgery.

Caution: When you apply the Indian Herb or a similar bloodroot salve, be very careful not to use too much of it or put it on parts of the skin that don't require any treatment. The zinc chloride it contains can cause damage to healthy skin. The Bloodroot Paste doesn't contain zinc and may be less aggressive. Once a mole or skin cancer has been removed, that part of the skin may be lighter in color because their presence has diminished or destroyed any melanin-producing cells. For more information and to purchase these herbal products see *Product Information* at the end of the book.

Another, but more expensive approach to remove skin blemishes such as freckles, age spots, liver spots, sun spots, moles, warts, skin tags, etc. is called 'Blemish-free' (see *Product Information*). The do-it-yourself home kit uses the same treatment method dermatologists use, i.e. liquid nitrogen, an FDA approved method of freezing blemishes to safely remove them. There are no scars left, but the skin may also be lighter where the blemishes once were.

Pfaffia, Black Cohosh and Evening Primrose (For Women)

Pfaffia (also known as Brazilian Ginseng or Suma) is very effective for menstrual problems, menopausal symptoms, diabetes and any other hormonal problems. *Black cohosh* is one of the most effective natural products for menopause. It helps reduce and even stop hot flushes and other discomforts during a woman's hormonal changes. There were some anecdotal cases where the use of Black Cohosh was linked with liver problems, but the real cause was not clear. To avoid complications, it is important to discontinue taking hormone replacements while taking Black Cohosh, or best wait at least two months before starting the Black Cohosh regimen. Evening Primrose oil is another great natural product for female health issues (see also *The Purpose of Menopause* in Chapter 16).

Detoxified Iodine - For Thyroid Disorders and Other Conditions

Detoxified Iodine can end a stubborn bladder infection, dissolve ovarian cysts and excessive cholesterol, and even flatten hemorrhoids when mixed with a vegetable oil and applied topically before bedtime. It can be used for nail fungus, too. For resistant infections, prostate cancer and other estrogen-caused illnesses, use 10 drops of detoxified iodine three times daily, for four to six weeks.

A few drops of detoxified iodine added to germ-infested water a few minutes before drinking it makes it safe to drink. To avoid getting sick after a long airline-flight, drink some water mixed with a few drops of iodine. The iodine travels quickly to the ears, nose and sinuses, thereby zapping hoards of bacteria and viruses circulating in the cabin air. Other applications include removal of toenail fungus, reduced flatulence and zapping of new acne.

A note on thyroid disease/goiter: About 96 percent of goiters are caused by an iodine deficiency. If you medicate with regular iodine, it should best be done under careful supervision because, if overused, iodine can lead to hypothyroidism (see below). However, eating iodine-rich foods, such as dulse and kelp (sea vegetation), is a more indirect and safe way to increase iodine and shrink goiters. Detoxified iodine is certainly a better choice, since it has not shown to produce hypothyroidism.

The famous Edgar Cayce used to treat goiter and other thyroid conditions very successfully by giving his patients detoxified iodine. There are three products that meet his requirements; *Magnascent, Atomic Iodine*, and *Atomidine* (see Product Information). The latter two seem to be nearly identical. Magnascent has shown some excellent results with hypothyroidism, menopausal symptoms, cancer, arthritis, and other illnesses.

While treating the thyroid, it is important to remove any congestion from blood vessel walls and lymphatic vessels, which are major reasons behind the poor nutrient supply (including iodine) and waste drainage from the neck area and thyroid gland. Trapped lymphatic waste, consisting of metabolic waste products and dead cells, causes nodule formation and general thickening of the tissues there. This requires an overhaul of the digestive system, including the removal of all bile stones from the bile ducts of the liver, (see also *The Amazing Liver & Gallbladder Flush*) cleansing of the colon, and changing one's diet/lifestyle according to body type requirements.

And yes, it is essential to avoid all dairy foods (except unsalted butter), meat, and especially foods that contain soy (hundreds of processed foods contain soy).

Caution: Although lack of iodine can cause thyroid disease, iodine can also suppress thyroid function when taken for long periods of time, such as several months or years. If you suffer from a thyroid condition, you need to take special care in monitoring thyroid function while using this treatment. I recommend that you consult with your doctor or a naturopathic healthcare professional before using any of the above products. Although very few people are allergic to iodine, those who are should avoid it in any form.

Green Tea - A Tea for Life

For more than 30 years, Western researchers have known that the occurrence of solid tumor cancers is far less in countries where populations consume large amounts of green tea. Cultures that are endowed with a long tea tradition have much to contribute to individual and global health. However, this applies only to green tea. Regular black tea, presently very popular almost everywhere, has not much to do with *real tea.* Real tea is derived from the tea plant *Thea sinensis* or *Thea asoncica,* not to be confused with herb teas such as peppermint, chamomile or fennel.

Both black and green teas originate from the same tea plant, but their methods of processing are different. The breaking of the leaves of the plants and exposing them to the oxygen of the air produces black tea. The resulting natural fermentation process destroys the most important biological ingredients of the tea—the tannins. By contrast, during the production of green tea, the leaves are stabilized through exposure to both humid and dry heat. This eliminates fermentation-producing enzymes and safeguards the nutrients.

Due to fermentation, black tea assumes drug-like qualities. Since tannins and other important nutrients are no longer present in the tea, its caffeine appears in free and unbound form. The stimulating effect of the quickly released caffeine causes the addictive effect of black tea. It triggers a 'fight or flight' response in the body. Since the body treats the ingested caffeine as a nerve toxin, the adrenal glands naturally respond by secreting the antidote *adrenaline.* This defense response by the body has a stimulating and enlivening effect. However, as the effects of the caffeine and adrenaline diminish, the body starts feeling tired and may end up exhausted.

Green tea works in a different way. The large amounts of *tannins* in green tea make certain that the caffeine is taken to the brain in only small and well-dosed amounts, which actually harmonizes the energies in the body. Unlike black tea, the original green version of the tea makes the body's own energy-use more efficient. This helps the consumer of green tea improve his vitality and stamina without having to experience the 'up and down' effect so often accompanied with the consumption of black tea.

The value of tannin has been studied for centuries all over the world. Besides its ability to bind caffeine, it also has healing properties. Green tea is particularly helpful with intestinal disorders and high blood pressure. It has been shown to be 20 times more effective in slowing the aging process than vitamin E. Studies have demonstrated that the success rate of green tea in reducing oxidants in the body (considered responsible for aging) is 74 percent compared to 4 percent with vitamin E. The vitamin C content of green tea is four times higher than in lemon juice and it contains more B-vitamins than any other known plant. This makes green tea useful for facial skin conditions such as rosacea/acne. Apart from drinking green tea, you may apply it directly to the skin before bedtime and after washing your face in the morning.

Since green tea is highly alkaline it naturally helps combat hyperacidity. People who drink green tea also suffer less from arteriosclerosis. It also keeps the blood thin and prevents coronary heart disease, heart attacks and strokes. Furthermore, researchers from the University of Osaka, Japan, have been able to prove that green tea kills microbes responsible for cholera and tooth decay; it also destroys salmonella germs before they even have the chance to enter the stomach. A substance called 'EGCG' has been found to retard tumor growth. The Botikin Hospital in Moscow reported that green tea is more effective against infection than antibiotics, without producing any harmful side effects.

Green tea has over 100 ingredients that have been found useful for a number of conditions, it

- inhibits cell mutations leading to cancer
- reduces blood fats
- balances serum cholesterol levels
- prevents high blood pressure
- increases heart efficiency
- improves brain functions
- enhances metabolism
- improves vision
- supports secretion of saliva
- increases growth of hair
- reduces body fat and weight
- stimulates digestion
- helps clear urinary tract obstructions

In a study testing the preventative action of green tea, a team of researchers from the Department of Preventive Medicine at the University of Southern California (U.S.C.) found that green tea prevented breast cancer in women by 30 percent if they consumed about ½ cup per day. If they drank more than that, their risk of developing breast cancer was further reduced. Women who regularly drank black tea, on the other hand, didn't have a reduction in their breast cancer risk. The good news is that this study revealed that you don't need to drink buckets full of green tea to benefit from it.

The best green tea comes from the *Shizuoka* area in Japan; it grows organically and has no additives. People living in this area have a much lower cancer rate than those living in other areas of Japan. A reliable brand is *Sencha* sold by Kurimoto Trading Co., Japan. With over 130 ingredients, it is the richest of all green teas. Other brands are *Ocha* or *Bancha*; you should be able to find at least one of them at a good health food store.

<u>Note</u>: The effectiveness of green tea depends on how you prepare it. Take 1½ teaspoons of green tea for two cups of tea. Bring water to a boil and turn the heat off. Put the tea into a pot and pour the boiled water over the tea as soon as the water has stopped bubbling. After no longer than 35-45 seconds, pour the tea through a sieve into a teapot, otherwise the tea loses much of its effectiveness. You may use the same leaves a second time by applying the same procedure.

Does Green Tea Contain Toxins?

Some web sites on the Internet claim that tea is very high in *fluoride* content. Fluoride in tea is supposedly much higher than the Maximum Contaminant Level (MCL) set for fluoride in drinking water. Another site confirms that information, adding that the typical cup of tea exceeds one milligram of fluoride, which is well over the recommended amount for fluoridated drinking water. On yet another site, it says that *fluorine* and its compounds in food are entirely different from chemically-produced sodium fluoride. It states that once an element is extracted from the soil and incorporated into plant life, its properties change greatly. All this can be greatly confusing for those concerned about fluoride poisoning.

Yes, fluoride is found in tea and also in mother's milk. This applies also to areas where there is no fluoride in the drinking water or air. Numerous plants contain naturally occurring fluorine or fluoride compounds. The hideous version of fluoride that is added to drinking water in so many parts of the world is the poison we ought to protect ourselves against. "Fluoride, once touted as an osteoporosis treatment, is, in fact, toxic to bone cells," says John R. Lee M.D. Thankfully, the American Dental Association, which has for many years been one of fluoride's biggest advocates, changed course when it alerted its members in 2006 that parents of infants younger than a year old "should consider using water that has no or low levels of fluoride" when mixing baby formula.

If the naturally occurring fluoride in green tea were even remotely toxic (like the fluoride added to drinking water), it would not have shown to have such a wide range of preventive and curative effects. The body's immune system would reactively respond to it and become weakened in the process, yet quite the opposite is true. Green tea inhibits cell mutation, stimulates digestion and enhances brain functions. Synthetic fluoride has the exact opposite effects.

The fluoride - or fluorine - that occurs naturally in tea and other foods is so volatile that most of it evaporates in the heating process. The synthetic sodium fluoride added to water, on the other hand, remains stable when heated. So the sodium fluoride in your cup of tea is of much greater concern than the natural fluoride in the tea itself. Excessive fluoride intake can lead to hyperthyroidism. If you have been diagnosed with this disorder you should consult with a doctor of Ayurveda, Chinese Medicine or an ND (doctor of naturopathic medicine) who is knowledgeable about nutrition and its effects on the body's endocrine glands.

Gingko Biloba - Brain Food; And Coenzyme Q10

I also recommend *Gingko Biloba*, available at most health food stores. Guarana and Gingko seem to complement each other. Gingko is considered brain food. It apparently increases blood flow to the brain, thereby improving memory and brain function. It is known to improve all kinds of circulatory problems and it especially increases blood flow to the heart, extremities, skin, eyes, inner ear and other organs. Gingko is known to relieve anxiety and depression, vertigo, headaches, tinnitus, PMS, asthma, allergy symptoms, and hepatitis. It is also a natural mood-enhancer.

More than 300 studies by 200 scientists in 18 countries have proven that Coenzyme Q10 can help lower your blood pressure, revive a failing heart, and strengthen your immune system. The problem is to find a supplement that can actually be absorbed by the body; most powder or liquid forms on the market have a very low absorption rate. Since CoQ10 is a fat-soluble nutrient, it requires a fat-soluble medium to digest and absorb it. You may search the Internet for one that includes fat molecules in the capsules, such as, Ultimate CoQ10 Formula™.

Aloe Vera - An Ancient Healer

Throughout the ages, *aloe vera* has been known as the 'medicine plant', 'burn plant', 'first-aid plant' or 'miracle plant'. Even today, aloe vera is one of the most effective plants for treating burns, healing wounds and relieving aches and pains. It is recommended for psoriasis, where, when used regularly, it reduces scaling and itching and greatly improves appearance.

Aloe vera became very popular for its use in combating the severe burning effects caused by x-rays and nuclear disasters. Radiation burns cause skin ulcerations that had been nearly incurable until physicians began trying the old folk remedy of the aloe vera leaf.

Today, aloe vera has gained such great popularity that it is being used in many cosmetics and health products. Aloe vera juice that is taken internally has been found to be effective in almost every illness, including cancer, heart disease and AIDS. In fact, there is hardly any disease or health problem for which aloe vera has not been proven successful. It is helpful for all kinds of allergies, skin diseases, blood disorders, arthritis, infections, yeast overgrowth, cysts, diabetes, eye problems, digestive disorders, ulcers, liver diseases, hemorrhoids, high blood pressure, kidney stones and stroke, to name a few. Its use is most beneficial if treatments are applied both internally and externally. Aloe vera contains over 200 nutrients, including the vitamins B1, B2, B3, B6, C, E, Folic acid, iron, calcium, magnesium, zinc, manganese, copper, barium, sulphate, 18 amino acids, important enzymes, glycosides, polysaccharides, etc.

There are an estimated 500 published independent research studies conducted by doctors and scientists on the healing agent found in the aloe vera plant and it's non-toxic benefits. That is many more studies than one would find on any other natural substance, and hundreds of times the confirmation of safety and effectiveness of any drug available.

Watch out for the frauds: Since the consumer market has created a great demand for aloe vera juice, production is increasing rapidly. Unfortunately, many brands contain inadequate amounts of aloe vera juice to be effective. According to the law, if you take a 10,000-gallon vat and put 9,999 gallons of water in it and then add one gallon of aloe vera juice, you are allowed to advertise that it contains '100 percent pure stabilized aloe vera'. You are not required to mention how much extra water has been added to the 100 percent aloe vera juice. Hence many people are disappointed because they do not receive the acclaimed benefits. Before using any brand it is good to check out the exact table of contents as mentioned in a company's brochure or better ask the company to give you the exact figures of contents.

Also, don't be tempted to buy the cheapest aloe vera juice. Aloe vera juice is expensive. If you are not getting any benefits from it, you may have chosen the wrong product. Try other brands until you are satisfied. Tests have shown that less than one percent of readily available brands contain acceptable levels of aloe vera to be of any medicinal value. From the over 1,000 brands of aloe vera available on the market today, some hardly have a trace of aloe vera in them. Their labels contain such phrases 'it tastes like mineral water' and 'no additives or preservatives'. Chemical analysis reveals that these 'products' contain almost nothing but plain mineral water.

The good news is that more and more people have begun to see through the fraud business; hence, many other companies are now also introducing the real thing.

There is an excellent new aloe vera product in powdered form, which dissolves in water. It is sold by goodcausewellness.com (see *Product Information*). It is more convenient than having to buy bottled aloe vera juice. It is completely free of additives.

Caution: With regular drinking of aloe vera, diabetics may improve the ability of the pancreas to produce more of its own insulin. Since too much insulin is dangerous, diabetics should consult their physician to monitor their need for extra insulin. Many diabetics report a reduction in the amount of insulin required.

Also if you experience diarrhea or intestinal cramping for more than two to three days, discontinue. This is due to irritants the aloe plant contains. Instead, you may choose a product that has all irritants removed.

Ionic Liquid Minerals

Your body is like *living soil*. If it has sufficient minerals and trace elements to work with, it is able to nurture you and produce everything you need to live and grow. These essential materials, however, can get easily depleted when you are not getting enough of them through your food. Centuries of constant use and overuse of the same agricultural fields have led to foods that are highly nutrient-deficient. The situation worsened with the onset of chemical fertilizers that manipulate crops into growing more rapidly, with no regard to nutrient availability. When minerals and trace elements run low in the body, important functions can no longer be sustained, or become subdued. Disease is generally accompanied by lack of one or more of these important substances.

Because of the unnatural situation of mineral depletion in our soil today and, therefore, in our bodies, it may be useful for certain individuals (especially Vata and Pitta types who suffer from chronic health problems) to supplement with natural minerals. The crucial question is whether the minerals sold in nutrition stores or pharmacies are capable of replenishing the mineral supply to the cells of the body. The answer is: "Highly unlikely!"

Minerals are commonly made available in three basic forms: capsules, tablets and colloidal mineral water. Before the depletion of soils, plant foods and the mineral-rich water they absorbed were our best source of minerals. When a plant grows in a healthy soil environment, it absorbs existing colloidal minerals and changes them into an ionic, water-soluble form. The ionic minerals come in the minute size known as *angstrom*, whereas the colloidal minerals, also known as inorganic, metallic minerals, are

Timeless Secrets of Health and Rejuvenation

about 10,000 times larger (micron-size). Ionic, water-soluble, plant minerals are absorbed readily by our body cells. In contrast, the absorption rate for colloid particles packed into complex compounds and delivered is less than 1 percent. The minerals found in colloidal mineral waters are not any better absorbed. These are not water-soluble, just suspended between water molecules.

Common mineral compounds include calcium carbonate and zinc picolinate. These colloid particles tend to get caught in the bloodstream and subsequently are deposited in different parts of the body. As deposits, they can cause major mechanic and structural damage. Many health problems today, including osteoporosis, heart disease, cancer, arthritis, brain disorders, kidney stones, gallstones, etc. are the direct result of ingesting large quantities of such metallic minerals.

Fortunately, there is a very efficient way to obtain minerals in the size and with the characteristic of plant minerals. By vaporizing minerals in a vacuum chamber (without oxygen), they are prevented from oxidizing and forming into complex states. Once vaporized, the minerals can be combined with purified water and be made readily available to the cells of the body. One company located in Minnesota, U.S.A. has managed to create a delivery process capable of converting colloids into 99.9 percent water-soluble, ionic minerals. The company, ENIVA, makes these minerals available via distributorship.[18] I recommend VIBE, their most balanced and effective product. I have seen very obvious effects in one woman whose skin used to be absolutely covered with liver spots. After two months on VIBE, over 60 percent of the spots had faded away, or were about to disappear. The natural vitamins in the products are part of the juices or their extracts. Another good brand is 'WaterOz & Angstrom Ionic Minerals'. Their prices for some of their products appear to be more competitive and products can be purchased directly from the Internet without having to go through a sponsor[19] (See *Product Information* for more details). There are more details about minerals and vitamins in Chapter 11, Section 1.

Miracle Mineral Supplement (MMS)
An Instant Healer of Malaria, AIDS, Cancer, Hepatitis and More?

The following is a quote from a book by Jim Humble, the discoverer of MMS and the author of the book, *Breakthrough . . . Miracle Mineral Supplement of the 21st Century:*

"While first developed to address Malaria in Africa, it has now been shown to address any disease condition that is directly or indirectly related to pathogens. There is documentation of over 75,000 cases of Malaria being overcome in Africa. Often in as little as four hours all symptoms are gone, and the patient is tested clear of Malaria. It is now known that MMS can be used to overcome the symptoms of AIDS, Hepatitis A, B & C, Typhoid, most cancers, herpes, pneumonia, food poisoning, tuberculosis, asthma, colds, flu and a host of other conditions. Even conditions not directly related to pathogens seem to be helped due to the huge boost to the body's immune system, for example, macular degeneration, allergies, lupus, inflammatory bowel disorders, diabetes, snake bites, abscessed teeth and fibromyalgia. Please note that MMS doesn't cure anything, but rather it allows our body to heal itself. Notice how I carefully step around the words 'cure' and 'heal', even though that is what is really happening."

"Separate tests conducted by the Malawi government produced 99% cure results for malaria. Over 60% of AIDS victims treated with MMS in Uganda were well in three days, with 98% well within one month. More than 90% of the malaria victims were well in four to eight hours. Dozens of other diseases were successfully treated and can be controlled with this new mineral supplement."

---

[18] To order any products from Eniva (www.eniva.com), you require a sponsor name and ID. You may use the name and ID of the author, Andreas Moritz, #13462. He does not benefit from your order.
[19] WaterOZ products can be ordered from Kornax (www.kornax.com).

The inventor believes that this information is too important to the world that any one person or any group should have control. The free e-book (digital book) download gives complete details of this discovery. Please help make sure that it gets to the world free. There are many medical facts that have been suppressed and this invention must not be added to that list. The name of the e-book is *The Miracle Mineral Supplement of the 21st Century*. You can download it (for free) or ask a friend to download and print it for you if you don't have a computer. The web site address is www.miraclemineral.org. Jim Humble's book tells the story of the discovery, and how to make and use it. I recommend every person to read it. Jim has no personal, vested interest in making MMS available to the world, except to end disease and poverty. For a short description of how MMS works, please see '*Should we kill Intestinal Parasites?*' Chapter 4.). To purchase MMS, *see Product Details*).

A general note of advice about taking supplements: As always, while any or all of these products may be very beneficial, don't forget to take care of the root causes of your ailments. Merely relieving symptoms of disease can actually be detrimental to your health unless you also remove whatever causes them. In most cases, cleansing the liver, kidneys and colon and adjusting one's diet/lifestyle are sufficient to take care of most physical health problems.

To deal with the psychological, energetic and emotional issues that are behind most physical disorders, I suggest using *Sacred Santémony* and *Ener-chi Art* (see details below), and reading *Lifting the Veil of Duality* and *It's Time to Come Alive* (see *Other Books, Products and Services by the Author* at the end of the book).

Waterless Stainless Steel Cookware

Since 1985, I have been using *Surgical Stainless Steel Waterless Cookware* for all my cooking. In my opinion and experience, this is by far the most uncomplicated and least time-consuming method of preparing cooked meals while preventing the loss of valuable vitamins, enzymes and flavor. This five, seven or nine-ply surgical stainless steel cookware allows you to cook your food in less than half the time and with one-fourth the heat.

There is no more pouring the nutrients down the drain when boiling vegetables. There is no more cooking in hot oil and robbing the food of its vital nutrition and fiber. The tight vapor-seal created during cooking allows the flavor and nutrients to remain in the food. Unlike with pressure cookers, waterless cookware involves no steam-pressure buildup inside the cookware. The temperature generated inside the cookware is much less of what is required for boiling water, yet the food cooks much faster than with ordinary cookware.

There is also no need to keep checking on the food. In fact, if you do, the cooking process will be interrupted and will take longer than necessary. While the food is being cooked, you can prepare other foods, such as salad. Within 20 minutes you can serve a meal consisting of three cooked items, such as vegetables, rice and beans. A light evening meal consisting of vegetables or a vegetable soup can be fixed in a matter of 10 minutes. Cooking from scratch must no longer be a burden. Since I do this every day, I can personally attest to that.

Waterless cooking cannot be accomplished with Teflon, iron, aluminum, glass, porcelain and department store lightweight stainless steel. In the United States, you can buy 15-piece sets of 9-ply stainless steel cookware for as little as $180. Waterless cookware not only costs hundreds of dollars less than the cookware you see in cooking shows, but it also comes with a Lifetime Warranty (search for 'Waterless Cookware' on the Internet or see *Product Information*). Please note there may be other metals in some parts of the cookware to make the steel extra hard and resistant to corrosion. However, the parts of the cookware that come into contact with food should only be made of pure extra heavy 304 surgical steel.

Basic Rules of Cooking with Waterless Cookware:

> **Always use the right pan**
> Select the pan the food will most nearly fill, as air pockets created by 'too large for the food quantity' pans may destroy vitamins, dry your foods and possibly burn them.

> **Rinse prepared fruits and vegetables**
> Rinsing in cold water and then draining is important for two reasons: it removes harmful chemicals and allows water to cling to the food, combining with the natural juices to cook in its own steam. You may add spices, salt, vegetable bouillon, oil or butter, salt, coconut milk or other ingredients. This is waterless, nutritional cooking. Until you get used to this new method, you may want to add several tablespoons of water.

> **Control the heat**
> Always control the heat throughout the cooking process. If you have heat that is too high, it evaporates the steam and your food burns. With waterless cookware, the control is never on higher than medium heat.

> **Get a vapor seal**
> Start the cooking process on medium heat until the steam control valve whistles in the open position. Then turn the heat down to low or simmer and close the valve. After you do this, the lid will form an airtight heat seal.
> When cooking watery type food such as apples and cabbage, it takes about three minutes to create a water seal. More solid food such as potatoes and carrots take about five minutes for the lid to seal after turning the heat to low and closing the steam control valve.

> **Don't peek**
> Resist that urge to peek! When the cover is removed during the cooking period, heat and steam are allowed to escape. This lengthens the cooking time and dries out the food.

Caution: AVOID non-stick pans: The chemical perfluorooctanoic acid (PFOA) used in non-stick pans, fast-food containers, carpets, furniture and a host of other everyday household products accumulates in the umbilical cords of babies and is retarding their growth and brain development, according to two new studies published in the prestigious journal Environmental Health Perspectives (August 2007). Babies whose umbilical cords had the highest concentrations of PFOA were born lighter, thinner and with smaller head circumferences than others. This chemical - produced in the United States by DuPont - has been used so widely and is so persistent in the environment that it has been found all over the world. It is now found even in the Arctic and in remote Pacific atolls - in rain and water supplies, food, wildlife and human blood. DuPont 'agreed' to phase out this chemical in **2015!** In other words, it's up to you to protect you and your family by choosing to use only chemical-free products.

Water Ionizers

Water Ionizers are machines that can turn normal tap water into a good cleanser that has antioxidant effects. Water with a negative charge (ORP) is known to retard the aging process. A high or rising ORP, on the other hand, causes oxidation and therefore aging. Machine-ionized water counteracts this rising ORP and has a rejuvenating effect on a cellular level. For instance, freshly squeezed orange juice has a negative ORP of -250. Although we can only drink comparatively small amounts of orange juice in a day without becoming overburdened by the sugar it contains, we *can* drink as much ionized water as we wish in a day (although it is generally best not to exceed 8 glasses per day).

Ionized water also contains hydroxyl ions. These are oxygen molecules with an extra electron attached to them, as are such antioxidants vitamins A, C and E. You can see these molecules in the form of thousands of tiny bubbles when you slow down the water flow on the water ionizer. Hydroxyl ions scavenge free oxygen radicals and provide us with extra oxygen and energy. Oxygen carries away acid waste from body tissue. It inhibits cancer cells and protects us against bacteria and viruses invading the body. Oxygen is the body's most essential nutrient.

Ionized water also helps balance the body's pH which tends to become acidic when on a diet comprised of processed, refined and preserved foods. Besides meat and highly acid-forming foods, medical drugs and soft drinks contain the most acidifying substances you can consume. Because it is alkaline, ionized water can help dissolve accumulated acid waste and protect the body against acidity-related illness (most diseases are a form of acidosis).

The human body consists mostly of water. Ionized water is fundamentally different from conventional water. In ionized water, the size and shape of the water molecule cluster is smaller, which allows it to pass through intestinal walls, blood capillary walls, and cell walls more easily and remove toxins and acidic waste matter more effectively. This makes ionized water an excellent detoxifier. Water ionizers have several levels of strength. Accordingly, people who have accumulated a lot of toxins in the body may begin by drinking 'mild' ionized water (lower alkaline pH) and gradually increase ionization levels as they get used to it. Besides its health benefits, ionized water also improves the taste of foods and beverages. It also ionizes the minerals in the food, which helps make them more biologically available.

One of the primary causes of disease is chronic cellular dehydration, a condition which leaves the body's cells in a perpetual state of weakness and defense. Ionized water is up to six times more hydrating than conventional water. In other words, by drinking less or the same amount of water but in ionized form, you will actually hydrate your cells much more effectively. (The hot ionized water described earlier is used to remove toxins from the tissues and therefore rarely hydrates cells directly. However, once the toxins are removed, the cells become more efficiently hydrated than before)

The water ionizers separate alkaline water from acid water. The alkaline water is good for drinking and the acid water is good for external applications. When applied topically, the ionized acid water tightens skin, and helps remove wrinkles, acne and other blemishes. At its strongest level, ionized acid water kills most harmful bacteria on contact. It improves hair and skin conditions of any kind, including removal of fungus, healing of cuts, scrapes, and even serious wounds. It takes the itch out of mosquito bites, and the sting out of other insect bites. You can also use it to remove pesticides from fruits and vegetables. Lastly, ionized acid water promotes substantially healthier plant growth. *Tyent USA* offers one of the most efficient, precise and user-friendly water ionizers, and I can recommend it to anyone who is interested in using water as a healing method or as an enhancement of health and well being. I am so convinced of Tyent's superior performance that I decided to make it avaialble through my web site www.ener-chi.com.

Body Odor? - A Good Reason Not to Use Deodorants

Most people are not aware of why they perspire. Antiperspirants and perfumes have become so much a part of our lives that we rarely think about why we need them or whether we really need them. It may even be more important to find out if they can be harmful to us.

Deodorants and antiperspirants were invented because more and more people began to perspire excessively and develop body odor. It now appears to be the normal thing to do to give the underarms a spray in the morning and forget about this 'smelly nuisance' for the rest of the day. But sweating is not a nuisance; it is the body's natural way of ridding itself of certain waste products and keeping itself cool. Like the bowels, liver, urinary system and lungs, our sweat glands are also meant to help keep the body clean. Why else would we have them?

To make your body sweat once a day even for a few minutes is a good way to stay healthy. Conversely, clogging up the skin's pores with chemicals (makeup, beauty creams, sun-blocks, antiperspirants, etc.) harms the skin. Trying to prevent the sweat glands from releasing bodily waste is rather like trying to run a car while blocking its exhaust pipe.

Many people today feel that they need chemical products to control their body odor. This is because other eliminative organs, such as the colon, liver, lungs and kidneys, are badly congested, which coerces the body to dump some of the excess toxic waste into the skin. The chemical products block its excretion of toxins through the skin, which may please the nose, but causes a steady buildup of toxins in the skin and underlying connective tissues; it also increases bacterial development and the risk for skin diseases, even skin cancer.

Body odor is not caused by sweat. Sweat is an odorless fluid consisting of 99 percent water. Normal sweat evaporates from the skin very quickly and leaves no unpleasant odor behind. A slightly unpleasant smell under the armpits or on the skin occurs only when your body needs to employ bacteria to eliminate excessive sweat that could not be removed by fresh air, usually because of wearing synthetic clothes that do not permit proper aeration. There can be as many as ½ million bacteria occupying a square inch of skin. In addition, when there are excessive amounts of toxins that need to be *digested* by bacteria, a strong, putrid smell occurs. Destructive microbes naturally produce bad-smelling gases while digesting waste. The odor on the skin may be a sign of constipation accompanied by poor breath. It also indicates poor performance of liver and kidneys. The body is crying out for help as toxins are 'bursting at the seams'. But instead of reading the body's symptoms as a sign of imbalance and taking care of it, most people merely search for ways to shut down the symptoms. If body odor occurs only occasionally, it may be due to indigestion or chemicals in foods.

To combat the bacteria most people use deodorants, and to tackle the excessive underarm wetness, they apply antiperspirants. Deodorants contain germicides that kill the microbes and, as is the case with most of the brands, a synthetic perfume to mask the smell of the germicide. The two most common active ingredients in commercial deodorants/antiperspirants are *chlorohydrate* or *aluminum zirconium chlorohydrate*. These chemicals react with the protein contained in the sweat and form a gel that partially blocks the sweat gland's ability to excrete liquid. These chemicals are easily absorbed by the skin. There is increasing evidence that people who suffer from Alzheimer's disease have large amounts of aluminum in their bodies, which may result from the use of deodorants.

Fruits and vegetables naturally synthesize aluminum. This organic, ionic mineral is not only harmless, but also essential for the human body. By contrast, synthetically derived aluminum is highly toxic. The argument by the industry that aluminum can be found almost everywhere in nature is highly misleading because these two types of aluminum have completely opposite effects on the body. The same applies, of course, to almost all minerals and trace elements, including gold, silver, lead, and even arsenic. In their ionic, angstrom-size state (processed by plants), these substances are essential for our bodies, but when taken in their inorganic, metallic forms they can lead to serious poisoning and numerous disorders. Antiperspirants and deodorants are packed with heavy metals and poisonous chemicals. By applying them to your skin they enter the blood and end up accumulating in the liver, kidneys, breast and brain tissue.

These products may not be as damaging to the brain and other parts of the body if all other causes of metal accumulation were excluded. The average person absorbs anywhere from 10 to 100 mg of aluminum every day through aluminum cookware, baking soda, antacids, and numerous other sources. And although the cause of Alzheimer''s disease remains unclear, research indicates that aluminum toxicity may be one of the primary culprits.

A natural deodorant stone costs only about $10 and lasts at least two to five years. It works wonderfully and has no nasty side effects. When you check the ingredient list of a deodorant stone, don't get alarmed when you see the word 'alum' written there. Alum isn't the same thing as aluminum chlorhydrate. Alum is a natural mineral salt, and is unrelated to aluminum chlorohydrate or aluminum zirconium chlorohydrate. The mineral salts in the deodorant stone don't block perspiration, they mainly just cover ordor.

Tips to effectively deal with body odor:

- Pitta and Pitta-Vata types are the most prone to develop body odor. Follow the Ayurvedic regimen and cleansing procedures. Remove all gallstones from your liver and cleanse your kidneys. Avoid too many acid-forming foods such animal proteins, fats and starches. The more refined and processed the foods are, the more likely the skin will have to eliminate toxic waste. The digestion of toxins by skin bacteria causes an unpleasant smell of skin. Meat eaters especially have a tendency to develop bad body odor. Stick to fruits, vegetables, and salads as your main source of alkaline-forming foods. They also work as natural cleansers.
- Stop using deodorants and antiperspirants; they only reinforce the problem by blocking off part of your lymphatic system and dispersing the toxins together with the chemicals contained in these products into other parts of your body, including the breasts. This can cause lumps and cancer of the breast!
- Wash the afflicted areas in the morning with a natural soap that contains no harmful chemicals and finish off with a splash of cold water on your underarms.
- Make sure to wear loose-fitting cotton clothes. Synthetics will prevent your skin from breathing and eliminating toxins.
- You may want to make a solution of your most favorite essential oil (one to two drops in an ounce of water; shake well to disperse the oil!) and dab it on your underarms (you may want to use the Kinesiology muscle test to determine which oil or oils are most suitable for you).
- I recommend deodorant stones that are made from non-toxic and natural materials such as potassium sulphate and other colloidal minerals. They are pure and harmless and stop bacteria from spreading if applied right after washing. They are available from most health food stores.

A note on colognes or perfumes: They can lead to serious allergies, birth defects, and even cancer. A major loophole in U.S. Federal law allows fragrance makers to include potentially hazardous chemicals in their products, including the highly toxic phthalates and artificial musk. Most fragrances contain phthalates. They are added to plastic to soften it. When absorbed by the skin, they act as the most powerful estrogens ever known. And abnormal estrogen levels cause cancer. Synthetically produced musk is linked to skin irritation, hormone disruption, and cancer as well. Natural fragrances emitted from aroma oils are beneficial for the body. Synthetic aromas, on the other hand, disrupt hormonal communication, and they accumulate in your body.

Ener-Chi Art

Ener-Chi Art is a unique tool for rejuvenation (based on energized oil paintings by Andreas Moritz) that helps restore a balanced flow of chi (vital energy) through the organs and systems in the body, within less than a minute. When seen in the context of physical cleansing and healing, I consider this healing approach to be a profound addition to all other natural healing methods in facilitating a more successful outcome.

When chi flows properly through the cells of the body, the cells can more efficiently remove their metabolic waste products, they more readily absorb all the oxygen, water, and nutrients they need, and they conduct any necessary repair work more swiftly. The body can restore its health and vitality much more easily when there is constant, unrestricted availability of chi. Although I consider the liver flush to be one of the most effective tools to help the body return to balanced functioning, by itself it may not be able to restore the body's overall vital energy, as a result of many years of congestion and deterioration. Test results have shown that Ener-Chi Art may very well fill this gap.

Its rate of effectiveness so far has been 100 percent for every person who has been exposed to it. Due to its unique healing benefits, all the pictures of Ener-chi Art were once exhibited for over one month at the prestigious Abbot Northwestern Hospital in Minneapolis, Minnesota, for all the patients to view. Viewing the pictures is all that is required to achieve the desired results.

Please note that Ener-Chi Art is not designed to influence physical conditions per se but to balance life energy 'chi' which underlies all physical and mental activities. Other methods aiming to restore chi include acupuncture, Shiatsu, Tai-Chi, and Yoga. Ener-Chi Art is perhaps one of the most profound and instantly effective healing programs to balance the life force chi in the following organs, parts and systems in the body.

- Back
- Blood
- Brain & Nervous System
- Ears
- Eyes
- Endocrine System
- Heart
- Immune System
- Joints
- Kidneys and Bladder
- Large Intestine

- Liver
- Lymphatic System
- Muscular System
- Neck & Shoulders
- Nose & Sinuses
- Respiratory System
- Small Intestine & Circulation
- Skeletal System
- Skin
- Spleen
- Stomach

There is also one picture for General Health, one for transmuting emotional and physical trauma, called 'Beyond the Horizon', and pictures to balance our relationship with the water and air elements, the rocks & mountains, the animal kingdom, the plant kingdom, and the world of nature spirits.

Ener-Chi Art involves viewing of the various photographic pictures for about 30 seconds each.

(For more information on Ener-Chi Art, see *Other Books, Products and Services by the Author* at the end of this book.)

Ener-Chi Ionized Stones

Ener-Chi Ionized Stones are stones and crystals that have been energized, activated, and imbued with life force through a special process I was very fortunate to introduce as part of the healing system of Ener-Chi Art.

Stone activation has not been attempted before because stones and rocks have rarely been considered useful in the field of healing. Yet, stones have the inherent power to hold and release vast amounts of information and energy. Once ionized, energized or activated, they exert a balancing influence on everything with which they come into contact. The energizing of stones may be an important key to survival in a world that is experiencing high-level pollution and destruction of its eco-balance.

In the early evolutionary stages of Earth, every particle of matter within the mantle of the planet contained within it the blueprint of the entire planet, just as every cell of our body contains, within its DNA structure, the blueprint of our entire body. The blueprint information within every particle of matter is still there - it has simply fallen into a dormant state. The ionization process 'reawakens' this original blueprint information and enables the associated energies to be released. In this sense, Ener-Chi Ionized Stones are alive and conscious, and are able to energize and balance any natural substance with which they come into contact.

Potential Uses for Ionized Stones

Drinking Ionized Water
Placing an Ionized Stone next to a glass of water for about half a minute ionizes the water. Ionized water is a powerful cleanser that aids digestion and metabolism, and energizes the entire body.

Eating Ionized Foods
Placing an Ionized Stone next to your food for about half a minute ionizes and balances it. Due to the pollution particles in our atmosphere and soil, even natural organic foods are usually somewhat polluted. Such foods are also impacted by ozone depletion and exposure to electro-magnetic radiation in our planetary environment. These negative effects tend to be neutralized through the specified use of Ionized Stones.

Ionized Foot Bath
By placing Ionized Stones (preferably pebbles with rounded surfaces) under the soles of the feet, while the feet are immersed in water, the body begins to break down toxins and waste materials into harmless organic substances. This can be done as often as one desires, but for at least 20 minutes each time.

Enhancing Healing Therapies
Ionized Stones are ideal for enhancing the effects of any healing therapy. For example, 'LaStone Therapy' is a popular new therapy that is offered in some innovative health spas. This involves placing warm stones on key energy points of the body. If these stones were ionized prior to being placed on the body, the healing effects would be enhanced. In fact, placing Ionized Stones on any weak or painful part of the body, including the corresponding chakra, has healthful benefits. If crystals play a role in the therapy, ionizing them first greatly amplifies their positive effects.

Aura and Chakra Balancing

Holding an Ionized Stone or Ionized Crystal in the middle section of the spinal column for about one-half minute balances all of the chakras, or energy centers, and tends to keep them in balance for several weeks or even months. Since energy imbalances in the chakras and auric field are one of the major causes of health problems, this balancing procedure is a powerful way to enhance health and well-being.

Attach to Main Water Pipe in Your Home

Attaching a stone to the main water pipe will ionize your water and make it more absorbable and energized.

Place in or near the Electrical Fuse Box in Your Home

By placing a larger Ionized Stone in, above, or below the fuse box in your house, the harmful effects of electromagnetic radiation become nullified. You can verify this by doing the muscle test (as shown on the instruction sheet for Ener-Chi Art) in front of a TV or computer, both before and after placing the stone on the fuse box. If you don't have a fuse box that is readily accessible, you can place a stone next to the electrical cable of your appliances or near their power sockets.

Use in Conjunction with Ener-Chi Art

Ionized Stones may be used to enhance the effects of Ener-Chi Art pictures. Simply place an Ionized Stone over the related area of the body while viewing an Ener-Chi Art picture. For example, if you are viewing the Ener-Chi Art picture related to the heart, hold an ionized stone over the heart area while viewing the picture. The nature of the energies involved in the pictures and the stones is similar. Accordingly, if the stones are used in combination with the pictures, a resonance is created which greatly enhances the overall effect.

Creating an Enhanced Environment

Placing an Ionized Stone near the various items that surround you for about half a minute helps to create a more energized and balanced environment. The Ionized Stones affect virtually all natural materials, such as wood floors, wood or metal furniture, stone walls, and brick or stone fireplaces. In work areas, especially near computers, it is a good idea to place one or more Ionized Stones in strategic locations. The same applies to sleeping areas, such as putting stones under your bed or pillow.

Improving Plant Growth

Placing Ionized Stones next to a plant or flowerpot may increase their health and beauty. This automatically ionizes the water they receive, whether they are indoor or outdoor plants. The same applies to vegetable plants and organic gardens.

Creating More Ionized Stones

Make any number of ionized stones by simply holding your 'seed stone' against any other stones or crystals for 40-50 seconds. Your new stones will have the same effects as the seed stone.

Sacred Santémony - Divine Chanting for Every Occasion

Sacred Santémony is a unique healing system that uses sounds from specific words to balance deep emotional/spiritual imbalances. The powerful words produced in Sacred Santémony are made from whole-brain use of the letters of the *ancient language* – a language that is comprised of the basic sounds that underlie and bring forth all physical manifestation. The letters of the ancient language vibrate at a much higher level than our modern languages, and when combined to form whole words, they generate feelings of peace and harmony (Santémony) to calm the storms of unrest, violence, and turmoil, both internal and external.

In April 2002 I spontaneously began to chant sounds that are meant to improve certain health conditions. These sounds resembled chants by Native Americans, Tibetan monks, Vedic pundits (Sanskrit), and languages from other star systems (not known on planet Earth). Within two weeks, I was able to bring forth sounds that would instantly remove emotional blocks and resistance or aversion to certain situations and people, foods, chemicals, thought forms, beliefs, etc. The following are but a few examples of what Sacred Santémony is able to assist you with:

⇒ Reducing or removing fear that is related to death, disease, the body, foods, harmful chemicals, parents and other people, lack of abundance, impoverishment, phobias, environmental threats, the future and the past, unstable economic trends, political unrest, etc.

⇒ Clearing or reducing a recent or current hurt, disappointment, or anger resulting from past emotional trauma or negative experiences in life.

⇒ Cleansing of the *Akashic Records* (a recording in consciousness of all experiences the soul has gathered throughout all life streams) from persistent fearful elements, including the idea and concept that we are separate from and not one with Spirit, God, or our Higher Self.

⇒ Setting the preconditions for you to resolve your karmic issues, not through pain and suffering, but through creativity and joy.

⇒ Improving or clearing up allergies and intolerances to foods, chemical substances, pesticides, herbicides, air pollutants, radiation, medical drugs, pharmaceutical byproducts, etc.

⇒ Balancing the psycho-emotional root causes of any chronic illness, including cancer, heart disease, MS, diabetes, arthritis, brain disorders, depression, etc.

⇒ Resolving other difficulties or barriers in life by helping to 'convert' them into the useful blessings that they really are.

(For more details, and to book a personal session with Andreas Moritz, visit his website or see contact details at the end of the book.)

Beeswax - For Asthma, Allergies and Sinus Problems

Hundreds of years ago, most candles were made of beeswax. But over the past few centuries, beeswax candles were gradually replaced by tallow candles (made from animal fat), and in the last century by paraffin candles. Paraffin is made from the sludge that sits at the bottom of barrels of crude oil. The sludge is then bleached with benzene and treated with other chemical solvents. When you burn paraffin candles, they put out soot and smoke, along with toxins and carcinogens, including very harmful chemicals dispersed by the commonly used lead-core wicks (as studied & reported by the University of Michigan). You would probably never burn paraffin candles unless the bad smell they produce (comparable to diesel fumes) were not covered up by synthetic fragrances, many of which are irritants or toxins themselves. And if you had known that the soot, smoke and chemical residue from these candles can stick to the walls, ceiling, and ventilation ducts and get circulated whenever you turn on your healing/cooling system, you would probably never have lit them. Now you know. Pure beeswax candles don't cause any of those problems. Quite to the contrary, they actually exert amazing healing effects on the respiratory system.

Just by lighting a beeswax candle, people suffering from asthma, allergies and sinus problems have reported significant improvements in their symptoms. Their breathing became much easier and their sleep less disturbed after burning pure beeswax candles in their bedrooms for a few hours before bedtime. Some asthmatics claim that their symptoms vanished completely after burning beeswax candles all day long for several days or weeks.

Apparently, burning beeswax produces negative ions. Negative ions are nature's vacuum cleaners. They clean the air of dust, mold, viruses, bacteria and other pollutants responsible for numerous chemical sensitivities. For candles to have this air-purifying effect, though, they must consist of 100 percent beeswax. Many beeswax candles contain only 51 percent beeswax, which is enough to allow producers to label them as beeswax candles. When you burn a beeswax candle it has a refreshing smell and hardly produces any smoke. Although beeswax candles are more expensive than regular paraffin-based candles, they last a lot longer and, of course, improve your health rather than weaken it. Beeswax is recommended by the American Lung Association as a therapeutic product. For a reliable source of 100 percent pure beeswax candles see *Product Information* at the end of the book.

How to Deal With Electro-Pollution

Environmental changes, earth changes, and living in unhealthy homes and congested cities have all lowered our intake of magnetic energy. Magnetic energy keeps our cells alive and our minds coherent. In addition to living in a disturbed magnetic field, we are also exposed to the harmful low frequency Electromagnetic (EM) fields of 50-60 cycles per second (Hz) that are generated by electricity. This man-made electric current produces 'electro-pollution' emitted by computer equipment, TV transmissions, AM radio waves, mobile telephones, and the various home and industrial appliances such as hairdryers, electric toasters, and microwave ovens.

If you happen to sleep in a room that has a television set connected to the power circuit, your body may be building up an electric charge of up to 105 Volts! The same occurs when you lie next to an electronic alarm clock or a bedside light. A switched-on electric blanket can even double or triple the electric charge in your body. While lying in your bed, your feet are not in direct contact with the floor. This practically prevents you from dispersing that charge. Regular exposure to such abnormal voltages can create chaos in the body's electric circuitry, suppress proper immune activity and lead to disorders such as cancer.

Badly shielded electric cables within the walls or under the floor can have similar effects. Therefore, it is best to move all electrical appliances or equipment out of the bedroom, or ideally turn off the fuse for the entire room during the night, especially if you have trouble sleeping. If you are not sure whether your electric cables are safe or not, choose the latter solution, or otherwise you may want to hire an expert who can measure the safety of your most immediate environment. When I tested for electro-pollution in one of my previous homes, I was surprised that the worst culprit wasn't my computer but the ungrounded electrical strip lights. The use of Ener-chi Ionized Stones as explained in section 13 can help protect you against the harmful effects of a low frequency EM field and also balance the magnetic field around you.

Electromagnetic disturbance in the body can also be triggered by overexposure to chemical pollution. As you may know, the degree of indoor pollution in most modern homes and work places is many times higher than outdoor pollution. Add to these pollutants the harmful chemicals contained in the cosmetics, deodorants and perfumes, clothes, food, water and air that enter our bodies every day, and even a healthy body will eventually succumb to the overdose of such forms of stress and duress. Although many of us cannot completely avoid living in a polluted environment, we still can reduce our direct exposure to it to the least possible degree We have control over what we wear, eat, drink, put on our skin and hair, and how much time we spend outside in the fresh air. [For more in-depth information on Electromagnetic Fields please read the author's book: *It's Time to Come Alive*]

How to Avoid the Negative Effects of Ley Lines

If you suffer from unexplainable recurring health problems such as headaches, irritability, depression or any other persistent ailment, you may be working or sleeping on or above a ley line. Ley lines are a source of potentially harmful 'slow' frequency energy.

Slow frequency energies can easily infiltrate and distort the body's electromagnetic field. Some of these energies are generated outside our home and others originate from within our home or work environment. These include geographic stress points, ley lines and distorted ground energies.

Sleeping on a ley line can be particularly harmful since such a source of energy can disrupt the body's biochemical processes and energy systems for as many as 8-10 hours each day. Disharmony in relationships and diseases of body and mind are more likely to occur if you are exposed to such disruptive energies for extended periods of time, such as several years. Genetic weaknesses or latent physical problems can suddenly manifest themselves as migraines, ulcers, varicose veins or cancer. Placing a small mirror that faces the current and direction of a ley line or moving the bed away from such a stress line can lead to sudden recovery. The following are some examples of ley line problems that were resolved by simply moving the bed:

- A 55-year-old widow experienced an unexplainable loss of weight from 154 to 97 pounds within two years. She suffered from severe diarrhea, which became very painful and was accompanied with blood. All medical treatments failed. Her condition became life threatening. A search of ley lines in her house revealed two ley lines crossing her bed. The bed was moved by six feet. One week later her intestinal bleeding stopped. After one month all pain ceased and she steadily began to put on weight again.

- A young woman had been suffering from severe nightmares and sleeping problems for many years. After moving her bed sideways by 1.5 feet, her nightmares stopped and sleep returned to normal.

- A 40-year-old businessman had a chronic heart complaint with heart cramping, panic attacks and circulatory problems. All complaints spontaneously disappeared within two weeks after his bed was moved away from a ley line.

Over the past few years I have visited many homes and offices where ley lines have caused physical and psychological problems. In most cases, just placing a small mirror to neutralize the effects of a ley line, or slightly moving the bed or office chair, led to marked improvements of these conditions, and in some cases even to complete recovery. I consider it important to have one's home or working place checked for such disturbances as they may not only contribute to ill health but also cause it. There are an increasing number of experts who are able to identify the exact position of ley lines, although the method of mirror placement is less known. You may contact your nearest center for alternative therapies; they may be able to put you in touch with a reliable and trustworthy ley line specialist. If in doubt, whether or not a ley line affects your health, you may move your bed and/or desk chair by one to two feet for a few days. If this makes a difference in how you feel, you have given yourself a great gift of health.

Preconditions Necessary For Healing An Illness

Your body's healing power is always present within you - the conscious being who uses the physical body as an instrument to express his/her individuality and purpose. True healing, which has nothing to do with suppressing symptoms of disease, cannot be enforced by even the best of treatments unless the preconditions for healing are already in place. The following are some of the most important clues about how this healing power can become activated in you:

1. Before you can heal an illness, you have to accept it. Acceptance of your illness is not a sign of resignation or passiveness that would just result in depression and fear. Acceptance of your illness rather shows that you are willing to take responsibility for yourself and your situation. This will help you infuse your body with feelings of compassion, love, tenderness and energy. Accepting what is will allow your own healing energies to stream into your body and provide it with the calm, relaxed state it requires to return to a balanced condition (equilibrium).

For as long as you feel you are a victim of some misfortune, food, medicine, or even karma (effect of past actions), you are far from being healed. Rejecting an illness only energizes your resistance to it, which is stressful for the body and mind and puts all the cells of your body into a mode of self-defense. Stress undermines immune functions and prevents the healing response. By accepting your illness, you are no longer subjected to fear and insecurity but in control of yourself. This will also help you to understand the true reasons behind your illness.

2. Instead of seeing an illness as a negative event that you need to fight against, you will need to perceive it as an opportunity to become stronger in areas that have been weak and underdeveloped. 'Detours' can lead you into important areas that you would otherwise miss out on. Rejecting or fighting disease also repels the opportunities that disease always brings along. Since disease has no power or agenda except to heal your body and mind, it is wise to work with the illness, not against it.

Physical healing involves repair of damaged cells and growth of new ones. At the same time, while undergoing the process of healing, you have the opportunity to grow stronger, become more relaxed, peaceful, and content. Growing spiritually and emotionally as a result of an illness greatly minimizes the necessity for further detours, such as repeated or new physical disorders.

3. Since your illness is only your body's attempt to redirect your life in a more supportive and fulfilling direction, there is no reason to fear it or to be upset about it. Your body is doing the very best it can to make it easier for you and help you return to a state of balance. Therefore, you may greatly benefit from not judging yourself or your body for going through such a healing crisis. You are certainly not a victim of some kind. Your body is totally on your side, never against you. Make your body your friend and stop treating it as an enemy.

Don't be fooled by the medical concept that there are autoimmune diseases which supposedly make the body attack itself! By design, the body is not suicidal unless you are (consciously or unconsciously). Instead, the body is merely attacking toxins that have settled in the joints, blood vessels, lymph ducts, or cells. The resulting inflammation merely is a survival response and should not be mistaken for a disease, even if it involves pain, infection or proliferation of cancer cells.

Remain positive and peaceful about your own healing ability, and trust that the body is always engaged in trying to make you well again. Your illness can be your personal guide for a new purpose or orientation in life. A wise man once said: "Illness is God's way of getting your attention!" Once you pay attention to your illness and accept it as a blessing in disguise rather than a nuisance or threat, it will reveal its inherent blessing to you and surely help you live your life in a gentler, more nurturing way.

4. Avoid making physical wellness your goal in life; instead, let it be your process each moment. Seeing health as being a goal you have to fight for implies the idea that there is something fundamentally wrong with you. For example, if you suffer from pain, don't perceive this as a sign of sickness, but rather as a healthy response by your body to deal with an imbalanced situation. Sickness is but a process of healing that the body is going through. Trying to escape the present and reach a better future merely drains your energies, which makes it difficult for the body to heal itself. Being well is a matter of being in the present moment, and not a fictional, futuristic dream. The current moment is the only sure thing you can possibly own in life, and it is perfectly suited for you, even if it doesn't feel that way. If you resist or reject something such as an illness, you will be stuck with it until it is able to remove the fear that lurks behind your resistance. Accepting the illness, on the other hand, makes it useful for you, regardless of its appearance. Attending to your goal of becoming well some time in the future is unrealistic because it takes you outside the present reality into one that hasn't happened yet. Life is not about attaining a perfect physical body, but being able to live perfectly well with its imperfections. This is true health.

Energy follows thought. Living for a goal, such as trying to get rid of a disease, robs the body of your attention, and therefore, also of the energy necessary to heal and sustain itself. By living from moment to moment, your full attention is present in the body. This is all the cells of your body need to know and feel in order to do or resume the job assigned to them. Cells that are 'fed' with loving, caring attention believe that you are present and alive. By contrast, cells that are being attacked for 'making you suffer', either through harsh words, anger, and threats or drugs, surgery, and radiation, are paralyzed in their healing capacity because they believe you dislike or hate them and want them to die. Cells are living, conscious beings just like you are. By attending to the present moment of being ill without any judgments, but with loving acceptance, you automatically program your cells to carry out a healing response.

Multi-Purpose Healing Bath with Salt

Directions:
- Place a cup of pure sea salt (or Himalayan salt) into a cooking pot (Pyrex glass or stainless steel) and heat it on low heat over the stovetop.
- While heating the salt, gently and continuously stir, preferably with a wooden utensil (the salt will become hot). Make sure to keep the heat on low. The heat will break the capsule of energy that is inside the salt and release it. This may take about 10 minutes. If you are sensitive to energies, you will notice when the capsule of energy will be opened and released. At this point, turn off the heat, remove the pot from the stovetop and empty the salt into a small glass bowl (must be glass).
- Now pour some water into the bowl while gently moving the salt around in the bowl. Stir for about 5-10 seconds.
- Fill your bathtub (or Jacuzzi) with warm water, and then empty the glass bowl with the moistened salt into the bathtub. Move the bathwater with your hands. Make sure that no one except you touches the bathwater.
- In addition to the above, add a little salt (1/2 teaspoon) to a glass or bowl of water (4-6 ounces) and place it near the tub where you can easily reach it while taking the bath. Then enter the bathtub and stay there for half an hour (30 minutes). When you are inside the tub, relax and visualize how the energy coming from the salt embraces you, enters your cells, atoms, aura,

mind, etc, thereby cleansing your thoughts, feelings, and physical body. Keep your feet and neck submerged in the water.

- Discordant, harmful energies will start coming out of you. Perhaps you will feel some dizziness or pain; that is good. These are things coming out of you; sometimes they can be heavy and uncomfortable. Be prepared for this, in case it happens.
- If at any time you feel that something heavy or dark is coming out of you, place one of your hands over the glass of salt next to you until this feeling or sensation has passed. The salt in the glass of water will absorb these energies.
- Once you have finished your bath, pour the saltwater that you have kept in the glass next to you into the toilet. Wash the bowl and empty your tub. Make certain the entire tub is clean and no salt residue remains.
- You may repeat this healing bath anytime you feel the need for it. You may also use salt for other situations. It is good to keep a plate or small bowl of glass with salt in the place where you work or spend a lot of time. Because salt absorbs negative energies, it is important to change it, ideally, every day. Avoid covering the glass. If you wish, you can communicate with the salt molecules using your mind, and order them to absorb any discordant energies that may be present in your home, office, etc. Salt has an amazing power that most people are not aware of.
- If placed around the house, salt keeps harmful energies at bay. You can also purify objects (including cloth) by submerging them in saltwater for a little while.

CHAPTER 8

Healing Secrets of the Sun -
And Why They Boost Your Energy, Strength, and Happiness

The Sun—The Ultimate Source of Life on Earth

Regular exposure of your body to the germicidal wavelength of ultraviolet light (UV) of the sun successfully controls germs, mites, mold, bacteria, and viruses. Its powerful, immune-stimulating effect makes sunlight one of the most important disease-inhibitors. But this is only one of the many benefits sunlight has to offer for enhancing and sustaining human health.

Throughout the ages, the electromagnetic waves generated by the sun have kept the planet habitable for humans, animals, and plants. The sun is, in fact, the only true source of energy on planet Earth. It provides the perfect amount of energy for plants to synthesize all of the products required for growth and reproduction. Sun energy is stored by plants in the form of carbohydrates, proteins, and fat. When ingested, plant foods provide us with the vital energy we need in order to lead active and healthy lives. The processes of digestion, assimilation, and metabolism of food in the body are mainly used to break down, transfer, store, and utilize these various forms of encapsulated solar energy. The lowest level of the food chain, where foods are manufactured directly by sunlight, makes available the most sun energy. In contrast, products that are high on the food chain contain little or no sun energy and are practically useless, if not harmful, for the body. These include products made from dead animals, fish, junk foods, microwaved foods, frozen, irradiated, genetically engineered[20], and other highly processed foods.

Wood, fuel, and minerals, too, are merely various forms of locked-up sun energy. In fact, all matter is 'frozen' light. Our body cells are bundles of sun energy. The glucose and oxygen we feed them are products of the sun. We couldn't think or process a single thought without the molecules of sun-energized glucose and oxygen.

Air, which is warmed by the sun, is capable of absorbing water from the oceans while passing over them. As this moisture-laden air moves over land masses up to higher elevations, it starts to cool down and thereby releases some of its absorbed water. This water falls on the earth as rain or snow, feeding the rivers, and through them, the land and the vegetation.

Depending on its position in relation to the earth's rotation, the position of the moon, and the sun's internal cyclic activities (sun spot cycles), the sun masterminds the entire earth's climate and seasonal changes down to the smallest details, including temperature, amount of rainfall, cloud formation, periods of dryness, etc.

---

[20] In 1998 scientists have found the first evidence that genetically-modified food may damage human health. Researchers at the prestigious Rowett Research Institute in Aberdeen, U.K., found that genetically-modified foods could damage the immune systems of rats. Around 60 percent of the processed food products found in supermarkets—from hamburgers to ice cream—may contain ingredients that have been genetically tampered with.

The planet is not a home for human beings alone. The sun also has to support the growth of all the other species, including plants, animals, insects, and especially microbes, without which life here would not be possible. The mathematical complexity that stands behind a system of organization so infinitely diverse and intricate as planetary life cannot be fathomed, even by a trillion supercomputers. But the sun, without making mistakes, 'calculates' what each species, whether it is an ant, a tree, or a human being, requires in order to fulfill its evolutionary purpose and cycle.

The electromagnetic waves generated by the sun come in a variety of lengths, which determine their specific course of action and responsibility. They range from a 0.00001 nanometer for cosmic rays (a nanometer is one billionth of a meter) to about 4,990 kilometers for electric waves. There are cosmic rays, gamma rays, x-rays, various kinds of Ultraviolet rays, the visible light spectrum, consisting of seven color rays, short-wave infrared, infrared, radio waves, and electric waves.

Most of these energy waves are absorbed and used for various processes in the layers of atmosphere that surround the earth. Only a small portion of them - the electromagnetic spectrum - reach the surface of the earth. The human eye, though, can perceive just about one percent of this spectrum. Although we are unable to see any of the ultraviolet and infrared waves, they exert a very strong influence on us. In fact, ultraviolet light has proved to be the most biologically active among the various rays. Depending on the location of the earth and the season, ultraviolet light and all the other portions of light vary in intensity. This permits all life forms to go through constant cycles of change necessary for growth and renewal.

The Miraculous Healing Powers of UV Light

The time when one's immediate natural impulse on the first sunny spring day was to get outside and enjoy it is long gone. Only the very courageous or 'careless' who defy the grim warnings from medical mandarins and cancer specialists, wholeheartedly endorsed by the sunscreen industry, dare to venture forth into the 'dangerous' sun. Unless they are covered head to toe with sun protection factor 60, they gamble with their lives, or so they are made to believe, by those who serve their own vested interests. Fortunately, this view is beginning to crumble in the blatant absence of scientific proof that sunlight causes disease. What is being discovered instead is that lack of sun exposure is one of the greatest risk factors for disease. Very few people know that not getting enough sun kills 50,000 people from cancer deaths every year in the U.S. alone. As shown later, these are deaths that are easily preventable through the Vitamin D produced by the body in response to regular sun exposure.

Unfortunately, it is the ultraviolet portion of sunlight that is the most easily eliminated by windows, houses, spectacles, sunglasses, sun lotions, and clothing. Before antibiotic drugs were discovered in the 1930s - penicillin having been the first one - the healing power of sunlight was favored by the medical community, at least in Europe. Sunlight therapy, called heliotherapy, was indeed considered to be the most successful treatment for infectious diseases from the late 19th to the mid 20th century.

Studies revealed that exposing patients to controlled amounts of sunlight dramatically lowered elevated blood pressure (up to 40 mm Hg drop), decreased *cholesterol* in the bloodstream, lowered abnormally high blood sugar in diabetics, and increased the number of white blood cells, which people need to help resist disease. Patients suffering from gout, rheumatoid arthritis, colitis, arteriosclerosis, anemia, cystitis, eczema, acne, psoriasis, herpes, lupus, sciatica, kidney problems, asthma, and even burns, have all received great benefits from the healing rays of the sun.

The medical doctor and author, Dr. Auguste Rollier, was the most famous heliotherapist of his day. At his peak, he operated 36 clinics with over 1,000 beds in Leysin, Switzerland. His clinics were situated 5,000 feet above sea level, the high altitude allowing his patients to catch a lot more UV light than was possible at the lower levels of the atmosphere. Dr. Rollier used the UV rays of sunlight to treat diseases such as tuberculosis (TB), rickets, smallpox, lupus vulgaris (skin tuberculosis), and wounds. He followed in the footsteps of Danish physician Dr. Niels Finsen, who won a Nobel Prize in 1903 for his treatment of TB using ultraviolet light. Rollier found that sunbathing early in the morning, in conjunction with a nutritious diet, produced the best effects.

The miraculous complete cures of tuberculosis and other diseases facilitated by these doctors made headlines at the time. What surprised the medical community most was the fact that the sun's healing rays remained ineffective if the patients wore sunglasses. [Sunglasses block out important rays of the light spectrum which the body requires for essential biological functions.] Note: your eyes receive these rays even if you are in the shade.

By the year 1933, there were over 165 different diseases for which sunlight proved to be a beneficial treatment. However, with the death of Rollier in 1954 and the growing power of the pharmaceutical industry, heliotherapy fell into disuse. By the 1960s, man-made 'miracle drugs' had replaced medicine's fascination with the sun's healing powers, and by the 1980s the public was increasingly being bombarded with warnings about sunbathing and the risks of skin cancer.

Today, the sun is considered the main culprit for causing skin cancer, certain cataracts leading to blindness, and aging of the skin. Only those who take the 'risk'" of exposing themselves to sunlight find that the sun makes them feel better, provided they don't use sunscreens or burn their skin. The UV-rays in sunlight actually stimulate the thyroid gland to increase hormone production, which in turn increases the body's basal metabolic rate. This assists both in weight loss and improved muscle development. Farm animals fatten much faster when kept indoors, and so do people who stay out of the sun. Therefore, if you want to lose weight or increase your muscle tone, expose your body to the sun on a regular basis.

The use of antibiotics, which has practically replaced heliotherapy, has in recent years led to the development of drug-resistant strains of bacteria, which defy any treatment other than the balanced use of sun, water, air, and food. Cutting out or substantially reducing any of these four essential constituents of life results in disease.

Any person who misses out on sunlight becomes weak and suffers mental and physical problems as a result. His vital energy diminishes in due time, which is reflected in his quality of life. The populations in Northern European countries like Norway and Finland, which experience months of darkness every year, have a higher incidence of irritability, fatigue, illness, insomnia, depression, alcoholism, and suicide than those living in the sunny parts of the world. Their skin cancer rates are higher, too. For example, the incidence of *melanoma* (skin cancer) on the Orkney and Shetland Isles, north of Scotland, is 10 times that of Mediterranean islands.

UV light is known to activate an important skin hormone called *solitrol*. Solitrol influences our immune system and many of our body's regulatory centers, and, in conjunction with the pineal hormone *melatonin*, causes changes in mood and daily biological rhythms. *The hemoglobin* in our red blood cells requires ultraviolet (UV) light to bind to the oxygen needed for all cellular functions. Lack of sunlight can, therefore, be held co-responsible for almost any kind of illness, including skin cancer and other forms of cancer. As you are about to find out, it may be highly detrimental to your health to miss out on sunlight.

Can UV-Radiation Prevent and Cure Skin Cancer?

A major concern of our scientists today is the dramatic increase of skin cancers around the world. There are three main types of skin cancer, two of which, basal cell and squamous cell carcinoma (non-melanomas), are increasingly prevalent, whereas the third, malignant melanoma, is much rarer, but far more lethal.[21] The most pressing question is why would the sun suddenly become so vicious and try to kill scores of people after thousands of years of harmlessness?

The medical community claims that ultraviolet light (UV) is the major cause of skin cancers. This theory is based on the assumption that our thinning ozone layer permits too much of the germicidal UV to penetrate to the surface of the earth and causes destruction of all kinds, including damage to our skin and eye cells. Yet the theory has major flaws and no scientific backing. Contrary to general belief, there is no evidence that reduction in the ozone layer, observed at the poles, has caused any increase in melanomas.

The germicidal frequency of UV is destroyed or is filtered out by the ozone layer in the Earth's stratosphere, and only small amounts - necessary to purify the air we breathe and the water we drink - actually reach the surface of the earth. To that effect, a study of Punta Arenas, the largest South American city close to the Antarctic ozone hole, showed no increase in health problems related to depleted ozone. In fact, UV measures were too small to have any noticeable effect. Actual measurements taken in the United States since 1974 show that the amount of UV radiation reaching the surface of the earth is decreasing and continues to decrease slightly each year. This research was conducted to detect the frequency of UV radiation that causes sunburn. UV radiation had dropped an average of 0.7 percent per year over the period from 1974 to 1985 and continued to do so afterwards.

The fact that the number of skin cancers in the United States had doubled within this period of 11 years contradicts the theory that UV light is the reason behind the skin cancer epidemic. The number of malignant skin cancers (melanomas) discovered in 1980 in the United States was 8,000, and eight years later it had increased by 350 percent to 28,000. In 1930, the expectancy of developing melanoma was as low as 1 in 1,300 people. Since 2003, 45,000 to 50,000 new cases are diagnosed every year in the United States. Melanomas, which account for 75 percent of all skin cancer deaths, make up only 5 percent of all reported skin cancers. The most striking fact about this lethal form of cancer is that it can occur in parts of the body that are not necessarily exposed to the sun such as the eye, the rectum, vulva, vagina, mouth, respiratory tract, GI tract and urinary bladder.

Overall, since the beginning of the new millennium, each year one million Americans are being diagnosed with some form of skin cancer. There are millions of sufferers now, all of whom have been made to believe that the sun is the culprit for their skin diseases. But since UV radiation is decreasing every year and skin cancers were extremely rare 100 years ago when UV intensity was much higher and people spent much more time outdoors, what other factor could be held responsible for causing skin cancer?

The More UV, the Less Cancer

Even if UV penetration to the surface of the Earth did actually increase by, for example, one percent each year (which is not the case), such slight increases would still be hundreds, if not thousands, of times less than the normal variations which people experience because of differences in geography.

---

[21] **Basal cell carcinoma (BCC)** is the most common form, but does not spread. Untreated, it burrows deeply into underlying tissues causing disfigurement and serious damage.

    Squamous cell carcinoma (SCC) is considered to be more dangerous than BCC because it can spread to other parts of the body.

    Malignant melanoma is the most dangerous form of skin cancer. It can spread very quickly and, unless caught early, can be very difficult to treat. It develops from cells called melanocytes in the outer layer of the skin. Melanomas usually start in moles or in areas of abnormal-looking skin

Let's assume that you move from an area near either one of the Polar Regions, for instance Iceland or Finland, toward the equator, for instance. Kenya or Uganda in East Africa. By the time you reach the equator, you will have increased your body's exposure to UV light by a whooping 5,000 percent! If you live in England and decide to move to Northern Australia you will increase your exposure by 600 percent! Calculations show that for every six miles you move closer to the equator, you increase your exposure to UV light by one percent.

Today, millions of people around the world travel from low exposure places to areas of high exposure near the equator. Many thousands of tourists travel to areas that are located at much higher altitudes than where they normally live. For every 100 feet of elevation there is a significant increase in UV radiation. But this does not prevent people from climbing mountains or living in countries like Switzerland or at the high altitudes of the Himalayan Mountains. According to the UV/cancer theory, most Kenyan, Tibetan, or Swiss residents should be afflicted with skin cancer today. Yet this is not the case at all. The fact is that those who reside at high altitudes or near the equator where UV radiation is the most concentrated are virtually free of all cancers, not just skin cancers! This shows that UV radiation does not cause cancer; in fact, it can even prevent it.

The human body has a unique ability to become accustomed to all kinds of variations in the environment. It is equipped with perfect self-regulating mechanisms that protect it against damage from the natural elements. Overexposure to swimming in the sea or in a lake can lead to extensive skin swelling, shivering, and circulatory problems. Our body will let us know when it is time to get out of the water. Getting too close to a fire will heat us up and encourage us to move away from it. Rainwater is natural, but standing in the rain for too long can drain our immune system and make us susceptible to catching a cold. Eating sustains our lives, but overeating can lead to obesity, diabetes, heart disease, and cancer. Sleeping 'recharges our batteries' and revitalizes the body and mind, yet too much of it makes us sluggish, depressed, and ill. Likewise, sunlight has healing properties unless we use it to burn holes into our skin. Why should any of these natural elements or processes cause us harm unless we abuse or overuse them?

Wouldn't it make more sense to say that a preference for unnatural things like junk food, stimulants, alcohol, drugs, medical intervention (unless it is for an emergency), as well as pollution, irregular sleeping and eating habits, stress, excessive greed for money and power, and the lack of contact with nature, are more likely to cause such diseases as skin cancer and cataracts than natural phenomena that have ensured continued growth and evolution on the planet throughout the ages?

It is very encouraging to see that new treatments using light are increasingly being recognized as breakthrough methods for cancer and many other diseases. The U.S. Food and Drug Administration recently approved 'light therapy' to fight advanced esophageal cancer and early lung cancer - with fewer risks than are found with the use of surgery and chemotherapy. Although it has been known for over 100 years that light can kill diseased cells, it is only since a number of convincing research studies have been conducted that there has been a sudden resurgence of interest in light therapy. There is promising success with bladder cancer, infertility-causing endometriosis, advanced lung and esophageal cancers, skin cancer, and diseases leading to blindness, psoriasis, and autoimmune disorders. In one study, light therapy eliminated 79 percent of early lung cancers. Regular exposure to sunlight still seems to be one of the best measures one can take to prevent cancer, including cancers of the skin.

Now Even Doctors and Scientists Say: "It's Not True!"

Like myself, there have always been some health practitioners who didn't buy into the theory that the sun causes deadly diseases. It warms my heart to hear that now even some of the top authorities in the field are standing up for the truth, despite intense criticism from their colleagues. In an article written in the *New York Times* in August 2004, a high-profile dermatologist, Dr. Bernard Ackerman (a recent winner of the American Academy of Dermatology's prestigious, once-yearly Master Award), publicly questioned the commonly accepted assumption about the sunlight/melanoma link. According to Dr. Ackerman, who in 1999 founded the world's largest center for dermatopathology training, there is no proof whatsoever that sun exposure causes melanoma. To substantiate his arguments, he cites a recently published article in the *Archives of Dermatology* concluding that no evidence exists supporting the notion that sunscreen prevents melanoma, a claim the mega-million dollar sunscreen industry and those in the medical mainstream have falsely made for decades.

Dr. Ackerman didn't stop at exposing this decades-long deception of the masses; he also cast doubt on the increase in the incidence of melanoma cases medical mainstream doctors insist is happening. He found that an expansion of the diagnostic definition of 'melanoma' has allowed a much broader array of symptoms to be classified as the deadly disease compared to just 30 years ago. Melanoma has to a large extent 'grown' to epidemic proportions because of statistical manipulations. In other words, if the same diagnostic definition applied 30 years ago were applied today, melanomas would have increased only insignificantly.

Furthermore, this respected physician challenged the medical mainstream to explain why nearly all cases of melanoma among certain races (black African, Asian and South American) occur in areas of the body that are almost never exposed to sunlight—places like the palms, soles of the feet, and mucous membranes[22]. Should it not raise doubts among physicians and patients alike when even among pale-faces, the most common sites for melanoma (legs in women, torso in men) get significantly less sunlight exposure than other parts of the body? To make a point, based on this and other evidence, your best chance of avoiding melanoma is to move to areas of higher UV-concentration, such as mountainous regions or the equatorial tropics and become a nudist! Since sunlight boosts the immune system, you may find that such a move would also help with many other health issues from which you may be suffering. Naturally, all this data raises the question, what actually causes skin cancer? The answer may surprise you greatly.

Skin Cancer Caused By Sun Protection

The sun is completely harmless unless we expose our bodies to it for unduly long periods of time, especially between 10:00 a.m. and 3:00 p.m. (during the summer). Overexposure to sunlight makes most people feel very hot and bothered and burns their skin. To avoid being burned and to find relief, our body's natural instinct urges us to look for a shady place or to take a cold shower. Sunscreen, however, interferes with this natural response to sunlight.

Sunscreens usually block UV rays in two ways: either by using a physical sun filter, such as talc, titanium oxide or zinc oxide, or by using chemicals, whose active ingredients include *methoxycinnamate, p-aminobenzoic acid, benzophenone* and other agents that absorb certain sun-burning UV frequencies while allowing others to pass through. Sunscreen lotions containing *para-aminobenzoic acid* (PABA), for example, not only block out the therapeutic and healing effects of sunlight, but may also cause genetic damage to the skin. A recent report issued by the U.S. Food and

---

[22] Although melanoma has been rising among pale-skinned populations (who use sun-screens) worldwide, there has been no corresponding rise among native, dark-skinned populations, who have only one-tenth to one-third the incidence. Their skin's higher melanin level may protect them, but they also tend to spend much more time outdoors in normally higher concentrations of UV light.

Drug Administration included evidence that fourteen out of seventeen suntan lotions containing PABA may be carcinogenic, i.e., cause cancer. Further research has shown that PABA causes increased genetic damage to the DNA in skin cells during exposure to sunlight. The damage done to the genes and chromosomes impairs the cell's ability to properly reproduce itself. UV light induces damage to the DNA in the presence of PABA, but to implicate UV light for this effect is tantamount to saying oxygen is dangerous because when it reacts with carbon atoms it turns into a harmful waste product in our blood.

Most sunscreens normally protect against UVA, UVB, or both[23]. They are also rated according to a sun protection factor (SPF), which indicates the time of burn protection when compared to sun exposure without lotion. For example, an SPF of 15 indicates that it should provide 300 minutes of protection for someone who could normally stay in the sun for 20 minutes without burning. SPFs only apply to protection rating against UVB, not UVA. But since the effectiveness of sunscreen usually wears off well before the calculated time, unsuspecting sunbathers keep applying very large amounts of these chemical poisons to their skin. The skin is not made of plastic, but of living cells. The constant biochemical warfare fought on the surface of the skin interferes with and destroys its own protective mechanisms, and makes it susceptible to permanent damage and abnormal cell growth. Such suspicions have caused some chemicals found in sun lotions, such as 5-methoxypsoralen, to be discontinued.

The main problem with using sunscreens is, however, that they may seduce sunbathers to stay in the sun much longer than it would normally be wise to do. A British medical report, released in July 1996 and published as the lead article in the prestigious British Medical Journal, showed that the use of sunscreens might indeed encourage skin cancer because they prompt people to stay in the sun far too long. Their use can postpone the onset of sunburn by many hours. Most people think that this is advantageous, whereas in fact it puts their lives at risk. The doctors who edited the report cited studies conducted in 1995 in Western Europe and Scandinavia that showed frequent users of sunscreen lotion actually suffered disproportionately higher rates of skin cancer. The report states: "Sunscreens containing only ultraviolet B blocks protect against sunburn and therefore enable greater exposure to ultraviolet A (UVA) than would otherwise be possible to obtain." In other words, many sunbathers expose themselves to much more UVA than they would if they didn't use screens. Sunburn, in fact, is the body's natural defense response against more serious damage, such as skin cancer.

Without sunscreen your skin begins to itch uncomfortably when exposed to too much sun. In contrast, with the use of sunscreen you would not notice when your body has had enough sun because your first line of defense - unbearable sunburn - has been undermined. Overexposure to UVA combined with external harmful chemicals and, perhaps, internal toxins, is the perfect recipe to damage skin cells and cause malignancies. Under normal conditions (without sunscreen), you would never get too much UVA even if you lay in the sun for many hours. Although you would burn your skin through overexposure to UVB, you would still be protected against too much UVA.

As Dr. Ackerman discovered, although sunburn may temporarily impair immune functions and damage the skin, there is no proof that it can cause skin cancer. The British Medical Journal concluded that medical experts know "little about the precise relation between sunburn and skin cancer." This fact refers to all skin cancers, especially the fatal type of skin cancer - melanoma. Despite the colossal

---

[23]
   Of the three UV rays, UVA is mainly responsible for the tanning response, UVB activates the synthesis of vitamin D which is crucial for the absorption of calcium and other minerals, while UVC, almost completely filtered out by the Earth's ozone layer, is germicidal and kills bacteria, viruses and other disease-causing germs.

               Timeless Secrets of Health and Rejuvenation

amount of research done on skin cancers, there has been no indication that malignant melanoma has any links with UV exposure. But what is known for sure is that sunscreen not only fails to prevent skin cancer but, on the contrary, encourages it by amplifying UVA absorption. This makes sunscreens far more dangerous than sunlight could ever be.

The question remains: Can sunscreens that are made to block out both UVA and UVB radiation solve this problem? Research has shown that they don't prevent skin cancer either. First, the skin still has to deal with the acid assault that occurs when applying the lotion. Second, shutting out UVAs and UVBs deprives the body of the most important rays of the sun responsible for maintaining proper immunity and numerous essential processes. The body requires UVB, for example, for the synthesis of vitamin D, without which we cannot survive. Is it surprising, then, to find that there are many people suffering from skin cancer today who have had either very little or no exposure to sunlight?

Deficient Sunlight – A Death Trap

It has been known for several decades that those living mostly in the outdoors, at high altitudes, or near the equator, have the lowest incidence of skin cancers. And as the evidence suggests, those who work under artificial lighting have the highest incidence of skin cancers. In a study conducted on U.S. Navy personnel between 1974 and 1984, researchers found a higher incidence of skin cancers among sailors who had indoor jobs than those working outside. Those working both indoors and outdoors showed the most protection, with a rate 24 percent below the U.S. national average. Since none of the sailors spent their entire day outside, it could not be determined whether being outside all day would offer the highest degree of protection.

It is interesting to note that some of the hottest places in the U.S., such as Phoenix, Arizona, have the highest rates of skin cancers, but not because residents of Phoenix overly expose their skin to the sun. The extreme heat throughout much of the year keeps most people indoors during the day. In addition, the dry, hot air while outside, and the dry, cold air produced by air conditioners inside the home, office building, and car quickly removes any moisture from the skin, thereby leaving the skin with very little natural protection against the elements, fungi, and bacteria. Even during the night, because of constant air-conditioning, the skin is rarely able to breathe natural, moist air. The lack of moisture in the skin greatly reduces its ability to remove harmful waste products from the connective tissues and other parts of the body. In addition, the dehydrated skin readily absorbs the harmful chemicals contained in most moisturizers and sunscreen lotions, both of which are used more frequently in hot, dry places such as Phoenix. All this can lead to increasingly weak and damaged skin cells, which in many cases become cancerous.

The average city-dwelling American spends twenty-two hours a day indoors, most of that time beneath and around artificial light. Children, too, are increasingly spending less time outside in nature, and more of their time indoors at home, in school, on the computer, and in front of the television set. During the winter season, most of the working population in the cities never even sees daylight, except through windows that reflect UV light. Incandescent light has a narrow band compared to sunlight, and exposure to it is known to weaken one's natural immunity. (A Russian study showed that workers who were exposed to UV light during working hours suffered 50 percent fewer colds.) A weak immune system cannot properly defend itself against disease, and that includes skin cancer!

Researcher Dr. Helen Shaw and her team conducted a melanoma study at the London School of Hygiene and Tropical Medicine, and at the Sydney Melanoma Clinic in Sydney Hospital. They found that office workers had twice the incidence of the deadly cancer as people who worked outdoors. The results of the study were published in 1982 by the British medical journal *Lancet*. Dr. Shaw proved that those who spent most of their time exposed to natural sunlight had by far the lowest risk of developing skin cancer. In sharp contrast to those living or working outdoors, office workers who were exposed to artificial light during most of their working hours had the highest risk of developing melanomas. She also discovered that fluorescent lights cause mutations in cultures of animal cells.

Dr. Shaw's research led to the conclusion that both in Australia and Great Britain, melanoma rates were high among professional and office workers and low in people working outdoors. In other words, the Australians and British (and the rest of us) would be better off spending more time outside where there is plenty of UV light! Similar controlled studies were conducted at the New York University School of Medicine, which confirmed and substantiated Dr. Shaw's research results.

People with brown to black Afro-Caribbean skin and hair can spend long periods in the sun without burning. They rarely suffer from skin cancer while living in their native lands where sunshine is plentiful. Their skins' high melanin level filters out a lot of UV but still provides them with enough of the beneficial rays. The problem arises once they move to more moderate or colder climates, like the U.K. or Sweden. This requires that they get extra exposure to the sun to maintain normal vitamin D levels. In the U.S., 42 percent of African-American women of childbearing age are deficient in vitamin D. If the darker races don't get these extra amounts of sunlight, they are the ones who are most likely to develop skin cancer. The reason for their higher cancer risk is not *too much* sunlight, but *too little* of it.

In support of previous findings that Vitamin D prevents cancer, the American Journal of Clinical Nutrition, in its June 2007 issue [85(6):1586-91], published the first large-scale, randomized, placebo-controlled study on vitamin D and cancer. It showed that vitamin D can cut cancer risks by as much as 60 percent. The study observed nearly 1,200 women, aged 55 and older, over the course of four years. The women were divided into two groups. One group was given supplemental calcium and vitamin D, the other group received a placebo. Those in the first group had a 60 percent lower risk for all cancers compared with those who were in the placebo group.

This previous study was further substantiated by research from Stanford University. Exposure to sunlight may reduce your risk of advanced breast cancer, according to a new study published in the *American Journal of Epidemiology* October 12, 2007. The study followed 4,000 women between the ages of 35 and 79, and evaluated the effects of long-term sun exposure. It found that women with a light skin color who had high sun exposure had half the risk of developing advanced breast cancer (cancer that has spread beyond the breast) as women with low sun exposure. In other words, the more regularly you expose your skin to the sun, the less likely will you develop cancer of the breast or other types of cancer.

In response to these most recent cancer-breakthrough studies, the Canadian Cancer Society is now recommending vitamin D for all adults, the first time a major public-health organization has endorsed the vitamin as a cancer-prevention therapy. Although Vitamin D is available in some food sources and supplements, about 90 percent of the vitamin is produced by the body in direct response to sun exposure. In fact, the quickest and most efficient way top obtain enough cancer-preventing Vitamin D is sun exposure. Although direct contact with sunlight has prevented cancer and many other diseases for thousands of years, it is discouraged and even warned against by today's health care industry.

As is so often the case, the purely symptom-oriented medical theories fall short in explaining the causes of disease. In fact, they are likely to make you ill. Beware of any advice given to you by any doctor, company, or organization who wants to protect you against a supposed threat while at the same time trying to sell you something else, such as sunscreen lotions.

Pittas -Watch Out!

Australians who are not Aboriginals usually have fair and often freckled skin, reddish-blond hair, and light-colored eyes. Most Australians are Pitta types, which means that UV light penetrates deeper into their skin than among those who have darker skin or are Vata or Kapha types. In addition, many Australians are fond of drinking beer, which has a strong diuretic effect and draws water from the skin, leaving it unprotected against heat rays. Both are risk factors for damaging skin cells.

Our skin has *melanocyte* cells that release *melanin* when exposed to sunlight. *Melanin* is the skin's protective darkening pigment whose presence we refer to as a tan. Pitta types are very sensitive to heat, and their bodies will quickly tell them if the amount of *melanin* produced is not sufficient to protect them against burning. Pitta types should, therefore, *not* use sunscreens. Blocking out UVB may be disastrous for their skin. Blocking out both UVB and UVA altogether can undermine proper vitamin D synthesis and upset some of the most basic functions in their body. Pitta types are also the first to react to the presence of harmful chemicals and poisons, developing multiple chemical sensitivities and allergies.

If Pittas expose themselves to the direct sun (avoid the sun from 10:00 a.m. to 3:00 p.m.) for just a few minutes a day, they will soon be able to increase their body's exposure to a maximum of twenty minutes a day without having any signs of reddening. Their skin will improve and *melanin* production will increase. This exposure to the sun will give them enough UV light to remain healthy, provided they do *not* use devices and solutions that alter or filter out light, including sunscreens or sunglasses. Exposing their skin to the sun under the influence of alcohol or other diuretics, such as coffee, tea, and soft drinks greatly increases the chance of damaging the skin.

No Sun, No Health!

A balanced diet of sunlight, which varies according to body type and racial color[24], includes all the various frequency bands of ultraviolet light reaching the earth. Along with nutritious food and a balanced lifestyle, sunlight still offers the best protection against all types of diseases. Solar research from all over the world has shown that exposure to ultraviolet light is probably the most comprehensive and impressive healing method there is. With all of the tremendous benefits that sunlight has been proven to bestow upon us, it is truly astonishing that most of the sick people in the world still rely on expensive and poisonous medical drugs that do not offer nearly as many benefits. The following are a few examples of what ultraviolet light can do for you.

Ultraviolet light
- improves electrocardiogram readings
- lowers blood pressure and resting heart rate
- improves cardiac output when needed (not contradictory to lower resting heart rate)
- reduces cholesterol, if required
- increases glycogen stores in the liver
- balances blood sugar

---

[24] People with a dark skin, such as black Africans, block out the most rays and may need several hours of sun exposure each day to stay healthy. Fair-skinned people need less time (from 20-60 minutes each day) in the sun to receive the necessary amount of the beneficial rays. Being creatures of the Earth, we were designed to live in a natural environment. Being deprived of sunlight for long periods of time each day, therefore, poses a significant health risk.

- enhances energy, endurance, and muscular strength
- improves the body's resistance to infections due to an increase of lymphocytes and phagocytic index (the average number of bacteria ingested per leukocyte of the patient's blood)
- enhances the oxygen-carrying capacity of the blood
- increases sex hormones
- improves resistance of the skin to infections
- raises one's tolerance to stress and reduces depression

Sunlight not only purifies seawater to a depth of 12 feet, but it also disinfects the skin from harmful germs. The longer the ultraviolet wavelength, the deeper it penetrates the skin. At 290nm (one nanometer or nm equals one billionth of a meter) about 50 percent of the ultraviolet light penetrates a little deeper than to the superficial layers of the skin, whereas at 400nm, 50 percent reaches the deeper layers. The deeper-reaching rays can even penetrate the brain. The human body was designed to absorb UV light for very good reasons; otherwise we would have been born with a natural sunscreen for UV light on our skin and in our eyes. One of the most important reasons is that UV radiation is necessary for normal cell division. A lack of UV light disturbs normal cell growth, which can lead to cancer, as confirmed by Dr. Shaw's research. The use of sunglasses, including regular UV reflecting spectacles and contact lenses, are co-responsible for certain degenerative eye diseases such as macular degeneration. Most people who use sunglasses report continuously weakening eyesight. The solution is to this problem is simple: Stop wearing them. You will soon discover that your eyes are getting used to sunlight again. There are other ways to improve eyesight and reduce sensitivity to sunlight. These include eye-exercise (see my book, It's Time to Come Alive), good nutrition (consisting of mostly alkaline-forming foods), and avoiding eyestrain and watching too many hours of television.

Our typical indoor lifestyle, coupled with excessive overstimulation through highly acid-forming foods and beverages, the cholesterol-increasing and dehydrating effects of television, and various other stress factors, are sufficient cause for damage to body cells, including those that make up the eyes. By regularly shutting out much-needed UV light (even children and some pets are given sunglasses to wear nowadays), the eyes are unable to properly repair themselves and replace worn out eye cells. The increased incidence of blindness and eye diseases in the industrialized world may result, to a large extent, from the misinformation that the sun is dangerous. Please be aware that in sunny parts of the world almost everyone wears sunglasses nowadays. This may very well account for the increase of cataracts in these places. There may also be other factors involved, such as malnutrition (diarrhea can lead to severe demineralization), smoking, pollution, and poor diet. To keep your eyes healthy, be sure to allow enough direct or indirect sunlight to enter your eyes, ideally no less than one hour every day.

The reason so many people are attracted to being in the sun or long for it when it doesn't shine is inherent in the natural instinct of the body to expose itself to the healing and cleansing properties of sunlight. Without being tricked into overexposure by 'protective' sunscreens, the body will naturally know how much sunlight is good for its balanced growth. And even if circumstances lead to sunburn, the human body is perfectly equipped to handle that.

Chemical interference in this process of self-protection, however, can have serious consequences. By regularly using any of the following drugs or chemicals internally or externally, both skin and eyes become oversensitive to sunlight, and the skin may badly burn, even after a few minutes of exposure. Among these are antibacterial agents such as Sulfa, the aforementioned PABAs and other sun lotion ingredients, hypoglycemic agents used by diabetics, diuretics for control of high blood pressure, tranquillizers and anti-depressants, broad-spectrum antibiotics, anti-arrhythmic Quinidine used to suppress abnormal heart rhythms, halogenated, antiseptic compounds used in cosmetics, many types of soaps, synthetic ingredients in most commercial beauty products[25], and antihistamines used for colds and allergies.

In addition, gallstones in the liver prevent the liver from sufficiently detoxifying pharmaceutical drugs, alcohol, and other noxious substances. Whatever the liver cannot remove from the blood ends up in the kidneys and skin. Once overburdened with these internal, highly acidic toxins, the skin becomes vulnerable to the natural elements, including sunlight. Skin cancer and cataracts only occur if the liver is and the blood vessel walls are congested.

It is much easier to treat the cause of a physical problem than to suppress its symptoms. If you are taking any of the above drugs and wish to treat the cause rather than the effect of an illness, consult with your doctor about how to phase them out gradually, cleanse your elimination organs, and at the same time begin exposing your body to the sun, starting with one to two minutes and building up a few more minutes each day. (See directions below) Make certain, though, that your skin doesn't get burned. If you wear sunglasses, expose your eyes to natural light for as long as it is comfortable. Gradually you will wean yourself from sunglasses and no longer require them. To avoid dehydration of the skin, drink fresh water before and after exposure to the sun.

Sunlight Prevents Cancer, MS, Heart Disease, Arthritis, Diabetes...

According to a study published in the prominent *Cancer* journal *(March 2002; 94:1867-75)* insufficient exposure to ultraviolet radiation may be an important risk factor for cancer in Western Europe and North America. The findings, covering mortality rates from cancer in North America, directly contradict official advice about sunlight. The research showed that deaths from a range of cancers of the reproductive and digestive systems were approximately twice as high in New England as in the Southwest, despite a diet that varied little between the two regions.

An examination of 506 regions found a close inverse correlation between cancer mortality and levels of UVB light. The likeliest mechanism proposed by scientists for a protective effect from sunlight is vitamin D, which is synthesized by the body when exposed to ultraviolet B rays. According to the study's author, Dr William Grant, the northern parts of the United States may be dark enough during the winter months that vitamin D synthesis shuts down completely.

While the study focused mainly on white Americans, it also found that the same geographical trend affects black or darker skinned Americans, whose overall cancer rates are significantly higher. As explained earlier, darker skinned people require more sunlight to synthesize vitamin D.

The study showed at least 13 malignancies affected by lack of sunlight, mostly reproductive and digestive cancers. The strongest inverse correlation is with breast, colon, and ovarian cancer, followed by tumors of the bladder, uterus, esophagus, rectum, and stomach.

The Sun Cuts Cancer Risk by Half or More!
In the 1940s, Frank Apperly demonstrated a link between latitude and deaths from cancer. He suggested that sunlight provided people with a relative cancer immunity. This is now a proven fact. According to two recent studies conducted at the University of San Diego, increasing blood levels of

---

[25] Women who use synthetic make-up products on a daily basis can absorb up to 5 pounds of chemicals into their bodies each year. These chemicals are absorbed straight into the blood and enter the soft tissues of organs. Side effects range from skin irritation to cancer. The National Institute of Occupational Safety and Health stated that nearly 900 of the chemicals used in cosmetics are toxic. One class of cosmetic chemicals is *parabens*, which have been linked to cancer.

vitamin D through sunlight may decrease a person's risk of developing breast cancer by 50 percent and of developing colorectal cancer by more than 65 percent.

To increase the precision and accuracy of the study, researchers used meta-analysis to pool data from multiple previous studies. They divided subjects into groups based on their blood levels of vitamin D and compared the incidence of cancer between groups. The collected data showed that individuals in the group with the lowest blood levels of vitamin D had the highest rates of breast cancer, and the breast cancer rates dropped as the blood levels increased. The most astounding finding in this study is that the blood level associated with a 50 percent lower risk of breast cancer could be reached by spending as little as 25 minutes in the sun for darker skinned people, and no more than 10 to 15 minutes for lighter skinned individuals. This practically makes the sun an instant healer, far more effective than even the most aggressively hyped cancer drugs, such as Herceptin.

The second study showed that the same amount of sunlight corresponded with a two-thirds lower risk of contracting colorectal cancer. For any doctor or friend who asks for proof for the 'outrageous' claim that sunlight can prevent or cure cancer, you may want to refer him or her to the *Journal of Steroid Biochemistry and Molecular Biology* (doi: 10.1016/j.jsbmb.2006.12.007; 'Vitamin D and prevention of breast cancer: Pooled analysis') and to the *American Journal of Preventive Medicine* (Volume 32, Number 3, Pages 210-216; 'Optimal vitamin D status for colorectal cancer prevention - A quantitative meta-analysis').

Unlike drugs, surgery, or radiation, sunlight costs nothing, has no harmful side effects, and can prevent numerous other diseases at the same time.

Not dissimilar to the study on cancers, researchers found a strong correlation between geography and multiple sclerosis (MS). As it turns out, the incidence of MS decreases the closer to the equator (where the most UV sunlight is) one resides. Another study (2007) shows that exposing children to healthful levels of sunlight can significantly reduce their risk of falling victim to MS as adults. The University of Southern California team claim UV rays offer protection by altering the cell immune responses or by boosting vitamin D levels. MS is among the most common neurological diseases affecting around two million people worldwide. The research team noted that MS is more common at higher latitudes, which generally have lower levels of ultraviolet radiation - the type produced by the sun. Sunlight triggers a chemical reaction in the body leading to vitamin D production.

The American National Institute of Health (NIH) has linked deficiencies of the sun-made vitamin D to rising rates of many diseases, including osteoporosis, rheumatoid arthritis, heart disease, and diabetes, just to name a few. Today, up to 60 percent of all hospital patients and up to 80 percent of all nursing home patients are vitamin D deficient. What's worse, 76 percent of pregnant mothers are severely vitamin D deficient. To get the disease-curbing benefits of sunlight, you need to get outside at least three times a week, for a minimum of 15-20 minutes each time.

Pharmaceutical companies have also recognized the importance of vitamin D in the cure of cancer and other illnesses and now produce expensive drugs that contain synthetic Vitamin D. However, synthetic vitamin D has little or no effect when compared with vitamin D produced by sunlight. In addition, vitamin D added to foods such as milk, can cause serious side effects that include death (see details in 'Vitamin Euphoria', Chapter 14).

The Amazing Sunlight/Exercise Combination

Sunlight and exercise each seem to have excellent health and fitness benefits, but when used together, the effects are multiplied. Tuberculosis patients who are being treated with sunlight therapy alone (regular exposure to sunlight) experience a significant increase in muscle tone with very little fat, even if they don't exercise. The same happens to a person who is on a regular fitness program. But if sun exposure and exercise are combined, muscular tone and muscular strength increase much more than if either one is used alone.

In the male physiology, muscular development is linked to the production of the male hormone, *testosterone*. The old Greek practice of exercising nude on a warm sandy beach was used to develop a healthy muscular body. When sunlight falls on any part of the body, *testosterone* production increases substantially, but when it strikes the male genitals directly, secretion of the hormone is greatest. A study at Boston State Hospital proved that ultraviolet light increases the level of *testosterone* by 120 percent when the chest or back is exposed to sunlight. The hormone, however, increases by a whooping 200 percent when genital skin is exposed to the sun!

Regular sunbathing increases the strength and size of all muscle groups in the male physique. The combination of sun and exercise is, therefore, ideal to develop a strong and healthy body with optimal reproductive abilities. Given these findings, it may well be that constant lack of sun exposure along with physical congestion, is the main cause of the increased infertility problems among the city populations in the world. If you want to improve your sex life or fertility rates, rather than using one of the currently available costly treatments and risking your health due to their serious side effects, I would recommend that you first try the sun.

Women, of course, benefit from sunlight, too. Their levels of female hormones rise when they are exposed to particularly one specific portion of UV light, i.e., 290-340 nanometers (UVB), which is *assumed* to be dangerous and useless. Women who have only very little exposure to sunlight often suffer from menstrual problems or have no menstrual periods at all. They can re-establish a healthy menstrual cycle by sunbathing regularly and spending several hours of the day outdoors. Normalization of the menstrual cycle can occur within a few weeks after starting sunlight therapy.

In addition to assisting with the regulation of the menstrual cycle, sunlight therapy can also help those who suffer from high blood pressure. Several independent studies have demonstrated that hypertensive patients who followed a vigorous exercise program for six months lowered their blood pressure by 15 percent, whereas those who had one single exposure to the ultraviolet light of the sun had markedly lower blood pressure readings for five to six days. Exercising in the sun could, therefore, be one of the best non-medical treatments for hypertension, cost-free, and without any side effects. At the same time, both exercise and sunbathing increase the heart's efficiency, which is measured by the amount of blood pumped by the heart at each beat. A single exposure to the ultraviolet rays of the sun increases heart efficiency by an average of 39 percent, again lasting for as long as five to six days. Such an approach could effectively replace drugs currently used to stimulate the heart. It should be noted that sunlight does not act like a drug that merely suppresses the symptoms of disease but rather restores balance in body and mind.

Diabetics, too, can benefit from exercise and sunlight. Their blood sugar levels drop when they exercise or sunbathe. A single exposure to sunlight stimulates the production of the enzyme *phosphorylase*, which decreases the amount of stored glycogen. Two hours after sun exposure, another enzyme, *glycogen synthesize*, increases storage of glycogen in the tissues, while lowering blood sugar levels. Thus, sunlight acts just like insulin. The effect may last for days. It is important for diabetics to know that they may need to adjust their insulin dose and should, therefore, regularly consult their doctor while gradually increasing their body's exposure to sunlight.

Furthermore, both sunlight and exercise have beneficial effects on reducing stress levels. These include a decrease of nervousness, anxiety, and emotional imbalance; an increase of stress tolerance, self-confidence, imagination, and creativity; positive changes in personality and moods; and a reduction of unhealthy habits such as cigarette smoking and alcoholism. Studies from Russia also show that duodenal ulcers greatly improve through regular exposure to the sun.

American research found that when exposure to sunlight was added to fitness programs, subjects had a 19 percent increase in performance as measured by physical fitness tests. In addition, those exposed to UV light had 50 percent fewer incidences of colds than those who weren't. Their immune systems were maintained at a high level of efficiency. Also, children who received extra UV light during wintertime had a marked increase in physical fitness. Taking a vacation to a sunny locale, for example, can help balance the immune system during wintertime. Spending some time outside every day, even if it is cold, also helps to fill one's UV requirements. UV lamps can also be very useful. The *UV Lamp Module* sold on Dr. Mercola's website, www.mercola.com, produces hydroxyl radicals and other elements that neutralize toxins and effectively destroy microbes up to .001 microns that come in contact with its powerful UV-C rays.

And if you are on pain medication, check this out: A recent hospital study found that patients in sunnier rooms needed fewer painkillers than patients in darker rooms. In fact, they were able to cut their drug costs by 21 percent.

What Makes the Sun so 'Dangerous' - The Fat Connection!

Sunlight is most beneficial for those who eat a balanced diet according to their individual requirements and body type. Sunbathing may be dangerous, however, for those who live on a diet rich in acid-forming, highly processed foods and refined fats or products made with them. Alcohol, cigarettes, and other mineral and vitamin depleting substances, such as allopathic and hallucinogenic drugs, can also make the skin highly vulnerable to ultraviolet radiation. In particular, polyunsaturated fats as contained in refined and vitamin E depleted products, such as thin vegetable oil, mayonnaise, salad dressings, and most brands of margarine, pose a particularly high risk in the development of skin cancer and most other cancers. According to *Archives of Internal Medicine*, 1998, polyunsaturated fats increase a woman's risk of breast cancer by 69 percent. In contrast, monounsaturated fats, as found in olive oil, reduce breast cancer risk by 45 percent.

Untreated, expeller-pressed oils contain both types of fats, with varying ratios. Both kinds of fat are useful for the body. Sesame oil, for example has 50 percent polyunsaturated fats and 50 percent monounsaturated fats. If the monounsaturated fats are removed from the oil through the refining process, its polyunsaturated fats become highly reactive and damaging to cells.

This phenomenon is quite easy to understand. Polyunsaturated fats are more vulnerable to lipid per-oxidation (rancidity) than monounsaturated fats. In other words, they rapidly attract a large number of oxygen free radicals and become oxidized. Oxygen radicals are generated when oxygen molecules lose an electron. This makes them highly reactive. These free radicals may quickly attack and damage cells, tissues, and organs. They can be formed in refined, polyunsaturated fats when these are exposed to sunlight before consumption. Free radicals may also form in the tissues after the oil has been eaten. The polyunsaturated fats in refined oils are difficult to digest, since they are deprived of their natural bulk and are no longer protected against free radicals by their natural protector, vitamin E, a powerful anti-oxidant (vitamin E interferes with the oxidation process). Vitamin E and many other valuable nutrients are filtered out or destroyed during the refining process. Eating a hamburger and French fries can flood your body with free radicals. Both foods are heated with refined oils. Heating these oils greatly increases their oxidation and, therefore, tissue-damaging effects.

Most people have no idea what happens to the oil when it is extracted from a nut or seed. To extend the oil's shelf life, create a clear color and remove its natural scent, it is bathed in a petroleum solvent, then 'degummed' or placed in hot water and swirled at a high speed to separate out various substances. To further refine the oil, it is mixed with an alkali such as lye or caustic soda; then it is agitated, heated again, bleached, hydrogenated to stabilize it and finally deodorized. To increase shelf-life further, manufacturers add preservatives and other food additives. Although all of that improves the oil's shelf life, it does not prevent it from turning rancid before the expiration date. The chemical treatments it undergoes disguises signs of rancidity, which makes these oils so dangerous to the unsuspecting consumer.

Saturated fats are solid, and found in products such as lard and butter. They contain large quantities of natural antioxidants, which make them much safer against oxidation by free radicals. They are also digested quite easily. The polyunsaturated fats in refined oils (stripped of their monounsaturated fats), on the other hand, are virtually indigestible and thereby become dangerous to the body. Margarine, for example, is just one molecule away from plastic, and therefore extremely difficult to digest. Free radicals, the natural cleansers of the body, try to get rid of the fatty culprit which attaches itself to the cells' walls. But when the radicals digest these harmful fats, they also damage the cell walls. This is considered to be one of the main causes of aging and degenerative disease. This also shows how something so useful as oxygen radicals can become harmful when we expose the body to unnatural foods and chemicals.

Research has shown that out of 100 people who consumed large quantities of polyunsaturated fats, 78 showed marked clinical signs of premature aging. They also looked much older than others of the same age did. By contrast, in a recent study on the relationship between dietary fats and the risk for Alzheimer's disease, researchers were surprised to learn that the natural, healthy fats can actually reduce the risk for Alzheimer's by up to 80 percent. The study showed that the group with the lowest rate of Alzheimer's ate approximately 38 grams of these healthy fats every day, while those with the highest incidence of this disease consumed only about half of that amount.

Tissue cells that have been damaged by abnormal free radical activity are unable to reproduce properly. This can impair major functions in the body, including those of the immune, digestive, nervous, and endocrine systems. Ever since refined polyunsaturated fats have been introduced to the population on a large scale during and after WWII, degenerative diseases have increased dramatically, skin cancer being one of them. In fact, polyunsaturated fats have made sunlight 'dangerous', something that would never have been the case if foods hadn't been altered and manipulated, as they are today. When polyunsaturated fats are removed from their natural foods, they need to be refined, deodorized, and even hydrogenated, depending on the food product for which they are used. During this process some of the polyunsaturated fats undergo chemical transformations, which turns them into *trans fatty acids* (trans fats), often referred to as 'hydrogenated vegetable oils'. Margarine can contain up to 54 percent of them, vegetable shortening up to 58 percent.

You can detect hydrogenated vegetable oils in foods by reading the food labels. Most processed foods contain them, including breads, crisps, chips, doughnuts, crackers, biscuits, pastries, all baked goods, cake and frosting mixes, baking mixes, frozen dinners, sauces, frozen vegetables, and breakfast cereals. In other words, nearly all shelf foods that are processed, refined, preserved, and not fresh can contain trans fats. Trans fats inhibit the cell's ability to use oxygen, which is required to burn foodstuffs to carbon dioxide and water. Cells, which are inhibited in completing their metabolic processes, may thus become cancerous. The current movement to get trans fats out of foods has merely led to the replacement of one harmful fat with another harmful, artificially produced fat. For all practical purposes, the new man-made fats, called 'interestified' fats, are not better than the old trans fats. Research, published in *Nutrition & Metabolism* (January 15, 2007) indicates that a new method of modifying fat in commercial products raises blood glucose, depresses insulin, and reduces levels of beneficial HDL-cholesterol.

The trans fats also make the blood thicker by increasing the stickiness of the platelets. This multiplies the chances of blood clots and the buildup of fatty deposits, which can lead to heart disease. Research at Harvard Medical School, in which the dietary habits of 85,000 women were observed for over eight years, found that those eating margarine had an increased risk of coronary heart disease. Further studies have shown that trans fatty acids prevent the body from processing *Low Density Lipo Protein* (LDL) or bad cholesterol, thereby raising blood cholesterol to abnormal levels. A Welsh study linked the concentration of these artificial trans fats in body fat with death from heart disease. The Dutch government has already banned any products containing trans fatty acids.

Polyunsaturated fats have also been shown to suppress immunity. For this reason, they are used today in patients who have undergone kidney transplant operations or skin grafts taken from other people. This helps the patient's immune system not to reject the foreign tissue, but of course it also leaves the person vulnerable to infection and other disorders. The same approach is used in the so-called *autoimmune diseases* where the immune system attempts to kill off some of the body's own cells, i.e. those that have become toxic and are a risk to the survival of the body. The tragedy in all of this is that such treatments don't change overall mortality rates; only the cause of death becomes altered. The message here is that if you don't want to damage or destroy your immune system, don't eat refined, processed fats and oils.

What Really Burns and Damages the Skin

A person who consumes polyunsaturated fats in his diet and exposes his skin to ultraviolet light to the point of reddening produces hormone-like substances called *prostaglandins* from the linoleic acid contained in the fats. *Prostraglandins* suppress the immune system, thereby contributing to tumor growth. In addition, polyunsaturated fats are accompanied by free radical production, which can damage cells. If you add sunscreens to the skin, you have the right combination of chemicals to produce skin cancer, especially on areas that are more exposed to the sun than others.

In nature, oils never occur in large quantities. To obtain one tablespoon of corn oil in natural form you would have to eat 12-18 ears of corn. Since oil extraction from corn, grains, and seeds became possible 80-90 years ago, consumption of polyunsaturated and unsaturated fats (thicker oils) as salad and cooking oils has increased dramatically in the industrialized world. The average person today consumes 16 times more of these fats than a person did 90 years ago[26]. That does not include all the other fats contained in today's foods. The lack of exercise, fresh air, and foods rich in nutrients make it even less possible for a human being to cope with such large amounts of unnatural fats. They impair the digestive power and lead to a buildup of toxins and subsequent crises of toxicity. The presence of excessive amounts of free radicals indicates that the body is full of toxins. Once they enter the skin tissue, even short-term exposure to ultraviolet light can burn and damage skin cells.

If your eyes and skin are sensitive to sunlight, this indicates that your body is toxic. Your subsequent effort to avoid the sun may result in serious light deficiency, which can lead to serious health problems. The fact that cancer of all kinds increased when sunscreens were introduced is hardly surprising. The UV light entering through the eyes also stimulates the immune system. Today, more than 50 percent of the U.S. population wears prescription or sun-protective glasses, which are able to block out most UV light. The latest fashion is to wear plastic glasses, which also block out all UV light. The

---

[26] It easier for the digestive system to deal with oils that are expelled from foods with a higher concentration of oil, such as olives, coconuts, avocados etc., than from small nuts and seeds , such as almonds and linseeds.

same holds true for plastic contact lenses. Indoor activities, sunscreens, clothing, UV-repelling windows, etc. make certain that we receive very little of it. Without regular exposure to sunlight, however, the immune system decreases its effectiveness with every year of age. With sunlight, the use of oxygen in the body tissues increases, but without it, our cells begin to starve for oxygen. This leads to cellular malfunction, premature aging, and even death.

Starved of a balanced sunlight diet, we tend to look for help elsewhere, even though nature is ready to cure us at any time. It is very unfortunate that sick people are mostly kept indoors, often with curtains drawn and windows closed. One of nature's most potent preventive and curative powers is there for everyone to use.

Guidelines for Increasing Sun Exposure

If you wish to benefit from the sun but cannot afford much time to be outdoors, there are several ways to increase your exposure to sunlight:

- Windows should consist of glass that permits all the types of UV rays to enter
- Have as many such windows as possible
- Keep your curtains pushed back so that you have maximum exposure
- Depending on weather and the season, keep your windows open
- Install as many full spectrum lights as possible (the best alternative to natural sunlight)

Those living in a moderate climate can sunbathe regularly. In very hot countries or states, it is best to avoid the sun between 11.00 a.m. and 3.00 p.m. during summer, whereas in northern countries or states and during winter, spring, and fall, this time is actually more beenficial. During winter you can sunbathe if you lie in a totally wind protected place. You can build your own sunbathing area against a wall facing the sun. The sidewalls should be made of material that can serve as a good windbreak. The wall pointing toward the sun should be at an angle slanted toward the sun so that the low winter rays can shine into the sunbathing area. Lying on a blanket, you will be warmer than if you were indoors. Another, perhaps, more practical way is to open a window on a sunny day when there is no breeze. I have done this many times in my life, even in countries where winters can be very cold.

If for any reason you are going to be exposed to the sun for unduly long periods, you may apply Aloe Vera gel, coconut oil, or olive oil.

For maximum benefits, though, and to wash off any natural oiliness, it is best to take a shower before sunbathing. Start your sunlight treatment by exposing your entire body (if possible) for a few minutes, and then increase the time each day by a few more minutes until you reach 20-30 minutes. Alternatively, walking in the sun for 40-60 minutes several times per week minutes has similar benefits. This will give you enough sunlight to keep your body and mind healthy, provided you incorporate the basic measures of a balanced diet, lifestyle, and daily routine as outlined in the earlier chapters. Your body can store up a certain amount of vitamin D, which may last you through 4-6 weeks of wintry weather, but it is always good to recharge your 'vitamin D battery' whenever possible by exposing yourself to direct sunlight.

Note: Avoid sunlamps, tanning beds, and tanning booths. According to a study published in the *International Journal of Cancer* (Vol 120, No 5, March 1, 2007; 1116-1122), exposure to tanning beds before age 35 increases melanoma risk by 75 percent. Many young people now use tanning beds, which may be responsible for the recent sharp increase of melanomas in their age group. There is also a link between tanning bed use and squamous cell carcinoma, a less-deadly type of skin cancer. Conventional tanning equipment uses *magnetic ballasts* that emit powerful electromagnetic fields (EMFs) responsible for cancer growth. Their high concentration of UVA may also play a role. Electronic ballasts are safer than magnetic ballasts, but very few parlors use these. There are a few safe tanning devices I do recommend, such as the ones made available on www.mercola.com, and "vitamin D" lamps found on the internet.

The Ancient Practice of Sun Gazing

Sun energy is the source that powers the brain. It enters the body through the elements of air, water, fire, and earth. Sunlight enters and leaves the human body most easily and directly through the human eye, provided it isn't filtered out by colored lenses. Sun gazing is an ancient practice that can induce healing of body and mind.

The eyes are very complex organs, consisting of 5 billion parts. Acting as a photo lens, the human eye is able to break down the entire spectrum of sunlight into the different color rays. In a camera, the various rays of light react with the chemicals of the film and encode the pictures you take. Likewise, upon entering the pineal gland in the brain, the different rays are chemically encoded in the brain and passed on to the organs and systems in the body. The vital organs of the body are dependent on specific colors of the light spectrum. For kidney cells to function properly, for example, they require red light. Heart cells need yellow light, and liver cells require green light. Light deficiencies in any of the organs and systems of the body can lead to disease. Regular sun gazing can help restore balance and efficiency to all cells in the body.

One should gaze at the sun only in the morning or evening hours, about one or two hours after sunrise or before sunset. Look at the rising or setting sun once per day. On the first day, look at the sun in a relaxed manner for a maximum of 10 seconds. On the second day, look at it for 20 seconds, adding about ten seconds every succeeding day. After ten continuous days of sun gazing you will be looking at the sun for about 100 seconds. The eyes can blink or flicker and don't need to be steady.

To receive the main benefits of sun gazing, you need to increase the duration in the above manner until you reach three months. This brings you up to the length of 15 minutes of gazing at a time. At this stage, the sun energy of the sun's rays passing through the human eye will be charging the hypothalamus tract - the pathway behind the retina leading to the human brain. As the brain increasingly receives extra power through this pathway, you will find a drastic reduction of mental tension and worries. With access to this additional source of energy, you are likely to develop a more positive mindset and increased self-confidence. If you suffer from anxieties and depression, you will find that these go away. Sadness and depression are known to increase with reduced or lack of exposure to sunlight. With fewer worries and fears, your brain may use the saved and additionally supplied energy for healing and improvement of mental and physical wellbeing. One of the most frequently reported benefits of regular sun-gazing is improvement of eyesight.

I would like to conclude this important topic on sunlight by quoting a reader's observation he made at Sydney airport: "Some years back while waiting for a flight out of Sydney I remained in the terminal for several hours. Many flights came and went. There was a great difference in the people's facial expression of new arrivals. The ones who arrived from a colder part, (not much sun) did not smile, did not appear happy, and basically kept to themselves. People arriving from warmer, sunny parts of Australia radiated warmth and friendliness, and it was very notably etched on their faces. This observation I have never forgotten. So, you see what sunshine does to people..." ~ *Roger Sorokoput*

CHAPTER 9

The Secret Cause of Heart Disease - And Why It is So Easily Reversed

Less than one hundred years ago, heart disease was an extremely rare disease. Today, it kills more people in the developed world than all other causes of death combined, with the exception of doctor-caused, iatrogenic diseases (see Chapter 14). According to the *New England Journal of Medicine*, sudden cardiac arrest claims 350,000 to 450,000 lives per year in the United States (over 1,000 per day) and is responsible for more than half of all deaths attributed to cardiovascular disease. Each year, 865,000 Americans suffer a heart attack. As of 2004, 7.8 million people in the U.S. had survived heart attacks. Direct (medical costs) and indirect (lost productivity) costs related to coronary heart disease totaled about $133 billion in 2004. And a recent study concludes that 85 percent of people over 50 and 71 percent of people over 40 already have artery blockages!

Although the ability to recognize patients who are at high risk for cardiac arrest has greatly improved over the past 20 years, 90 percent of sudden deaths from cardiac causes occur in patients without identified risk factors. It is known that the majority of sudden deaths from cardiac causes involve patients with pre-existing coronary heart disease. Yet cardiac arrest is the first manifestation of this underlying problem in 50 percent of patients.

The most common underlying cause of sudden cardiac arrest is a heart attack which causes irregular heart rhythm and subsequent stoppage of the heart. In several industrialized nations, mortality rates from heart attacks have slightly decreased due to a generation of breakthroughs in heart care. These include new medicines, the bypass operations, and the angioplasties. But now the 'beneficiaries' of this kind of heart care are living with unexpected, often devastating consequences; their damaged hearts still beat, but not strong enough to enjoy a decent quality of life. Many wish they had died swiftly rather than suffering a slow and torturous death.

The unintended result of better cardiac care is an unprecedented increase in a debilitating disease called *chronic heart failure*, which could very well be called an epidemic. Heart failure is described as a gradual ebbing of the heart's power to pump blood and supply the body with oxygen. "Heart failure is a product of our success in dealing with heart disease and hypertension," said Dr. Michael Bristow of the University of Colorado. Treating the symptoms of heart disease and hypertension, rather than their causes, has led to more hardship and suffering than anticipated. It is the call of our time to take a more holistic look at the causes of this greatest of killer diseases in the modern world and to apply natural methods to restore heart functions swiftly and permanently, without side effects.

The Beginning Stages of Heart Disease

Our cardiovascular system is composed of a central pumping device, the heart muscles, and a blood vessel pipeline consisting of arteries, veins and capillaries. The heart muscles pump blood through the blood vessel system to deliver oxygen and nutrients to all parts of the body. The blood vessel system is over 60,000 miles long and has a surface of more than half an acre. The 60-100 trillion cells in the body depend on the frictionless flow of blood through this vast network of ducts and channels of circulation.

The tiny blood capillaries, which have the thickness of one tenth of a human hair, are of particular importance to the body. Unlike the arteries, capillaries permit oxygen, water, and nutrients to pass through their thin walls to bring nourishment to the designated tissues. At the same time, they allow for certain cellular waste to return to the blood so that it can be excreted from the body. If the capillary network becomes congested for the reasons explained below, the heart has to pump the blood with greater pressure to reach all parts of the body. This considerably increases the heart's workload and makes its muscles tense and tired. This also weakens the blood vessel walls, making them less elastic. In due time, the exertion of the heart leads to stress and fatigue and impairs all major functions in the body.

Since the blood capillaries are also responsible for nourishing the muscle cells of the arteries, a reduced supply of oxygen, water and nutrients will eventually injure and destroy arteries. To counteract this unintended self-destruction, the body responds with inflammation. The inflammation response, which is often mistaken for and treated as a disease, is actually one of the body's best methods to increase the blood supply and deliver vital nutrients to promote the growth of new cells and help repair damaged connective tissue. However, continuous inflammatory responses eventually generate sizable lesions in the arteries which, in turn, lead to the development of atherosclerotic deposits. Hardening of arteries is commonly believed to be the main cause of heart disease, although this is, as new studies have shown, not entirely true.

Major Contributing Factors

Most heart attacks are believed to be triggered by the clogging of the heart arteries, which destroys millions of heart cells, while strokes are assumed to be caused by the clogging of the brain arteries, which causes the death of millions of brain cells. Since brain cells coordinate the activities and movements of every part of the body, their death can lead to partial or complete paralysis and death. A stroke is considered to be merely a consequence of advanced arteriosclerosis.

The brain arteries are located in close proximity to the heart. The blood pressure in both the brain and heart arteries is relatively higher than in other arteries of the body; hence the difference of blood pressure in the different arteries of the circulatory system. If turbulence and congestion occur in the branching areas of the arteries, the blood pressure begins to rise. This particularly stresses the coronary, carotid (neck), and cerebral (brain) arteries to the point of injury. Blood vessels that are already weakened by internal congestion and nutritional deficiencies are the first to become damaged. All this can turn high blood pressure into a major risk factor for strokes and heart disease.

Lowering an elevated blood pressure through medication, however, is not a solution, but a mere postponement and further aggravation of the problem. According to recent research, such blood pressure mediation can actually lead to chronic heart failure. Without removing the root cause(s) of elevated blood pressure, the standard treatment for hypertension can cause severe cellular dehydration and sharply reduce the blood's main functions to deliver oxygen to the heart muscles and to remove acidic waste from the body's cells and tissues. This further increases the risk of heart disease, kidney and liver disorders and many other diseases.

The Western Hemisphere leads the world in the percentage of population with heart disease. For many years now, doctors have blamed eating the wrong type of food, overeating, too little exercise, smoking, and stress as the major risk factors. The latest research has added a few more, such as free radicals, pollution, poor circulation, certain drugs and chemicals, and a decreased ability of the blood to digest protein, which may lead to the formation of blood clots. When protein is no longer able to be broken down due to insufficient proteolytic enzymes (bromelain, trypsin, and chymotrypsin), the most likely consequences are heart attacks, phlebitis, and strokes.

The major physical cause of coronary heart disease, however, is the overeating of animal proteins. When stored in the body, protein becomes one of the greatest risk factors for heart disease and most other diseases as well. One of the latest finds as to the cause of arterial damage and inflammation is the protein homocysteine, found in high concentrations in meat. This substance is now believed to be the main reason behind blood clots triggering a heart attack.

Meat Consumption and Heart Disease

To illustrate the development of heart disease from virtual non-existence to the biggest killer disease in the Western Hemisphere, I have used statistical trends describing disease development in Germany, a typical, modern industrialized nation. In the year 1800, meat consumption in Germany was about 13 kg (28 pounds) per person per year. One hundred years later, meat consumption was nearly three times as high, at 38 kg per person per year. By 1979 it had reached 94.2 kg, which is an increase of 725 percent in less than 180 years. During the period of 1946-1978, meat consumption in Germany increased by 90 percent and heart attacks rose by 20 times. These figures do not include the consumption of fats. During the same period, fat consumption remained the same, whereas consumption of cereals and potatoes, which are major suppliers of vegetable protein, decreased by 45 percent. Therefore, fats, carbohydrates, and vegetable proteins cannot be considered as causes of coronary heart disease. This leaves meat as the main factor responsible for the dramatic upsurge of this degenerative blood vessel disease.

In consideration of the fact that at least 50 percent of the German population is overweight and most overweight people eat more meat than those with normal weight, meat consumption among the overweight must have at least quadrupled in the 33 years after World War II. Being overweight is considered a major risk for high blood pressure and heart disease.

According to statistics published by the World Health Organization (WHO) in 1978, the yearly increases in heart attacks in Western European countries were accompanied by a continuous increase in meat consumption, as much as 4 kg per person annually. This shows that eating habits after World War II shifted from a healthy mixed diet to one very high in animal protein but low in carbohydrates such as fruits, vegetables and grains. According to the WHO, fat consumption remained virtually unchanged. Heart attacks and arteriosclerosis began to increase dramatically in Germany and other industrialized nations soon after the war. Today these conditions account for over 50 percent of all deaths, excluding those caused by medical treatment.

Although fat consumption among vegetarians is not lower than among meat eaters, vegetarians have the lowest death rates from heart disease. The *Journal of the American Medical Association* reported that a vegetarian diet could prevent 97 percent of all coronary occlusions. The reason for the virtual absence of coronary heart disease among vegetarians is their more balanced carbohydrate consumption and low intake or complete absence of animal protein. Fat consumption is, therefore, merely an accomplice of the disease, but not its cause. (As was already explained, the highly toxic trans-fats found in refined oils and margarines are the exception). The constantly recycled mass hysteria that declares fat, generally associated with cholesterol, to be the main dietary culprit of heart disease, is completely unfounded, outdated, and has no scientific basis.

The incredibly popular high protein, low-carbohydrate *Atkins Diet* and *South Beach Diet* have the unfortunate side effect of starving a person by clogging his capillary and artery walls with excessive proteins and by greatly limiting his fuel intake from carbohydrates. This can certainly make a person lose weight, but not without also damaging his kidneys, liver and heart. Both the late Dr. Atkins, a heart disease and obesity victim, and former U.S. President Bill Clinton, a keen follower of the South Beach Diet and recipient of a quadruple bypass, suffered the consequences of the high protein diet (for details, see next section). Millions of Americans are following in their footsteps.

A study by Scottish researchers, published in the journal *Applied and Environmental Microbiology*, examined the prolonged use of exceptionally low-carbohydrate weight-loss diets on gut health. The scientists at Aberdeen's Rowett Research Institute found that prolonged adherence to the low-carb diet may adversely affect the gut bacterial populations that beneficially produce a substance called butyrate, which is important for keeping the gut healthy and preventing colorectal cancer. Thankfully, low-carb diets recently lost popularity with the public since the approach has been shown to put followers at a higher risk for clogged arteries, heart attack, and possibly colorectal cancer as well.

Yes, Your Body Can Store Protein!

Meat and meat products have 5 to 10 times the protein concentration of plant food proteins. Whereas you can easily overeat on animal protein, it is much less likely to overeat on proteins contained in vegetables, grains and nuts. The stomach would have to be at least five times larger to accommodate such large portions of food. It is common knowledge that the body is able to store unused sugar and other carbohydrates in the form of fat, but it is lesser known that the body also has a large 'storage' capacity for protein. The body's (unintended) protein stores are the *connective tissue*, notably the fluid between the capillaries and the cells, and the *basal membrane* of the blood vessel walls. The basal membrane supports the cells of the blood capillaries and arteries and keeps them in place (see **illustration 19**). Without this membrane, the blood vessels would collapse and fall apart. The basal membrane has the capacity to accommodate excessive protein by increasing its thickness up to eight times.

When this protein storage is filled to capacity, the protein-congested blood capillaries can no longer deliver enough oxygen and nutrients to the organs and arteries. The cells that make up these parts of the body begin to suffocate in their own metabolic waste products. The resulting toxicity crisis prompts an inflammatory process by the body, which is necessary to increase blood flow and to make nutrients available for the growth of new cells and the repair of damaged tissues. Repeated bouts of inflammation in the artery walls can involve bleeding and the subsequent formation of blood clots. Blood clots are the number one cause of strokes and heart attacks (see **illustrations 20a/b**).

As a first aid measure to avert potential heart attacks or strokes, the body attempts to contain the bleeding wounds. It does this by dispatching the glue-like *lipoprotein, LP5*, into the blood. LP5 attaches itself to the open wounds, thereby sealing them. To promote the wounds healing and to prevent them from repeated bleeding, the sticky LP5 catches the relatively large lipoprotein molecules, such as LDL and VLDL cholesterol molecules (or 'bad' cholesterol), and builds them into the artery walls. The resulting protective 'bandage' saves the person's life, at least for a while. It prevents blot clots from escaping into the blood and causing a heart attack or stroke. If this survival mechanism occurs in the coronary arteries, it is called *hardening of arteries* or *coronary heart disease*. As you can see, there is nothing bad about 'bad' cholesterol. Cholesterol is a stress and healing hormone that the body dispatches to any injured parts of the body.

Thickening of Blood Capillary Wall

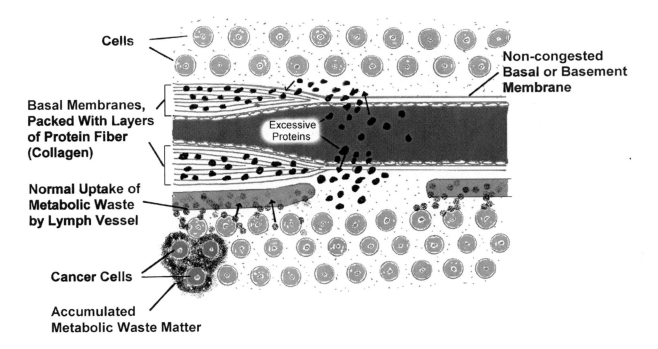

Cells

Non-congested
Basal or Basement
Membrane

Basal Membranes,
Packed With Layers
of Protein Fiber
(Collagen)

Excessive
Proteins

Normal Uptake of
Metabolic Waste
by Lymph Vessel

Cancer Cells

Accumulated
Metabolic Waste Matter

Hardening of Artery

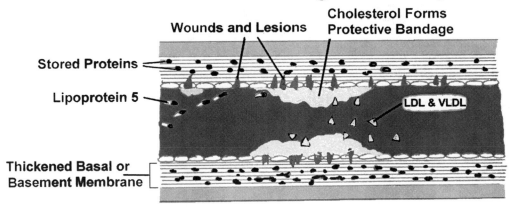

Wounds and Lesions

Cholesterol Forms
Protective Bandage

Stored Proteins

Lipoprotein 5

LDL & VLDL

Thickened Basal or
Basement Membrane

Illustration 19: Congestion of Blood Vessel Walls with Excessive Protein

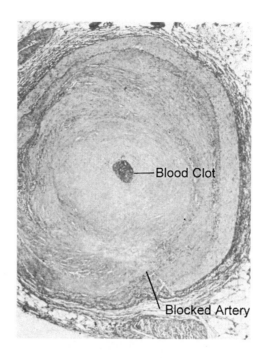

Illustration 20a: Blood clot that caused heart attack in 54-year old man

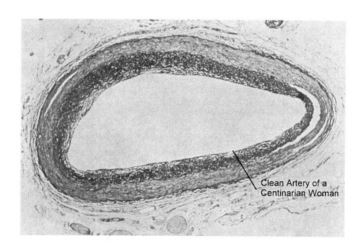

Illustration 20b: Healthy, open artery of a 100-year old woman

A person who eats too many simple carbohydrate foods (sugar, bread and pasta) or fats in a particular meal may have elevated concentrations of these substances and the cholesterol-containing lipoproteins in his blood. But a blood test would also reveal a higher concentration of proteins if he ate a large protein meal. Nutritional science assumes that protein is completely burned during the digestive process, despite the fact that no scientific evidence supports such an assumption. The current hypothesis is that whatever protein the cells don't use or need continues to circulate in the blood until it is broken down by liver enzymes and excreted as urea.

A major problem arises when a person does not have enough of these enzymes to remove the excessive protein from the bloodstream. The liver of a Kapha or Pitta type, for example, requires only very few food proteins to sustain the body, and therefore has only a limited capacity to break down food proteins. If liver bile ducts are congested with stones, this also greatly diminishes the liver's ability to break down proteins. The same applies to people who regularly eat too many proteins. In all these situations, the extra protein not broken down and eliminated by the liver is instead absorbed by the connective tissue under the skin, which for the short-term is the least harmful solution. It will also end up in the intercellular, connective tissue of the organs, which can potentially be fatal. If large amounts of food protein are continuously ingested, the intercellular connective tissue and basal membranes of the capillaries start filling up with protein and begin to thicken. Unless protein intake is discontinued, the cells of the capillary walls become progressively weaker and damaged. The body responds with inflammation to help destroy damaged cells and remove dead cells. The inflammatory response, though, has side effects. This is the beginning stage of diet-caused arteriosclerosis.

It was first discovered in 1955 that people who avoid eating animal protein for a certain length of time do not produce extra urea following their first few protein meals. Urea results from the breakdown of protein in the body. The lack of extra urea means that their connective tissues contain no abnormal amounts of protein yet. The blood levels also rise with protein consumption. A blood urea nitrogen (BUN) test measures the amount of nitrogen in the blood that comes from urea. This test is done to see how well the kidneys are working. If the kidneys are not able to remove all urea from the blood normally, the BUN level rises. A diet high in protein makes the BUN level higher, which can easily overtax the kidneys. Vegetarians whose source of protein is purely vegetarian (grains, legumes, nuts, seeds, etc.) rarely have high BUN levels. Because they hardly ever develop a surplus of protein in the connective tissues and blood vessel walls, their risk of developing atherosclerotic deposits is virtually non-existent. This has been confirmed by the American Medical Association.

It is a commonly accepted medical theory that all unused calories, whether they occur in the form of carbohydrates, fat, or protein, are converted into fat and deposited in the body's fat cells. This would make fat to be the only storage molecule responsible for obesity and related illnesses, including coronary heart disease and Type 2 diabetes (see chapter 11). Yet there is overwhelming evidence to show that stored fat alone cannot be held responsible for causing coronary heart disease. The only other substance that the body can store in large amounts is protein. And much of it ends up in the blood vessel walls.

It is important to know that proteins accumulating in the wrong places can be fatal. In 1961, research published by a journal of the American Medical Association showed that even the body's own blood proteins, which continuously enter the connective tissue of organs and systems, can kill a person within 24 hours if they are not swiftly removed and returned to the blood stream by the lymphatic system. If the lymphatic system is severely congested, these proteins have to be also stored in the basal membranes of the blood vessel walls.

A well-trained athlete can utilize no more than 40 grams of protein per day. The average American eats up to 200 grams of protein per day. The body converts any proteins it cannot store in the blood vessel walls into nitric, sulfuric and phosphoric acids, similar to the acids found in your car battery. This is very likely to occur if more than 30-40 grams of protein is eaten each day. The kidneys try to eliminate some of these strong acids by attaching a basic mineral to every acid molecule. As a result, the major basic minerals sodium, potassium, magnesium as well as others become depleted. All this pushes your body toward an incidence of *acidosis*, which is another name for a toxicity crisis. Heart disease is a typical symptom of chronic acidosis.

Protein Storage - A Time Bomb

Obese people have both high concentrations of fats and excessive amounts of protein in the blood. The blood's tendency towards clotting, considered to be the greatest cause for heart attack or stroke, stems almost exclusively from the saturation of proteins in the blood. (Note that smoking also increases blood protein concentrations, as shown below). Fats, on the other hand, have *no* blood-clotting ability. In their attempt to avert a heart attack, the capillary cells absorb the excessive protein, convert it into *collagen fiber*, and store it in their basal membranes. Although this emergency response has a blood-thinning and, therefore, life-saving effect, it also makes the blood walls thicker and more vulnerable to injury.

Examinations of connective tissue in obese people have proved that it contains not only plump fat cells, but also large amounts of dense collagen-fiber. Collagen is 100 percent pure protein. Building more collagen-fiber than normally needed is one of the main emergency measures the body takes to deal with dangerously high protein concentrations in the blood. By removing the protein from the blood and thereby putting it out of circulation, the blood becomes thin and a major crisis is avoided. But the situation changes drastically when the body's 'protein stores' are all filled up to capacity, and protein consumption continues. This time, the blood becomes and remains saturated with protein. In such a case, the blood begins to permanently thicken and develop a tendency towards clotting.

Unless the afflicted person takes aspirin, which has a blood-thinning effect, a stroke or heart attack may occur. Yet in the long term, aspirin not only fails to prevent such an incidence but strongly encourages it. A heightened risk of deadly uncontrolled bleeding may also result from regular or excessive use of aspirin. In addition, once aspirin treatment discontinues, the risk of suffering a heart attack is greatly increased.

Warning: If you suffer from *macular degeneration*, the #1 cause of blindness in people over 55 years old, avoid taking aspirin. Also avoid smoking.

Recent research found that smoking is the leading cause of macular degeneration; half of all smokers develop it. As soon as a person stops smoking, the risk lessens by one third. A major study linked aspirin to America's epidemic of macular degeneration. The often prescribed one-aspirin-a-day routine makes the retinas more likely to hemorrhage. Besides, aspirin belongs to the same class of painkillers as Vioxx, Celebrex and Aleve, all of which were found to increase heart attack and stroke risk by over 50 percent.

Tests have shown that abstaining from food for a periodic length of time reduces the size and amount of both fat cells and collagen fiber deposits. This also demonstrates that overeating protein does, in fact, increase protein tissue in the body. As explained before, and to emphasize this crucial point, the protein deposits accumulate in the basal membranes of the capillary walls and the connective tissues that surround the cells. As a direct consequence of this development, the thickened blood vessel walls are no longer capable of absorbing sufficient amounts of oxygen, water, and nutrients, and hence they cannot remove all the metabolic waste products that the cells produce. Therefore, the cells that make up these blood vessels become injured and eventually die from malnutrition, suffocation and dehydration.

In a young person, the main blood vessels of the heart have a diameter of about 3mm. By regularly overeating protein foods, the normally smooth and polished inner wall of a blood vessel becomes uneven, and the blood vessel as a whole thickens and loses its elasticity. This leads to a deterioration of blood flow throughout the circulatory system and may culminate in a complete blockage. Coronary arteries that are totally blocked resemble old rusty, calcified water pipes. Their walls are brownish-red and are clogged with yellowish, calcified material.

The Revealing Role of Homocysteine

Researchers discovered that the toxic, sulphur-containing amino acid *homocysteine* (HC) promotes the tiny clots that initiate arterial damage and the catastrophic clots that precipitate most heart attacks and strokes (Ann Clin & Lab Sci, 1991 and *Lancet* 1981). HC is a consequence of the normal metabolism of the amino acid *methionine*, which is abundant in red meat and dairy products. Normally, your body has a built-in defense mechanism against homocysteine buildup; it transforms it into a harmless substance called *cystathionine*, which is flushed from the body in the urine. However, regularly overeating proteins greatly undermines this ability. Foods that are high in folic acid (see chapter 7) have been shown to drastically lower homocysteine levels and thereby reduce the risk of cardiovascular disease.

Although increased homocysteine levels as a major risk factor of heart disease has been common knowledge in the medical research field for many years, it is only now being recognized as such in the field of applied medicine. The presence of unsafe levels of homocysteine in the body was thought to be associated with people genetically unable to convert homocysteine at a sufficient rate. But the enormous incidence of abnormal homocysteine levels among heart disease patients suggests that the genetic factor is secondary, or may rather be a response to continuously overwhelming the body with protein foods (similar to the phenomenon of genetic mutation in cancerous growths, see chapter 10). In one recent study, a group of people participated in a week-long program that included a strict vegan diet, stress management and spirituality enhancement sessions, group support, and exclusion of tobacco, alcohol, and caffeine. Just within one week on this program, the average homocysteine level fell 13 percent.

Conclusion: If you regularly consume large quantities of animal protein, including meat, pork, poultry, fish, eggs, milk, cheese, etc., your body's ability to break down and safely remove all the protein or homocysteine becomes increasingly impaired, if it is not already naturally low by constitution. Since excessive protein consumption thickens the blood and increases its risk of clotting, the body is forced to store the extra protein and the byproducts of protein metabolism in the connective tissues under the skin as well as in the connective tissue of the organs and basal membranes of the capillary network. When the storage capacity of these membranes is exhausted, no more protein can be deposited in the capillaries. If overconsumption of animal protein continues, the body begins to store the excessive protein in the walls of the arteries (see **illustration 19**). At this stage, the main coronary arteries become thickened, damaged and inefficient. As they become occluded and cut off the oxygen supply to the heart, breathing becomes difficult, and pain and numbness may occur. Suddenly a heart attack occurs. Thus, the storage of excessive protein in the body acts like a 'time bomb', ready to explode at any moment.

C-Reactive Protein Reveals the Truth

Continuous storage of excessive proteins in the blood vessel walls will eventually damage them. To help repair the damage and remove weak and injured cells, the body responds with inflammation. Inflammation is not a disease, but the body's basic emergency response system to heal itself. The blood vessels are the body's lifelines. When threatened by a build-up of harmful proteins in the basal membranes of the blood vessel walls, the body will attempt to save itself by allowing the formation of protective fatty plaque in the arteries.

The body takes drastic measures to deal with potentially life-threatening obstructions in its blood vessels, similar to the immune system sending out swarms of specialized cells to fight off invading germs. In the process of trying to fix the problem through inflammation, the immune cells cause multiple lesions that become increasingly unstable and may eventually rupture. When the body is unable to contain the bleeding from a ruptured lesion and fails to seal off the wound, a heart attack or stroke occurs.

In a groundbreaking study published in the *New England Journal of Medicine* in 2002, doctors from Boston's Brigham and Women's Hospital showed that a simple blood test, called C-Reactive Protein

(CRP), was able to predict which patients are most likely to suffer a heart attack or stroke. CRP is a protein produced by the liver in reaction to the immune system's inflammatory response. This blood test measures the presence and intensity of inflammation in the walls of the blood vessels. Inflammation in the blood vessel walls is a much more accurate indicator of imminent heart trouble than measuring the concentrations of the 'good' cholesterol (HDL) and 'bad' cholesterol (LDL) in the blood. This finding is very significant because half of all heart attacks occur in people with normal cholesterol levels. It not only shows that inflammation plays a key role in heart disease, but also in a wide range of other disorders involving the circulatory system, including arthritis, diabetes and cancer.

In the above study, the research team tracked the levels of both CRP and LDL ('bad' cholesterol) in nearly 28,000 women for eight years. According to the results of the study, women with high levels of CRP were twice as likely to have heart disease as those with high LDL. It also showed that many women who later suffered heart attacks would have been given a clean bill of health on the basis of their low LDL. Simply testing a person's cholesterol levels is not enough, and, in fact, may endanger his/her life.

CRP cannot be considered the ultimate test for heart disease either, because it can jump as much as 10-fold when a person is fighting a cold or the flu. Infection includes an inflammatory response, and, therefore, the C-reactive protein is most likely to show up in the blood. However, this important piece of research shows that cholesterol testing is not the correct focus if we want to save the lives of people who are at risk of heart disease. This is further substantiated by the most recent research showing that elevated blood cholesterol level cannot even be considered to be a major risk factor for heart attack (see *Risk Indications of a Heart Attack* below). Instead, focusing on the very causes of the inflammatory response will help us eradicate the incidence of heart disease, as well as arthritis and cancer.

How and Why Heart Attacks Really Occur

Merely cutting off the oxygen supply to the heart may not be enough to destroy it. The heart is one of the most innovative and resilient organs in the body and it requires excessive abuse to cause it to die. When the basal membranes of the capillaries and arteries can no longer guarantee sufficient supplies of oxygen, sugar and insulin to the cells of the heart muscles, their ability to contract and pump blood is greatly reduced. To continue their work with less oxygen, the heart cells begin to ferment glucose to produce energy, but this (anaerobic) process produces lactic acid, which subsequently acidifies the muscle tissues.

To further maintain its pumping action, the heart employs an additional emergency tool to obtain energy; it mobilizes and breaks down fats. Yet, without using oxygen in the process, these fats turn into harmful, cell-destroying acids. Proteins are then used to provide energy but the byproducts of this process are harmful fatty acids. Since the thickening of the connective tissues, lymph, and blood capillaries in the heart begins obstructing normal elimination of metabolic waste, the heart muscles become intensely saturated with harmful, acidic material. This may cause intense pain in the heart.

When uric acid, a waste product resulting from the breakdown of old, worn-out cells, accumulates in the connective tissues, gout occurs. Gout is a painful condition, similar to arthritis. Congestion in the connective tissues leads to dehydration in the muscle cells, which prompts a group of cells known as mast cells to secrete the hormone *histamine*, a major water-regulating hormone in the body. When histamine passes over the sensitive pain nerves in the muscle tissues, strong muscle pain results. If this form of muscle rheumatism occurs in the heart, it is called *Angina Pectoris*. Both the acid accumulation (gout) and the lack of oxygen lead to the death of heart cells.

Heart attacks can occur in a number of ways:

- The connective tissues surrounding the heart cells may become so densely congested that the heart cells simply die a painless death of suffocation.
- An angina attack may occur, meaning that acidification and low oxygenation have destroyed the heart muscles.
- The basal membranes of the capillaries and arteries are blocked and can no longer supply oxygen to the heart. A heart attack then occurs at the location where the storage capacity for protein was first exceeded.
- A blood clot breaks loose from a congested and injured blood vessel, enters the heart and blocks its oxygen supply. The same scenario can cause a stroke.

New Studies Question Value of Opening Arteries

The emerging understanding of the causes of heart attack raises the question of the value or usefulness of opening blocked arteries. For one thing, the increasingly popular aggressive treatments of opening arteries with bypass surgery, angioplasty[27] and stents[28] do little or nothing to prevent the recurrence of an occlusion. Although bypass surgery was found to extend the lives of some patients with severe illness, it does nothing to prevent heart attacks. As we shall see, heart attacks don't occur because of an arterial blockage, as most people assume, but because of one of the four reasons mentioned above. Overall, none of the currently used surgical procedures have been shown to significantly lower the mortality rate from heart disease.

One of the main reasons for the poor success rate of these treatments is that the vast majority of heart attacks do not originate with obstructions that narrow arteries. To tackle the heart disease epidemic, which is spreading like wildfire in most industrialized nations and now also in developing nations, we need to rely mostly on preventative strategies. However, these approaches cost next to nothing and are therefore not financially lucrative for those in charge of health care. The preventative measures include eating less protein, regular exercise, early bedtimes, regular mealtimes and balanced meals, drinking enough water, avoiding junk foods, giving up smoking, reducing alcohol consumption, removing stress sources, etc.

The old model of understanding heart disease is rapidly falling apart, much to the surprise of heart specialists. "There has been a culture in cardiology that the narrowings were the problem and that if you fix them the patient does better." said Dr. David Waters, a cardiologist at the University of California at San Francisco. This theory made so much sense to the surgeons, cardiologists and laypeople that for decades hardly anyone questioned it, except those few (including myself) who were more interested in discovering the true causes of heart disease. The newest scientific discoveries now finally expose this theory's major flaws, with little room for discussion.

Until recently[29], it was believed that coronary disease evolved like sludge building up in a pipe. Plaque accumulates slowly, over decades, and once a coronary artery is blocked completely, no blood can get through to the heart and the patient suffers a heart attack. In order to prevent this catastrophe

---

[27]Opening of arteries by pushing plaque back with a tiny balloon and then, often, holding it open with a stent

[28] Stents consist of wire cages that hold plaque against an artery wall; they can alleviate crushing chest pain. They can also rescue someone in the midst of a heart attack by holding the closed artery open.

[29] This is not quite true, since as long ago as 1986, Dr. Greg Brown of the University of Washington at Seattle published a paper showing that heart attacks originated in areas of coronary arteries where there was too little plaque to be stented or bypassed.

from happening, the most apparent rational 'solution' to this problem was to perform bypass surgery or angioplasty to replace or open the narrowed artery before it would close completely. The assumption that this would avert heart attacks and prolong life seemed indisputable. But as medical research shows, this theory is no longer valid (it actually never was) and therefore, is misleading. A study published in the *New England Journal of Medicine* by the *Coronary Artery Bypass Surgery Cooperative Study Group* clearly demonstrated that the three-year survival rate for heart disease patients undergoing bypass surgery is almost the same as for patients who have no surgery.

According to numerous heart disease studies, most heart attacks do not occur because an artery is narrowed by plaque. Instead, researchers say, heart attacks occur when an area of plaque bursts in a coronary artery, causing formation of blood clots that abruptly block blood flow to the heart. In fact, in 75 to 80 percent of cases, the hardened plaque obstructing an artery is not a culprit and should not even be considered for bypass surgery or stenting. The most dangerous type of plaque is soft and fragile. It produces no symptoms and would not even be seen as an obstruction to blood flow. The soft, newly-formed patches of plaque are much more likely to break off than old, hard ones; and when they do, blood clots are formed that enter the heart, causing a heart attack. Therefore, creating a bypass around the hardened parts of an artery does nothing to lower the risk of a future heart attack. For this reason, many heart attacks occur in people who don't have any arterial occlusions. Accordingly, a person may have no problem jogging one day, but suffer a heart attack (or stroke) the next day. If a narrowed artery were the culprit, the person would not even be able to exercise due to severe chest pain or breathing restriction.

Most heart patients have hundreds of vulnerable plaque sites in their arteries. Since it is impossible to replace all these injured, plaque-ridden sections, the currently applied interventional procedures are unable to prevent heart attacks. Regardless, this doesn't mean that fewer bypasses or stent operations are performed. The multi-billion dollar stent business seems, in fact, unstoppable.

Heart researchers and some cardiologists are becoming increasingly frustrated with the fact that their findings are not being taken seriously enough by the health practitioners and their patients. "There is just this embedded belief that fixing an artery is a good thing," said Dr. Eric Topol, an interventional cardiologist at the Cleveland Clinic in Ohio. It has almost become fashionable to have one's arteries fixed, just in case. Dr. Topol points out that more and more people with no symptoms are now getting stents. In 2004, over one million Americans opted for a stent operation.

Although many doctors know that the old heart disease theory no longer holds true, they feel pressured to open blocked arteries anyway, regardless of whether patients have symptoms or not. Dr. David Hillis, an interventional cardiologist at the University of Texas Southwestern Medical Center in Dallas, explained: "If you're an invasive cardiologist and Joe Smith, the local internist, is sending you patients, and if you tell them they don't need the procedure, pretty soon Joe Smith doesn't send patients any more. Sometimes you can talk yourself into doing it even though in your heart of hearts you don't think it's right."

According to Dr. Topol, a patient typically goes to a cardiologist with a vague complaint like indigestion or shortness of breath, or because a scan of the heart indicated calcium deposits or a buildup of plaque. Doing his job, the cardiologist follows the standard procedures and puts the patient in the cardiac catheterization room, examining the arteries with an angiogram. If you live in a developed country like America and are middle-aged or older, you are most likely to have arteriosclerosis, and the angiogram will show a narrowing. It won't take much convincing to tell you that you need a stent. "It's this train where you can't get off at any station along the way," Dr. Topol said. "Once you get on the train, you're getting the stents. Once you get in the cath lab, it's pretty likely that something will get done."

Dr. Hillis believes the American psyche is convinced that the worth of medical care is directly related to its aggressiveness. Hillis has tried to explain the evidence to his patients, but with little success. "You end up reaching a level of frustration,' he said. "I think they have talked to someone along the line who convinced them that this procedure will save their life. They are told if you don't have it done you are, quote, a walking time bomb."

Even more disquieting, Dr. Topol said, is that stenting can actually cause minor heart attacks in about 4 percent of patients. This means that, out of the 1 million stent patients in 2004, 40,000 ended up suffering heart damage from a procedure meant to prevent it, heart damage that they may never have developed without undergoing the procedure. According to a report published in the *New England Journal of Medicine* (October 15, 2004), the two stents that are currently approved by the Food and Drug Administration (FDA), the Cordis Cypher sirolimus-eluting stent and the Boston Scientific Taxus Express paclitaxel-eluting stent, have been associated with highly publicized adverse events after they were approved for marketing.

Bypass, angioplasty and stent operations are really not about preventing heart attacks per se. The obvious purpose of these procedures is symptom relief. Patients are satisfied that "something" was done, relieved of the anxiety of dying from a sudden heart attack. And the doctors are satisfied that their patients are happy. The drug industry is satisfied because the patients are doomed to taking expensive drugs for the rest of their lives.

Risk Indications of a Heart Attack

Most food-related blood vessel diseases, including heart attacks, stroke, rheumatism and angina pectoris, are not primarily disorders of sugar and fat metabolism, but diseases resulting from protein storage. Eating too much protein food is considered to be one of the greatest risk factors for developing any kind of disease, especially heart disease, cancer, diabetes (see chapter 10) and rheumatoid arthritis. The thickening of the basal membranes of blood vessels and connective tissues caused by the storage of protein affects all cells in the body. Whenever and wherever such congestion occurs in the body, premature aging of cells and organs result. On the other hand, wherever the capillary walls maintain their porous, flexible nature and original thinness, cell nourishment and organ vitality continue throughout life, regardless of age.

Fat and *cholesterol* are not the primary blocking agents of blood vessel walls and can, therefore, not be considered the main cause of heart disease or any other disease in the body. Storage of protein in the blood vessel walls, on the other hand, is the common factor in all patients who suffer from alimentary (food-caused) arteriosclerosis. Since most people in the industrialized nations have consistently been consuming excessively large quantities of protein, particularly since World War II, coronary heart disease has become a leading cause of death in the developed world. As you will be able to see below, most of the major risk elements of suffering a heart attack are either directly or indirectly linked with high protein consumption and protein deposits in the blood vessel walls. Following are the indications of such risks:

1. *Thickening of blood as measured by Hematocrit*

The *Hematocrit* is the volume of red blood cells in one liter of whole blood and can be determined by a simple and inexpensive blood test. If it is above 42 percent, the risk of a heart attack increases. A healthy person has a Hematocrit of 35 to 40 percent. Under the assumption that the presence of larger quantities of protein in the blood is harmless, many doctors consider a volume of 44-50 percent to still be in the normal range. Research, however, has shown that heart attacks were twice as high when the Hematocrit reached 49 percent compared to a level of 42 percent. Simply said, the higher the Hematocrit rises, the greater is the risk of suffering a heart attack.

The question arises, why would the volume of red blood increase beyond 40 percent? When the basal membranes and the intercellular tissues become thickened because of the storage of excessive protein, blood flow slows down and eventually becomes obstructed. This 'naturally' increases the concentration of all blood values, including proteins, fats, and sugar. The thickening of the blood poses a great risk that affects all parts of the body. To deal with the dangerously high concentration of protein in the blood, the pancreas secretes extra insulin, but in doing so, the insulin may further injure and weaken the blood vessel walls. The cells making up the capillary walls start to absorb some of the excessive protein, convert it into collagen fiber, and deposit it in the basal membranes. Although this has a much-needed thinning effect on the blood, it also reduces proper nutrient delivery to the cells. Consequently, when the cells signal malnutrition, the blood nutrient levels begin to rise until the pressure of diffusion is high enough to again deliver sufficient quantities of nutrients to the cells.

Meanwhile, this constant maneuvering raises the number of red blood cells, which contain the red-colored *hemoglobin*. Hemoglobin combines with oxygen in the lungs and transports it to all the body cells. With increased thickness of the basal membranes, the oxygen supply to the cells also becomes restricted. The resulting increased need for oxygen by the cells raises hemoglobin concentrations in the red blood cells. However, this makes the red blood cells swell up. Eventually, they are too large to pass through the tiny capillaries, blocking them altogether.

This even more drastically cuts down the nutrient and water supplies to the cells, causing them to suffer dehydration. To signal dehydration, the cells release their water deficiency enzyme *renin* into the tissue fluid which, through a myriad of chemical events, leads to an increase of heartbeat and cardiac output. This emergency measure increases water supply to the cells and alleviates their predicament but also raises the blood pressure. Known as *essential hypertension*, this situation causes additional stress and damage to the blood vessels. The vicious cycle is closed. The preconditions of suffering a heart attack are now in place.

Conclusion: The combination of both factors - an increased Hematocrit which indicates increased blood thickening and a higher hemoglobin concentration in the red blood cells - reduces blood circulation. A round, red-colored face and chest are typical indications of an abnormally high blood volume and diminished blood circulation in the adult hypertensive and diabetic patient. The cell tissues begin to dehydrate as water distribution becomes increasingly difficult. The rate and force of contraction of the heart muscle increases to help maintain the cardiac output against a sustained rise in congestion throughout the circulatory system. Eventually, the heart can no longer afford such strenuous activity and collapses.

2. *Eating too much Animal Protein*

The majority of heart attack patients confirm that they have been eating large quantities of animal protein, including, meat, chicken, fish, eggs, or cheese throughout their lives or at least for many years. By contrast, virtually no heart attacks occur among vegetarians eating a balanced plant food diet.

Most people know that eating the wrong kind of fat damages the heart and other organs in the body. Now researchers from the University of Alberta have discovered that trans fats can also wreak havoc with the electricity in your heart, worsening the severity of heart attacks and increasing the risk of death. They discovered these unnatural fats also affect the cells of the heart, causing an excessive build-up of calcium within the cells and disrupting the rhythm of electricity flow in your heart.

3. *Cigarette Smoking*

The risk of cardiovascular diseases increases greatly with smoking. This, however, is not so much due to the nerve toxin *nicotine*, which is completely broken down within a few hours after smoking, but is rather caused by the *carbon oxide* (CO) contained in cigarette smoke. *Carbon oxide* or *monoxide* diffuses from the lungs into the blood where it attaches itself to the hemoglobin of the red cells about 300 times faster and tighter than oxygen does. All the CO of the inhaled smoke combines with hemoglobin and thereby blocks off oxygen transport to the cells. The red blood cells thus loaded with carbon monoxide-hemoglobin burst and shed their defective protein particles into the plasma of the blood. Many of these protein particles are now deposited in the basal membranes of the capillary walls. When the capillaries' storage capacity has reached its saturation point, the arteries begin to deposit the protein debris in their walls as well.

This makes the carbon monoxide of cigarette smoke a slow-working but lethal poison that, by forming excessive amounts of protein debris, destroys the body's circulatory network and heart muscles. Also, passive smokers inhale large amounts of carbon monoxide, which explains why they share a similar risk of developing coronary heart disease as active smokers.

4. *Constitutional (genetic) Disposition toward Reduced Protein Digestion*

People whose constitution does not require extra food protein in order to be healthy (especially the Kapha and Pitta types) don't have a very efficient digestive system for breaking down animal protein. Since constitutional body types are mostly hereditary, this genetically determined 'inefficiency' is passed on from parents to children. Those with a family history of heart attacks **appear** to be at risk because of possible hereditary factors, but the role of genetics in heart disease is only marginal, if it exists at all. The primary connection is that family members share a similar diet, lifestyle and constitutional body type, with possibly the same 'inefficient' enzyme systems for destroying excess, unused proteins.

5. *Women during and after Menopause*

Women who consume large quantities of protein foods and/or smoke cigarettes are at risk once their menstrual cycles become irregular or end. The regular discharge of menstrual blood protects a woman (before menopause) from accumulating dangerous amounts of protein in the body, as long as the reproductive system functions normally. This may explain why menstruating women before age 40 are generally not at risk of suffering a heart attack, whereas men of that age are. All the different blood values in women under 40 are lower than among men in the same age group. These include red blood cells, hemoglobin, Hematocrit, and the total amount of protein. Research has shown that men between the ages of 30 and 40 years are six times more likely to die from a heart attack than women of the same age. In fact, heart attacks among menstruating women are extremely rare.

Once a woman's menstrual cycles subside, her continued ingestion of animal protein will steadily raise the level of protein concentration in the blood. By the time she is about 50 years old, her risk of suffering a heart attack is nearly the same as it is for a man of the same age. The earlier that menopause begins, the greater the risk. Women whose ovaries have been removed before age 35 have a seven times greater risk of a heart attack than those who have yet to enter menopause.

The hot flushes and reddening of the face, which many women experience during menopause, are often signs of higher blood values. They indicate that the body has stored excessive amounts of protein which it can no longer expel with the menstrual blood. It has now been found that a diet consisting of large quantities of dairy products hastens the forming of atherosclerotic deposits in a woman's body and, as I will explain later, also causes osteoporosis.

6. *Not eating enough fruit and vegetables, smoking, and not exercising*

It was a wakeup call for Baby Boomers when newscasters reported in 2004 that former President Bill Clinton had to undergo emergency heart surgery. Unfortunately, the message conveyed to the world wasn't really focused on improving heart health but on taking the right drugs. It was by mere coincidence that just one week before President Clinton was admitted to the hospital, the prestigious medical journal *The Lancet* sounded a wakeup call with a different meaning. A major new study on heart disease risk published by *The Lancet* had this message for those concerned about their hearts: "Wake up and get heart healthy. You don't need medicine for that."

When President Clinton left office in 2001, he was still on the cholesterol-lowering statin drug *Zocor*. But once his excessive weight came off and his cholesterol levels dropped, he discontinued taking the statin drug. So when mainstream doctors heard about Clinton's heart condition, they immediately pointed the finger at the lack of statins as being the culprit. "See what happens when you don't take your pills?" Their words carried a warning for the rest of us who perhaps are just as careless when it comes to keeping our cholesterol levels in check. Some cardiologists believe that Clinton will now have to be on a much higher dose of a cholesterol-lowering drug for the rest of his life. This is certainly not unusual after undergoing a heart bypass operation, but it rarely if ever makes sense.

In a *Newsday* report, Dr. Valavanur Subramanian, chairman of cardiovascular surgery at New York's Lenox Hill Hospital, noted that two of the three arteries used in Clinton's operation were mammary arteries, taken from his chest. Dr. Subramanian described these arteries as 'extraordinarily resistant to cholesterol buildup'. The question arises: why put a man on potentially dangerous statin drugs when his arteries are virtually incapable of accumulating cholesterol deposits? Clinton is also most likely sentenced to a lifetime of taking a daily aspirin, a diuretic drug (to prevent buildup of fluid), and a beta blocker (to help regulate heartbeat). This potentially hazardous drug cocktail is going to be his 'crutch' for the rest of his life, unnecessarily, though.

According to the editors of *The Lancet*, the new study titled INTERHEART is one of the most robust studies ever done on heart disease risk factors. The 260 researchers closely observed and rigorously tested 15,000 heart attack patients for about a decade, matching them with the same number of subjects who had not experienced any heart problems. The worldwide study included male and female subjects with a wide range of ages, cultural backgrounds and dietary habits. The result may come as a shock to those who believe that high LDL cholesterol (the 'bad' cholesterol), is a major risk factor for heart attacks. The study shows that this isn't the case at all.

According to INTERHEART, the number one physical risk factor of heart attack is an abnormal ratio of *apolipoproteinB* (*apoB*) to *apoA1*. Apolipoprotein is cholesterol's protein component. ApoB is the protein found in LDL and apoA1 is found in HDL. The ideal apo ratio is one apoB to two apoA1. In other words, elevated bad cholesterol (LDL) alone poses no major risk for the heart. Yet, high LDL is the very condition for which cholesterol-lowering statin drugs are prescribed. The whole focus has been on getting the cholesterol down and keeping it low. When doing this with drugs, trouble can be expected. Thus, due to the numerous harmful side effects of statin drugs, millions of unsuspecting healthy people have already been turned into real patients with real (drug-caused) diseases. They have never been told that elevated cholesterol poses no major risk to their heart. Certainly, no patient I know has heard from his doctor about the apo ratio.

The INTERHEART study was launched in 1994, at a time that other major risk factors were not yet widely known, factors such as triglycerides, homocysteine and C-reactive protein. In their report, the INTERHEART team listed the most important risks of heart attack after apo ratio as (from greater to lesser risk) cigarette smoking, diabetes, high blood pressure, excessive abdominal fat, stress, inadequate intake of fruits and vegetables, and lack of exercise. Much to the surprise of the cholesterol/heart disease lobbyists, elevated cholesterol wasn't among these risks. In the concluding remarks of the 10-year study, researchers wrote that the relative risk for heart attack can be lowered by about 80 percent just by doing three things: eating plenty of fruits and vegetables, getting regular exercise, and avoiding smoking. Since cholesterol-lowering drugs have not been shown to lower the risk of heart attack, they were notably absent in the study's list of recommendations, much to the annoyance of the major statin producers.

INTERHEART isn't the only large study that discovered the significance of the apo ratio. During a Swedish study, researchers tracked more than 175,000 men and women for about five and a half years. The average age of the subjects was 48. Researchers studied all the main markers believed to be a risk, including total cholesterol, LDL and HDL cholesterol, triglycerides, and concentrations of apoB and apoA1. Over the course of the study, 864 men and 359 women died from heart attacks. While comparing the blood profiles of these heart attack victims to the remainder of the participants, the researchers found that an unbalanced apo ratio was the strongest predictor of heart attack death among all of the markers studied. Apo ratio was the only marker consistent over all age groups. They also found that an abnormal apo ratio continued to pose the same heart attack risk even when total cholesterol, LDL cholesterol, and triglycerides were within normal ranges.

It is my experience with hundreds of heart disease patients that eliminating animal proteins from their diet has helped restore normal heart functions, sometimes within a matter of six weeks. I, therefore, have come to the conclusion that eating a high protein diet, which is among the most acid-forming diets anyone can eat, greatly upsets the apo ratio and induces an inflammatory response in the coronary arteries. Both factors go hand in hand and, as we now know, pose the greatest physical risks to the health of the heart.

7. *Kidney Disease*

While many people live with stones obstructing the liver's bile ducts and the gallbladder, many people also live with undetected chronic kidney disease. When symptoms finally begin to appear, it is often too late to reverse the damage. Health officials estimate that as many as 10 to 20 million people in the U.S. have serious kidney problems. But what has this to do with heart disease? Two new studies, published in September 2004 in the *New England Journal of Medicine (NEJM)*, found a clear correlation between chronic kidney disease (even non-severe) and cardiovascular disease, which makes prevention of kidney disease more important than ever.

In one of the studies, researchers examined three years of data covering the medical records of over one million patients (data made available by the Kaiser Permanente Renal Registry in San Francisco). The average age of the subjects was 52 years. The research team specifically looked at the results of a blood test that measures the rate at which kidneys are able to filter waste from the bloodstream (glomerular filtration rate or GFR). The findings revealed that as GFR dropped, the risks of cardiovascular disease, stroke, hospitalization and death all increased sharply. In those patients where the GFR was below 45, the risk of death jumped by 17 percent and the risk of a cardiovascular event increased by more than 40 percent.

In the second study, conducted in the cardiovascular division of Boston's Brigham and Women's Hospital, researchers showed that heart attack patients with a GFR below 45 boosted their death risk to more than 45 percent. Noting that factors common to kidney disease - such as protein albumin in the urine, high homocysteine levels, inflammation and anemia - may boost the risk of cardiovascular disease and death, the researchers concluded that even mild kidney disease should be considered a major risk factor for cardiovascular complications after a heart attack.

To ensure that your kidneys continue functioning properly, keep your colon, liver and kidneys clean (see chapter 7). Kidney health largely depends on efficient performance of the digestive system. In addition, to allow the kidneys do their important job of blood filtering, the basal membranes of the capillaries and arteries supplying blood to the kidney cells must be free of any protein deposits. Kidney health also depends on the ability of the lymphatic ducts to drain the kidneys' metabolic waste products and millions of dead kidney cells each day. Congestion in the body's largest lymph vessel (the thoracic duct) leads to backwashing of waste in the kidneys, which slowly suffocates them in their own waste and cell debris (see also the kidney-liver connection in my book *The Amazing Liver & Gallbladder Flush*). Among the most lymph-congesting foods are animal proteins, milk and cheese, sugar and trans fatty acids, as well as highly processed and fat-deprived foods.

Besides keeping the main eliminative organs clean, other ways to prevent kidney disease are a low-protein diet, regular nutritious meals, sleeping between 10 p.m-6 a.m. to permit the liver and kidneys to do their respective work, taking care of one's emotional health, and most other advice provided in this book. If you keep your kidneys healthy, your heart may have little to fear.

8. *Antibiotics and other synthetic drugs*

It is becoming increasingly evident that medical drugs with a suppressive effect on any symptoms of disease diminish heart health. Every time your body tries to clear out accumulated toxins and waste through a cold, a viral infection, or any other disease process that includes inflammation, your heart is burdened with the difficult task of pushing the harmful waste material released from the tissues back where it came from. With each new attempt to subdue pain, infection, cholesterol, etc., less and less of this waste finds its way out of the body. Some of it ends up congesting the lymph ducts responsible for draining the heart muscles of their metabolic waste products. Antibiotics are one of the leading culprits for this form of heart damage.

For many years, antibiotics have been over-prescribed, often for simple infections such as the common cold and flu on which they have no effect at all. It is common knowledge that antibiotics don't kill viruses, only bacteria. A more recent study shows that the popular antibiotic erythromycin, which has been widely used since the 1950s, may actually trigger cardiac arrest.

Heart doctors have been aware of a risk of cardiac arrest when erythromycin is used intravenously, but this risk has been less well-known among family practitioners who often prescribe the same antibiotic in pill form to treat a wide variety of infections. This new study, conducted by researchers from Vanderbilt University, examined the risk of cardiac arrest when oral erythromycin is used alone or with other medications. Their report, which was published in the *New England Journal of Medicine* in October 2004, covered the medical records of more than 4,400 Medicaid patients, averaging 15 years per patient. Approximately 1,475 subjects suffered cardiac arrest during the study period. When the complete medication use of each subject was analyzed, researchers came up with these results:

- The rate of sudden death from cardiac causes was twice as high among patients using erythromycin compared to subjects that didn't use the antibiotic.

- Two blood pressure medications, sold generically as verapamil and diltiazem, were both associated with an additional increased risk of cardiac arrest when taken with erythromycin.
- Other drugs associated with increased cardiac attack risk when taken with erythromycin include the antibiotic clarithromycin, the vaginal yeast infection drug fluconazole, and two antifungal drugs, itraconazole and ketoconazole.

According to the researchers, blood levels of these additional drugs may be boosted by erythromycin, making the blood thick and sluggish. This can result in a slower heart rate, which in turn may trigger irregular rhythms, setting in motion a cardiac arrest. In an interview with *The Associated Press*, the lead researcher of the study, Wayne A. Ray, Ph.D., warned that erythromycin levels may also be increased by drinking grapefruit juice or by taking protease inhibitors also used to treat AIDS.

Just because your doctor prescribes a medical drug does not mean it is safe for you. Very few tests have been done on drug interactions with other drugs or with common foods. Drug prescriptions can be a gamble of life and death that you are risking when you enter your doctor's office. The bottom line is that all pharmaceutical drugs contain poisons that have a detrimental effect on your health. Your heart pays the ultimate price for these constantly offered and highly praised 'shortcuts' to health; they cut your life short.

The fact is no disease control agency or Federal Drug Administration (FDA) can protect you from developing a serious illness or dying as a result of using prescribed drugs. The Vioxx scandal of September 2004 has taught us that no safe drugs are out there. Vioxx, a leading arthritis drug, was withdrawn by its producer, Merck & Co., after evidence leaked out that its use doubled the risk of heart attack and stroke. [As per the end of 2007, Merck was faced with 4,200 state and federal Vioxx-related lawsuits pending across the U.S.] According to documentation, both the drug producer and the FDA knew of this risk since the mid-nineties. The result of this well-kept secret was that a minimum of 27,000 people suffered a heart attack or died because of it. Given the high number of unreported side effects, this number may well exceed hundreds of thousands.

More and more drugs are coming under suspicion of being killer drugs. Bextra is next. According to a study of more than 1,500 patients who had previously undergone cardiac surgery, those who were treated for pain with Bextra were more likely to have heart and blood-clotting problems than those who received no drug at all. Stroke, heart attack, blood clots in the lung, deep vein blood clots in the leg, all can result just from taking this drug. Arthritis drugs have never been properly tested for safety. Vioxx, Celebrex, Bextra, Aleve, and aspirin are just plain poisons. Another arthritis drug, *infliximab* (Remicade), is on alert for causing cancer.

Amazingly, many people have been so blinded by clever advertising campaigns and brainwashing that they have no clue they are being methodically poisoned in order to support and sustain the most lucrative business in the world besides oil, the pharma-medical industry. An investigation made public by CNN on 26 September 2007 discovered that 56 million prescriptions each year are handed out by doctors for drugs that are not even approved by the FDA. Two percent of all prescription drugs in the U.S. are not backed by any scientific research and can be fatal to unsuspecting patients. As shocking as it is, the FDA acknowledges that it hands out licenses to any drug producer who wants to sell a drug, regardless of whether it has been proven safe or effective.

The main question is how could anyone possibly want to entrust his life to drug producers whose only objective is to keep the sickness business going by making sure their products create more health problems than they resolve? In the majority of cases, attempting to prescribe medications that claim to offer relief to the symptoms of disease is not only a dangerous approach, but also an unscientific and unethical one.

Ending the Cholesterol-Heart Disease Myth

Why has there never been a record of cholesterol having blocked a vein in the body? What is it about arteries that makes cholesterol attach itself to their walls, while leaving the veins alone? It is really the sticky nature of cholesterol that is behind the blockage of healthy blood vessel walls?

The answers to these questions may surprise you. The body actually uses the lipoprotein cholesterol as a kind of bandage to cover abrasions and tears in damaged arterial walls just as it does it for any other wound. Cholesterol is nothing less than a life-saver. However, for the past thirty-eight years, this lipoprotein has been stigmatized to be the number one cause of deaths in the rich nations - heart disease.

This is how the theory goes: For reasons not really known, a form of cholesterol that has earned the name 'bad' somehow increases in the bloodstream of millions of people today; it sticks to the walls of arteries, and eventually, it will starve the heart muscles of oxygen and nutrients. Accordingly, the masses are urged to reduce or ban cholesterol-containing fats from their diet so that they can live without the fear of arterial occlusion and dying from a heart attack. The tremendous concern of being attacked by this 'vicious' lipoprotein has finally led to innovative technologies that can even extract cholesterol from cheese, eggs, and sausages, thus making these 'deadly' foods 'consumer-safe'. Products that claim to be low in cholesterol, such as margarine and light foods, have become a popular choice of 'healthy eating'.

Cholesterol is Not the Culprit After All

But as INTERHEART and other studies have shown, cholesterol isn't a serious risk factor for heart disease at all. An earlier study sponsored by the German Ministry of Research and Technology showed that no exact link exists between food cholesterol and blood cholesterol. Even more surprising, in Japan, the cholesterol levels have risen during recent years, yet the number of heart attacks has dropped. The largest health study ever conducted on the risks of heart disease took place in China. Like so many similar studies, the Chinese study found no connection between heart disease and the consumption of animal fats.

In an 8-year long heart study, researchers observed 10,000 people with high cholesterol levels. Half of them received a best-selling statin drug. The other half were simply told to eat a normal diet and get enough exercise. The results stunned the researchers. Although the statin drug did indeed lower serum cholesterol, this had no impact whatsoever on death rate, non-fatal heart attacks and fatal arterial disease. In other words, the statin-users had zero advantage over those who received no treatment at all. However, they had just spent eight years taking a costly drug with hideous side effects - risking liver failure, muscle wasting, even sudden death. Lowering cholesterol either through drugs or low fat diets does not lower the risk of developing heart disease.

All the major European long-term cholesterol studies have confirmed that a low-fat diet did not reduce cholesterol levels by more than 4 percent, in most cases merely 1-2 percent. Since measurement mistakes are usually higher than 4 percent and cholesterol levels naturally increase by 20 percent in autumn and drop again during the wintertime, the anti-cholesterol campaigns since the late 1980s have been very misleading, to say the least. A more recent study from Denmark involving 20,000 men and women, in fact, demonstrated that most heart disease patients have normal cholesterol levels. The bottom line is that cholesterol hasn't been proved a risk factor for anything.

The current medical understanding of the cholesterol issue is more than incomplete. The argument that animal tests on rabbits have confirmed that fatty foods cause hardening of the arteries sounds convincing, but only when the following facts are omitted:

- Rabbits respond 3,000 times more sensitively to cholesterol than humans do.
- Rabbits, which are non-carnivorous animals by nature, are force-fed excessive quantities of egg yolk and brain for the sake of proving that cholesterol-containing foods are harmful.
- The DNA and enzyme systems of rabbits are not designed for consumption of fatty foods, and if given a choice, these animals would never eat eggs or brains.

It is obvious that the arteries of these animals have only an extremely limited ability to respond to the damage caused by such unsuitable diets. For over three and half decades, Western civilization assumed that animal fats were the main cause of dietary heart disease. This misinformation is highlighted by the fact that heart attacks began to rise when consumption of animal fats actually decreased. This was verified by British research, which revealed that those areas in the U.K. where people consumed more margarine and less butter had the highest numbers of heart attacks. Further studies revealed that heart attack patients had consumed the least amounts of animal fats.

In this context, it is important to differentiate between processed and unprocessed fats. It has been discovered that people who died from a heart attack were found to have many more of the harmful fatty acids derived from the partially hydrogenated vegetable oils in their fat tissue than those who survived. These so-called 'faulty' fats (trans-fatty acids) envelop and congest the membranes of cells, including those that make up the heart and coronary arteries. This practically starves the cells of oxygen, nutrients, and water, and eventually kills them. In another more comprehensive study, 85,000 nurses working in American hospitals observed a higher risk for heart disease in patients who consumed margarine, crisps, potato chips, biscuits, cookies, cakes, and white bread, all of which contain trans fats.

Eating margarine can increase heart disease in women by 53 percent over eating the same amount of butter, according to a recent Harvard Medical Study. While actually increasing LDL cholesterol, margarine lowers the beneficial HDL cholesterol. It also increases the risk of cancers up to five times. Margarine suppresses both the immune response and insulin response. This highly processed and artificial product is practically resistant to destruction, being one molecule away from plastic. Flies, bacteria, fungi, etc. won't go near it because it has no nutritional value and cannot be broken down by them. It can last for years, not just outside the body, but inside as well. It is very apparent that eating damaged, rancid fats or trans-fats can destroy any healthy organism and should be avoided by anyone. In 2007 New York City banned the use of trans fats in its restaurants; however, the trans fats are merely being replaced with new artificial fats that have the same or worse effects.

Healthy Today - Sick Tomorrow

Unfortunately, high cholesterol (*hypercholesterolemia*) has become the dominating health concern of the 21st century. It is actually an invented disease that doesn't show up as one. Even the healthiest people may have elevated serum cholesterol and yet their health remains perfect. But they are instantly turned into patients when a routine blood test reveals that they have a 'cholesterol problem'.

Since feeling good is actually a symptom of high cholesterol, the cholesterol issue has confused millions of people. To be declared sick when you actually feel great is a hard nut to swallow. So it may take a lot of effort on behalf of a practicing physician to convince his patients that they are sick and need to take one or more expensive drugs for the rest of their lives. These healthy individuals may become depressed when they are being told they will need to take potentially harmful drugs to lower their cholesterol levels on a long-term, daily basis. When they also learn that they will require regular checkups and blood tests, their worry-free, good life is now over.

These doctors cannot be blamed for the blunder of converting healthy people into patients. Behind them stands the full force of the U.S. government, the media, the medical establishment, agencies, and of course, the pharmaceutical companies. All of them have collaborated to create relentless pressure in disseminating the cholesterol myth and convincing the population that high cholesterol is its number one enemy. We are told that we need to combat it by all means possible to keep us safe from the dreadful consequences of hypercholesterolemia.

The definition of a 'healthy' level of cholesterol has been repeatedly adjusted during the past 30 years, which certainly does not give me much confidence in a system of medicine that professes to be founded on sound scientific principles. In the early days of measuring cholesterol levels, a person at risk was any middle-aged man whose cholesterol was over 240 and possessed other risk factors, such as smoking or being overweight.

After the adjustment of parameters during the Cholesterol Consensus Conference in 1984, the population was hit by a shock wave. Now, anyone (male or female) with overall cholesterol readings of 200 mg percent (200 mg per 100 ml) could receive the dreaded diagnosis and a prescription for pills. The claim that 200 blood serum cholesterol is normal and everything above is dangerous was scientifically unfounded, though. At least, this was the consensus of all the major cholesterol studies. In fact, a report in a 1995 issue of the *Journal of the American Medical Association* showed no evidence linking high cholesterol levels in women with heart conditions later in life. Although it is considered completely normal for a 55-year-old woman to have a cholesterol level of 260 mg percent, most women that age are not told about this. Also healthy employees are found to have an average of 250 mg percent with high fluctuations in both directions.

The lack of evidence linking elevated cholesterol with increased risk of heart disease, however, didn't stop the brainwashing of the masses. In the U.S. 84 percent of all men and 93 percent of all women aged 50-59 with high cholesterol levels were suddenly told they needed treatment for heart disease. The totally unproved but aggressively promoted cholesterol theories turned most of us into patients for a disease that we probably will never develop. Fortunately, not everyone has followed the advice to have their cholesterol levels checked but, unfortunately, millions of people have fallen into the trap of misinformation.

To make matters worse, the official, acceptable cholesterol level has now been moved down to 180. If you have already had one heart attack, your cardiologist will tell you to take cholesterol-lowering statins even if your cholesterol is very low. From the viewpoint of conventional medicine, having a heart attack implies that your cholesterol must be too high. Hence you are being sentenced to a lifetime of statins and a boring low-fat diet. But even if you have not experienced any heart trouble yet, you are already being considered for possible treatment. Since so many children now show signs of elevated cholesterol, we have a whole new generation of candidates for medical treatment. So yes, current edicts stipulate cholesterol testing and treatment for young adults and even children! The statin drugs that doctors use to push cholesterol levels down are Lipitor (atorvastatin), *Zocor* (simvastatin), *Mevacor* (lovastatin), and *Pravachol* (pravastatin). If you decide to follow your doctor's advice and take one of these drugs, make certain to read the list of side effects so that you know the risks you are taking.

If you want to obtain objective and untainted information on cholesterol, agencies like the National Institutes of Health and the American College of Cardiology are certainly not the places from which to obtain it. Until recently, they wanted you to keep your overall cholesterol level below 150. Then, in 2001, they finally admitted that measuring overall cholesterol levels makes no sense at all, so they began recommending an LDL level below 100. Now their aim is to keep LDL lower than 70. Every time they lower the target, the number of 'patients' requiring treatment jumps dramatically, much to the benefit of the drug producers. Being officially backed by these agencies, doctors feel motivated, if not obliged, to prescribe these expensive drugs to their new patients. The extensive promotional campaigns by the pharmaceutical giants have already brainwashed the masses to believe they need these drugs to be safe from sudden heart attack. Even if a doctor knows the truth about the cholesterol deception, these anxious patients will demand a prescription from him. This is not just affecting their health, but everyone's economic future. The massive sales of these best-selling drugs of all time drive up health care costs to levels that undermine economic growth and make basic health care unaffordable to an ever-increasing number of people. The masses have been so brainwashed with misinformation that this lurking financial crisis doesn't seem to be their immediate concern.

In 2004, there were already 36 million statin candidates in the U.S., with 16 million using Lipitor alone. When the official LDL target level drops to 70, another 5 million people will be eligible for their use. At the consumer markup price of $272.37 and an actual cost of $5.80 for a month's supply of Lipitor, you can understand the incentive that the pharmaceutical industry has to push their products and make them a mass commodity.

What Statins May do to You!

Statins are drugs that inhibit the production of cholesterol. Now, most people would think that this is a good thing. The statins manage to lower cholesterol by inhibiting the body's production of *mevalonate*, which is a precursor of cholesterol. When the body makes less mevalonate, less cholesterol is produced by the cells and thus blood cholesterol goes down as well. This sounds good to most people. But mevalonate is a precursor of other substances also, substances with many important biologic functions that you definitely don't want to disrupt (see side effects below).

Through the mass media and doctors' advice, people are being told that the most important objective is to get rid of the excessive cholesterol so that it doesn't clog up arteries and cause a heart attack. However, this rather simplistic train of thought got us into trouble in the first place. Contrary to what we know about the true value of cholesterol, we are made to believe this essential substance to be a dangerous nuisance that only makes our lives miserable.

The fact is that each cell in your body requires cholesterol to make it waterproof and prevent its membrane from becoming leaky or porous. Although this is a very important role of cholesterol, the following one is absolutely essential for preventing a heart attack.

If your diet contains a lot of acidic compounds, such as meat protein, sugar and trans fats, your cell membranes become easily damaged and require repair. To fulfill the repair request by the cells, the body releases a flood of corticoid hormones that cause extra amounts of cholesterol to be taken to them. As you can see, one of cholesterol's many roles is to repair tissue damage. Scar tissue is known to contain high levels of cholesterol, including scar tissue in the arteries. In other words, whenever an artery becomes injured due to acid attacks and buildup of proteins in their walls, you can expect cholesterol to be there to help repair the damage. The increased demand for more cholesterol is naturally met by the liver, which can raise production by 400 percent if necessary. That this emergency response leads to elevated cholesterol levels in the blood is not only common sense but desirable. Obviously, this may change any negative preconceived notions that you may have had about the role of cholesterol in your body. Cholesterol is not your worst enemy, but your best friend.

Apart from cholesterol protecting your health, there are many more reasons why we need to avoid meddling with the finely-tuned cholesterol-producing mechanism in the body (explained in following sections). A real problem arises when we lower cholesterol by bypassing or disturbing this life-essential mechanism. The cholesterol-lowering statin drugs do just that. If your body has reasons to increase cholesterol levels in your blood, it is for your protection only. Artificially lowering blood cholesterol with synthetic drugs removes that protection and can generate an entire host of health problems, starting with disrupting the production of adrenal hormones. This, in turn, can lead to:

- Blood sugar problems
- Edema
- Mineral deficiencies
- Chronic inflammation
- Difficulty in healing
- Allergies
- Asthma
- Reduced libido
- Infertility
- Various reproductive disorders
- Brain damage

The last side effect on the list - brain damage - may be one of the most disturbing side effects resulting from long-term use of statins. A case-control study published in 2002 by the American Academy of Neurology found that long-term exposure to statins may substantially increase the risk of polyneuropathy, a neurological disorder that occurs when many peripheral nerves throughout the body malfunction simultaneously.

The problem with the new statin drugs is that they **don't** cause immediate side effects like the older cholesterol-lowering drugs did. The old cholesterol-reducing drugs prevented its absorption from the gut, which led to nausea, indigestion and constipation. But their success rate was minimal and patient compliance was very low. The new statin drugs became an overnight success story because they were able to lower cholesterol levels by 50 points or more with no immediately known major side effects. On the false notion that cholesterol causes heart disease, statins have become the miracle drugs of the 21st century as well as the best-selling drugs of all time. The promise of the drug giants is that, if you keep taking their drugs for the rest of your life, you will forever be protected against man's greatest killer disease. This equation, however, has two major flaws in it. One, cholesterol has never been proved to cause heart disease. Two, by lowering cholesterol with the help of statins, you can actually make your body gravely ill. The industry is now faced with an ever-growing number of reports listing the side effects that manifest many months after the commencement of treatment.

A 1999 study at St. Thomas' Hospital in London found that 36 percent of patients on Lipitor's highest dose reported side effects and 10 percent of the patients at the lowest dose also reported side effects. The steady increase of obvious and hidden side effects (such as liver damage) isn't at all surprising. The 'benefits' of Lipitor seen early in the approval-process study were so convincing that the study was halted approximately two years ahead of schedule. The trial was never long enough to show that Lipitor had long-term side effects that could devastate people's lives. Side effects from using Lipitor include gas, stomach pain or cramps, diarrhea, constipation, heartburn, headache, blurred vision, dizziness, rash or itching, upset stomach, muscle pain, tenderness, muscle cramps or weakness with or without a fever. Anything that constantly interferes with the digestion of food can practically cause any type of illness, including, heart disease, cancer, diabetes, multiple sclerosis, Alzheimer's disease, skin disorders, rheumatism, and so forth.

The most commonly experienced side effects are muscle pain and weakness. Dr. Beatrice Golomb of San Diego, California is currently conducting a series of studies on statin side effects. Golomb found that 98 percent of patients taking Lipitor and one-third of the patients taking Mevachor (a lower-dose statin) suffered from muscle problems, such as severe calf pain and foot pain. An increasing number of long-term patients (after three years) develop slurred speech, balance problems and severe fatigue. These side effects often begin with restless sleep patterns. A new study (October 2007), announced by the media, found that fat soluble statins, such Zocor and Pravachol can cause sleep deprivation, resulting in obesity and mental disturbances. Fine motor skills can be affected and cognitive functions decline. Memory loss is not uncommon. Usually, when patients discontinue taking the statins, the symptoms weaken or disappear.

A more recent German study, published in the July 25, 2005 issue of *The New England Journal of Medicine*, found that not only do cholesterol-lowering statin drugs fail to help patients with severe diabetes, but statins may also double their risk of experiencing a deadly stroke.

In fact, they can also greatly increase your risk of heart attack because they lower an important liver enzyme, CoQ10. This enzyme protects your body against heart conditions, muscular dystrophies, Parkinson's disease, cancer and diabetes. Taking CoQ10, though, as a supplement has shown very little benefit. In other words, taking statins may send you down a spiral of degeneration that you cannot stop unless you stop using these dangerous drugs.

I found in my own practice that regular statin users accumulate an excessive amount of cholesterol stones in the bile ducts of their liver and gallbladder, which can lead to a vast number of chronic diseases (see *The Amazing Liver & Gallbladder Flush* for details).

Before you decide to take Lipitor or other statins, consider these basic points:

- You need to tell your doctor and pharmacist if you are allergic to any other drugs. *This obviously raises the question of the number of patients who follow that advice.*

- You are supposed to tell your doctor and pharmacist the prescription and nonprescription medications you are taking, especially antacids, antifungal medications such as itraconazole (Sporanox) and ketoconazole (Nizoral); digoxin (Lanoxin), erythromycin, medications that suppress the immune system such as cyclosporine (Neoral, Sandimmune), oral contraceptives (birth control pills), other cholesterol-lowering medications such as cholestyramine (Questran), colestipol (Colestid), gemfibrozil (Lopid), and niacin (nicotinic acid), and vitamins. *You may wonder how many people follow that advice and how many doctors ask this information of their patients.*

- You need to tell your doctor if you have or previously had liver or kidney disease, a severe infection, low blood pressure, or seizures. *How many people actually know if their liver's bile ducts are packed with stones, whether their kidneys have major stone deposits in them, or if their blood pressure is below acceptable?*

- Tell your doctor if you are pregnant, plan to become pregnant, or are breast-feeding. If you become pregnant while taking Lipitor/Atorvastatin, you are supposed to stop taking this drug and call your doctor immediately as it can harm the fetus. *If the drug can harm the fetus, you may need to ask what else it can harm.*

- If you are having surgery, including dental surgery, tell the doctor or dentist that you are taking Lipitor/Atorvastatin. *How many people remember to do that?*

- Talk to your doctor about the safe use of alcohol while taking this Lipitor drug. Alcohol increases the side effects caused by Lipitor /Atorvastatin. *Many doctors forget to tell their patients about the potential risks regarding alcohol, and many patients just ignore that warning, often with severe consequences.*

- Plan to avoid unnecessary or prolonged exposure to sunlight and to wear protective clothing, sunglasses, and sunscreen. Lipitor /Atorvastatin may make your skin sensitive to sunlight. *It is a pretty serious condition when the sun becomes so dangerous that you have to hide from it. Not getting enough sunlight lowers your vitamin D levels and thereby increases your risk of cancer and many other illnesses.*

- For the drugs to be effective, you *must* eat a low-cholesterol, low-fat diet. This kind of diet includes cottage cheese, fat-free milk, fish (not canned in oil), vegetables, poultry, egg whites, and polyunsaturated oils and margarines (corn, safflower, canola, and soybean oils). You are supposed to avoid foods with excess fat in them such as meat (especially liver and fatty meat), egg yolks, whole milk, cream, butter, shortening, lard, pastries, cakes, cookies, gravy, peanut butter, chocolate, olives, potato chips, coconut, cheese (other than cottage cheese), coconut oil, palm oil, and fried foods. *How many patients receive such dietary advice from their doctor or even stick to it?* Most patients assume the drug will do its job regardless of what they eat. Please see Chapter 14 about the damaging side effects that arise from being on a prolonged low-fat diet or light food diet.

But Doesn't Aspirin Protect Against Heart Disease?

If you are diagnosed with heart failure and follow the recommended treatment of taking blood thinners such as *aspirin* or *coumadin*, you could seriously endanger your health. In a recent study, researchers compared blood-thinning therapies to not receiving any antithrombotic treatment. The researchers not only found no advantage in undergoing such treatments, but risks of further complications. Participants included 279 patients who were diagnosed with heart failure that required diuretic therapy. The subjects were divided into three groups, aspirin therapy, warfarin therapy and no antithrombotic therapy.

Results of the Study

- Aspirin and warfarin didn't provide the patients with any valuable health benefits.
- There didn't appear to be any substantial differences of incidences of death, nonfatal heart attacks or nonfatal stroke in the three groups of the study.
- Patients in the aspirin group had increased chances of experiencing serious gastrointestinal problems.
- Cases of minor bleeding complications were primarily seen among the aspirin and warfarin group.
- Patients in the aspirin therapy group were twice as likely as the patients in the warfarin group to face hospitalization for cardiovascular complications, particularly worsening cases of heart failure during the first 12 months following the study.
- Warfarin proved to be ineffective and should be eliminated as a treatment option.

Popular medications such as aspirin, ibuprofen and acetaminophen can raise blood pressure and raise the risk of heart disease among men, according to findings published in the *Archives of Internal Medicine*. Men who took such drugs for most days in a week were about one-third more likely to be diagnosed with high blood pressure than men not taking them, the researchers found. The new findings reinforce a study published in 2002 that these drugs raise blood pressure in women. "This is a potentially preventable cause of high blood pressure," Dr. John Forman of Brigham and Women's Hospital in Boston, who led the study, said in a statement.

The main problem with aspirin is that millions of people take it for all sort of reasons, such as to 'treat' every day headaches, arthritis, muscle pulls, blood and other aches and pains, as well as to 'reduce' the risk of heart attack and stroke. Aspirin and other NSAIDs can affect the ability of blood vessels to expand, and may also cause sodium retention - two factors that can both raise blood pressure. In the same context, COX-2 inhibitors - prescription arthritis drugs designed to be safer than NSAIDS - have been found to actually raise heart attack risk and cause strokes.

Based on the results from these studies, the treatment of heart failure should **not** involve the use of drug-based blood thinners, such as aspirin. It is relatively easy to keep the blood thin through a balanced vegetarian diet, drinking sufficient quantities of water, avoiding diuretic foods and beverages, keeping regular mealtimes and bedtimes, and cleansing the liver, kidneys and colon.

Dangers of Low Cholesterol

Instead of being concerned about high cholesterol, it seems we rather need to be concerned about low cholesterol, which constitutes a major risk for cancer, mental illness, stroke, suicide, liver diseases, anemia and AIDS. Studies conducted in major German hospitals verified that low cholesterol levels are linked to high mortality rates. When cholesterol levels dropped to 150 mg percent, two out of three patients died. Most of the patients with high cholesterol levels recovered from whatever they suffered. Also, longevity in retirement homes is linked with higher levels of cholesterol. Recent studies published in the *British Medical Journal (BMJ)* indicate that a low level of overall blood cholesterol could increase a person's risk of suicide.

A study published in *The Lancet* in 1997 showed that high total cholesterol levels are associated with longevity, particularly among the elderly. The research suggests that elderly people with elevated cholesterol levels live longer and are less likely to die from cancer or infection. Doctors at Reykjavik Hospital and Heart Preventive Clinic in Iceland noted that the major epidemiological studies on cholesterol had not included the elderly. So when they studied total mortality and blood cholesterol in those over 80, they found men with cholesterol levels over 6.5 to have less than half the mortality of those whose cholesterol level was around 5.2, the 'healthy' level. In support of this discovery, scientists working at the Leiden University Medical Centre found that "each 1 mmol/l increase in total cholesterol corresponded to a 15 percent decrease in mortality". A study of the Maori people in New Zealand showed that those with the lowest levels of blood cholesterol had the *highest* mortality rates.

Similar findings were also borne out by the Framingham Heart Study. Forty years after the Framingham Heart Study began, its researchers looked at total mortality and cholesterol. They found *"no increased overall mortality with either high or low serum cholesterol levels"* among men over forty-seven years of age. In addition, no relationship was found in women older than forty-seven or younger than forty. But the researchers concluded that people whose cholesterol levels are falling may be at an increased risk.

The same also applies to children. Research on seven- to nine-year-old boys from six countries revealed a strong correlation between low blood cholesterol and childhood deaths in those countries. The death rate rose dramatically as blood cholesterol levels fell. So, for children too, low blood cholesterol is clearly unhealthy. And once again, the official line is for parents to reduce their children's fat intake in order to lower their cholesterol or keep it low. Parents should instead be told that it is better to let cholesterol rise naturally. This effectively lowers their children's risk of disease and death.

The low-cholesterol-cancer connection has been known for many years. Although no convincing evidence has emerged that high levels of cholesterol have any causal relationship with coronary heart disease, this hasn't stopped the drug giants from advertising statin drugs as a safe approach to protect the masses against heart disease. The extremist attempt to indiscriminately lower cholesterol levels, especially among the elderly where elevated cholesterol levels are normal and very necessary, has led to numerous cancers in the U.S. and worldwide. As most studies have shown, high serum cholesterol is a weak risk factor or no risk factor at all for men above fifty, and actually increases longevity in those over eighty.

Women, in particular should be cautious about using statins. Most studies have shown that high serum cholesterol is not a risk factor for women at all and, therefore, should not be lowered by any means. The bottom line is that cholesterol protects the body against cancer. Removing this natural protection is synonymous with 'involuntary suicide'. Both animal and human trials have demonstrated increases in cancers when cholesterol was lowered through fibrates and statins. In the CARE trial, for example, breast cancer increased a whooping 1,400 percent!

An important connection also exists between low cholesterol and strokes. On Christmas Eve, 1997, a very important study made the headlines in the press. Researchers heading the famous Framingham study (still ongoing) said that *"Serum cholesterol level is not related to incidence of stroke..."* and showed that for every three percent more energy from fat eaten, strokes would be cut by fifteen percent. They conclude: "Intakes of fat and type of fat were not related to the incidence of the combined outcome of all cardiovascular diseases or to total of cardiovascular mortality."

All this published evidence, of course, does not deter the big pharmaceutical industry from coming up with more and increasingly 'smarter' drugs. Soon doctors will be recommending one pill to lower your LDL level and another drug to raise your HDL level and lower your triglycerides. Some already do so. This will not only double the already high cost many people are paying for their current statin drugs, but also greatly increase the risk of suffering a stroke or dying from cancer or any other disease.

Even aggressive behavior and suicides are now linked with lower cholesterol levels. Since 1992, researchers have noted increases in suicides among those undertaking cholesterol-lowering treatment or dietary regimes. By lowering blood cholesterol you also reduce serotonin receptors leading to increased micro viscosity and affecting the balance of cerebral lipid metabolism. This is believed to have profound effects on brain function. Data from mental institutions have revealed that aggressive people and those with antisocial personalities have lower blood cholesterol levels than average. Mental patients with high blood cholesterol levels were found to be less regressed and withdrawn than those with lower levels.

After many years of researching heart disease and its risk factors, no evidence has appeared to date linking high cholesterol levels to heart disease, stroke or any other disease as a cause-and-effect relationship although, in some cases, both may occur together. The decision to embark on lifelong cholesterol-lowering drug treatment in patients with primary hypercholesterolemia depends on the doctor's interpretation of available evidence. However, such evidence exists only for those who have a vested interest in keeping the cholesterol myth alive. At the same time, the true culprits or contributing factors of vascular diseases remain largely concealed from the public eye. Yet it is becoming increasingly evident that a diet high in animal proteins poses, perhaps, the greatest physical risk for arterial damage and subsequent buildup of cholesterol-containing plaque.

Cholesterol - Your Life and Blood

A newborn baby that is being breastfed by its mother receives a high dose of cholesterol right from the beginning of its life. Mother's milk contains twice the cholesterol of cow's milk! Nature certainly has no intention of destroying a baby's heart by giving it such high amounts of cholesterol. On the contrary, a healthy heart consists of 10 percent pure cholesterol (all water removed). Our brain is made of even more cholesterol than the heart and half of our adrenal glands consist of it. Cholesterol is an essential building block of all our body cells and is needed for every metabolic process. Because cholesterol is such an important substance for the body, every single cell is capable of producing it. We could not even live a single day without it.

Cholesterol

- is needed to form bile acids to help digestion of fats and keep us lean.
- is important for brain development.
- protects the nerves against damage or injury.
- repairs damaged arteries (seals off lesions).
- supports immune functions.
- gives elasticity to red blood cells.
- stabilizes and protects cell membranes.
- is the basic ingredient of most sexual hormones.
- helps to form the skin.
- is the essential substance which the skin uses to make vitamin D.
- is the basic ingredient used to manufacture the body's stress hormones.
- helps to prevent kidney damage in diabetes.

Cholesterol plays a vital role in every living being. Microbes, bacteria, viruses, plants, animals, and human beings all depend on it. Since cholesterol is so important for our body, we cannot solely depend on its supply from external sources, but must be able to produce it internally as well. Normally, our body makes about half a gram to one gram of cholesterol a day, depending on the amount required by the body at the time. The main cholesterol producers are the liver and the small intestines. These organs release the cholesterol into the bloodstream where it is instantly tied to blood proteins that will transport it to their designated areas for the purposes listed above. Cholesterol basically consists of fat and protein molecules, which gives it the name 'lipoprotein'. Only about five percent of our cholesterol circulates in the blood, while the rest is used for numerous activities in the body's cells.

If a healthy person consumed 100 g of butter a day (the average European eats 18 g a day), he would ingest 240 mg of cholesterol, of which only 30-60 percent would be absorbed through his intestines. This would give him about 90 mg of cholesterol each day. Yet of this amount, only 12 mg would eventually end up in his blood and raise the cholesterol level by as little as 0.2 percent. In comparison, our body is able to produce 400 times more cholesterol than we could obtain from eating 100 g butter. In other words, if you eat more than the usual amount of cholesterol in your food, your blood cholesterol levels will naturally rise. However, to balance this increase, your body will automatically reduce its own cholesterol production. This self-regulating mechanism ensures that cholesterol remains at the exact level that your body requires to sustain optimal functions and equilibrium.

If eating fatty foods does not significantly increase cholesterol levels to meet the body's demands for this vital substance, the body must take other more drastic measures. One of them is the stress response. If your body runs low on cholesterol, you are likely going to feel stressed. You will lose your calm and patience, and feel tense and anxious instead. This can occur without any external reason. Stress is a powerful trigger for cholesterol production in the body. Since cholesterol is the basic constituent of all stress hormones, any unsettling situation will use up large quantities of cholesterol. To make up for the loss or increased demand of cholesterol, the liver starts making more of it.

Take the example of the cholesterol-increasing effect of television. Research has shown that watching television for several hours at a time can drive up blood cholesterol more dramatically than any other so-called risk factors, including diet, sedentary lifestyle or genetic disposition. Exposure to television is a great challenge for the brain. It is far beyond the brain's capacity to process the flood of incoming stimuli that emanate from the overwhelming number of picture frames appearing on the TV screen every second. The resulting strain takes its toll. Blood pressure rises to help move more oxygen, glucose, cholesterol, vitamins, and other nutrients around the body and to the brain, all of which are used up rapidly by the heavy brainwork. Add violence, suspense and the noise of gunshots etc. to the spectacle and the adrenal glands respond with shots of adrenaline to prepare the body for a 'fight or flight' reaction. This causes the contraction of many large and small blood vessels in the body, leading to shortage of water, sugar and other nutrients in the cells.

The signs for this stress-response can be several. You may feel shattered, exhausted, stiff in the neck and shoulders, very thirsty, lethargic, depressed, and even 'too tired' to go to sleep. If the body did not bother to increase cholesterol levels during such stress encounters, we would have millions of television deaths by now. Thanks to rising cholesterol levels for saving TV watchers!

When Cholesterol Signals SOS

The self-regulating cholesterol mechanism that keeps the body healthy even in stressful situations is disrupted when the body has begun to store excessive amounts of protein in the liver capillaries. The liver capillaries, called *sinusoids*, are grid-shaped. Their thin basal membranes have sizable pores that normally permit larger molecules, and even the relatively large blood cells, to leave the bloodstream and enter the fluids surrounding liver cells. Unlike other cells, liver cells are thus able to work directly with the blood and its contents.

The High Density Lipoproteins (HDL), also known as 'good' cholesterol, are much smaller molecules than the Low Density Lipoprotein (LDL) as well as Very Low Density Lipoprotein (VLDL), termed 'bad' cholesterol. Despite their larger size, the latter two are still able to pass through the sinusoids and enter the liver cells where they are rebuilt, sent to the gall bladder for storage, or excreted into the intestines. In fact, most of these large cholesterol molecules cannot 'escape' the bloodstream anywhere else but through the liver sinusoids. Only the small HDL molecules, which make up 80 percent of all lipoproteins, are small enough to pass through ordinary capillaries in different parts of the body. For this reason, HDL is hardly ever found to reach abnormally high levels in the blood. LDL and VLDL, on the other hand, may rise to levels that reflect an underlying disorder (congestion) of some sort.

Under normal circumstances, most of the cholesterol eaten in a meal is absorbed by the small intestine and sent to the liver. Once the larger LDL and VLDL molecules enter the liver, they are removed from the blood in the manner described above. This mechanism, which keeps the cholesterol concentration of the blood balanced, becomes defective when the grid fibers of the sinusoids become blocked by excessive amounts of stored proteins. Consequently, LDL and VLDL concentrations begin to rise in the blood to levels indicative of blockages and, possibly, inflammatory processes in the sinusoids and coronary arteries. The 'bad' cholesterol is trapped in the circulatory system because its escape routes, the liver sinusoids, are congested. The liver's sinusoids become congested with proteins whenever the capillary and artery walls in the rest of the body are congested. The injuries caused by these acidic protein deposits require that much of the bad cholesterol be used as a band aid to prevent multiple occurrences of heart attack. Eventually, however, the arteries become increasingly hard, rigid and occluded. This may raise arterial blood pressure and further stress the heart.

The vicious cycle completes when the liver cells are no longer able to receive enough of the LDL and VLDL cholesterol. They naturally assume that the blood does not contain sufficient amounts of cholesterol. The liver cells subsequently begin to produce extra quantities of cholesterol which they pass into the bile ducts. Much of the cholesterol intermixes with other bile constituents and is then dispatched to the intestines where it combines with fats and enters the bloodstream. This may raise the blood cholesterol levels even further. Affected individuals may produce up to twice as much LDL as a healthy person does.

In the presence of toxic substances and due to the lack of bile salts resulting from poor digestion, some of the excessive cholesterol forms intrahepatic stones, so-called because they are produced inside the liver. These stones decrease bile flow and further reduce the body's ability to digest protein and fat-containing foods. As a result, every meal that contains cholesterol, a natural constituent of numerous foods, adds more of the 'bad' cholesterol to the quantity already trapped in the bloodstream. The body's final attempt to stay alive consists of accommodating more and more cholesterol in the bile ducts and tissue of the liver, which leads to an enlarged, fatty liver, and of sticking as much cholesterol as possible on the damaged walls of the arteries.

In many cases, the liver's sinusoids become so congested with proteins that they do not even allow enough water and sugar to reach the liver cells. As a result, many of the liver cells simply die off. The dead liver cells are replaced with fibrous tissue, leading to portal hypertension, diabetes and, possibly, liver failure. Because the protein storage does not only occur in the liver sinusoids but also in the capillaries and arteries throughout the body, the risk of a heart attack or stroke increases dramatically.

Cholesterol cannot be considered a culprit for heart disease or any other illness. Because of protein deposits in the sinusoids, liver cells are increasingly cut off from the daily necessary cholesterol supplies, and are therefore forced to synthesize more and more cholesterol. Lowering blood cholesterol by cutting out fats in the diet and/or artificially reducing it through statin drugs has little or no benefit in the control of heart disease. The most helpful action is cutting out all animal protein (meat, fish, poultry, eggs, cheese, milk) from the diet until the condition has been completely normalized. If any of these foods are being reintroduced, they should only be eaten occasionally and very sparingly. At the same time, all gallstones in the liver bile ducts and gallbladder should be removed through a series of liver cleanses, and the colon should be cleansed from any existing waste deposits. Additional essential measures include drinking enough water (6-8 glasses per day), maintaining a healthy diet and lifestyle, and, if necessary, giving blood to reduce the excessive amounts of protein in the blood and to lower the Hematocrit value. All this can effectively reverse arteriosclerosis and prevent a heart attack or stroke.

Balancing Cholesterol Levels Naturally

Apart from the above methods, a number of herbal substances and foods have powerful cleansing effects on the blood vessels and lymphatic ducts. When ingested regularly, they naturally balance blood cholesterol concentrations to their appropriate levels for the body to function optimally. Take, for example, the extract from a common Indian tree known as the *mukul myrrh* or *guggul*. Guggul is no strange medicine in India. It has been used for over 3,000 years to treat a variety of diseases. One side benefit happens to be the lowering of cholesterol and triglycerides in those who suffer from a congestive illness, an indication that this herb works holistically on many levels at the same time. Double blind clinical trials in India have proven that the extract of this small thorny tree is just as effective for these conditions as some common prescription drugs. Of course, substances that heal common ailments naturally are unattractive to big drug companies and, therefore, stand no chance of making it into the field of mainstream medicine, at least not in countries where health care is dominated by the pharmaceutical giants.

Dozens of herbs and common foods have similar effects to guggul. Green tea alone has shown to have great benefits for cholesterol health. Most fruits and vegetables, including apples, citrus fruit, berries, carrots, apricots, cabbage, and sweet potatoes have also shown to be helpful in naturally balancing cholesterol. Almonds, walnuts, pumpkin seeds, olive oil, coconut oil, oats, barley, etc. are just as effective. It is important to understand that natural food or herbs can only balance cholesterol levels when the underlying conditions responsible for such elevated levels are also improved.

Recently, the drug giants declared war on red yeast rice and succeeded in having it banned in the U.S. Several studies show that this ancient Asian rice slashed cholesterol an average of 40 points in just 3 months, without any side effects whatsoever. As its reputation increased, it became a serious threat to the greatest drug money-maker of all time, the statins. To ensure the continuance of the big pharma business, red yeast rice was eliminated, thanks to the FDA.

Lemon rind and orange peel also contain a substance that lowers cholesterol quite dramatically. Even the researchers were shocked when they tested *policosanol*, a safe, natural substance found in citrus peels. In one study, 244 women with high cholesterol received either a placebo or policosanol. Researchers saw the bad cholesterol of the policosanol group plunge by 25 percent. Total cholesterol fell 17 percent. And their ratio of total to good cholesterol (the most important risk factor) improved by a whopping 27.2 percent! Another study compared policosanol against a popular statin drug. Those given policosanol lowered their bad cholesterol by an average of 19.3 percent, versus just 15.6 percent for the statin subjects. Most importantly, policosanol improved the most crucial ratio, total cholesterol to good cholesterol, by 24.4 percent, while the statin drug only improved it by 15.9 percent. Just chewing on organic lemon rind once daily may be enough to balance cholesterol.

Nuts pack a powerful nutritional punch. They contain monounsaturated fats which help lower low-density lipoprotein (LDL) cholesterol and may raise high-density lipoprotein (HDL) cholesterol when substituted for saturated fats in the diet. Several major studies have found that eating nuts significantly reduces the risk of coronary heart disease by 25-50% in both men and women. One of these studies, the Nurses' Health Study, also found that regularly eating nuts reduces the chance of developing Type 2 diabetes by 21-27%. Besides monounsaturated fats, nuts are rich in vitamins, minerals, and other substances that are beneficial to your health. For example, walnuts contain a type of omega-3 fat similar to fish oil, and almonds contain calcium and vitamin E. Nuts are also good sources of digestible protein and beneficial fiber. Research shows that people who eat nuts tend to weigh less than those who don't eat nuts, despite the fact they are calorie dense (160-200 calories per oz). Nut eaters may follow a healthier diet (lower in animal proteins and junk foods) than people who abstain from nuts, and those who are overweight may shun nuts because of their high-calorie content. Richer foods like nuts require more energy to digest, so more calories may be used in the digestion process.

Food is still by far the best medicine for most ailments plaguing the human body. If used wisely and prepared carefully before its consumption, food can create miraculous cures of the most common diseases. I have discussed a number of such healing foods and herbs in Chapter 7. When choosing the right healing foods for you, please refer to the food lists shown in Chapter 6. Foods that harmonize with one's body type have the most healing properties, whereas foods that aren't in harmony may actually interfere with the body's own effort to restore health and vitality.

Overcoming Heart Disease - Two Encouraging Stories

Over the years I have seen hundreds of patients with 'heart' conditions that, in fact, were not heart conditions at all. Most people actually had simple indigestion, causing strong sensations of pain in the chest and stomach. Their stomachs were usually hard and swollen, filled with pockets of gas exerting great pressure on the diaphragm and heart. Trapped gas and 'heartburn' more often than not are the reason for the false alarm of a heart condition. Other patients, however, did have serious heart trouble, in addition to suffering chronic indigestion, or, as I see it, because of it. George, age 64, was one of them.

George had received medical treatment for thirty years for what his cardiologist called 'progressive heart disease'. During the same period, he had been on a large variety of drugs to relieve the symptoms. One of them was an anti-hypertensive drug. The drug's diuretic effects helped to drain excess fluids from his body, but also caused severe cellular dehydration and damaged his kidneys and liver. Other side effects included impotence, increase of angina pain, stomach upset, eye pains, muscle weakness, depression, and nightmares.

Despite taking these drugs regularly, he was advised to undergo a bypass operation since several of his heart arteries were almost completely blocked. A few years after the operation, at age 62, his 'new' coronary arteries also showed strong signs of damage, causing chest pain and severe tiredness. His heart was no longer able to perform sufficiently well and he was informed that, as a last resort, only a heart replacement could prolong his life. That when I saw George for the first time. He said this to me: "I feel more dead than alive. My energy level is only a fraction of what it used to be. There is not much I can do now except wait for a heart replacement, but considering my general condition, I am not sure whether I even can make it through such an operation."

After applying the diagnostic tools of Ayurvedic Pulse Reading and Eye Interpretation, I explained to him that his real problem wasn't his heart, but the amassed and toxic undigested food in his intestines (I was pointing to his grossly protruded belly) and the stored animal protein throughout his blood vessel system. The toxic material was suffocating the cells of his body and causing a gradual poisoning of his liver, kidneys and heart cells. His liver bile ducts were congested with thousands of gallstones. I suggested to him that he remove all the toxic waste which his body had collected over the past 40 years in his small and large intestines through intestinal cleansing and stimulate the digestive power through a series of liver cleanses. Thereby, he could directly relieve his heart from the heavy burden of having to deliver nutrients to a body that was blocked and overtaxed with harmful material. His heart was obviously exhausted from pumping blood through a congested body.

George quickly began to implement a program that included eating a specific body-type diet, cleansing of his intestines and liver, carrying out the daily and seasonal Ayurvedic routine, doing a regular full-body oil massage, meditating, and doing yoga and walking near the beachfront.

Within three days of his first colonic irrigation session and after strict avoidance of any protein foods, George felt a huge burden had been lifted from his heart. His energy began to return, but he still did not feel strong enough to go back to work. Two weeks later, though, he was back at his desk with great enthusiasm. Being the director of his own successful insurance company, he no longer felt as stressed at work as he had felt before the treatment. He was also asleep by 10 p.m. and meditating each day, which made him feel refreshed and calm, and able to handle the difficulties at work with a more relaxed attitude.

Three months later, George visited his cardiologist who took him through a series of tests to determine the condition of his heart. George was not surprised to hear his doctor confirm that he no longer needed a heart transplant operation. He saved himself the $750,000 that the heart transplant would have cost. Over a period of time, he reduced and finally stopped all of his medication. Fifteen years later, he is still very active and enjoys an excellent state of health.

"Just thought you would like to hear the latest report from my cardiologist, whom I went to see on Monday, just because it has now been over one year since my heart attack." This was the beginning of an e-mail message that Susan, a 62-year old friend of mine from Arizona, sent me a few years ago. "He was a bit disturbed when I first saw him," she continued, "because I said I was not taking any medications and had not since last August. As he was talking with me, he said he would probably prescribe a couple of medications for me to start taking again, but first he wanted to do an echocardiogram and a stress test."

"I agreed to them both and they were done in his office. While I was on the treadmill, I became tired, so I told his assistants I was getting tired and they said 'You may be, but your heart is not!' They said the echocardiogram and stress test were well within normal limits. When the cardiologist came back into the room, he said, 'I am totally surprised, just totally surprised. These tests show a healthy heart, no muscle damage at all! So you can go home, continue doing what you have been doing and come back to see me in six months.' He did not mention anything else about medications."

Her message ended by saying how grateful she was for all the advice and recommendations that had given her the power to reclaim a healthy normal heart. Susan is one of thousands of people diagnosed as having incurable heart disease but, through liver cleansing and changes in diet and lifestyle, has returned to a healthy active life.

Non-dietary Causes of Heart Disease

A Lacking Social Support System

Traditionally, Japanese people living in Japan have very low rates of heart disease and cancer. But when Japanese began immigrating in large numbers to the United States, their newly adopted lifestyle and diet often proved disastrous for their health. By the second generation in their new home, their health advantage over the American population was completely gone. First it was hypothesized that the typical American diet rich in fats was responsible for this development. But soon the *heart disease-diet-cholesterol* theory received a severe blow.

One subgroup among the Japanese immigrants in California continued to have very low rates of heart disease, irrespective of whether their blood cholesterol levels were high or low. The group consisted of males who retained their sense of being Japanese by growing up in a Japanese neighborhood, by participating in traditional Japanese cultural and social events, and by learning and speaking their mother tongue. The close family ties and social support system were the only factors that prevented them from developing degenerative heart disease. Even if they had personal problems at home or financial difficulties, they had a large family to lean on and to give them moral and often financial support.

A Swedish study confirmed that frequent social interactions among men, such as friendships, golf outings, poker nights, etc. translated into a higher than 50 percent reduction in heart disease among test subjects. As far as I know, no prescription drug can come close to boasting such results. The feeling of being rejected, left behind, and lonely can be a 'heart-breaking' event that easily can turn a healthy heart into a sick heart.

It is well known that women are in greater need of support and understanding during pregnancy. An epidemiological study on pregnant women showed that 91 percent of those who felt unsupported by family and friends suffered serious complications during pregnancy. The women reported that they were leading stressful lives with little or no social support. Similar studies on unemployed men have revealed that those men who felt strong support from family, relatives and friends were less likely to develop physical or mental problems.

Greatest Risk Factors: Job Satisfaction and Happiness Rating

One the most important discoveries ever made about man's number one killer disease is rarely mentioned in reports on heart disease and its contributing risks, but this doesn't make it less real. The greatest risk factors of developing heart disease are job satisfaction and the happiness rating. These unexpected risk factors turned up when American researchers looked once more for clues to the causes of heart disease.

If you ask a man on the street whether he is satisfied with his job and generally happy with his life, his answer will give you a fairly accurate prognosis about his heart health. It would be too simplistic to assume that heart disease is *only* caused by stress, cigarette smoking, overeating, alcohol abuse, etc. These risk factors are not the ultimate causes of a dysfunctional heart, but rather the effects or symptoms of plain dissatisfaction in life. The origins of all major causes of heart disease (lack of happiness and contentment) may still be there after all the other risk factors or causes have been eliminated. A large number of people have died from heart attacks with perfectly clean arteries and no other tangible, physical reasons. Many of them have never even smoked, abused alcohol or led a particularly stressful life. But they were unhappy within themselves.

One 1998 study by the Johns Hopkins School of Medicine has confirmed what 10 other surveys have found: Men who are clinically depressed are twice as likely as those who aren't to suffer heart attacks or develop other heart illnesses. If the 'heartache' is severe enough, several ways will appear to shut down the arteries and, in fact, the entire energy system in the body. Gene research has shown that the double strands of the DNA, which controls the health of every cell in your body, will instantly contract and shorten whenever you feel fear, frustration, anger, jealously or hatred. It's like the malfunctioning of a computer's software program that renders the computer incapable of performing properly. By applying the procedure of Kinesiology (muscling testing) to a depressed or unhappy person, you find that all the muscles in his body are weak, especially while he ponders his personal problems. His discontent also affects the muscles of his heart and arteries. If unhappiness persists, disease is inevitable, and whatever part of his body is the weakest will succumb first to the chronic shortage of energy. If it happens to be the heart, then heart disease may result.

Even if such a person doses himself with antioxidants, which are believed to protect the arteries against oxygen radical attacks, they will neither be digested and assimilated, nor be successfully delivered to the damaged arteries. Lack of satisfaction in life paralyzes the body's functions of digestion, metabolism and elimination. This causes congestion, high toxicity, and damage to all cell tissues. People who have blocked coronary arteries are not just sick in the area of the heart, they are sick throughout the body, and they are sick in their sense of self. The most important determinant factor of disease appears to be the inability to live a happy, satisfying life. A new study on women published in the medical journal *General Psychiatry* and reported by the mass media in September 2007 showed that women suffering a panic attack have a three times higher risk of suffering a heart attack or stroke within five years.

How does a prolonged state of anger, depression or anxiety damage the heart? That's a question researchers have been asking for years. A research team led by Dr. Boyle, Duke University North Carolina, wanted to find out if a troubled mind might trigger the type of inflammation that could damage the heart and blood vessels. In a group of more than 300 healthy middle-age men, between 1972 and 2002, the Duke researchers monitored blood levels of two key inflammation markers known as C3 and C4. C3 has been particularly linked to a higher risk of heart disease. Depression, anger, and hostility were also assessed. In a recent issue of the journal *Brain, Behavior and Immunity*, the Duke team reports that the highest increases in C3 between 1992 and 2002 were seen in men who displayed the highest levels of depression, anger and hostility.

A new study funded by health agencies in the British and U.S. governments finds that those who think they've been treated unfairly are more likely to have coronary problems. The main message taken from this study is that if you believe life to be unfair, your heart may be failing you. The study found that people who thought they were treated unfairly were more likely to suffer a heart attack or chest pain. Those who believed they were victims of the worst injustice were 55 percent more likely to experience a coronary event than people who thought life was fair. According to this report published in the *Journal of Epidemiology and Community Health* (Vol. 61, No. 6, June 2007: 513-518), people who think they are victims of discrimination often respond by drinking, smoking or overeating. The researchers suggested that the question of unfairness be raised with patients at routine medical checkups.

The reason modern medicine is so helpless in providing lasting cures for heart disease is because not much in the current medical approach can increase happiness in a patient. Yet there is hardly any other primary risk factor for disease, including coronary heart disease, other than lack of happiness and satisfaction. It is the absence of inner happiness and peace of heart and mind that makes a person feel stressed, take drugs, overeat protein and other foods, abuse alcohol and cigarettes, drink excessive amounts of coffee, become a workaholic, or dislike his job or himself.

Your Need to Love

Satisfaction in life increases spontaneously when we devote time to meeting our spiritual needs, apart from developing our physical and mental aspects. The human self cries out to be recognized as a spiritual being whose innate nature is unconditional happiness. A truly happy person finds deep inner satisfaction in sharing whatever he likes about himself with others - this is called love. Love is the most basic characteristic of a human being. Love is the life force that makes the heart beat, the cells thrive and the spirit soars. This is the meaning of living a spiritual life, a life filled with spirit and meaning. However, at times love becomes overshadowed or remains unexpressed. If it is unable to flow inside and outside the body, it causes deep sadness and frustration in the heart center.

Having a doctor identify a few risks of disease and 'treating them away' does nothing for a person's profound inner need to open his heart to others and to himself. Such an approach is futile because it ignores the fact that human feelings are far more powerful than any physical effect could ever be. If unhappiness continues to prevail in a patient's life, no amount of vitamin C or E will stop free radicals from creating havoc in the body.

The continual emphasis on the risk factors for disease today may divert people's attention from the real issues in life. The fact that happiness rating and job satisfaction are the leading causes of heart disease is hardly being publicized because there doesn't seem to be a magic formula to deal with them. The pharmaceutical industry possesses no drugs that can make people happy; all it can offer is drugs that deal with the physical symptoms of the disease. If you are troubled with heart disease, you may need to ask yourself a few basic questions, such as these:

Am I living a lifestyle that is detrimental to my health, and if yes, why would I do that? Do I feel that no one really likes or loves me? Am I afraid of being rejected by my partner? Is it up to me or others to see myself as a victim of some sort? Do I believe that I have a deeper purpose in my life but cannot find it? Am I feeling frustrated because I am not able to get out of life what I really want? And most importantly, am I afraid to love, out of fear of being hurt? Loving others who don't know how to love themselves heals the heart. Helping those who cry out for help opens and relaxes your heart. This prevents heart disease. You can always find someone who needs your help. When you make a difference in someone else's life, you will automatically feel loved, too.

What a Loving Spouse Can Do

Major research on male heart attack patients has shown that the men's feeling of being loved by their wives was the most crucial element that determined whether they survived an attack or not. Heart attacks often turn into a revelation for estranged couples who have forgotten how to love and care about each other. The sudden closeness which couples often experience after one partner suffers a heart attack can serve as an incentive for many of the patients to continue wanting to live, and the chances are that they *will* live.

Surveys of male heart attack victims revealed that most men felt lonely or misunderstood before their attack. Minor attacks led to death only in those men who felt that their wives no longer loved them. If a relationship was brought back to 'life' as a result of the attack, then even a massive heart attack could not take the person's life. Most men are quite sensitive at heart, even though they may not necessarily admit it. They generally tend to put on a brave face and suffer silently when they have 'heartache'. Most men tend to consider it a sign of weakness to shed tears, especially if it is in front of a woman. Yet the male's tendency to repress feelings of weakness makes him a likely candidate for heart disease. A heart attack can reveal his deep vulnerability and yearning for support and comfort. If he allows his partner to see this 'new' side of him, it can trigger love, compassion, a new sense of intimacy, and a new lease on life for both of them.

A new European study from the U.K. confirmed all of the above. It showed that having loving, close relationships with spouses, relatives or close friends helped to measurably lower heart attack victims' risk of suffering a second cardiovascular event in the future. In fact, heart attack survivors that don't have an intimate relationship for emotional support or social interaction are twice as likely to suffer major heart problems within one year of their initial heart attack.

The Healing Power of 'Loving Touch'

Every time someone touches us with loving care or we do the same for someone else, an emotional exchange takes place that profoundly nourishes the heart. The expressions "He touched my heart", "I felt so touched by his words", or "It was so touching to see my old friend again" show that the sense of touch is closely related to our physical and emotional heart, which is also the center of our being. To touch and to be touched is as essential to health as a balanced diet, if not more.

When American researchers discovered that prematurely born babies who are stroked three times a day increased their weight by 49 percent, they had unintentionally discovered the power of *loving touch*. As it turned out, loving touch, or 'kinesthetic tactile stimulation' to scientists, became recognized as an effective method for reducing the time and cost of a baby's stay in hospital. Loving touch (I prefer to use the less sterile and more human term for this precious healing gift) stimulated the babies' production of growth hormones and thereby improved utilization of nutrients from the daily food ratio. The researchers did not realize that they had stumbled upon a major technique of healing that could be applied successfully to the young and the old, the healthy and the sick, and not only for prevention, but also for cure.

In the human body, the sense of touch is so highly developed that it can detect or sense everything with which it comes into contact, like radar. By (unconsciously) picking up other people's *pheromones*[30] and/or 'touching' their aura, your body can identify who is friendly, honest and loving or cold-hearted, deceitful, and aggressive. The body may instantly translate all that information into powerful chemical responses that can make you either feel well or ill. These internal responses, however, also depend on your interpretation of the experience. Muscle testing can verify whether your interpretation is correct. You may think of a person and check with your muscles whether this person has a positive influence on

---

[30]Chemicals produced by the body that signals its presence to others. Pheromones play a particularly important role in sexual behavior. It has become crystal clear that human pheromones affect us more than most people can imagine. Our knowledge of visual input, and of how vision might influence our sexual behavior, pales by comparison.

you or not. A weak muscle indicates that your relationship with this person may disturb your balance and energy field. Merely thinking of a person gives you enough physical responses to decide whether you want to be with that person or not.

Multiple forms of touch can have profound healing effects. The Ayurvedic oil massage, for example, has been proven to open clogged arteries because of its deeply penetrating and detoxifying action. However, the purely physical part of this kind of touch is only partly responsible for this healing phenomenon. By touching your body with the intention to improve its health, the body automatically senses that you love and appreciate yourself and your life, otherwise you wouldn't do it. Love carries the highest frequency of energy, and, when present in the depth of your heart, it triggers a strong healing response by releasing *endorphins*[31], serotonin and other happiness/healing drugs throughout the body, similar to the ones a breastfed baby receives from its mother.

If you want to help a sick person but do not know how, hold his/her hand in yours or gently hold or massage his/her feet. This does more to help the person's condition than any amount of sympathetic words could do. The body remembers a loving touch more vividly than spoken words and it reproduces the same drugs whenever it links into the 'touching' feeling through remembering. Heart patients especially need to feel that they are loved and cared for because their hearts have lost the sweetness of life that is naturally present in a committed and loving relationship where emotional exchange is most common. Many heart disease victims isolated themselves from such intimacy before they became ill, by overloading themselves with work, commitments, deadlines and too many social engagements. By rediscovering the secrets of loving touch, they can once again connect to the circuit of love that supplies the only frequency the heart needs in order to function properly and efficiently, i.e. the love frequency.

If it is impossible for you to have a meaningful loving exchange with other human beings, you may consider getting a pet. Pets can open your heart and make you feel better about yourself. They have been known to lower blood pressure and reduce the risk of suffering a heart attack. This is called 'pet therapy'. Psychiatrists have added pet therapy to their treatment repertoire. Therapy pets are now are used in schools, mental institutions, nursing homes, rehabilitation facilities and children's hospitals.

Loving touch opens the heart. It is the kind of touch that gives without expecting anything in return. It is the kind of touch that can create miracles. Each one of us has this healing gift; it is only a matter of acknowledging that you have it, which is a prerequisite for being able to use it. Give your touch freely and without reservations, for it is one of the few gifts that can make you truly happy, too. It may feel nice to be loved by someone, but it is most important to express love to others, in whatever form is possible. You always have the choice to touch someone with your kindness, generosity, and honesty and feel so much better for it. This opens your heart. Only a closed heart can be broken or attacked. Living your whole life without the danger of suffering a heart attack is more your choice than something that just happens to you. Take care of your heart and it will take care of you.

---

[31] Endorphins are hormones produced by the body that stop pain and make you feel good (pleasure drugs).

Chapter 10

Why Cancer Is a Not a Disease -
And Why That's the Good News

"It is more important to know what sort of person has a disease than to know what sort of disease a person has." ~ ***Hippocrates (460-377 B.C.).***

What you are about to read may rock or even dismantle the very foundation of your beliefs about your body, health and healing. In 2006 I published a book titled *Cancer is not a Disease - It's a Survival Mechanism*. The title may be provocative to most, unsettling for many and encouraging for a mere few. I wrote this book for those who are sufficiently open-minded to consider the possibility that cancer and other debilitating illnesses are not actual diseases, but desperate and final attempts by the body to stay alive for as long as circumstances permit. It will perhaps astound you to learn that a person who is afflicted with the main causes of cancer (which constitute the real illness) would most likely die quickly unless he actually grew cancer cells. In the book *Cancer is not a Disease*, I will provide evidence to this effect. This chapter establishes the foundation for understanding the true causes, purpose and role of cancer.

I further claim that cancer will only occur after all other defense or healing mechanisms in the body have failed. In extreme circumstances, exposure to large amounts of cancer-producing agents (carcinogens) can bring about a collapse of the body's defenses within several weeks or months and allow for rapid and aggressive growth of a cancerous tumor. Usually, though, it takes many years, or even decades, for these so-called 'malignant' tumors to form.

Unfortunately, basic misconceptions or complete lack of knowledge about the reasons behind tumor growth have turned 'malignant' tumors into vicious monsters that have no other purpose but to kill us in retaliation for our sins or abusing the body. However, as you are about to find out, cancer is on our side, not against us. Unless we change our perception of what cancer really is, it will continue to resist healing, even through the best of treatments. If you have cancer, and cancer is indeed part of the body's complex survival responses and not a disease, as I suggest it is, you must find answers to the following pressing questions:

- What reasons coerce your body into developing cancer cells?
- Once you have identified these reasons, will you be able to change them?
- What determines the type and severity of cancer with which you are afflicted?
- If cancer is a survival mechanism, what needs to be done to prevent the body from taking recourse to such drastic defense measures?

- Since the body's original genetic design always favors the preservation of life and protection against adversities of any kind, why would the body permit self-destruction?
- Why do almost all cancers disappear by themselves, without medical intervention?
- Do radiation, chemotherapy and surgery actually cure cancer, or do cancer survivors heal due to other reasons, *despite* these radical, side-effect-loaded treatments?
- What roles do fear, frustration, low self-worth and repressed anger play in the origination and outcome of cancer?
- What is the spiritual growth lesson behind cancer?

To deal with the root causes of cancer, you must find satisfying and practical answers to the above questions. If you feel the inner urge to make sense of this life-changing event, cancer that is, you will greatly benefit from continuing to read this book. Cancer can be your greatest opportunity to help restore balance to all aspects of your life, but on the other hand, it can also be the harbinger of severe trauma and suffering. Either way, you will discover that you are always in control of your body. To live in a human body, you must have access to a certain amount of life-sustaining energy. You may either use this inherent energy in a nourishing and self-sustaining or in a destructive and debilitating way. In case you consciously or unconsciously choose negligence or self-abuse over loving attention and self-respect, your body will likely end up having to fight for its life.

Cancer is but one of the many ways the body tries to change the way you see and treat yourself, including your body. This inevitably brings up the subject of spiritual health, which plays at least as important a role in cancer as physical and emotional reasons do.

Cancer appears to be a highly confusing and unpredictable disorder. It seems to strike the very happy and the very sad, the rich and the poor, the smokers and the non-smokers, the very healthy and the not so healthy. People from all backgrounds and occupations can have cancer. However, if you dare look behind the mask of its physical symptoms, such as the type, appearance and behavior of cancer cells, you will find that cancer is not as coincidental or unpredictable as it seems to be.

What makes 50% of the American population so prone to developing cancer, when the other half has no risk at all? Blaming the genes for that is but an excuse to cover up ignorance of the real causes. Besides, any good genetic researcher would tell you that such a belief is void of any logic and outright unscientific.

Cancer has always been an extremely rare illness, except in industrialized nations during the past 40-50 years. Human genes have not significantly changed for thousands of years. Why would they change so drastically now, and suddenly decide to kill scores of people? The answer to this question, which I will further elaborate on in this book, is amazingly simple: Damaged or faulty genes do not kill anyone. Cancer does not kill a person afflicted with it! What kills a cancer patient is not the tumor, but the numerous reasons behind cell mutation and tumor growth. These root causes should be the focus of every cancer treatment, yet most oncologists typically ignore them. Constant conflicts, guilt and shame, for example, can easily paralyze the body's most basic functions, and lead to the growth of a cancerous tumor.

After having seen hundreds of cancer patients over a period of two decades, I began to recognize a certain pattern of thinking, believing and feeling that was common to most of them. To be more specific, I have yet to meet a cancer patient who does not feel burdened by some poor self-image, unresolved conflict and worries, or past emotional trauma that still lingers in his subconscious. Cancer, the physical disease, cannot occur unless there is a strong undercurrent of emotional uneasiness and deep-seated frustration.

Cancer patients typically suffer from lack of self-respect or worthiness, and often have what I call an 'unfinished business' or 'unresolved conflict' in their life. Cancer can actually be a way of revealing the source of such inner conflict. Furthermore, cancer can help them come to terms with such a conflict, and even heal it altogether. The way to take out weeds is to pull them out along with their roots. This is how we must treat cancer; otherwise, it may recur eventually.

The following statement, which runs like a red thread through this chapter, is very important in the consideration of cancer: "**Cancer does not cause a person to be sick; it is the sickness of the person that causes the cancer.**" To treat cancer successfully requires the patient to become whole again on all levels of his body, mind, and spirit. Once the cancer causes have been properly identified, it will become apparent what needs to be done to achieve complete recovery. The approaches provided in this book offer to deal with the causes of cancer while giving very little importance to the symptoms of cancer, that is, cancer cells.

It is a medical fact that every person has cancer cells in the body at all times. These cancer cells remain undetectable through standard tests until they have multiplied to several billion. When doctors announce to their cancer patients that the treatments they prescribed had successfully eliminated all cancer cells, they merely refer to tests that are able to identify the detectable size of cancer tumors. Standard cancer treatments may lower the number of cancer cells to an undetectable level, but this certainly cannot eradicate all cancer cells. As the long the causes of tumor growth remain intact, it may me redevelop at any time and at any rate.

Curing cancer has little to do with getting rid of a group of detectable cancer cells. Treatments like chemotherapy and radiation are certainly capable of poisoning or burning many cancer cells, but they also destroy healthy cells in the bone marrow, gastro-intestinal tract, liver, kidneys, heart, lungs, etc., which often leads to permanent irreparable damage of entire organs and systems in the body. A real cure of cancer does not occur at the expense of destroying other vital parts of the body. It is achievable only when the causes of excessive growth of cancer cells have been removed or stopped. This entire book is dedicated to dealing with the causes of illness, including cancer.

Cancer's Main Characteristics

1. Its Physical Side

Mary visited me when she was 39 years old. One year earlier, she was diagnosed with advanced breast cancer. Her oncologist prescribed the standard routine treatments for cancer - radiation and chemotherapy - but to no avail. Shortly afterwards he submitted her for surgery to amputate her right breast. The operation took place shortly before her menstrual period. Much to her relief, her doctors informed her that they 'got all the cancer' and the situation was now under control. Little did her doctors know that, according to the science of *chronobiology*[32], there is a four times higher risk for recurrence of cancer in women who undergo surgery for breast cancer one week before or during menstruation. While menstruating, a woman's immunity and iron levels are measurably low. And her body is, therefore, not able to destroy all the cancer cells left over from surgery. Hence, there is a high risk of cancer cells developing in other parts of the body.

---

[32] Chonobiology is the science of 'body clocks,' attuned to the earth's cycles and encoded in our cells. The human body is endowed with at least 100 'clocks' unrelated to our watch time. The Circadian rhythm, for example, is responsible for numerous hormonal cycles that determine our hungers, moods, metabolism, rate of growth and aging. For more information, see chapter 5.

Not surprisingly, one year after her mastectomy, Mary complained of severe pain in the lower spine and in her left knee. Ten years earlier she had been diagnosed as having *cervical spondylosis*[33] in her lower spine, caused by abnormal outgrowth and ossified cartilage around the margins of joints of the vertebral column. This time, however, the examinations revealed that she had developed bone cancer in her lower spine and left knee. The breast surgery and resulting suppression of the immune system had, as so often is the case, encouraged millions of cancer cells to develop in other already weakened parts of the body. Therefore, cancer cells began to grow in her lower spine where the resistance to cancer formation was particularly low.

Mary had also been suffering from severe menstrual problems as long as she remembered. In addition, she was diagnosed with having anemia. However, despite taking iron tablets regularly for years, which caused her frequent nausea and stomach cramps, she remained anemic. She told me that her digestive system had 'never worked properly' and constipation often lasted for as many as three to five days in a row. My examination revealed that her liver was filled with thousands of intrahepatic stones.

Mary also mentioned that she had received multiple treatments of antibiotics over the years for all kinds of infections. It is a well-established fact that regular use of antibiotics sharply increases breast cancer risk. According to cancer research, the risk of breast cancer is twice as high among women who receive 25 or more prescriptions for antibiotics of any variety over a 17-year period, in comparison with women who use no antibiotics at all.

Mary was brought up with a lot of candy, cakes, ice cream and chocolate. A number of recent studies linked a greater risk of breast cancer among women to a diet high in sugar (especially soft drinks and popular sweet desserts). Scientists now believe that the extra insulin released to process the simple starches and sugars found in these foods cause cells to divide and estrogens in the blood to rise. Both of these factors (cellular division and blood estrogens) can contribute to cancer growth.

2. Its Emotional Side

Mary experienced a very sad childhood because her parents had great problems relating with one another. When I asked her, she could not remember even one single instance when there had not been tension between her parents. Being a very sensitive person at heart, she took everything more seriously than her more extrovert brother, and consequently felt insecure, frightened and depressed. With a painful smile on her face, she said that she always felt torn between her mother and father and could not make a choice between which one to favor.

Eating her meals with the parents was particularly difficult for her. She was forced to sit and eat with them while being tormented by a very tense atmosphere. Sometimes everyone would keep quiet so as to not arouse any new conflicts. Today, she has a strong aversion to, and fear of, food and she gobbles it down very quickly, often while standing or driving.

Mary also faces great difficulties at work. In her job as a teacher, she feels that her students are allowed to take their frustrations out on her, but she has to keep it all inside. When she returns home, though, she shouts at her own children, which creates much guilt in her. She wants to be a good mother, but believes she is not; she just doesn't know how to be kind to her children. Mary also told me that she never wanted to be a teacher; she always dreamt of becoming a gymnastics teacher.

The frustration of not fulfilling her desires was a major cause of Mary's cancer. Right from the beginning of her life she was taught to conform to the social system, which meant for her that she

---

[33] Spondylosis is spinal degeneration and deformity of the joint(s) of two or more vertebrae.

always had to do what she was told. Deep inside herself she had dreams that she could never fulfill because she did not want to stir up tension or make other people think badly of her.

In order to keep the peace, Mary went along with what her parents demanded of her, but inside herself she was boiling with rage. When Mary walked into my office that morning, she gave me a beautiful smile which did not reveal the pain she was feeling inside. She had learned to conceal her inner world from the outer world. It was not so much the physical pain in her body that hurt her, it was all the bottled-up frustration, fear and insecurity that threatened the sensitive feelings of love and peace in her heart. The physical pains merely reminded her of the profound emotional heartache she had been suffering from for so long. All the endless attempts of suppressing or hiding her true inner feelings during her childhood and adulthood shaped a personality that eventually required a disease to bring it all to some kind of conclusion.

Torn between her parents for many years and trying to please both of them, Mary was never bold enough to make a choice that would please her and her only. The division within her heart sapped all her energy and happiness. The cancer started in her divided heart, in all the unexpressed grief and frustration that filled her early life.

It's All Psychosomatic

Whatever happens in our emotional body also occurs in our physical body. The real cancer is a trapped and isolated emotion, a feeling of 'having no choice'. Through the mind/body connection, any repressed feelings of wanting and deserving harmony, peace, stability and a simple sense of joy in life are translated into appropriate biochemical responses in the body. This effectively deprives the body cells of all these positive qualities as well. Cells are not physical machines that have no feelings, no sense of I-ness, or no reaction to external or threats. The emotional suffocation caused so much anger and frustration in Mary, that for fear of not being loved or liked by others, including her parents, she targeted these negative emotions at her own body. Her 'toxic' mind translated into a toxic body, and it threatened Mary's very survival. She threatened the cells of her body by keeping her most important thoughts and feelings to herself.

Whatever you keep to yourself out of fear of being criticized or hurt actually turns into poisons in the body. These poisons are so strong that if you cried and put your tears on a snakeskin, they would burn holes into it. Tears of joy, on the other hand, do not have any poison in them.

The constant tension, which Mary experienced during dinnertime at her parental home, had greatly impaired her digestive functions. Under stress or tension, the blood vessels supplying the organs of the digestive system become tight and restricted, preventing them to digest even the healthiest of foods. Furthermore, to eat while you are emotionally upset suppresses the secretion of balanced amounts of digestive juices. Whenever you feel angry or upset, your bile flora (beneficial bacteria that keep bile balanced) is altered, which predisposes it to coagulate. Constant emotional strain leads to stone formation in the bile ducts of the liver and in the gallbladder. The resulting curbed secretion of bile lowers *Agni*, the digestive fire. Mary still associates the eating of her meals with the tension she experienced while sitting at the parental dinner table. Her unconscious attempt to avoid everything that has to do with food and eating programs her body to do the same. The body cannot properly digest and absorb foods that are eaten in a hurry, hence the accumulation of large quantities of toxic waste in her small and large intestines. Chronic constipation and the poor absorption of nutrients, including fats, calcium, zinc, magnesium, and vitamins had increasingly depleted and weakened her bone tissue, bone marrow and reproductive functions.

When the reproductive tissue, which maintains the genetic blueprint (DNA) of the cells, is starved of oxygen and nutrients, it is only a matter of time before normal and healthy cells begin to mutate their genes and abnormally divide in order to survive the 'famine.' Normally, a host of immune cells, pancreatic enzymes and vitamins break down cancer cells in the body, wherever they appear. However, most of the digestive enzymes are 'used up' quickly when the diet is rich in animal protein, such as meat, pork, poultry, fish, eggs, cheese and milk, as well sugar-enriched foods. Mary practically lived on these foods. Having suffered from poor digestion and constipation for nearly all her life, Mary's body was practically deprived all of these natural antidotes to cancer cells. Cancers are much more likely to occur among those whose digestive functions are continually disturbed and who are deprived of a sense of emotional well-being than in those whose digestive system is efficient and who generally have a happy disposition.

The spondylosis of Mary's lower spine signifies weakening of her internal and external support system; it manifested in direct response to the lack of support and encouragement by her parents. Mary's body slumps forward while she sits, and looks half its size. She looks like a scared child, without confidence and trust. Her posture suggests that she is trying to protect her heart from being hurt again. In addition, her breathing is shallow and insufficient, as if she does not want to be noticed and possibly be criticized or disapproved of by her parents. The knees serve as a support system for the entire body. A lifetime of 'giving in' and 'not standing up for herself and her desires' manifested as the knee problems she developed over the years.

Mary's Personal Remedies

Japanese research has shown that cancer patients whose cancerous tumors went into spontaneous remission, often within less than 24 hours, experienced a profound transformation in their attitude towards themselves before the sudden cure occurred. Mary needed to make several major changes in her life - one of which was to change her job, even if this meant fewer earnings for her and her children. While Mary was still highly susceptible to stressful situations and chaotic noise, the tense atmosphere present at her school was hardly conducive to the healing process. She also needed to spend more time in nature, walk in the sun and on the beach, paint her impressions, listen to her favorite music and devote some time in quietness and meditation every day.

Apart from following an Ayurvedic daily routine and diet, Mary began to use a number of cleansing procedures to rid her colon of stagnant, old fecal matter and to purify the blood, liver, and connective tissue from accumulated toxins. The liver flush produced thousands of stones that had affected both her liver and gallbladder for at least 15 - 20 years.

The most important thing for Mary was to become more conscious about everything in her life. This included eating, emotional releases, listening to the body's signals of thirst, hunger, tiredness, etc. She needed to become aware of her needs and desires and begin to fulfill them whenever possible. The most important realization she had to make was that she did not need to do anything that did not please her. Giving herself the permission to make mistakes, and not judge herself if she made them, was essential therapy for her.

Mary's friends and family also needed to understand that she was at a very crucial stage of recovery where every positive thought and feeling towards her could serve as a tremendous support system, one that she never had when she was young. Mary started to improve steadily six months after she adopted about 60% percent of my recommended advice. Today she feels that the disease has brought her a deeper understanding of life and has led to an inner awakening she had never experienced before. Today, while free of cancer, Mary continues to improve and grow in confidence and self-acceptance.

Cancer - A Response to Rejection

Jeromy has *Hodgkin's* disease, which is the most common *lymphoma*. Lymphomas are malignant neoplasms of lymphoid tissue that vary in growth rate, also known as lymph cancer. Contemporary medicine has no explanation as to what causes the disease. Hodgkin's disease usually begins in adolescence or between 50 and 70 years of age.

When Jeromy was 22 years old, he noticed two enlarged lymph nodes in his neck. A few days later, he was diagnosed with Hodgkin's disease. In some people, the disease leads to death within a few months, but others have few signs of it for many years. Jeromy was one of them. Being a Kapha type[34], he has a very athletic and strong body and is naturally endowed with a lot of stamina and physical endurance. His naturally slow metabolic rate can be considered responsible for the slow advancement of the illness.

Jeromy received his first chemotherapy treatment in 1979, soon after diagnosis of the lymphoma, but there was no detectible improvement of his condition. In 1982, his doctors added multiple radiation treatments to the regular chemotherapy, but these produced severe side effects, including loss of all body hair and his sense of taste. His distress was considerable. Yet, despite the traumatic experiences caused by the various treatments during the following fourteen years, Jeromy was not willing to give into depression and desperation. His strong fighting spirit permitted him to continue his work as a general manager of a successful business enterprise.

Through the Ayurvedic Pulse Reading method and Eye Interpretation (Iridology)[35] I was able to determine that from a very early age Jeromy's digestive functions and lymph drainage had begun to decline rapidly. His liver showed presence of a large number of intrahepatic stones. As it turned out, Jeromy went through a very traumatic experience when he was four years old, although at first he had difficulties remembering it. According to Jeromy, the most traumatic event for him occurred at age 21 when his long-term girlfriend suddenly left him for another man. Exactly one year after she left him he discovered the lymph swellings in his neck. The rejection by his girlfriend was one of the most heart-breaking experiences of his life. Yet this experience merely triggered the memory of an even more traumatic rejection.

Fighting the Ghost of Memory

Jeromy was born in a developing country with an unstable political situation. When he reached the age of four, his parents sent him to a boarding school in another developing country, for his own safety. Unable to understand the reasons behind this move, he felt that his parents had stopped loving him and no longer wanted him around. All he remembers is the feeling of being cut off from what he considered his lifeline - the closeness with his parents. Although his parents believed that sending him away was in Jeromy's best interest, he suddenly lost the love of the most important people in his life, at an age when he needed it most. His little world had collapsed on this first 'black' day in his life, and his body's main functions subsequently began to decline.

Jeromy dedicated the major part of his life trying to prove to his parents that he was worthy of their love. He was not aware, however, of his incessant drive to succeed in life. He proudly told me that he never gives up in life and that he would not allow anything to get him down. One part of him never

---

[34] See details about the Ayurvedic body types, Vata, Pitta and Kapha, in chapters 5 and 6. The Kapha type has the strongest bones and muscles among all the types.

[35] Diagnostic methods used to determine any existing imbalances in the body and mind.

acknowledged that he was gravely ill. His physical appearance, except for being bald, would not reveal the battle his body was fighting. He spent all his energy and time in his work and he was very good at it.

To heal himself physically, though, Jeromy needed to become aware of the 'rejected child' within him. He had buried that part of him in the most hidden depths of his subconscious when he was four years old, and a second time, when he was 21 years old and his girlfriend left him. This second rejection further amplified the already profound deep hurt caused by what he considered a rejection by his parents.

The body stores all experiences we have in some kind of invisible 'filing cabinets'. Accordingly, all the feelings of anger we have in life go into one file, sad events into another, and rejections are deposited in yet a different file, and so on. These impressions are not recorded and stored according to linear time, but compiled in terms of similarity. They feed 'the ghost of memory' and give it more and more energy. Once a file is 'filled up,' even a small event can trigger a devastating eruption and awaken the ghost of memory, thereby giving it a life of its own. This happened in Jeromy's life.

The abandonment that Jeromy experienced as a four-year-old reawakened in his awareness when his girlfriend left him. By ignoring or denying the fact that this rejection ever took place, he unconsciously directed his body to create the identical response, which was a cancer in the very system that is responsible for neutralizing and removing harmful waste in the body - the lymphatic system. Unable to get rid of the ghost of memory, which consisted of deep-seated fear and anger from feeling abandoned, Jeromy was also no longer able to free himself of dead, turned-over cells and metabolic waste products[36]. Both his liver and gallbladder had accumulated thousands of gallstones, which nearly suffocated him. His body had no other choice, but to give physical expression to the cancer that had tortured his heart and mind for so many years.

Letting Go of the Need to Fight

All events in life that appear to be negative are in fact unique opportunities to become more complete and whole inside, and to move forward in life. Whenever we need to give ourselves more love, time and appreciation, but fail to fulfill these essential needs, there will be someone or something in our life that pushes us in that direction. Feeling rejected by or being disappointed and angry with another person highlights a lack in taking responsibility for the negative things that happen to us. Blaming someone else or oneself for an unfortunate situation results in the feeling of being a victim of sorts and is likely to manifest as disease. Moreover, if we cannot understand its accompanying message we may even have to face death to appreciate life or living.

Cancer, in an unconventional way, is a way out of a deadlock situation that paralyses the heart of a person. It helps to break down old rigid patterns of guilt and shame that keep it imprisoned and bound by constant poor self-worthiness. The current medical approach does not target this major issue behind cancer, but the 'disease process' does, provided it is allowed to take its course. Chemotherapy, radiation and surgery encourage a victim mentality in the patient and are unlikely to heal the root causes of this affliction. Miracle cures happen when the patient frees himself/herself of the need for victim-hood and self-attack, and when external problems fail to have a major impact on the person's inner wellbeing and self-acceptance. Just removing the external problems in life may not be sufficient to induce a spontaneous remission.

---

[36] To be healthy, the human body has to remove daily over 30 billion dead, worn-out cells and a large amount of metabolic waste.

Jeromy needed to give himself the love and appreciation he did not feel he was getting from his parents. He also needed to make room for enjoyment and pleasure, and take time for himself, for meditation, for self-reflection, for being in nature and sensing the joy and energy it is able to evoke in us. Cancer cells are cells fighting to survive in a 'hostile,' toxic environment. Letting go of the need to fight in life reprograms the DNA of the body, changing its course of warfare and eventual annihilation to one of healthy reproduction. Not needing to fight for their survival gives the cancer cells a chance to be accepted again by the entire 'family' of cells in the body. Cancer cells are normal cells that are rejected by what they consider home. They are deprived of proper nourishment and support. In their desperation to survive, they grab everything they can find to live on, even cellular waste products and toxins. This practically turns them into 'outcasts'.

However, just as *we* want to be loved, cancer cells also need to know that they are loved. Cutting them out of the body through surgery, or destroying them with poisonous drugs or deadly radiation just adds even more violence to the body than it already has to deal with. To live in health and peace, we especially need to be friends with the cells of the body, including cancer cells. The saying 'love thy enemy' applies to cancer cells just as it applies to people. Jeromy's cause of cancer was a lack of self-appreciation, a feeling of not being loved and wanted and not being worthy or good enough. By waiting for his parents to show him their love, he effectively denied this love to himself. Jeromy realized that his disease was, in fact, a great blessing in disguise that could help him find and love himself, for the very first time. If we could only see that what we call disease is a perfect representation of our inner world, we would pay more attention to what is going on inside rather than trying to fix something that does not really need fixing. Cancer, as hard as this may be to understand, has profound meaning to it. Its purpose is not to destroy but to heal what is not whole anymore.

Cancer Cannot Kill You

Cancer, like any other disease, is not a clearly definable phenomenon that suddenly and randomly appears in some part(s) of the body like mushrooms popping up out of the ground. Cancer is rather the result of many crises of toxicity that have as their common origin one or more energy-depleting influences. Stimulants, emotional trauma, repressed emotions, irregular lifestyle, dehydration, nutritional deficiency, overeating, stress reactions, lack of sleep, accumulation of heavy metals (especially from metal fillings) and chemicals, etc. all hinder the body in its effort to remove metabolic waste, toxins and 30 billion dead cells each day. When these accumulate in any part of the body, they naturally lead to a number of progressive responses that include irritation, swelling, hardening, inflammation, ulceration and abnormal growth of cells. Like every other disease, cancer is but a toxicity crisis and marks the body's final attempt to rid itself of septic poisons and acidic compounds that result from not being able to properly remove metabolic waste, toxins and putrefying dead cells in the body.

Cancer cannot be its own cause. Treating it as if it were its own cause is like cleaning a dirty pot with filthy mud; it will never get clean. Of course, you can throw away the pot and thereby solve the problem, but when it comes to preparing a new meal, you will face an even bigger problem: you have nothing to cook your food in. Similarly, by killing the cancer we also kill the patient; perhaps not right away, but gradually.

Despite the huge effort and expenditure on behalf of the medical establishment, mortality rates from cancer remain unchanged. Although radiation, chemotherapy drugs or surgery can certainly help neutralize or eliminate a lot of the septic poison kept in check by a tumor mass and in a good number of cases improve the condition, these procedures nevertheless fail to remove the cause(s) of cancer. A cancer patient may return home after a 'successful' treatment, relieved and obviously 'cured', but continue depleting his body's energy and gathering toxins as he did before. The immune system, already battered by one traumatic intervention, may not make it through a second one. However, if the patient dies, it is not the cancer that killed him but its untreated cause(s). Given the extremely small remission rate for most cancers (7%), the promises made to cancer patients that by destroying their tumors they will also be cured are deceptive, to say the least. Patients are not being told what turns a normal, robust cell into a weak, damaged and abnormal cell.

Tumor cells are cells that 'panic' due to lack of food, water, oxygen, and space. Survival is their basic genetic instinct, just as it is ours. To survive in such an acidic, unsupportive environment, the defective cells are forced to mutate and begin devouring everything they can get hold of to sustain them, including toxins. They leach more nutrients such as glucose, magnesium and calcium from the connective tissue than they would need to if they were normally growing cells. Their healthier neighboring cells, however, begin to gradually waste away in the process, and eventually an entire organ becomes dysfunctional due to exhaustion, malnutrition or wasting. Cancerous tumors always look for more energy to divide and multiply cells. Sugar is one of their favorite energy-supplying foods. Craving sugar reflects excessive cell activity, and many people who eat lots of sugar end up growing tumors in their body.

It seems so obvious that the cancer cells must be responsible for the death of a person - the main reason why almost the entire medical approach is so geared towards destroying them. However, cancer cells are far from being the culprits, just as blocked arteries are not the real reason for heart disease. In fact, cancer cells help a highly congested body survive a little longer than it would without them. In a body filled with toxic waste, what possible reason could the immune system have to ignore cancer cells that cluster together and form a tumor mass? Cancer cells are not at all vicious; in fact, they serve a good purpose. You wouldn't call a poisonous mushroom 'vicious' or 'evil' just because it could kill you if you ate it, or would you? Those mushrooms in the forest that attract and absorb poisons from the soil, water and air form an essential part of the ecologic system in our natural world. Although the cleansing effect produced by the mushrooms is hardly noticeable, yet it allows for the healthy growth of the forest and its natural inhabitants. It is not the primary choice of normal healthy cells to suddenly become 'poisonous' or malignant, but it is the next best choice they have to avoid an immediate catastrophe in the body. If the body dies, it is not because of cancer, but because of the reasons that lead up to it.

Cancer Is Not a Disease

To continue doing their increasingly difficult job, these tumor cells need to grow, even if it is at the expense of other healthy cells. Without their activity, an organ may suddenly lose its already weakened structure and collapse. Cancer theories make the assumption that cancer cells can leave a tumor site and enter lymph fluid carrying them to other parts of the body. However, if this were true (which has never been proved), it could only occur in parts of the body where there is an equally high concentration of toxicity or acidosis. The 'spreading' of cancer cells is known as *metastasis*. But to repeat, cancer cells are programmed to settle only where there is a 'fertile' ground of high toxicity (acidity) - a terrain in which they can survive and continue their unusual rescue mission. They have mutated to be able to live in a toxic, non-oxygenated environment, and to help neutralize at least some of the trapped metabolic waste, such as lactic acid, uric acid, urea and ammonia (highly caustic and hazardous), as well as decomposing cellular debris. Given these circumstances, it would be a fatal mistake by the immune system to destroy these types of 'estranged' cells as they are doing part of the immune system's work. Without the tumor's presence, large amounts of septic poison resulting from the accumulated corpses of decomposing cells would perforate the capillary walls, seep into the blood and kill the person within a matter of hours or days. Cancer cells are still the body's cells and if they were no longer needed, one simple command from the DNA would stop them from behaving like senseless lunatics. Cancer cells are anything but senseless lunatics.

The body has to exert a lot more effort in maintaining a tumor than eliminating it. If it were not forced to use cancer growth as one of its last survival tactics, the body would opt for this final attempt of self-preservation - final, because it could very well fail in its attempt to survive against the odds. As mentioned before, most tumors (about 90-95%) appear and disappear completely on their own, without any medical intervention. Millions of people walk around with cancers in their body and will never know they had them. There is no other cancer treatment that can even closely compete with the body's own healing mechanism, which we unfortunately label as disease. Cancer is not a disease; it is a very unusual, but apparently highly efficient mechanism of survival and self-protection.

We ought to give the most developed and complex system in the universe - the human body - a little more credit than it has so far received, and trust that it knows perfectly well how to conduct its own affairs, even under the grimmest of circumstances.

Cancer is 'Not Loving Yourself'

Many cancer patients have devoted their entire lives to helping and supporting others. Their selfless service can be very a noble quality, depending on the motivation behind it. If they sacrifice and neglect their own wellbeing to avoid facing any shame, guilt or unworthiness within them, they are actually cutting off the very limb they are hanging on. They are 'selflessly' devoted to please others so that, in return, they may be loved and appreciated for their contributions. This, however, serves as an unconscious acknowledgement of *not loving oneself.* This may lock up unresolved issues, fears, and feelings of unworthiness in the cellular memory of organs and tissues in the body.

'Love your neighbor as yourself' is one of the most basic requirements for curing cancer. This phrase means that we can only love others as much as we are able to love and appreciate ourselves, no less and no more. To be able to truly love someone without cords of attachment and possessiveness, one has to fully accept oneself with all the flaws, mistakes and inadequacies one may have. The degree to which we are able to care about the well-being of our body, mind, and spirit determines the degree to which we are able to care about other people, too. By being critical of ourselves, or disliking the way we look behave, or feel, we close down our heart and feel unworthy and ashamed. To avoid exposing our shadow self (the part of us we do not like) to others out of fear of rejection, we try to win over the love of others by pleasing them. This way, we assume, we can receive the love we are unable to give to ourselves. However, this approach fails to work in the long term.

Your body always follows the commands given by your mind. Your thoughts, emotions, feelings, desires, beliefs, drives, likes, dislikes, etc., serve as the software your cells are programmed with on a daily basis. Through the mind/body connection, your cells have no other choice but to obey the orders they receive via your subconscious or conscious mind. As DNA research has recently proved, you can literally alter your DNA's genetic setting and behavior within a matter of a moment. Your DNA listens to every word you utter to yourself and it feels every emotion you experience. Moreover, it responds to all of them. You program yourself every second of the day, consciously and unconsciously. If you choose to, you can rewrite the program in any way you want to, provided you are truly self-aware. Once you know who you truly are you cannot help but love yourself. You can no longer judge yourself for making mistakes in life, for not being perfect, for not always being how others want you to be. Seeing yourself in this light, you send a signal of love to your cells. The bonding effect of love unites differences and keeps everything together, including the cells of your body. When love, which should not be confused with neediness or attachment, is no longer a daily experience, the body begins to disintegrate and become sick.

It is the expansion of love that is the main purpose of our existence here on earth. Those who love themselves are also able to love others and vice versa. These two aspects of love always go hand in hand. People who accept themselves fully have no real fear of death; when their time comes to die, they leave peacefully without any regrets or remorse in their hearts.

Whenever we close our hearts to ourselves, we become lonely, and the body begins to become weak and diseased. It is known that widows and people who are socially isolated, or have nobody to share their deepest feelings with, are the most prone to developing cancer.

Your body cells are the most intimate 'neighbors' you can have and they need to feel your love and self-acceptance, to know that they are a part of you and that you care about them. Giving yourself an oil massage, going to sleep on time, eating nutritious foods, etc. are simple, but powerful messages of love that motivate your cells to function in harmony with each other. They are also messages that keep elimination of toxins flawless and efficient. There is nothing unscientific about this. You can go around a number of hospitals and ask all the patients whether they felt good about their life prior to falling ill. The overwhelming response would be a 'no'. Without being a medical researcher, you would have conducted one of the most important research studies anyone could ever do. You would have stumbled over the most common cause of ill health, which is 'not loving yourself', or, to use a different expression 'not being happy about how your life turned out to be'. Not being happy or satisfied in life is perhaps the most severe form of emotional stress you could possibly have. It is, in fact, a major risk factor for many diseases, including cancer.

A recently published study suggests that severe emotional stress can triple the risk of breast cancer. One hundred women who had a breast lump were interviewed before they knew that they had breast cancer. One in two who had the disease had suffered a major traumatic life event, such as bereavement, within the previous five years. The effects of emotional stress or unhappiness can severely impair digestion, elimination, and immunity, thus leading to a dangerously high level of toxicity in the body. Just ridding the body of cancer through 'weapons of mass destruction' doesn't remove the unresolved emotional pain behind it. (See Chapter 7 about my approaches for restoring emotional health.)

The Power of Resolving Conflict Situations

Unresolved conflict is mostly likely the starting point of any illness, including cancer. The body always uses the stress response to cope with the traumatizing effect of conflict. According to a study released by the Journal of Biological Chemistry, March 12, 2007, the stress hormone *epinephrine* changes prostate and breast cancer cells in ways that may make them resistant to cell death. The researchers found that epinephrine levels increase sharply in response to stressful situations, and can remain continuously elevated during long periods of stress or depression. They discovered that when cancer cells are exposed to epinephrine, a protein called BAD, which causes cell death, becomes inactive. This means that emotional stress may not only trigger or contribute to the development of cancer, but also undermine or reduce the effectiveness of cancer treatments.

The German university professor, Ryke Geerd Hamer, M.D., discovered during routine CT scans of over 20,000 cancer patients that each of them had a lesion in a certain part of the brain that looks like concentric rings on a shooting target or like the surface of water after a stone has been dropped into it. This distortion in the brain is known as 'HAMER herd'. Dr Hamer, now living in Spain, found that these lesions resulted from a serious, acute-dramatic and isolating conflict-shock-experience in the patient.

Whenever the conflict became resolved, the CT image changed, an edema developed, and finally scar tissue formed. Naturally, the cancers would stop growing, become inactive and disappear.

Simply by helping patients to resolve their acute conflicts and supporting the body during this healing phase, Dr Hamer achieved an exceptionally high success rate with his cancer therapy. According to public record, after 4 to 5 years of receiving his simple treatment, 6,000 out of 6,500 patients with mostly advanced cancer were still alive.

The Body's Desperate Attempt to Live

Nobody wants to be attacked by anyone; this also applies to the cells of the body. Cells only go into a defensive mode and turn malignant if they need to ensure their own survival, at least for as long as they can. A spontaneous remission occurs when cells no longer need to defend themselves. Like every other disease, cancer is a toxicity crisis that, when allowed to come to its natural conclusion, will naturally relinquish its symptoms.

Out of the 30 billion cells that a healthy body turns over each day, at least one percent are cancer cells. Does this mean, however, that all of us are destined to develop cancer - the disease? Certainly not! These cancer cells are products of 'programmed mutation' that keep your immune system alert, active and stimulated.

The situation changes, though, when due to constant energy-depleting influences the body can no longer adequately deal with the continual presence of worn out, damaged and cancerous cells. The result is a gradual build-up of congestion in the intercellular fluids. This can affect both the transportation of nutrients to the cells and the elimination of waste from the cells. Consequently, a large number of the corpses of dead cells begin to decompose, leaving behind a mass of degenerate protein fragments. To remove these harmful proteins, the body builds some of them into the basal membranes of the blood vessels and dumps the rest into the lymphatic ducts, which leads to lymphatic blockage. All this disrupts the normal metabolic processes and alienates some groups of cells to such a degree that they begin to become weak and damaged. Out of these cells, a number of them undergo genetic mutation and turn malignant. A cancerous tumor is born and the toxicity crisis has reached its peak.

With the correct approaches, a tumor as big as an egg can spontaneously regress and disappear, regardless of whether it is in the brain, the stomach, a breast or an ovary. The cure begins when the toxicity crisis stops. A toxicity crisis ends when we cease to deplete the body's energy (see chapters 3&4) and remove existing toxins from the blood, bile ducts, lymph ducts and cell tissues. Unless the body has been seriously damaged, it is perfectly capable of taking care of the rest. Medical intervention, on the other hand, reduces the possibility of a spontaneous remission to almost zero because of its suppressive and debilitating effects.

Most cancers occur after a number of repeated warnings. These may include: Headaches that you stop with pain killers; tiredness that you keep suppressing by having a cup of coffee, tea, or coke; nervousness you want to control through nicotine; medicines you take to ward off unwanted symptoms; seasonal head colds which you don't have time to let pass on their own; not giving yourself enough time to relax, laugh, and be quiet; conflicts that you keep avoiding; pretense that you are always fine when you are not; having a constant need to try pleasing everyone, but feeling unworthy and unloved by others; trying to constantly prove yourself to others; rewarding yourself with comfort foods, etc. All of these and similar symptoms are serious risk indicators for developing cancer or another illness.

There are no fundamental physiological differences between a simple cold and the occurrence of a cancerous tumor. Both are attempts by the body to rid itself of accumulated toxins, but with varied degrees of intensity. Taking drugs in an attempt to ward off a head cold or an upper respiratory infection before giving your body the chance to eliminate the accumulated toxins, has a strongly suffocating effect on the cells of the body. It coerces the body to keep large amounts of cellular waste products, acidic substances and, possibly, toxic chemicals from drug medicines, in the extra-cellular fluid (connective tissue) surrounding the cells. By repeatedly undermining the body's efforts of cleansing itself, the cells are increasingly shut off from their supply routes of oxygen and nutrients. This alters their basic metabolism and eventually affects the DNA molecule itself.

Located in the nucleus of every cell, the DNA makes use of its six billion genes to mastermind and control every single part and function of the body. Without the adequate supply of vital nutrients, the DNA has no other choice but to alter its genetic program in order to guarantee the cell's survival. Mutated cells can survive in an environment of toxic waste. Soon they begin to draw nutrients from other surrounding cells. For these nutrient-deprived cells to survive, they also need to subject themselves to genetic mutation, which leads to the spreading or enlargement of the cancer. Cancerous growths are anaerobic, which means that they develop and survive without the use of oxygen.

Nobel Prize winner Dr. Otto Warburg was one of the first scientists to demonstrate the principal difference between a normal cell and a cancer cell. Both derive energy from glucose, but the normal cell utilizes oxygen to combine with the glucose, whereas the cancer cell breaks down glucose without the use of oxygen, yielding only 1/15 the energy per glucose molecule that the normal cell produces. It is very obvious that cancer cells opt for this relatively inefficient and unproductive method of obtaining energy because they have no access to oxygen anymore. The capillaries supplying oxygen to a group of cells or to the connective tissue surrounding them (usually both) may be severely congested with harmful waste material, noxious substances such as food additives and chemicals, excessive proteins, or decomposing cellular debris, and unable to deliver enough oxygen and nutrients.

Because their oxygen and nutrient supply is blocked, cancer cells have an insatiable appetite for sugar. This may also explain why people with constant cravings for sugar foods have a higher risk for developing cancer cells or why cancer patients often want to eat large amounts of sweets. The main waste product resulting from the anaerobic breakdown of glucose by cancer cells is lactic acid, which may explain why the body of a cancer patient is so acidic, in contrast to the naturally alkaline body of a healthy person.

To deal with the dangerously high levels of lactic acid and to find another source of energy, the liver reconverts some of the lactic acid into glucose. In doing so, the liver uses 1/5 the energy per glucose molecule that a normal cell can derive from it, but that's three times the energy a cancer cell will get from it. To help feed the cancer cells, the body even grows new blood vessels, funneling more and more sugar towards them. This means that the more the damaged cancer cells multiply, the less energy is available to the normal cells, hence the sugar cravings. In a toxic body, the concentrations of both oxygen and energy tend to be very low. This creates an environment where cancer spreads most easily. Unless the toxins and the cancer's food source are eliminated, and oxygen levels are sharply increased, the wasteful metabolism associated with cancer becomes self-sustaining and the cancer spreads further. If death occurs it is not caused by the cancer, though; it is due to wasting of body tissues and final acidosis.

Genetic mutation is now believed to be the main **cause** of cancer, yet in truth it is only an **effect** of 'cellular famine' and nothing more or less than the body's desperate, but often unsuccessful, attempt to live and survive. Something similar occurs in a person's body when he uses antibiotics to fight an infection. Most of the infection-causing bacteria that are being attacked by the antibiotics will be killed, but some of them will survive and reprogram their own genes to become antibiotic-resistant.

Nobody really wants to die and this includes bacteria. The same law of nature applies to our body cells. *Cancer is the final attempt of the body to live, and not, as most people assume, to die.* Without gene mutation, those cells in the body that live in a toxic, anaerobic environment would simply suffocate and expire. Similar to bacteria that are attacked with antibiotics, many cells, in fact, succumb to the poison attack and die, but some manage to adjust to the abnormal changes of their natural environment. The cells know that they will eventually die, too, once their final survival tactics fail to keep the body alive.

To understand cancer and more successfully treat it than we currently do, we may have to radically alter our currently held views about it. We may also have to ask what its purpose is in the body and why the immune system fails to stop it from spreading. It is just not good enough to claim that cancer is an autoimmune disease that is out to kill the body. Such a notion (of the body trying to commit suicide) goes against the core principles of physical life. It makes so much more sense to say that cancer is nothing but the body's final attempt to live.

By removing all excessive waste from the gastrointestinal tract and any harmful deposits from the bile ducts, connective tissues, blood and lymph vessels, the cancer cells will have no other choice but to die or reverse their faulty genetic program. Unless they are too damaged, they certainly can become normal, healthy cells again. Those anaerobic cells and seriously damaged cells that cannot make the adjustment to live in a clean, oxygenated environment may simply die off. By thoroughly cleansing the liver and gallbladder from gallstones and other toxins, the body's digestive power improves considerably, thereby increasing the production of digestive enzymes. Digestive and metabolic enzymes possess very powerful anti-tumor properties. When the body is being decongested through major cleansing and is given proper nourishment, these powerful enzymes have easy access to the cells of the body. Permanently damaged cells or tumor particles are easily and quickly neutralized and removed.

There are many people in the world who cure their own cancers in this fashion. Some are aware of this because their diagnosed tumors went into spontaneous remission without any form of medical treatment, but most of them will never even know they had cancer because they never received a diagnosis. After passing through a bout of flu, a week of coughing up bad-smelling phlegm or a couple of days with high fever, many people eliminate massive amounts of toxins, and along with them, tumor tissue. Recent cancer research on gravely ill patients at M.D. Anderson Cancer Center in Houston, Texas revealed a promising treatment to kill cancer cells by giving them a cold, that is, injecting tumors with a cold virus. It may still take a while, though, before researchers will discover that catching a few colds can do the same job. This way, without interfering with the body's self-repair mechanisms, a person may experience a spontaneous remission of cancer, easily and only with relatively minor discomfort.

Prostate Cancer and Its Risky Treatments

There is, indeed, enough scientific evidence to suggest that most cancers disappear by themselves if left alone. A 1992 Swedish study found that of 223 men who had early prostate cancer but did not receive *any* kind of medical treatment, only 19 died within ten years of diagnosis. Considering that one third of men in the European Community have prostate cancer, but only one percent of them die (not necessarily from the cancer), it is very questionable to treat it at all. This is especially after research has revealed that treatment of the disease has not decreased mortality rates. On the contrary, survival rates are higher in groups of men whose 'treatment' consists merely of watchful waiting, compared with groups undergoing prostate surgery. In the Trans-Urethral Resection (TURP) Procedure, a 1/4-inch pipe is inserted into the penis to just below the base of the bladder and the prostate is then fried with a hot wire loop. Far from being a safe procedure, one study found that a year after the surgery, 41% of men had to wear diapers because of chronic leakage, and 88% were sexually impotent.

Even the screening procedure for prostate cancer can be dangerous. According to a number of studies, more men who are screened with the PSA (prostate-specific-antigen) screening test die from prostate cancer compared to those who are not tested. A recent editorial in the British Medical Journal sized up the value of the PSA test with this comment: "At present the one certainty about PSA testing is that it causes harm." A high enough positive PSA test is typically followed by a prostate biopsy - a painful procedure that can result in bleeding and infection. Recent evidence suggests that a large number of these biopsies are completely unnecessary. In fact, they may be life-endangering. Each year, 98,000 people die in the U.S. because of medical testing errors, PSA tests included.

Another serious problem with PSA tests is that they are notoriously unreliable. In a 2003 study undertaken by the Memorial Sloan-Kettering Cancer Center in New York City, researchers found that half of the men found to have PSA levels high enough to be recommended for a biopsy had follow-up tests with normal PSA levels. In fact, doctors at the Fred Hutchinson Cancer Research Center (FHCRC) in Seattle estimated that PSA screening may result in an over-diagnosis rate of more than 40 percent. To make matters worse, a disturbing new study finds that fully 15% of older men whose PSA readings were considered perfectly normal had prostate cancer - some even with relatively advanced tumors.

There is a much more reliable test than PSA. The less well-known AMAS (Anti-Malignin Antibody Screening) blood test is very safe, inexpensive, and more than 95% accurate at detecting cancer of any type. Anti-Malignin antibody levels become elevated when any cancer cells are present in the body, and can be detected several months before other clinical tests might find it (find out more about the AMAS test at the web site http://www.amascancertest.com).

If men learned how to avoid a buildup of toxins in the body, prostate cancer could perhaps be the least common and the least harmful of all cancers. Aggressive treatment of early prostate cancer is now a controversial issue, but it should be controversial for every type of cancer, at whatever stage of development.

About Prostate Enlargement

Prescription drugs for enlarged prostate encourage testosterone-to-estrogen conversion. This can greatly increase cancer risk. Men who take them have even grown female breasts. Also beware of estrogen-mimicking foods (soy products and others) that both men and women are advised to eat. There are better ways to prevent prostate enlargement. In a study published in a recent issue of the *British Journal of Urology International*, researchers from the University of Chicago reviewed the results of nearly 20 trials that tested Permixon, a commercial extract of saw palmetto. The results were overwhelmingly positive, including improved urine flow; reduction of urinary urgency and pain; improved emptying of the bladder; reduction in size of the prostate gland after two years; and significant improvement in quality of life. In one trial saw palmetto extract produced positive results similar to the drugs, but without the sexual dysfunction that accompanied the drug use. Permixon is manufactured in Europe and not yet available in the U.S., but there are other supplements available here that are just as effective. Look for prostate products that contain Beta-sitosterol, such as 'Prostate Care' by *Healthy Choice Nutritionals*, which is even more powerful than Saw Palmetto. If there are red blotches on the penis, massage it with pure Aloe Vera gel, twice daily. Many prostate problems are due to trapped urinary deposits/crystals in the penis and disappear when removed by the gel. You should notice a clearing of the skin irritation within a few days.

Why Most Cancers Disappear Naturally

Every toxicity crisis, such as a complex cancer or a simple head cold, is actually a healing crisis that, when supported by cleansing measures, leads to swift recovery. However, if interfered with by symptom-suppressive measures, a usually short-lived 'recovery' may easily turn into a chronic disease condition. Unfortunately, cancer researchers do not dare or do not care to find a natural cure for cancer; this is not what they are trained and paid for. Even if they did stumble over a natural cure, it would never be made public.

Rose Papac, M.D., a professor of oncology at Yale University School of Medicine, once pointed out that there is little opportunity these days to see what happens to cancers if left untreated. "Everyone feels impelled to treat immediately when they see these diseases," says Papac, who has studied cases of spontaneous remissions of cancer. Being stifled with fear, and in some cases being paranoid about finding a quick-acting remedy for the dreaded illness, many people don't give their bodies the chance to cure themselves, but instead choose to destroy what does not need to be destroyed. This may be one of the main reasons spontaneous remissions occur in just so few cancer patients nowadays.

On the other hand, numerous researchers have reported over the years that various conditions such as typhoid fever, coma, menopause, pneumonia, chickenpox and even hemorrhage can spark spontaneous remissions of cancer. However, there are no official explanations of how these remissions relate to the disappearance of the cancer. Because they are unexplained phenomena having no scientific basis, they are not used for further cancer research. Consequently, the scientific community's interest in discovering the mechanism for how the body cures itself of cancer remains almost nil. These 'miracle cures' seem to happen most frequently in certain types of malignancies: kidney cancer, melanoma (cancer of the skin), lymphomas (cancers of the lymph), and neuroblastoma (a nerve cell cancer that affects infants).

Considering that most of the body's organs have eliminative functions, it stands to reason that liver, kidney, colon, lungs, lymph, and skin cancers are more likely to disappear when these major organs and systems of elimination are no longer overloaded with toxins. Likewise, malignant tumors do not develop in a healthy body with intact defense and repair functions. They only thrive in a specific internal environment that promotes their growth. Cleansing such an environment by whatever means can make the difference when it comes to surviving cancer.

A toxicity crisis like pneumonia or chickenpox removes large amounts of toxins and helps the cells to 'breathe' freely again. Fever, sweat, loss of blood, mucus discharge, diarrhea, and vomiting are additional outlets for toxins to leave the body. After breaking down and removing the toxins in an unhindered way, the immune system receives a natural boost. A renewed immune stimulation based on reduced overall toxicity in the body can be sufficient to do away with a malignant tumor that no longer has a role to play in the survival of the body. The undesirable chickenpox, pneumonia, fever, etc. may actually be 'a gift from God' (to use another unscientific expression) that could save a person's life. Refusing to accept the gift could take his life. Many people die unnecessarily because they are prevented from going through the all the phases of an illness. Illness is nothing other than the body's many attempts attempt to create outlets for poisonous substances. Blocking the exits routes for these poisons, which happens when symptoms are being treated away, can suffocate the body and stop its vital functions.

The suppression of children's diseases through unnatural immunization programs can put the children at a high risk for eventually developing cancer. Chickenpox, measles, and other natural self-immunization programs (wrongly called 'children's diseases') help equip a child's immune system with the ability to counteract potential disease-causing agents more efficiently and without having to go through a major toxicity crisis.

With more than 550,000 annual cancer deaths in the United States alone, the justification of mandatory immunization programs in this country is very questionable. The standard approach of establishing immunity, which is unproved and unscientific, may undermine and override the body's own far superior programs of self-immunization. The body gains natural immunity through a healing crisis, which naturally eliminates cancer-producing toxins. Whether manufactured immunization directly or indirectly causes cancer is irrelevant. It is important to know, however, that conventional immunization programs can prevent the body from developing a potentially life-saving healing crisis.

Cancer—Who Cures It?

Those who have gone into complete remission of cancer and remained free from it are also the most likely candidates to reveal the mechanisms that cause and cure cancer.

Anne was 43 when she was diagnosed with an incurable form of lymphoma and was given only a short time to live. It was strongly recommended that she have radiation and chemotherapy treatments, the two most commonly used methods of combating cancer cells. Anne was aware that the treatments could not only substantially increase the risk of secondary cancer, but also have potentially severe side effects. She refused the treatment, arguing that if the cancer was incurable anyway, why treat it and suffer painful side effects.

Having accepted that she had an incurable disease, which meant that she came to terms with death, Anne felt free to look for alternative ways to make the 'transition' easier. Rather than passively accepting her fate, she decided to focus on feeling well and began taking an *active* role in improving her well-being. She tried everything from acupuncture and herbal medicine to meditation and visualization, which were all definite signals of *caring attention* sent to her body's cells. Anne's cancer went into remission a few months later. Within a year all apparent signs of cancer had disappeared, much to the astonishment of her oncologist. Now, over two decades later, she is not only without a trace of cancer, but she also feels that she has never been healthier and more vital as she is now.

Linda was diagnosed with a malignant melanoma (the most aggressive form of skin cancer) when she was just 38 years old. After several unsuccessful operations, she was informed that her cancer had progressed to the point that it was 'terminal' and that she had only about one year to live. Linda also refused treatment with chemotherapy and radiation and, instead, focused on the more positive approaches of healing, including yoga, praying, vegetarian diet, meditation and daily visualizations. Today, 22 years after having outlived her death sentence, she is as healthy as she can be with no trace of even a skin irritation.

Both Anne and Linda have changed their entire attitude to life from being passive victims of an uncontrollable 'invasive' disease, to being active participants in the creation of a healthy body and mind. Taking self-responsibility was their first step to remove the focus from cancer and direct it towards consciously creating healthfulness.

To call the remissions 'miracle cures' is certainly not correct. Today there is ample documentation of remarkable recoveries with every type of cancer and nearly every other disorder, from diabetes to warts and even AIDS. The fact that a spontaneous remission of cancer can occur even in the final stages of the illness shows that the immune system has not only the potential to quickly and effectively clear the body from existing tumors, but also to prevent new ones from forming, provided their causes are addressed. A shift in attitude from 'having' to attack and kill cancer cells to leaving them in peace and eliminating the energy-depleting influences in life may be a strong enough stimulant for the immune system to do away with the symptom (the cancerous tumor). Without its root causes, cancer is as harmless as a simple cold.

People like Anne and Linda don't have to be the exception, they can be the rule. When Michalis, a Cypriot businessman, came to me with kidney cancer, he told me that his doctors had given him only one month to live. They had already removed one of his kidneys and believed that his second one 'would not make it that much longer either'. Yet one month was sufficient for Michalis to remove enough toxins from his body to stop the cancer from growing. The cleansing procedures described in chapters 6 and 7 turned out to be very effective for him. Formerly a heavy drinker, meat eater, and late night reveler, he decided to stop depleting his energy from one day to the next. I have seen few people as determined to change his lifestyle as Michalis. The next visit to his cancer clinic in Germany three months later (much to the doctors' surprise, as they didn't expect to see him alive) revealed no trace of kidney cancer or any other disease, and after 14 years he is as healthy and active as ever.

Spontaneous remissions rarely occur spontaneously or for no apparent reason. The body regards cancer as an emotional and physical obstruction that can be overcome through a healing crisis and cleansing on all levels of body, mind and spirit. Active participation in the healing process and taking self-responsibility (an expression of love for oneself) is an absolute necessity in the treatment of every type of disorder, including cancer. Having cancer does not equate with being a helpless victim who is at the mercy of oncologists or surgeons.

Useful Tips to Remove the Need for Cancer

After I examined a large number of cancer patients in my European practice during the nineties, I discovered that all of them, regardless of the type of cancer, had accumulated large amounts of gallstones in the liver and gallbladder. By removing *all* stones from the liver and gallbladder through a series of liver cleanses, and cleansing the colon and kidneys before and after each liver flush[37], you create the physical preconditions for most every type of cancer to go into spontaneous remission. This also applies to cancers that are considered to be terminal.

If a healthy diet and lifestyle is maintained hence forward, the cure is likely to be permanent. There is plenty of evidence that fruits and vegetables have cancer-curing and cancer-preventive properties. Research carried out at Britain's Institute of Food Research has revealed that brassica vegetables such as cabbages, kale, broccoli and Brussels sprouts contain anticarcinogenic compounds, stimulating cancer cells to commit suicide. These vegetables have strong purifying effects on tissues and blood. Eating them regularly greatly reduces overall toxicity and eliminates the body's need for cancer cells.

In this context, Dr. Warburg's insights about the sugar-cravings of cancer cells are very helpful. Cancer cells are unable to multiply rapidly without it. If you have cancer, it is important that you stop eating refined, processed sugar immediately. Nutritionally, refined sugars contain none of the nutrients necessary for the assimilation of the sugar ingested. The eating of these sugars drains body stores of nutrients and energy (if any are still present), leaving less (or none) for other tasks. Cancer never kills a person; the wasting of organ tissues does. Cancer and wasting go hand in hand. Eating regular sugar feeds cancer cells, but starves healthy cells.

Natural sweeteners like stevia and xylitol do not rob the body's nutrient and energy resources. Stevia has zero calories, so it cannot serve as food for cancer cells. Xylitol, contains calories (about 40% less than sugar), but its slow release into the blood gives it a much lower glycemic index. If taken in moderation, xylitol is unlikely to pose a problem. However, refined carbohydrates, such as pasta, white bread, pastries and cakes are quickly broken down into glucose and act just as refined sugar does.

---

[37]See directions for these cleanses in *The Amazing Liver & Gallbladder Flush* or earlier chapters.

Obviously, sugar-rich foods and beverages, such as chocolate, ice cream, and sodas should be avoided. Milk, yoghurt and cheese should also be avoided. Cancer cells thrive on milk sugar (lactose).

Miracle Mineral Supplement/Solution (MMS)

All cancers have three things in common: 1. the immune system is weak and depleted; 2. the body is overwhelmed with toxins and waste matter; 3. there is a massive presence of pathogens (infecting agents) inside and around cancer cells, including parasites, viruses, bacteria, yeast, fungi, etc. One mineral substance - sodium chlorite - may have the most balanced and immediate effects on all these disease-causing factors. Apart from the topics already discussed, the main requirements for healing cancer and most other serious and minor illnesses are as follows:

1. Neutralize the toxins and poisons that weaken the immune system and feed pathogens.
2. Strengthen the immune system to remove all pathogens and keep them at bay.
3. Remove all harmful parasites, viruses, bacteria, fungi, molds, yeast and eliminate them from the body

To be successful, all these activities need to occur at the same time.

The product *Miracle Mineral Supplement* (MMS) is a stabilized oxygen solution of 28% sodium chlorite (not "chloride") in distilled water. When a small amount of lemon juice or citric acid solution is added to a few drops of MMS, chlorine dioxide is created. When ingested in this form, the chlorine dioxide instantly oxidizes harmful substances, parasites, bacteria, viruses, yeast, fungi, and molds, etc. within a matter of hours, while boosting the immune system by at least ten times. By doing so, MMS has shown to remove, for example, any strands of the malaria and HIV viruses from the blood within less than 24 hours in nearly every person tested. MMS has also been successfully used for many other serious illnesses, including Hepatitis A, B & C, Typhoid, most cancers, herpes, pneumonia, food poisoning, tuberculosis, asthma, influenza (for more details on MMS see Chapter 7 and *Product Information*).

Prevention is better than cure. This old saying applies to cancer as well. Whatever can prevent cancer can also cure it. The approaches and insights described in this book address the causes of nearly all illnesses, including cancer.

If you have cancer or wish to prevent it, make certain to avoid the following things: Chlorinated water; fluoridated water; pesticides and other chemical toxins as found in non-organic foods, commercial beauty products, chemical hair dyes, chemical shampoos and skin lotions; unnatural make-up products; artificial sweeteners such as Aspartame and Splenda; exposure to ionizing radiation (X-rays, mammograms, etc.); alcohol; cigarettes; sunscreens; microwave ovens; pharmaceutical drugs. (Almost all drugs are toxic for the body and can contribute to or directly cause cancer.)

The Early Puberty and Breast Cancer Link

Girls in the United States and other modern countries are reaching puberty at very early ages, which has been shown to increase their risk of breast cancer. Just decades ago, biological signs of female puberty - menstruation, breast development, and growth of pubic and underarm hair - typically occurred around 13 years of age or older. Today, girls as young as 8 are increasingly showing these signs. Apparently, African-American girls are particularly vulnerable to early puberty. Even 5- and 6-year-olds now go through precocious puberty (aka early sexual development). Early puberty exposes girls to more estrogen - a major risk of hormone-related breast cancers. According to data published by biologist Sandra Steingraber, girls that get their first period before age 12 have a 50 percent higher risk of developing breast cancer than those who get it at age 16. "For every year we could delay a girl's first menstrual period," she says, "we could prevent thousands of breast cancers."

Potential causes for this trend include rising childhood obesity rates and inactivity, cow's milk- and soy-infant-formula foods, bovine growth hormones commonly added to milk, hormones and antibiotics in flesh, non-fermented soy products such as soy milk and tofu (they mimic estrogens), bisphenol A and phthalates (found in many plastics such as baby containers, water bottles and the inner lining of soda cans), other man-made chemicals that affect hormonal balance (as found in cosmetics, toothpastes, shampoos and hair dyes), stress at home and at school, excessive TV viewing and media use, and more.

Electric Light and Cancer

As explained in chapter 5, there is a strong link between the hormone melatonin and cancer. Melatonin protects genetic material from mutation, according to Russell Reiter, professor of cellular and structural biology at the University of Texas. "Night light suppresses the body's production of melatonin and thus can increase the risk of cancer-related mutations," he told a gathering in London. Scott Davis, chairman of the department of epidemiology at the University of Washington, stated that "while the link between light at night and cancer may seem like a stretch on the surface, there is an underlying biological basis for it." Both Davis and Stevens have been studying how night lighting affects the production of female hormones, which, in turn, can affect the risk of breast cancer. "We have found a relationship between light at night and night-shift work to breast cancer risk," Davis said. "The studies indicate that night work disrupts the activity of melatonin, which leads to excessive production of hormones in women."

The message here is to get about 8 hours of regular sleep, starting before 10 p.m. (without any artificial lighting around you). In addition, get regular exposure of sunlight (without the use of sunglasses and sun lotions). Both constitute some of the most effective ways to treat and prevent cancer.

Exercise and Cancer

There have been controversial opinions about whether exercise is either beneficial or harmful for cancer patients. New research clears up any such doubts and points to the benefits of exercise as a means of fighting cancer, according to a new report issued by Johns Hopkins University. As far as cancer patients undergoing chemotherapy are concerned, exercise is one of the best ways to combat treatment-related fatigue. "It's not recommended that you begin an intense, new exercise regimen while undergoing chemotherapy, but if you exercised before your cancer diagnosis, try and maintain some level of activity," says Deborah Armstrong, M.D., Associate Professor of Oncology, Gynecology, and Obstetrics at Johns Hopkins, "If you haven't been exercising, try low-level exercise, such as walking or swimming."

The benefits of exercise are not limited to helping treatment-related fatigue, but they are actively contributing to curing cancer. Several groundbreaking studies attest to that. This hardly comes at a surprise since cancer cells are typically oxygen-deprived, and exercise is a direct way to deliver extra oxygen to cells throughout the body and to improve the immune response. Researchers also believe that exercise can regulate production of certain hormones that, unregulated, may spur tumor growth.

Exercise should not be strenuous, however. Exercising for half an hour each day or several hours a week is all that is needed to significantly increase cell-oxygenation (also refer to chapter 6 for proper guidance).

In one study, published in the *Journal of the American Medical Association*, researchers followed 2,987 women with breast cancer. Women who, for example, walked more than one hour a week after their cancer diagnosis were less likely to die of their breast cancer. In another study of 573 women with colon cancer, women who followed a moderate exercise program for more than six hours a week after their colon cancer diagnosis were 61% less likely to die of cancer-specific causes than women who exercised less than one hour a week. In all cases, exercise was found to be protective regardless of the patient's age, stage of cancer, or weight. A third study, published in the *Journal of Clinical Oncology*, confirmed the above findings after examining the effects of exercise on 832 men and women with stage III colon cancer.

The Truth about Conventional Cancer Treatments

If you still consider chemotherapy to be an option for treatment, be aware that you may develop far more serious illnesses than cancer (which can be naturally cured by removing its root causes). The following are common side effects:

This is what leading oncologists, university professors and MDs said about the effectiveness of modern cancer treatments:

⇒ Chemotherapy and radiation can increase the risk of developing a second cancer by up to 100 times, according to Dr. Samuel S. Epstein. ~ Congressional Record, Sept. 9, 1987.

⇒ If I contracted cancer, I would never go to a standard cancer treatment center. Cancer victims who live far from such centers have a chance. ~ Professor Georges Mathé, French cancer specialist.

⇒ ...As a chemist trained to interpret data, it is incomprehensible to me that physicians can ignore the clear evidence that chemotherapy does much, much more harm than good. ~ Alan C Nixon, Ph.D., former president of the American Chemical Society.

⇒ Most cancer patients in this country die of chemotherapy. Chemotherapy does not eliminate breast, colon, or lung cancers. This fact has been documented for over a decade, yet doctors still use chemotherapy for these tumors. ~ Allen Levin, M.D., UCSF The Healing of Cancer.

⇒ Cancer researchers, medical journals, and the popular media all have contributed to a situation in which many people with common malignancies are being treated with drugs not known to be effective. ~ Dr. Martin Shapiro, UCLA.

⇒ Except for two forms of cancer, chemotherapy does not cure. It tortures and may shorten life. ~ Dr. Candace Pert, Georgetown University School of Medicine.

⇒ Chemotherapy is basically ineffective in the vast majority of cases in which it is given. ~ Ralph Moss, Ph.D., former Director of Information for Sloan Kettering Cancer Research Center.

⇒ Many medical oncologists recommend chemotherapy for virtually any tumor, with a hopefulness undiscouraged by almost invariable failure. ~ Albert Braverman M.D. 1991 Lancet 1991 337 p 901 'Medical Oncology in the 90s'

⇒ There is no scientific evidence for its ability to extend in any appreciable way the lives of patients suffering from the most common organic cancer...chemotherapy for malignancies too advanced for surgery which accounts for 80% of all cancers is a scientific wasteland. ~ Professor Dr Ulrich Abel, University of Heidelberg, Germany.

⇒ More than 75 percent of oncologists said if they had cancer they would not participate in chemotherapy trials due to its ineffectiveness and its unacceptable toxicity. ~ Dr. Ulrich Abel, University of Heidelberg, Germany.

⇒ The percentage of people with cancer in the U.S. who receive chemotherapy is 75% ~ Oncologist John Robbins M.D.

⇒ The percentage of cancer patients whose lives are predictably saved by chemotherapy is 3%. To this day, there is no conclusive evidence (majority of cancers) that chemotherapy has any positive influence on survival or quality of life. Chemotherapy and radiation do not make the body well. They destroy, they do not heal. The hope of the doctor is that the cancer will be destroyed without destroying the entire patient. These therapies do kill cancer cells, but they kill a lot of good cells too including the cells of the immune system, the very system that one NEEDS to get well. If a cancer patient survives the treatment with enough immune system left intact, the patient may appear to get well at least temporarily, but he will have sustained major damage to his body and his immune system. How much better it is to nourish the immune system directly by the use of natural therapies to assist it in getting you well instead of destroying it by the use of these therapies. Then the immune system itself can kill the cancer cells without any side effects and heal your body at the same time. ~ Dr. Lorraine Day, M.D., University of California; Associate Professor San Francisco School of Medicine, and Vice Chairman of the Department of Orthopedic Surgery.

Any claims that surgery, radiotherapy and chemotherapy are effective are invalid for most types of cancer. Patients who don't receive any medical treatment at all still do better and have significantly higher survival rates than those who do. Yet, dozens of cancer trials, including some randomized ones, claim that these therapies are effective and save lives. In October 2007, the mass media spread the news that for the first time mortality rates for breast cancer and some other cancers had dropped by a few percent, indicating that real progress is being made in the fight against cancer. However, as explained below, survival figures are unreliable and misleading as a measure of the efficacy of conventional treatments for cancer.

The media cited early detection to be a major cause for the lower mortality rates. In a sense, they are actually right about this, but for the wrong reasons. Early detection has not been shown to change overall mortality rates from cancer. Earlier diagnosis following screening merely starts the survival clock earlier. In other words, a patient can still die at the same time but appear to have lived longer.

For example, two women at age 45 develop the same type of breast cancer. The tumor size is exactly the same - small and just about detectable. One of the two women (woman A) is diagnosed with and treated for her early-stage breast cancer. The other woman (woman B) is not aware of her cancer for another 3 years because she missed her routine exams. Her cancer has grown to a stage IV tumor. It can easily take 3 years for a cancer to grow from a stage I to a stage IV. Both women die at age 51. The question arises, who lived longer? According to what the cancer industry would want us believe, woman A lived three years longer than woman B; but of course this is not true, it just appears that way. That's where the deception comes into play.

Although cancer does not begin with its diagnosis, this is the way mortality rates are calculated. Since woman A lived for a full 6 years after her initial diagnosis, she would be considered a breast cancer survivor because she lived beyond the 5-year survival benchmark. She is being added to the 'success' list. It doesn't matter that she died a year later. Woman B, on the other hand, is being added to the 'mortality' list because she died 3 years after her cancer diagnosis. The net result of this number game is that, with early detection of cancers, mortality rates seem to go down, although the exact opposite is true. More and more people develop cancer each day, and this trend remains unchanged.

The cancer industry uses early detection methods as a way to 'extend' the number of years of cancer survival after treatment to beyond the crucial 5-year benchmark and thereby 'lower' mortality rates and 'increase' the number of survivors. As a result, orthodox cancer therapy is now being heralded as bringing about the medical 'breakthrough' we all have been waiting for. It is the hope of this industry to that the recent media blitz and sponsored cancer awareness campaigns will encourage more people to opt for the now successful medical treatments instead of seeking any of the alternative, less costly, treatment options (which have become a big threat to the medical industry). Almost everyone in the U.S. now knows someone who either had cancer and died or greatly suffered as a result of undergoing the conventional treatments of chemotherapy, radiation and surgery. Relatively few survive these treatments, not because of them but in spite of them. Still, the cancer business keeps growing bigger, while it continues to be the main obstacle for finding the real cure for cancer.

The masses are being brainwashed with the idea that a cancerous tumor is the real killer and must be destroyed at any cost, and as early as possible. Proving to the masses that the currently propagated approach of early cancer detection is working and has already shown to lower mortality rates is good enough a reason for many people to pursue the radical orthodox approaches. However, cancer is not a localized disorder that is unrelated to the rest of the body. Cancer is a 'systemic disorder' - one that affects a number of organs and tissues, or the body as a whole. Removing the symptom of cancer, such as a tumor, does not remove the underlying causes of cancer, regardless whether the tumor is removed at an early or late stage. As explained before, the tumor is not the problem; it is actually part for the solution. Early cancer detection and treatment almost never prevent a recurrence unless, of course, the patient also removes the causes of the cancer. With most cancers, the highly suppressive and destructive cancer treatments eventually lead to a far more aggressive and fast-spreading cancer (survival response) than the original one. The time 'gained' at the beginning will be lost at the end.

All current orthodox cancer treatments damage or destroy the immune system which causes inflammation and makes the body susceptible to other illnesses. If a man had a cancerous tumor removed from his colon and gone through several rounds of chemotherapy but died 4 weeks later from a staph-infection, the death certificate would state he died from an infection, not from cancer. Death resulting from the treatment of cancer occurs far more frequently than death through cancer. Cancer patients dying from something else than cancer lowers the number of cancer mortality further, which only benefits the cancer industry.

To heal cancer, we must let go of the idea that cancer is a disease and out to kill us. We also must learn to identify and remove the causes that force the body to take to recourse to such drastic survival mechanisms as cancer. To cure oneself of cancer is neither expensive nor difficult, but it requires that you trust, love and respect your body and yourself. The body is always ready and eager to heal itself, but it is in your hands to set the preconditions for the healing to occur.

Chapter 11

3 Secret Sources of Diabetes -
How to Quickly Heal From Them

At one time in our recent history, many of today's chronic diseases were understood to be symptoms of diabetes. Strokes, both ischemic and hemorrhagic, heart failure due to neuropathy, ischemic and hemorrhagic coronary events, obesity, arteriosclerosis, elevated blood pressure, high blood levels of cholesterol and triglycerides were all known to be common consequences of a disturbed metabolism as it occurs in diabetes. In addition to these symptoms, impotence, retinopathy, renal failure, liver failure, polycystic ovary syndrome, elevated blood sugar, systemic candida, poor wound healing, peripheral neuropathy etc. have since been turned into separate diseases, requiring specialized treatments and specialists to administer them. Although this may greatly serve the medical and pharmaceutical industries, it causes untold suffering and costs many lives.

Diabetes afflicts over 8 percent of the American population. Many of them have the belief that diabetes is inherited and the body is a victim of a genetic flaw. Although genetic reasons can play a certain role in the manifestation of diabetes, in most cases they don't, and they certainly don't explain why pancreatic cells one day suddenly decide to self-destruct (), or why common cells in people of age 50 or older suddenly decide to block out insulin-laden sugar (Type 2 diabetes).

Many patients and their doctors assume that diseases manifest when the body somehow makes a mistake and thus fails to do its job properly. This idea defies all sense of logic, and scientifically, it is incorrect. In this world every *effect* must have an underlying *cause*. Just because doctors are not aware of what causes certain pancreatic cells to stop producing insulin doesn't automatically imply that diabetes is an autoimmune disease - a condition where the body presumably tries to attack and destroy itself. By developing diabetes, the body is neither doing something wrong nor is it out to kill itself. It certainly finds no pleasure in making you suffer and feel miserable.

Instead of doubting the body's wisdom and intelligence, we need to understand the circumstances that cause the body to shut down its insulin-producing capability in , and increase it in Type 2 diabetes. With its vast resourcefulness of devising incredibly sophisticated survival mechanisms, the body makes every effort to protect you from further harm than has already been caused through inadequate nourishment, emotional pain, and/or a detrimental lifestyle. When seen in this light, disease becomes an integral part of the body's incessant effort to *prevent* the person from committing unintentional suicide. It can be firmly stated that your body is always on your side, never against you, even if it *appears* to attack itself (as in autoimmune disorders, such as , lupus, cancer, and rheumatoid arthritis).

Just as there is a mechanism to become diabetic, there is also one to reverse it. To call diabetes, regardless whether it is Type 1 or Type 2, an irreversible disease reflects a profound lack of understanding the true nature of the human body. Once the preconditions for restoring balance or homeostasis have been met, the body will be able to use its full repair and healing abilities.

Almost all of us know how to heal a wound or mend a broken bone. Some of us may 'lose' this ability when the immune system becomes impaired, when prescription drugs interfere with blood clotting mechanisms, or when the body becomes severely congested with toxic waste. In the case of , pancreatic cells don't just stop producing insulin because they are tired of doing their job. And in the case of Type 2 diabetes, the body's 60 trillion cells don't just reject insulin because they have developed a dislike to it. In both situations, the cells are prevented from doing their job for a number of reasons, all of which are basically under our control. If we stop destroying the cells directly or indirectly by the way we eat and live, they can just as easily be reprogrammed, nursed back to life or be replaced by new ones.

Healing the pancreas is not so much different than healing a broken bone. However, for healing to occur we must make certain changes that facilitate the healing, not counteract it. Treating diabetes on the symptom level is difficult and actually prevents its cure. On the other hand, it is not difficult to determine what causes the insulin-secreting pancreatic cells to malfunction in , and then to remove those causes. To perform properly, these specialized cells require adequate nourishment. Insulin is an all-important hormone that all of us need to take essential nutrients (proteins, sugar, fats), especially glucose, into the cells of the body. If there is not enough insulin available to deliver these nutrients to the cells, sugar in particular becomes trapped in the blood, causing it to rise to dangerously high levels.

In the case of insulin-dependent diabetes (which can apply to both types), it appears to make sense to inject insulin into the blood in order to remove the excessive sugar, fat and protein molecules from the bloodstream. However, without investigating and rectifying what has put the body into this awkward position in the first place, merely administering insulin shots to the patient to enforce a lower blood sugar does not only not solve the problem, but, as we will see, makes it worse. This quick-fix approach actually makes a true cure impossible and, at the same time, increases the risk of developing many other ailments.

It is now known to be a fact (again) that diabetics suffering from either type have an increased risk of heart disease, cancer, stroke, blindness and Alzheimer's disease, etc. Elevated levels of insulin can cause inflammation in the brain that may increase the risk of Alzheimer's disease (AD). This finding was reported in the Archive Of Neurology (Volume 62, page 1539).

More evidence has been uncovered that Alzheimer's disease may actually be a third form of diabetes, according to researchers from Northwestern University (Chicaco). Insulin and insulin receptors in your brain are crucial for learning and memory. For this reason, the brain makes its own insulin. In 2005, it was discovered that both insulin and insulin receptors are lower in people with Alzheimer's disease. In the brain, insulin binds to an insulin receptor at a synapse, which triggers a mechanism that allows nerve cells to survive and memories to form. The new research from Northwestern University discovered a toxic protein in the brain of Alzheimer's patients - called ADDL for 'amyloid ß-derived diffusible ligand' - that removes insulin receptors from nerve cells and renders those neurons insulin resistant. As a result, the neurons can no longer take up enough glucose and, thus, degenerate and block memory function. In 2004 researchers revealed that diabetics may have a 65 percent higher risk of developing Alzheimer's disease.

The question arises whether the higher risk of Alzheimer's disease, heart disease, stroke, cancer, blindness, etc. is really due to the diabetes itself or its treatments. I propose that diabetes has become such a dangerous ailment because it is treated on the symptom level rather than on the causal level. If a non-insulin dependant Type 2 diabetic gets an insulin shot, it can seriously harm or even kill him. And as surprising as it may be, a healthy person who receives insulin shots develops diabetes, which is not so uncommon, given the high percentage of false positive blood tests nowadays. 'Once a diabetic, always a diabetic' is a sad consequence of medical intervention. But it doesn't have to be this way.

For example, scientists at a Toronto hospital recently made a stunning discovery which could lead to a near-cure of . The researchers injected diabetic mice with capsaicin, the active ingredient in red pepper, which counteracted the effect of malfunctioning pain neurons in the pancreas. The mice became healthy practically overnight. Conventional wisdom stipulates that   is caused solely by the body's immune system attacking the pancreas. The new research, however, shows that this is not true. Apparently, our nerves secrete certain neuropeptides that are crucial to the proper functioning of the pancreas. Restoring proper nerve function through simple methods such as the above may be all that it takes to end . Capsaicin has already proven its healing properties in the treatment of joint pain and other inflammatory conditions. This shows that a cure doesn't have to be complicated and expensive.

With regard to Type 2 diabetes, there is ample evidence that it can be cured with natural methods and by avoiding foods that cause cells to resist the uptake of insulin.

Foods That Cause Diabetes

Refined Carbohydrates - A Cause of Insulin Resistance

One of the most common directions given to Type 2 diabetics is to reduce or even cut out their intake of carbohydrates. They are being told that the sugars they contain may raise their blood sugar to abnormal levels and endanger their lives. While there is basic truth to this statement, as we will see in the following section, it is also a highly misleading one. Let us first understand the true part of this statement.

It is certainly correct to say that refined, manufactured carbohydrates can seriously affect anyone's health, not just the health of diabetics. As a result of the normal digestion of plant foods, the body converts complex carbohydrates into complex sugars (glycogen), which it stores in the liver and muscles. Whenever required, the body converts glycogen into glucose for generation of cellular energy. On the other hand, if you eat refined carbohydrate foods (crisps, potato chips, cakes, candy, ice cream, pasta, white bread, soft drinks, etc.), you actually bypass this process and the sugars or starches (starch is sugar) enter the bloodstream within a matter of minutes. The more of these simple carbohydrates you consume, the higher your blood sugar rises. To keep the constantly rising blood sugar in check, your pancreas has to pump extra amounts of insulin into the blood. Insulin takes sugar out of the bloodstream and transports it to the cells. On the surface of the cells are insulin receptors which act like tiny doors that open and close to regulate the inflow of blood sugar.

There is a major difference between the highly valuable glucose the body makes available to the cells and the useless sugar forced into the bloodstream right after drinking a coke or eating a cone of ice cream. The cells don't like to absorb the acidic, bleached, processed, and energy-stripped sugar (empty calories) because they cannot make any use of it. To protect themselves against this cell poison, they put up a barrier that ignores the insulin when it knocks at their door, even as it tries to deliver proper, usable, quality glucose. As a result the sugar has no other choice than remain in the blood. The resulting buildup of blood sugar prompts even more insulin secretions by the pancreas, which in turn causes more and more cellular doors to close and blood sugar to rise further. This condition is known as 'insulin resistance'. When insulin production no longer keeps up with rising blood sugar, Type 2 diabetes results. This makes Type 2 diabetes a severe case of insulin resistance. Insulin resistance can lead to many complications in the body, including:

- Heart disease
- Hardening of the arteries
- Damage to artery walls

- Increased cholesterol levels
- Vitamin & mineral deficiencies
- Kidney disease
- Fat-burning mechanism turned off
- Accumulation & storage of fat
- Weight gain

Now, according to a report in the journal *Diabetes Care* (Volume 29, page 775), the kind of cereal you eat can help decrease your resistance to insulin. The more sensitive your body is to insulin, the more efficiently your cells take up glucose from the bloodstream, which is desirable for anyone with Type 2 diabetes. Earlier research showed that people who consume diets high in soluble and insoluble fiber have lower rates of Type 2 diabetes. To find out how insoluble fiber lowers diabetes risk, a team of German researchers designed a special bread that contained 10 g of insoluble fiber per slice. The researchers asked a group of 17 overweight and obese women to eat three slices of the bread daily, which placed their fiber intake well within the recommended 20–35 g per day. After only three days of eating the bread, the women's insulin sensitivity improved by 8 percent. You can naturally increase your insoluble and soluble fiber intake by eating mostly natural, unprocessed foods, such as fruit, vegetables, grains and legumes, nuts and seeds. Simple as this sounds, food is still the best medicine of all.

Animal Proteins - More Harmful Than Sugar

Without a question, foods that are nutritionally empty lead to malnutrition, eating disorders, and obesity. To avoid sudden, harmful blood sugar spikes, not even healthy individuals should eat refined sugar or starch-packed foods. Having a regular craving for sweets and starchy foods indicates there is a serious disturbance of cell metabolism. But sugar is actually not such a big concern when you compare its effects with those caused by eating animal proteins. Diabetes patients are almost never told that the amount of insulin the body needs to process, for example, one regular piece of steak equals the amount of insulin required for about 1/2 pound of white sugar. The reason no doctor is telling you about this is because eating the steak does not substantially raise your blood sugar levels, so it appears that meat is a safe food, especially for diabetics. And so the 'disease' can progress and worsen quietly and unnoticeably.

The insulin resistance in Type 2 diabetics describes the condition in which the pancreas is capable of producing insulin, but the cells are insensitive to it. Insulin acts as the 'key' that unlocks the 'gate' through which glucose and other nutrients must pass to enter cells. When there are too few 'gates' open, or the 'locks' on the gates are 'rusted shut' and difficult to open despite the presence of this hormone, insulin resistance results. Cells may actually become damaged and turn cancerous if insulin comes into contact with them too often and in too large amounts. Regular protein meals make the cells increasingly resistant to insulin, and, without at first raising blood sugar levels, eventually lead to Type 2 diabetes. Frequent snacks that contain sugars and refined fats also play a major role, but as already explained, to a much lesser extent.[38] Refined fats, though, play a major role in , as we will see in section 3.

---

[38] Apart from those conditions discussed here, there are other conditions which may predispose the body to the development of insulin-resistant diabetes or which may unmask a mild, sub-clinical, or transient diabetes that already exists. These include pregnancy, overproduction or overadministration of steroids like cortisone or prednisone, overproduction of growth hormone (acromegaly), infections, and prolonged or severe stress.

Even in a healthy body, pancreatic cells are unable to produce such large amounts of insulin required to deal with regularly consumed animal protein. Part of the unused protein is broken down by the liver, although this ability is greatly diminished in diabetics. The rest of the proteins circulate in the blood until they are taken into the intercellular fluids. But since the diabetic's cell membranes increasingly prevent insulin from entering the cells, sugar, proteins and fatty acids are also rejected. Whereas some of the excessive sugar can be converted into fats and fats can accumulate in the tissues, the protein must be removed from the intercellular tissue or connective tissue through different means. The process used by the body is the same one I have discussed in the last two chapters. The body converts the excessive proteins into collagen fiber which in turn is being built into the basal membranes of the blood capillary walls. This disappearance act of the protein makes it appear that protein poses no problem for the diabetic.

Sugar, on the other hand, doesn't have such a seemingly untraceable escape route. Once the intercellular fluid is saturated with the unutilized sugar, it naturally rises in the bloodstream. With continued protein consumption, the basal membranes accumulate so much protein fiber that simple sugars can no longer pass through them, even if the cells were to give up their insulin resistance and let the sugar pass through their membranes again.

Since the protein-diabetes connection is so important to understand, I will reiterate here what I already explained in chapter 6. If you eat concentrated protein foods such as meat or chicken, your body requires much insulin to synthesize proteins from the amino acids derived from these foods. According to research, the stimulation of protein synthesis is a classic action of insulin. Loss of the stimulatory effect of insulin on protein synthesis would reduce growth and result in weight loss, which are hallmarks of . To make certain that the amino acids derived from the protein meal are synthesized into proteins, the pancreas has to secrete insulin. In other words, the more protein you eat, the more insulin your body needs to make, thus increasing the chances of insulin resistance and Type 2 diabetes.

Accordingly, eating a normal-sized steak forces your pancreas to secrete more insulin than it would need to produce in response to eating 12 times the amount of sugar contained in one can of soda. In addition to that, if you also eat potatoes, a sweet desert, and drink a soda along with your meal, like most Americans do, you can expect to further increase insulin resistance. Currently, diabetes is the fastest growing epidemic in America, and it is easy to see why. (More on diabetes in Chapter 11)

The effect of insulin on protein metabolism is complex, and it involves changes in both the synthesis and degradation of protein. If protein intake is excessive, insulin secretions increase to help with its degradation. Protein synthesis and the control of carbohydrate and fat metabolism have now been linked in unexpected ways, and many of the same signaling systems utilized by insulin to control glucose metabolism, for example, have been found to be involved in the control of protein synthesis as well. The bottom line is that excessive intake of protein is a direct cause of insulin resistance and may lead to the onset of Type 2 diabetes.

Thus, overeating protein foods makes Type 2 diabetes a permanent condition, a chronic illness. But the progression of this illness doesn't stop there.

Refined Fats and Oils - Delicious Poison?

In the 1930s, physicians considered many of our degenerative diseases to be due to a failure of our endocrine system known as *insulin resistant diabetes*. The severe derangement of the body's blood sugar control system was understood to be the basic underlying disorder that could manifest itself as nearly any kind of illness. Although there are other reasons for bringing about such a profound imbalance, as discussed before, badly engineered fats and oils are among the biggest culprits. Although these fats and oils may be delicious to the taste buds, they act like poison in the body. Their destructive effects lead to severe nutritional deficiencies that prevent the body from maintaining normal cell metabolism.

In recent years, there has been a lot of publicity about good fats and bad fats. Although some food companies now claim to avoid bad fats, there are still thousands of common foods that contain them. The fats and oils industry still wants you to believe that the saturated fats are the bad ones, and the unsaturated fats are the good ones. This is false information. There are many highly beneficial saturated fats, and just as many unhealthy unsaturated fats. The only distinction that should be made when judging the value of fats is whether they are left in their natural form or are engineered. You cannot trust advertisements by the fats and oils industry that praise the amazing benefits of their unique flavorful spreads or low cholesterol cooking fats. Their smart ad campaigns have no interest in promoting your health; they are solely intended to create a market for cheap junk oils such as soy, cottonseed and rapeseed oil.

Until the early 1930s, manufactured food products were very unpopular and mostly rejected by the population because of their suspicion of them being of poor quality and not being fresh enough to be safe for consumption. The use of automated factory machinery to mass produce foods for immense potential profits was at first bitterly opposed by local farmers. But eventually, this resistance broke and gave way to an increasing interest in the 'new' foods that no one had ever seen before. When margarine and other refined and hydrogenated products were introduced into the U.S. food markets, the dairy industry was vehemently opposed to it, but the women found it to be more practical than the lard they had been using. Due to the shortage of dairy products during WW II, margarine became a common food among the civilian population, and the commonly used coconut oils, flax oils and fish oils disappeared from the shelves of America's grocery stores.

The campaign by the emerging food industry against natural oils and genuinely beneficial fats such as the very popular coconut oil became fueled by a massive media disinformation that blamed saturated fats for the wave of heart attacks that suddenly started to grip a large portion of the American population. For 30 or more years, coconut oil was nowhere to be found in grocery stores and has only recently re-emerged in health food stores. Coconut oil and other healthful oils were practically replaced by cheap junk oils, including soy oil, cottonseed oil and rapeseed oil. The coconut oil's powerful weight controlling effects helped prevent an obesity epidemic among the general population. Since eliminating it from the American diet, obesity has become the leading cause of illness in this country and the rest of the world.

If you are suffering from either type diabetes and wish to permanently restore your body's natural sugar-regulating mechanisms, for a certain period of time you will need to strictly avoid all artificially produced fats and oils, including those that are found in processed foods, restaurant foods, fast foods and are sold as 'healthy' foods in grocery stores. One of the more harmful oils is the genetically engineered canola oil made from rapeseeds. Rapeseeds are not suitable for human consumption. Produced in Canada (hence the name canola) this renamed, refined rapeseed oil found a huge and instant market in the U.S. during the height of the cholesterol mania (still going on). It is cheap and, therefore, widely used in restaurants and by people on a low food budget. The reason for its huge popularity is that it contains very little cholesterol. One of the main problems with this oil is that it should not be heated; yet heating it is a standard practice in the production process, and in restaurants and households. According to a January 26, 1998 Omega Nutrition press release: "heating distorts the omega-3 essential fatty acid found in canola, turning it into an unnatural trans form that raises total cholesterol levels and lowers HDL [good] cholesterol."

Japanese researchers found that the life spans of rats fed diets rich in canola oil were 40 percent shorter. Experimental rats that were fed canola oil 'developed fatty degeneration of the heart, kidney, adrenals, and thyroid gland'. Canadian federal scientists have spent several years and a lot of money to alleviate fears linking canola consumption to hypertension and stroke. The Health Ministry in Canada insists that although their tests match the Japanese data, canola poses no risks to humans. Yet canola oil consumption has been correlated with development of fibrotic lesions of the heart, lung cancer, prostate cancer, anemia and constipation. The long-chain fatty acids found in canola have been found to destroy the *sphingomyelin* surrounding nerve cells in the brain. Other illnesses and conditions that have been associated with canola oil consumption include loss of vision and a wide range of neurological disorders.

How can this government be so reassuring when Canola oil has been around for a short number of years and long-term effects may not develop before 3-5 years? Is it not also strange that the FDA allowed the canola industry to avoid the lengthy and expensive approval process, including medical research on humans? Given the alarming reactions that rats have to canola oil, could it at least be possible that a certain percentage of heart attack and stroke victims are actually due to regular canola oil consumption? Since canola oil is contained in the majority of manufactured foods, baked goods, frozen foods, and restaurant foods, is it any wonder why people are falling ill everywhere, at a rate that is absolutely stunning and unprecedented?

So what do refined and manufactured oils and fats actually do to the body? For one thing, they can cause severe gastrointestinal disturbances. The number of people in the U.S. suffering from acid reflux disease, irritable bowel syndrome, Crohn's disease, constipation, colon cancer, etc., exceeds the number of all other diseases taken together. Deep fried foods and other fast foods have become the popular choice of young people, aged 3-30. An ever-increasing number of them develop diabetes. Rape (Canola) oil also causes emphysema, respiratory distress, anemia, irritability, brain cancer and blindness.

The high temperatures used in canola refining and margarine production will damage many of the essential fatty acids, which are much more susceptible to damage by heat than saturated fats. As discussed earlier, heat is known to convert many of the unsaturated double bonds to the 'trans fatty acid' configuration. Although high-quality essential fatty acids as contained in some of these engineered foods are required for human health, in their damaged or rancid forms they become harmful. In fact, they may trigger powerful immune responses that may lead to autoimmune diseases such as Type 1 diabetes.

In order for cells to be healthy and functional, their plasma cell membrane, now known to be an active player in the glucose scenario, needs to contain a complement of *cis type w=3* unsaturated fatty acids. This makes the cell membranes slippery and fluid, thereby permitting glucose molecules to be able to pass through them and enter the cell interior for energy generation. This maintains balanced blood sugar levels. By regularly eating fats and oils that are heat-treated (in contrast with natural expeller-pressed oils and untreated fats) the cell membranes begin to lose their healthy fatty acids and replace them with harmful trans-fatty acids and short- and medium-chain saturated fatty acids. As a result, the cell membranes become thicker, stiffer, sticky, and inhibit the glucose transport mechanism, resulting in blood sugar rising.

The rest of the body suffers serious consequences of the clogging up of the cell membranes. To deal with the high blood sugar, the pancreas starts pumping out extra insulin, which can lead to inflammation throughout the body. The liver tries to convert some of the excess sugar into fat, stored by adipose cells. This can make the body fat. To get rid of the rest of the sugar in the blood, the urinary system goes into overdrive. Eventually, the body enters a condition of chronic exhaustion due to the lack of cellular energy. The adrenals respond by pumping extra amounts of stress hormones into the blood, creating mood swings, anxiety and depression. The endocrine glands malfunction. Overtaxed by the constant demand for extra insulin, the pancreas fails to produce enough. Body weight may increase a little more each day. The heart and lungs become congested and fail to deliver vital oxygen to all the cells in the body, including the brain. Each organ and system in the body is affected by this simple dietary mistake. All this and more is what we know to be diabetes, an acquired illness that can easily be avoided and even reversed by eating a natural diet consisting of natural, fresh foods that nature so generously provides for us. The idea that we can create better foods than nature is a fallacy that has turned into a weapon of mass destruction.

The Unfolding Drama of the Diabetes Syndrome

When sugar becomes trapped and begins to increase in the bloodstream, eating sugar at this point can be life-threatening. Not having enough glucose reaching the cells and organs of the body can also be fatal. If the heart cells run out of glucose, heart failure occurs. If the kidney cells run out of glucose, kidney failure occurs. If the eyes don't get their glucose, eyesight will fail. If the brain cells don't get enough glucose, Alzheimer's disease may result. The same fate of malfunctioning befalls a sugar-starved liver, pancreas, stomach, as well as fuel-deprived muscle and bone cells. By not receiving enough glucose, the body begins to crave food, especially sugars, sweets, starchy foods, sweet beverages, etc., which leads to overeating and further congestion, and possibly heart failure and cancer (see previous chapters).

Because Type 2 diabetes affects the health of each of the 60 trillion cells in the body, diabetics are predisposed to developing virtually every type of disorder there is. This has been denied by medical science for many years, but has recently been verified through major medical research. The majority of the chronic disorders plaguing our modern world today, including heart disease, cancer, arthritis, MS, Alzheimer's disease, Parkinson's, etc. may in actual fact not be separate diseases at all. We already know that Alzheimer's disease is the third form of diabetes 'Type 3 diabetes'. While sharing the same cause or causes, they manifest themselves in different parts of the body as unique symptoms of disease. There will come a time when the practicing physician will recognize that diabetes, cancer, heart disease, and dementia, for example, share the same underlying causes, and therefore require the same treatment.

At the beginning stages of Type 2 diabetes, the pancreas tries to respond to the increasing congestion of the blood vessel walls (with excessive proteins) and, possibly, to an excessive sugar or starch consumption, by secreting extra large amounts of insulin. By constantly producing disproportionate amounts of insulin, the cells become even further resistant to insulin. By blocking out insulin (along with vital nutrients) the cells attempt to protect themselves against the cell-damaging effects of too much insulin, or else they would have to face cell mutation. (Too much insulin in the body can cause cancer.) Eventually, though, through intricate hormonal feedback mechanisms and enzyme signals, the pancreas recognizes both the increase in blood sugar levels and the shortage of cellular sugar, proteins and fatty acids. So the pancreas begins to deactivate, destroy or 'put to sleep' a large number of its insulin-producing cells (pancreatic islets). This sets the stage for a non-insulin dependent diabetes to become an insulin-dependent diabetes.

There are a number of other reasons that may lead to reduced insulin secretions by the pancreas. When the basal membranes of blood capillaries supplying the pancreas with nutrients become congested with protein fiber, insulin production and other important functions, such as the production of digestive enzymes, become suppressed. The same occurs when stones in the bile ducts of the liver and gallbladder drastically reduce bile secretion. In an increasing number of individuals, bile sludge consisting of small cholesterol stones enters the common bile duct and gets caught up in the *Ampulla of Vater* (where the common bile duct and pancreatic duct meet and combine). Bile activates pancreatic enzymes before they enter the small intestine to aid in the digestion of foods. If bile flow is restricted, not all of the enzymes dispatched by the pancreas are activated. Any of these unused enzymes remaining in the pancreas can damage or destroy pancreatic cells, which leads to pancreatitis - a common cause of diabetes and pancreatic cancer. In any case, the inability of the pancreas to produce enough insulin can be a lifesaver, at least temporarily. The body often sacrifices one part to save another more vital part.

It is obvious, though, that this act of cancer-preventive self-preservation also means that there is not enough insulin around to transport the sugar out of the bloodstream. When Type 2 diabetics become insulin-deficient, doctors often prescribe insulin in addition to blood sugar medication, while letting them continue eating protein foods. Thus, a previously non-insulin-dependent diabetic now needs insulin shots, which greatly increases his health risks. This is completely unnecessary. I have had such insulin-dependent patients turn vegan, and within just six weeks become free of the main signs and symptoms of diabetes, for the first time in 20-30 years.

Chronic disease is only chronic for as long as its causes are intact. Insulin injection is the very thing that keeps the patient from recovering. It continues to increase the cells' resistance to insulin, and forces the pancreas to destroy an ever-increasing number of insulin-producing cells. There are plenty of natural things that can replace injection with insulin. Just one teaspoon of ground cinnamon per day can balance blood sugar. Turmeric is an amazing herb/spice with a similar effect. Broccoli and other vegetables, as well as regular full body exposure to sunlight (vitamin D-generating),[39] have superior blood sugar-regulating effects than potentially dangerous insulin injections.

Abstaining from proteins foods, cleansing the liver of stones (gallstones are a leading cause of diabetes, see details in The Amazing Liver and Gallbladder Flush), eating a balanced diet and living a balanced lifestyle as advocated in this book, are many more effective in restoring normal body functions than just trying to fix one symptom of disease. If you are a diabetic, by taking responsibility for your own health, and therefore your life, you have the opportunity to put the 'sweetness' back into your cells and, thus, into their life.

The Risk of Being Overweight

Approximately 16 million people in the United States are diagnosed with diabetes, according to national statistics. In reality, through, this figure is much higher. It is estimated that an additional 5.4 million people have this disorder and are not aware of it. Type 2 diabetes, also called *adult onset diabetes*, now appears routinely in children as early as six years old. Minorities are at particular risk, since their diet consists mainly of cheap fast foods, such as hamburgers, fried chicken, pasta, potatoes, refined sweets and other highly processed foods and beverages.[40] These foods typically cause a rapid

---

[39] Researchers at the University of California-Los Angeles School of Medicine (UCLA) found that compared to subjects with the highest vitamin D levels, those with the lowest levels had symptoms of Type 2 diabetes, including weaker pancreatic function and greater insulin resistance. When the skin is exposed to ultraviolet light, the body responds by manufacturing vitamin D.

[40] Researchers at the Harvard School of Public Health examined nine years of dietary and medical data on more than 51,000 women who participated in the Nurses' Health Study II. From this group, well over 700 cases of Type 2 diabetes were diagnosed during the study period. The Harvard team concluded that the excess calories and high levels of rapidly absorbable sugars found in non-diet soft drinks promote weight gain and a greater risk of developing Type 2 diabetes. In fact, women who drink one or more soft drinks per day may have an 80 percent increased risk of Type 2 diabetes compared to women who avoid this type of beverage. One sports drink a day can lead to 13 pounds of weight gain each year, according to a report issues by the University of California in Berkeley.

increase in blood sugar, which stimulates the production of large quantities of insulin. When there is too much insulin in the blood, the body reacts by producing the chemical *somatostatin,* which suppresses insulin release. In due time this natural response translates into diabetes. Compared with Caucasians, African Americans have a 60 percent higher risk of developing diabetes and Hispanics have a 90 percent increased risk. Considering the large number of undiagnosed diabetics, physicians are now losing more patients to diabetes than they are diagnosing.

An increasing number of American adults diagnosed with diabetes are obese, U.S. officials said in November 2004. A study by the Centers for Disease Control (CDC) and Prevention found that between 1999 and 2002, 54.8 percent of diabetics over the age of 19 were obese. That compared with 45.7 percent in the same age group between 1988 and 1994. When the category was expanded to include diabetics who were obese or overweight, the percentage surged to 85.2 percent in 1999-2002 compared with 78.5 percent in the earlier period. About 69 million people are obese or severely obese, according to the American Obesity Association.

In the CDC study, a person was considered overweight if their *body mass index* - the most commonly used method for calculating if a person weighs too much - was 25 to 29. Anyone with a body mass index of 30 or greater was categorized as obese. Using the body mass index to determine risk for diabetes is not completely reliable and can keep these numbers lower than they actually are. Taking averages in human statistic analysis always ends up distorting the true figures. A balanced Vata type, for example has a naturally lower weight than average. According to the body mass index Vatas are considered underweight. Their bones are much lighter and they have very little body fat on them. If a Vata type adds 25 pounds of body weight, it can cause him serious health problems, but according to the body mass index this extra weight would bring him up to the normal range. Kapha types, on the other hand, have a very heavy body structure already. They cannot afford to add 25 pounds without causing them to develop a typical Kapha disorder, such as diabetes, heart disease or cancer.

By removing the discrepancies that exist with currently used body mass calculations, it is likely that almost every diabetic is overweight or obese. Likewise, a person who is overweight or obese can actually be considered diabetic, or at least insulin resistant to some degree. Due to the accumulation of abnormal amounts of new cells in the overweight person, there is simply not enough insulin available to meet all the nutrient demands of these extra cells. And although the pancreas may still make a normal or a little extra amount of insulin, the added weight leads to a relative insulin shortage. Eventually, the pancreas suffers from being continuously overextended and stressed. The side effects of a relative insulin-deficiency can be just the same as an absolute insulin-deficiency where pancreatic cells stop producing insulin altogether.

According to the American Diabetes Association, diabetes accounts for 178,000 deaths (which may not be accurate[41]), 54,000 amputees, and 12,000-24,000 cases of blindness annually. Blindness is 25 times more common among diabetic patients compared to non-diabetics. Diabetic retinopathy, which can lead to blindness, affects more than 4.1 million Americans age 40 and older. It is the most common eye complication of diabetes. A report released by Johns Hopkins University (19 October 2007) stated that almost all people with Type 1 diabetes and more than 70% with Type 2 diabetes eventually develop diabetic retinopathy. Diabetic retinopathy is characterized by damage to the retina. Other long-term diabetes complications include abnormalities of small and large blood vessels; neuropathy (nerve damage); damage of the skin, gums and teeth.

---

[41] 1 "Fast Stats" National Center for Health Statistics, Deaths/Mortality Preliminary 2001 data shows that in 2001, the most recent year for which U.S. figures are posted, 934,550 Americans died from out-of-control symptoms of this disease.

It is estimated that by the year 2010 diabetes will actually exceed both heart disease and cancer as the leading cause of death through its many complications. It is my hope that more and more scientists and doctors begin to see the strong link that exists between all these "diseases." They are metabolic disorders that share a common cause, but show up as different symptoms.

Autoimmune (Type 1) Diabetes

Type 1 diabetes affects nearly 700,000 people in the United States. It is the most common chronic metabolic disorder to affect children. Caucasian populations, especially Scandinavians, have the greatest risk, and people of Asian or African descent have the lowest risk of developing this form of diabetes. Type 1 diabetes is usually diagnosed in children or adults under 30. The difference of risk is less due to genetic factors than to dietary ones, as I shall explain later. Type 1 diabetes can develop unnoticed for years. But then symptoms usually develop quickly, over a few days to weeks, and are caused by blood sugar levels rising above the normal range (hyperglycemia). Early symptoms include frequent urination, especially noticeable at night; possible bed wetting among young children; extreme thirst and a dry mouth; weight loss and sometimes, excessive hunger.

Type 1 diabetes is defined by the absence of insulin due to the destruction of insulin-producing cells in the pancreas—also called beta cells. Type 1 diabetics are dependent on insulin injections to control their blood sugar levels. The most common time for developing diabetes is during puberty, although it can occur at any age.

In Type 2 diabetes, due to insulin resistance, the cells in the body are unable to obtain glucose that they need for energy. In Type 1 diabetes, the cells are also deprived of glucose, but in this case it is because insulin is not available. When cells are glucose deprived, the body breaks down fat for energy. This results in *ketones* or fatty acids entering the bloodstream, causing the chemical imbalance (metabolic acidosis) called *diabetic ketoacidosis*. If left untreated, very high blood sugar would lead to flushed, hot, dry skin; labored breathing, restlessness, confusion, difficulty waking up, coma, and even death.

There is an increasing body of scientific evidence to suggest that cow's milk during childhood increases the risk of developing Type 1 diabetes. In a study published in *Diabetes* (2000), the journal of the American Diabetes Association, researchers found that children who had a sibling with diabetes were more than fives times as likely to develop the disorder if they drank more than half a liter (about two 8-ounce glasses) of cow's milk a day, compared with children who drank less milk.

While it is not clear which component of cow's milk may increase the risk of diabetes, researchers suspect that one of several proteins may be to blame by causing the immune system to attack insulin-producing cells in the pancreas. Hormones in dairy products so closely mimic human hormones that many times an autoimmune response is mounted. This may result in arthritis, irritable bowel, Crohn's disease, lymph edema and lymphatic congestion, phlegm in the throat, fatigue, cancer and many other disorders.

Although many Type 1 diabetics are known to be genetically susceptible to the disease (genetic variation), others with the same genetic variation will never develop diabetes. This suggests that dietary factors play a decisive role in who will become afflicted with the actual disorder. In fact, research showed that babies who breastfeed at least three months have a lower incidence of Type 1 diabetes and may be less likely to become obese as adults. This further supports and validates other research that has linked early exposure to cow's milk and cow's milk-based formula to the development of Type 1 diabetes. Clinical studies have also shown that women who breastfeed reduce the risk of their children developing Type 2 diabetes.

Risky Orthodox Medical Treatments

After the diagnosis of diabetes, doctors routinely prescribe either oral hypoglycemic agents or insulin. The causes of diabetes are rarely addressed, if known at all. Currently available oral hypoglycemic agents include *Biguanides, Glucosidase inhibitors, Meglitinides, Sulfonylureas,* and *Thiazolidinediones.*

The Biguanides lower blood sugar by inhibiting the normal release, by the liver, of its glucose stores, thereby interfering with intestinal absorption of glucose from ingested carbohydrates, and increasing peripheral uptake of glucose. All this can deverely disrupt the functions of all the organs and systems in the body.

The glucosidase inhibitors are designed to prevent the amylase enzymes produced by the pancreas to digest carbohydrates. The theory behind this is that if there is no digestion of carbohydrates the blood sugar wouldn't rise. That is approach can lead to starvation of cells throughout the body is obvious.

The meglitinides and sulfonylureas are engineered to stimulate the pancreas to produce extra insulin in a patient whose blood insulin is already elevated. Since most doctors don't measure insulin levels, this frequently prescribed drug is causing a lot of harmful side effects, including hypoglycemia. An insulin surplus in the blood can seriously injure blood vessels and lead to similar defects as high blood sugar.

The thiazolidinediones are known for causing liver cancer. One of them, Rezulin, was designed to stimulate the uptake of glucose from the bloodstream by the peripheral cells and inhibit the normal secretion of glucose by the liver. After the drug killed well over 100 diabetic patients and crippled many more, it was pulled off the market. Neither the oral hypoglycemic agents nor insulin injections have any effects on increasing the uptake of glucose by the cells of the body. This essentially means that the diabetic patient cannot expect to improve or become cured by any of these treatments. On the contrary, the prognosis with this orthodox treatment is an increasing disability and early death from heart or kidney failure, or failure of some other vital organ. Research has in fact shown that diabetes drugs increase your risk of heart attack by a whooping 250 percent!

Some diabetes drugs are less dangerous than others, but regardless, they are still dangerous enough to consider avoiding them. For example, the widely used diabetes drug Avandia has recently been linked to a greater risk of heart attack and, possibly, death, according to the New England Journal of Medicine (May 21, 2007). An analysis pooling the results of several dozen studies, encompassing some 28,000 patients, showed that Avandia, which is manufactured by GlaxoSmithKline, causes a 43 percent higher risk of heart attack. The U.S. government has issued a safety alert, but despite the enormous health risk imposed by the drug, the FDA has not requested a stronger warning label for the drug. I dare raise these simple questions: "Is it any wonder that 80 percent of diabetics die of heart disease?" and "Who benefits from downplaying these known and proven risks?"

Medical doctors don't treat you to cure your diseases. 'Cure' is not even a word they are permitted to use. Most practicing physicians and their patients want a quick fix, and in the case of Type 2 diabetes, it consists of glucose-lowering drugs. And although these drugs can temporarily control your symptoms and lower your blood sugar, they do nothing to address the *cause* of the disorder. One of the problems with glucose-lowering drugs is that they can lose their effectiveness over time. This can dramatically increase your chances of dying from a heart attack. If that is not bad enough, these drugs can also make your life more miserable. Common side effects are weight gain, elevated cholesterol and triglyceride levels, nausea, diarrhea, constipation, stomach pain, drowsiness and headache.

Healing the Causes

To help your body heal itself and remove the causes leading to the symptoms of diabetes (especially Type 2 and, possibly, Type 1), avoid eating animal proteins such as meat, fish, poultry, eggs, cheese and cow's milk. During the recovery phase, strictly refuse to consume cheap, refined oils or fats, such as those found in many restaurant foods and in nearly all processed foods. You may use healthful fats and oils such as expeller-pressed (cold-pressed) coconut oil, olive oil, sesame oil and ghee butter (see also your body type food list). Don't eat food that has been cooked in the microwave oven. Avoid frozen foods, canned products and leftover foods. Take *gymnema sylvestre* to heal damaged pancreas cells, and *evening primrose oil* to improve nerve function. Refer to chapter 7 for information on auto-urine therapy and blood-sugar-balancing foods, herbs and spices, including oils and cinnamon. Cleansing of the main organs of elimination (liver, colon and kidneys) is essential for reversing diabetes of both types.

Read labels. If a processed food contains more than two to three separate items on it, it is likely to be of no use for your body. Ideally, eat only foods produced by nature, such as fruits, fresh salads, cooked vegetables, grains, pulses, nuts, seeds, etc. With the exception of stevia, xylitol and D-mannose, some honey, etc., strictly avoid sugar and starchy foods such as pasta and potatoes. Much worse than sugar are artificial sweeteners and products that contain them; you should avoid these at any cost. Artificial sweeteners will reverse the recovery even if everything else is followed (see *Aspartame and Other Sweet Killer Drugs* in Chapter 14). Most vitamin supplements don't work for diabetics and may end up in the toilet, but not without first harming the kidneys (see chapter 14). Furthermore, avoid all manufactured beverages and fruit juices. Eat fruits whole, and separate from meals (see chapter 6).

While recovering, try to monitor blood sugar manually. For some time, you may want to use glycemic tables to help you in this regard. Make sure to work with a doctor who is aware of and supportive of the healing measures you are taking for yourself. Also avoid alcohol until blood sugar stabilizes in the normal range. The same applies to caffeine as well as other stimulants. Stimulants such as caffeine and nicotine prompt the liver to release sugar into the bloodstream.

Those who are on the verge of developing insulin resistance or are considered pre-diabetic should follow the same guidelines. If you don't ever want to risk developing diabetes, they apply for you also. For example, soft drinks are known to cause diabetes. Researchers at the Harvard School of Public Health examined nine years of dietary and medical data on more than 51,000 women who participated in the Nurses' Health Study II. From this group, well over 700 cases of Type 2 diabetes were diagnosed during the study period. The study found that women who drink one or more soft drinks per day may have an 80 percent increased risk of Type 2 diabetes compared to women who pass on this type of beverage.

Changing key lifestyle factors such as diet and physical activity may not be easy for everyone. But in the case of controlling blood sugar, you usually have a choice. In the above study, making the choice of drinking fresh water instead of soft drinks can make the difference between life and death. If you feel you cannot make that choice, please consider that becoming diabetic can make your lifestyle much more limited and complicated than following the simple suggestions made in this chapter.

Diabetes is not a disease; it is a complex mechanism of protection or survival that the body has no choice but to resort to in order to avoid the consequences of an unhealthful diet and lifestyle. Millions of people suffer or die unnecessarily from this non-disease. The diabetes epidemic is man-made, or shall I say, factory-made. It could be brought to a halt by more and more people refusing to eat foods that are not safe for human consumption.

CHAPTER 12

Banishing the Aids Myth -
Secrets for Understanding and
Healing From This So Called 'Disease'

THe first AIDS cases were diagnosed 1980, but despite the most colossal efforts by scientists and policy makers, AIDS has remained a mystery disease. Commonly believed to be caused by HIV - *Human Immune Deficiency Virus* - scientists still haven't found an antidote for the disease. To this day, there is no convincing medical knowledge as to *how* the pathogen HIV is supposed to cause AIDS. The current AIDS theory also falls short in predicting the kind of AIDS disease an infected person may be manifesting, and there is no accurate system to determine how long it will take for the disease to develop. The HIV/AIDS theory contains no information that can truly help identify those who are at risk of developing AIDS.

With regard to 'treating' AIDS, until recently, patients were able to choose between a small number of drugs that were originally developed as cancer chemotherapies, but had to bear with extreme side effects, such as loss of hair, anemia, muscle deterioration, nausea, and other immune suppressing effects. A newly introduced cocktail of three drugs (protease inhibitors), which are less toxic than the originally used drugs, seemed promising at first in being able to suppress HIV. Yet the cumulative failure rate of the new drugs has now reached 50 percent and continues to increase as strains of HIV develop resistance to them. Already between 20 and 30 percent of patients are now infected with viruses resistant to protease inhibitors, and the situation is worsening day by day. Although the drugs have given many AIDS patients a 'new lease of life' (not necessarily because the drugs suppress HIV, but because they also subdue most other disease-causing agents, at least for a while), the initial euphoria about the new AIDS treatment has died down and so has the hope of finding a cure, at least within the medical field.

The fact that there is no reliable latency period - the length of time from being infected with HIV and developing AIDS symptoms - makes it virtually impossible to predict the beginning of the disease. The first AIDS victims were told that they could expect to die within one year after infection, but today the grace period ranges from 12 to15 years, which makes immediate treatment after HIV infection dubious. This is certainly not the last revision. The majority of HIV infected people continue to be AIDS-free and only a fraction of them develop AIDS symptoms such as pneumonia, cancer of the blood, or dementia.

To add more confusion to the situation, health officials are unable to predict how many people will be afflicted with AIDS in the future, as only a small percentage of the one million HIV-infected Americans will get the disease. In the first 20 years or so of the epidemic, 95 percent of the AIDS cases were among the major health risk groups - highly active homosexuals, heroin addicts, or, in a few cases, hemophiliacs, and since then more and more heterosexual men and women are found to test HIV positive.

According to official estimates, two thirds of infected persons supposedly are in Africa, where the epidemic exploded during the 1990s, and one fifth are in Asia, where the epidemic has been growing rapidly in recent years. As of the end of 2003, an estimated 34.6 million to 42.3 million people throughout the world were living with HIV infection, and more than 20 million had died of AIDS. In that year alone, about 4.8 million people became infected with HIV, and about 2.9 million died of AIDS. However, as we shall see, these estimates are significantly flawed and manipulated.

Just four years earlier in 1999, the statistics showed figures that in no way support today's figures. With the officially proclaimed mortality rate of 50-100 percent among HIV infected people, we should have had many more deaths in Africa where the number of infected at that time was estimated to be as large as six to eight million, and also in Haiti, where over six percent of the population tested HIV-positive. Yet during the nineties, the African continent had only 250,000 AIDS cases, and Haiti had almost none. This leads to the simple, but most important and almost forsaken question regarding AIDS, which is "what causes it?"

So far, there is no scientific evidence that AIDS is a contagious disease, although it seems to be that way to most people. What *is* known from recently published research is that HIV only extremely rarely spreads heterosexually and can, therefore, not be responsible for an epidemic that involves millions of AIDS victims around the world. There is also no proof to show that HIV causes AIDS. On the other hand, it is an established fact that the retrovirus HIV, which is composed of human gene fragments, is incapable of destroying human cells - yet cell destruction is the main characteristic of every AIDS disease. Even the principal discoverer of HIV, Luc Montagnier, no longer believes that HIV is solely responsible for causing AIDS. In fact, he showed that HIV alone cannot cause AIDS. There is also increasing evidence that AIDS may be a toxicity syndrome or metabolic disorder that is caused by immunity risk factors, including heroin, sex drugs, antibiotics, commonly prescribed AIDS drugs, rectal intercourse, starvation, malnutrition and dehydration. Dozens of prominent scientists working at the forefront of the AIDS research are now openly questioning the virus hypothesis of AIDS.

HIV - A Harmless Passenger Virus?

If a germ or virus has infected a person, the disease-causing microbe is present in high concentrations within the patient's body. In the case of AIDS, there should be very large amounts of virus material in the affected tissues. Small amounts would not be sufficient to cause such extensive destruction, as is found in the body of an AIDS victim. Therefore, active virus material should be profusely present in the white cells of the immune system, particularly in the T-helper cells, as well as in lesions of *Kaposi's sarcoma* and in the brain neurons of those afflicted with dementia. Yet this is not the case at all. The HIV retrovirus cannot be found in *any* of the diseased tissues of AIDS patients. This fact alone should make anyone suspicious about the claim that HIV leads to the destruction of organs and system.

If HIV were capable of infecting T-cells or other parts of the immune system, then, as is the case with every other type of viral infections, the cell-free virus particles or *virions* would easily be detected in the bloodstream. However, in the majority of AIDS patients, there are no viruses found anywhere, and in the remaining few there are not even enough present in the blood to cause as much as a simple cold. This makes AIDS patients de facto HIV-negative. The 20 million deaths attributed to AIDS were, in fact, not caused by HIV, but other reasons.

Like other viruses, HIV becomes quickly inactivated by rapid antibody production of the host's immune system. When it first infects the body, HIV can achieve high levels of virus and for a brief period can cause mild flu-like symptoms, if any at all. The immune system then quickly neutralizes the retrovirus and puts it into a dormant state. Since AIDS patients who test HIV positive have been infected many years before they die, their HIV retrovirus remains inactive.

An HIV test can *only* detect either the dormant, inactive virus or antibodies that the immune system produces to remain immune to the virus in the future. Therefore, the HIV test itself proves the harmlessness of HIV. Although it is rarely mentioned in the medical literature, HIV has never been found in the lymph nodes, macrophage cells, dendritic cells, and elsewhere in the body of an AIDS victim; there has never been even a sign of a hidden virus infection. If the HIV were responsible for destroying the human immune system, it would have to be present where the destruction takes place. But this is not the case.

Flawed HIV Tests - The True Cause of the AIDS Epidemic

When Judith was diagnosed HIV positive she was told that there are a number of AIDS drugs that she could take to ward off the disease, at least for some time. But when she learned how sick these drugs could make her, she decided not to take them. About 18 months after the initial diagnosis, Judith showed no signs of being ill, and so her doctor recommended a retest. Since the new test came back negative, she did a second one, which turned out to be indeterminate. To further confuse an already very confusing situation, the thirst test she took turned out to be positive for HIV. Unable to figure out from the tests what was really going on, Judith began to investigate the medical literature and learned that HIV tests are highly inaccurate and even the HIV hypothesis was anything but correct.

Since testing positive, Judith gave birth to two children (now ages two and six) who, like herself, are the picture of health with no indications of a serious illness. She never had them tested for HIV. The whole family eats natural, organic foods and enjoys a completely normal life. Judith and her kids are not alone. There are thousands of healthy HIV-positive people who don't take AIDS drugs, and who show no sign of sickness. But only a few people escape the wrath of an unreliable testing procedure.

HIV can only be detected in the human body after the immune system has already killed the virus through its arsenal of antibodies. The presence of HIV antibodies proves that the virus has been rendered harmless, with no further role to play. This should make the HIV-testing procedure a method for informing infected people that **the virus has been successfully destroyed, rather** than delivering them a death sentence.

The most frequently used HIV test used today is ELISA and, in theory, it seems to be accurate. A sample of the patient's blood is added to a mixture of HIV proteins. If the blood contains HIV antibodies, they react to the proteins. This is supposed to be proof that the patient has been infected with HIV. Another test called Western Blot is often used as a confirmation. Besides being unable to detect actual virus in the blood of a patient, these tests are so unreliable that they are not only useless, but also the cause of unprecedented trauma and suffering in the world. In Russia, in 1990, after 20,000 'patients' had tested positive with the ELISA test, only 112 were confirmed using the Western Blot. The French government has recently withdrawn nine HIV tests because they were far too unreliable. If the true positive rates of these HIV tests, instead of their extreme failure rates, were applied to the alleged 40 million HIV infected population in the world, we would have a mere **total of 224,719 people infected with HIV**. Nobody could possibly call this a mass epidemic, especially since most HIV-infected people not undergoing drug treatments live normal, healthy lives like Judith and her children.

The above figure may, in fact, even be much lower. The only reason people are added to the ever-increasing list of HIV victims is because more and more people are tested for HIV. The most commonly used HIV tests are antibody tests, which means that they can cross-react with normal proteins in human blood. Both the ELISA and Western Blot tests react to proteins that are shared by all other retroviruses found to live in the human body. P24 is one of them. Considering the large number of retroviruses existing in the body, if a patient has produced antibodies to P24, which is generally accepted as proof for the presence of HIV, the chances that he is actually infected with HIV are very slim. In fact, **there are nearly 70 commonly occurring conditions** - all listed in the medical literature - **that are known to make the tests come up positive.** These include yeast infections, simple head or chest colds, influenza, rheumatoid arthritis, hepatitis, herpes, recent inoculations, drug use and pregnancy. There are literally hundreds of millions of people in the world who either have gone through such conditions or are currently experiencing them. Giving them an AIDS test would automatically sentence them to a disease they may not have. That is exactly what we are doing during the humanitarian AIDS campaigns promoted by the WHO and numerous charitable AIDS organizations.

Another class of HIV tests, called viral load tests, can produce dozens of conflicting results - even from the same blood sample. The general population is made to believe that an HIV test is a reliable method to determine whether they are infected with HIV or not. If they were to read the disclaimers on the HIV test kits they would perhaps become a little suspicious, at least enough to insist on further evidence, if such can ever be provided. This is what the disclaimers say: **"At present there is no recognized standard for establishing the presence or absence of HIV-1 antibody in human blood,"** or **"The AMPLICOR HIV-1 MONITOR [Viral Load] test is not intended to be used as a screening test for HIV or as a diagnostic test to confirm the presence of HIV infection,"** or **"Do not use this kit as the sole basis of diagnosis of HIV-1 infection"** (Abbott Laboratories HIV Test, Roche Viral Load Test and Epitope, Inc. Western Blot Test, respectively). And to top this fiasco, positive test results can occur due to **"prior pregnancy, blood transfusions...and other potential nonspecific reactions"** (Vironostika HIV Test, 2003).

If the screening tests for HIV are in fact not to be used for diagnostic purposes, what are they then used for, you may ask. Why are hundreds of millions of people in Africa and Asia subjected to AIDS tests if they shouldn't be used to confirm the presence of HIV infection? How many 'potential nonspecific reactions' could there be to influence the outcome of an HIV test? Moreover, why is the WHO proclaiming that there are nearly 40 million people infected with HIV when this worldwide organization knows so well that the tests used cannot be used to make such claims?

The AIDS tests are used to create statistics of an epidemic that has no scientific backing, but is blindly accepted as true by innocent people who have no reason to believe they are being deceived over something like a deadly disease. This information needs to be shared with every person who tests positive for HIV, yet it is being concealed from these 'patients'. Unless they do their own research, which cannot be expected by the vast majority of Africans, Asians and South Americans, these frightened, confused and unsuspecting people are misled to believe they are infected with a deadly virus. Most AIDS workers do not even know the scientific facts, or lack thereof, behind the HIV theory and these testing procedures.

In one study, 41 percent of patients with multiple sclerosis (MS) showed presence of antibodies to P24 in their blood. This didn't mean, however, that they were infected with HIV, although the ELISA test would have implied exactly that. As the co-discoverer of HIV and leading virologist Dr Robert Gallo[42] has repeatedly pointed out, P24 is not unique to HIV. If the ELISA test is applied to people who have been or are infected with the viruses that cause malaria, hepatitis B and C, tuberculosis, glandular fever, papilloma virus warts, syphilis, leprosy, and many other conditions, the chances they are declared AIDS victims are extremely high. In Africa and other developing countries, the HIV test is usually given to people who feel unwell or are already diagnosed with one of these diseases. Given the large number

---

[42] Dr. Gallo used the virus identified in his laboratory to make a blood test for AIDS that was patented by the United States Government. The patent earns millions of dollars in royalties annually for the United States Treasury and $100,000 a year each for Dr. Gallo and a former colleague, Dr. Mikulas Popovic.

of people affected by them, meaning, hundreds of millions, the number of possible false-positive results could well exceed 100 million, given the ever-expanding testing campaigns.

Take the striking example of worldwide malaria. In 1999, the World Health Organization (WHO) estimated that over 300 million clinical cases of malaria occur annually from among the 2.3 billion people (almost one-third of the world's population) who are at risk of infection with the malaria parasite. Accordingly, by 2004, over one billion people would have contracted malaria, all of whom will have developed antibodies for the harmless retrovirus P24 in their blood. Out of the 300 million annual malaria victims, an estimated 1.1 million people die from the disease. If you tested all the 300 million annually occurring malaria victims, you would automatically have about 299 million new cases of HIV. Moreover, most of the million who died from malaria would automatically be categorized as being AIDS victims because the ELISA test shows positive for P24.

While these numbers are shocking, they are probably underestimates of the world's malaria burden, given that only a fraction of malaria cases are reported each year and that deaths among children with chronic malaria are often attributed to other illnesses. These statistics may vary by a factor of three, depending on the method of estimation. In Africa alone, the 28 million reported cases of malaria are believed to represent only 5-10 percent of the total malaria incidence on the continent (Hamoudi & Sachs, 1999).

Dr. Max Essex, a highly respected and leading AIDS expert from the Harvard University School of Public Health, found that some 85 percent of Africans who tested HIV positive with the Western Blot test later tested negative.

Another source of false-positive results from HIV tests is the large variety of antibodies which people produce after undergoing blood transfusions, or when exposed to foreign semen and virus material during homosexual activity, and after taking drugs. Drug users and homosexuals are known to make many more antibodies than the average person does. The chances that they become victims of a false positive AIDS test are, therefore, more likely than not.

What all this basically means is that there is no reliable way of telling how many people are infected with the HIV virus. Nor can anything be said about how many of the so-called AIDS diseases, if any at all, are in fact HIV-related.

Nobel laureate Kary Mullis, who invented the first HIV test, has openly questioned the validity of the 'AIDS virus'. According to Mullis, his highly sensitive detection technique known as PCR can only be used to find **dormant, inactive HIV**, incapable of harming anyone. Mullis says: "I can't find a single virologist who will give me references which show that HIV is the probable cause of AIDS..." **PCR proves that AIDS cannot be caused by a virus!** This also means that the autoimmune deficiency syndrome (AIDS) can very well occur without the presence of virus.

HIV Cannot Cause as Much as the Flu

Contrary to the original HIV-AIDS hypothesis, which says there is a 50-100 percent probability of death from infection, there are only a few HIV infected people who actually die, at least not more than in any other category of disease. When blood from AIDS patients was injected into chimpanzees in 1983, all of them tested HIV positive but when tested 10 years later, none of them had developed any signs of sickness. In another experiment, over 150 chimpanzees received injections of purified (highly concentrated) HIV in 1984, but developed no symptoms of disease to this very day. However, what the experiments did show was that their immune systems had produced antibodies against the virus within a month, just as it happens in humans. The presence of antibodies ensures that immunity against the microbes has been secured on a permanent basis. Just as animals cannot get AIDS from HIV, so can human beings not get AIDS from HIV either.

Among other human viruses, such as those causing polio, flu, hepatitis, etc., HIV may be one of the most harmless ones; it is quickly and easily neutralized by our immune system. The incubation period for every known virus does not exceed more than a maximum of six weeks, as is the case with the human hepatitis virus. It is a well-established biological law that any germ that does not cause symptoms before it is cleared by the immune system cannot be considered a cause of disease. No virus is capable of surviving 10-15 years in a normal healthy body with an active immune system. And even if it were possible in theory that a few virus particles would survive a decade or longer, they still would have to overcome the immune system, and they would certainly not be enough in number to impair the person's immunity (unless of course the immune system is destroyed by other causes).

The AIDS theory suggests that HIV destroys the immune system's T4 cells, thereby leaving the body susceptible to all kinds of infections and diseases. It had already been discovered in the mid-eighties that the number of HIV infected T4 cells is far too small to cause widespread destruction and that the human body is perfectly capable of replacing T4 cells faster than HIV could destroy them.

Since the beginning of AIDS as we know it, many thousands of people, including medical workers and hemophiliacs, were accidentally infected with HIV, but only a few of them developed AIDS - in fact, not more than any other group in society. Among the health workers who developed AIDS, 90 percent belonged to the major risk group of AIDS cases - highly active homosexuals and intravenous drug users. Among hemophiliacs, who are 'naturally' immune-deficient, there are just as many HIV-negatives dying as there are HIV-positives dying. In other words, whether a hemophiliac is infected or not, his chances of developing an AIDS-type disease are exactly the same. Until now, there has not been even one human or animal that has developed AIDS after being infected only with HIV. This fact may be reason enough to reconsider the role of HIV as being the sole agent responsible for causing dozens of different kinds of (AIDS) diseases. Luc Montagnier, co-discoverer of the HIV virus, has already pointed out that, without another co-factor, HIV cannot cause AIDS.

HIV Behaves like Every Other Virus

Man lived with the HIV virus long before it was discovered and before large numbers of people underwent AIDS tests. The same applies to other types of viruses. For example, the *herpes* virus is present in 2 out of 3 Americans; another two thirds carry the herpes class *cytomegalovirus*. Four out of five Americans walk around with the *Eppstein-Barr virus,* which in few of them causes mononucleosis or 'kissing disease'. Even more people are host to the *papilloma virus*, which is known to cause warts. There is hardly anyone living on this planet who does not carry at least a dozen or so viruses in his body, each one related to a specific infectious disease. Yet no scientist in the world would use these facts to announce a mass outbreak of viral epidemics. Every experienced virologist knows that all these viruses are dormant, i.e. they have been neutralized by the immune system. He also knows that this makes the infected people immune against re-infection, *unless* of course the immune system is damaged or suppressed through other factors.

If HIV, herpes, and all the other types of viruses that are latent in humans and animals living on the planet were capable of killing people, there would hardly be anyone left to treat the billions of sufferers. HIV, being a human retrovirus (produced by the body itself), is totally benign to its host cells and is, therefore, incapable of destroying any cell it has infected. This applies especially to the cells of the immune system, which are equipped with highly sophisticated defense mechanisms. For HIV to have any destructive value, it would literally have to flood the body with active viral particles. Yet HIV can barely be detected even in late stage AIDS patients, despite using the most sensitive of tests. The traces of HIV virus found in some AIDS patients is inactive, which means, it is harmless, and therefore not responsible for the destruction of the body. If HIV *were* the cause of AIDS, it would have to do this during the two phases of HIV infection where blood levels of HIV are significant:

1. Soon after infection when the immune system produces antibodies.
2. At the very end stage of AIDS when the levels of *all* viral activity increase *because* the immune system has collapsed (due other reasons than HIV infection).

There is enough scientific data to show that HIV, being and remaining inactive even in AIDS patients, **does not kill T-cells** and, therefore, **cannot cause AIDS!**

Research under Scrutiny

There are numerous research studies which all seem to show that only HIV-infected persons can develop AIDS (in comparison with those who are not infected with the virus). This is but a correlation, not a cause and effect relation. Although there is no proof of it, this idea has become the most powerful and persuasive argument to convince both scientists and the general population to believe that HIV causes AIDS. And yet by analyzing any of these studies you will find that the HIV-infected groups consisted *only* of members who were in the AIDS risk category e.g. very active homosexuals, heroin addicts and patients with a history of major diseases. By contrast, the non-infected control groups consisted of healthy heterosexuals. In other words, AIDS seems to develop only in people whose immune system is already impaired due to other causes than HIV.

Official statistics from the 1990s revealed that 90 percent of all AIDS victims were men and 95 percent of all AIDS victims living in wealthy nations belonged to one or more of the above risk categories. But there exists no such distinction in the above studies. The only common factor between the two groups is age. Yet it is very obvious that a 25-year old immune deficient heroin addict is more likely to suffer an immune disease than a 25-year old healthy medical student, regardless of whether he has one or several inactive viruses in his body or not. That an increasing number of heterosexuals are now testing positive for HIV has less to do with a new trend, but with the expansion of the tests to that group. How many heterosexual Americans have virus-induced warts you may ask? Millions of them! And how many have had undergone blood transfusions or contracted once in their life a virus that causes malaria, hepatitis B and C, tuberculosis, glandular fever, syphilis, and many other conditions? Again, millions of them! All of these millions of people, if tested for HIV, are likely to test positive because they will have developed antibodies for the harmless retrovirus P24 in their blood. As we shall see, sexual intercourse between heterosexuals is not the reason for spreading HIV.

In the last 15 years, several scientists have proposed conducting a case-controlled study that would compare a large number of HIV-infected people with a similar number of uninfected people, all of whom would share the same health risks or medical history. Yet there hasn't been much interest in conducting such a study since the focus is still on destroying a virus rather than on eliminating immune-suppressive influences.

HIV + Pneumonia = AIDS?

In the meantime, more and more studies are being published to show that AIDS, which cannot be classified as a disease because every case displays a different combination of symptoms, occurs only in people who test HIV-positive. Before HIV was discovered, pneumonia, dementia, herpes-infections, weight loss, tuberculosis, *Kaposi's sarcoma*, chronic diarrhea, several lymphomas, yeast infection, and other opportunistic infections were considered separate diseases. Depending on whether a patient had already a deficient immune system or belonged to a certain health risk group, the symptoms of these diseases exactly matched those which are now considered AIDS diseases.

Before the HIV-AIDS hypothesis, a patient who died from pneumonia, tuberculosis, or a lymphoma died from the respective causes of these diseases. By contrast, a patient who dies from pneumonia today *and* happens to have antibodies to HIV or P24 in his blood, is automatically labeled and listed as an AIDS victim. People with a low T-cell count in their blood are considered immune deficient, but if they continue having the same condition after testing positive for HIV, they are routinely 'sentenced' to AIDS, with or without clinical symptoms.

There are already over 35 such diseases now that have been renamed 'AIDS' in this way. One of the latest ones is cervical cancer, which has become the first AIDS disease that can only affect the female gender. This may give the false impression that AIDS is now penetrating the heterosexual community as well. The inclusion of cervical cancer as an AIDS disease has 'increased' the number of AIDS victims among women quite dramatically, yet at the same time, it has 'decreased' the number of ordinary cervical cancers among women. Overall, the mortality rate of these diseases has not changed at all. The claim that more and more heterosexuals are now afflicted with AIDS is not based on real science, but ignorance or denial of the facts.

The renaming of old diseases as AIDS further supports the hypothesis that the AIDS syndrome is never found in anyone without presence of HIV. By definition, there is no AIDS without HIV, regardless how many non-HIV people may die from the very same symptoms. Accordingly, anything that even remotely resembles immune deficiency plus HIV now counts as an AIDS disease, despite the fact that AIDS patients with *Kaposi's sarcoma* have been reported to have normal immune systems. It has been argued that wherever there is HIV, AIDS will be the consequence. However, this argument is heavily flawed. AIDS-like indigenous diseases existed long before the testing of antibodies for HIV was introduced. What is different today is that the old diseases are renamed and 'become' AIDS diseases whenever HIV is found to be present as well. In real terms, though, there are not any more AIDS cases with HIV in the world than there are without HIV.

Grave Statistical Errors

In the United States alone, the estimated number of one million HIV-infected people has remained constant since the HIV test was made available in 1985. Given the fact that HIV tests produce far more false positives than correct positives, there may actually be very few HIV infected Americans. Of these, regardless of whether they are true positives or not, less than 1/3 had been diagnosed with AIDS by the year 1993 and 121,000 of them were still alive. Over two thirds of the HIV infected Americans have not developed any AIDS symptoms since 1985, and the already huge gap is widening each year. The number of new AIDS cases has actually been leveling off for several years and has dropped dramatically in 1996 despite the fact that the new yearly AIDS cases are always added to the totals of all AIDS victims so far. During the same period, although the new AIDS treatments were only made available in 1996, the number of AIDS deaths across the United States has dropped considerably, with a decrease of 44 percent during the first half of 1997. A similar trend occurred in Western Europe, also before new treatments were introduced. The new treatments had absolutely nothing to do with the reduction, although the extensive advertising campaigns by the drug companies may want to make the masses believe they did.

A contrived AIDS explosion took place at midnight, January 1, 1993. On New Year's Eve 1992, the Los Angeles Times reported: "As many as 40,000 Americans who are HIV-positive will wake up on

New Year's Day with a diagnosis of AIDS." As forecast, the number of new AIDS cases climbed by 204 percent within the first three months of 1993 compared to the same period of the previous year. This intended statistical error and similar ones occurred because much milder forms of diseases had been included in the official list of AIDS diseases.

The same manipulation of data has also influenced world AIDS figures. More and more indigenous types of disease occurring in developing countries are being added to the AIDS defined disease groups, thus giving the false impression that there is an AIDS explosion in the Third World. Statistics released by the WHO show that in 1995 AIDS soared by 25 percent, reaching 1.3 million. This figure, of course tripled ten years later, again due to intentional statistical error, false HIV tests, and the renaming of existing diseases as AIDS diseases.

In those areas of the world where there are more HIV infected people than in America, the actual number of AIDS cases is significantly less. For example, only 250,000 of the six to eight million Africans who were reportedly infected with HIV between 1985-1995 had contracted AIDS or whatever one may want to call the diseases formerly known as tuberculosis, glandular fever, diarrhea and slim disease (unlike our wasting syndrome). All of these old diseases have since been renamed AIDS diseases, and of course this catapulted AIDS into a mass epidemic in the developing world. Given the large number of people dying from tuberculosis alone (millions each year), and the high failure rate of AIDS tests in Africa (85 percent or more), it may well be that the number of real AIDS victims, if any, does not exceed 50,000.

Zaire alone, with its three million supposed HIV-infected people, has only a few hundred AIDS cases, or less than 0.02 percent. No scientific study would remotely consider AIDS to be caused by HIV when the number is this small. Her neighboring country Uganda, with its one million HIV-infected people, had only generated 8,000 AIDS cases. Out of the 360,000 HIV-infected Haitians, only a few hundred have AIDS. The Haitian AIDS patients, most of them undernourished, suffer from *toxoplasmosis,* which has *always* been a common cause of death. These figures may still be exaggerated, as the old HIV tests which were far less accurate and produced even more false positives than the extremely unreliable ELISA and Western Blot tests, were applied to millions of people worldwide.

Developing countries may have such low AIDS rates because they do not have such extraordinary health risks as the ones found among very active homosexuals, intravenous drug addicts, and hemophiliacs. Those who have long histories of various opportunistic infections or used 'poppers' regularly in the past, or had anal sex, received blood transfusions and took poisonous addictive drugs, belong to the risk group for AIDS, with or without HIV. Because all these factors severely damage the immune system, the individuals being in this risk group are the most likely candidates to 'acquire' the Human Immune Deficiency Syndrome.

The health risks specific for each group are responsible for the particular types of diseases. Heroin addicts are the most likely to develop tuberculosis, herpes infection and weight loss, and hemophiliacs produce pneumonia, regardless of whether they have HIV or not. This fact makes HIV a harmless passenger virus. There are as many cases of pneumonia and tuberculosis today *without* HIV as there are *with* HIV. *Kaposi's sarcoma* also is no longer an exclusive 'AIDS disease'. Slim disease is as common among Africans who test positive for HIV as it is for their HIV-negative counterparts. The lack of HIV test equipment in most parts of Africa compels doctors to diagnose prospective AIDS patients merely by symptoms, a very unreliable and unscientific practice. Yet the numbers of these cases are added to the overall 'statistical evidence' that AIDS is still continuing to spread.

The soaring AIDS epidemic is a product of mass deception based on faulty science, unreliable AIDS tests, and a greedy pharmaceutical industry that does everything in its power to have unrestricted access to the mostly untapped profit potential of Third World populations. Developing countries thus far have largely refused to rely on modern medicine to keep their people healthy. AIDS has profoundly scared them, and so they have given into the tremendous pressure exerted onto them by international organizations, such as the WHO and their generous sponsors - the drug giants. In the historic past, the developing world has been exploited by the wealthy nations. Today, this exploitation is concealed in the generous offer to help the AIDS-afflicted countries control the escalating crisis, a crisis that existed long before HIV was named a deadly virus.

HIV is not a New Virus

Most of the manipulated statistical evidence of an escalating AIDS epidemic occurred because of faulty testing procedures and the wrong assumption that HIV is a new virus. Everyone who tests HIV positive is believed to have acquired the virus from someone else. The HIV testing procedure reveals nothing about how long the virus has been in a person's body. So, in the assumption that HIV must be a new virus (because nobody has discovered it or tested for it before 1983), we have never even considered the possibility that HIV, like so many other human retroviruses, could have been around for decades or even centuries. If HIV is indeed an old virus - and there is ample evidence now to support this claim - we should be able to find its traces (antibodies for HIV) in large numbers of people, especially in developing countries.

HIV turns out to be a virus that has existed long before 1980. In 1998, research conducted at the Aaron Diamond AIDS Research Center at Rockefeller University, U.S.A proved through blood tests gathered in Africa between 1959 and 1982 that the HIV virus already existed in 1959. Based on this and other related research it is now estimated that the virus first got into people some time in the 1940s or early 1950s.

Since the HIV test was introduced to the Western Hemisphere in 1985, the number of HIV-infections has remained constant world-wide until the mid 1990s. But once the screening campaigns of HIV were extended to new countries in Africa, and in more recent years also in Asia, the number of infected people 'rose dramatically'. There is no information available on how long these people carried the HIV virus or even whether they had received it from their parents.

According to a previous version (1990) of the HIV/AIDS theory, HIV infected people would automatically contract AIDS within several years and subsequently die. This, however, is not and has never been correct, although it may apply to a small number of HIV infected persons whose immune system has been destroyed through major health risks that are listed below. Since major health risks exist almost everywhere in the world, a 'rise' in the number of HIV infected people in areas where no one had been tested before is more than likely, especially since HIV has been around since the 1940s. In its 'New World Health Report 1996', the World Health Organization (WHO) states that "there are now more than 21 million people infected with HIV." Eight years and 100 million ELISA tests later, the number has nearly doubled. The WHO reports omit the fact that this 'rise' in numbers stems mostly from the extension of this extremely inaccurate HIV-test to previously uncovered populations in the world. In actuality, HIV stopped spreading long ago. Besides, as the scientist who discovered HIV admitted, HIV cannot cause AIDS.

New Evidence: HIV Rarely Spreads Heterosexually

In the developing world, the virus has existed for at least 65 years **because** HIV is rarely spread heterosexually. Research that studied the wives of infected hemophiliacs showed that an HIV-positive person requires over 1,000 unprotected sexual contacts with an HIV-negative person from the opposite sex to pass along the virus just once. In another surprise study, published in the Lancet, 1997, 349:851-2, French doctors at the Cochin-Port Royal hospital in Paris looked at the risk of married couples wanting to conceive a baby where the man was HIV-positive. Their findings are in line with infection rates of 1 per 1000 acts of unprotected sex among stable heterosexual couples. According to this published research, it would take an HIV-infected heterosexual who has sexual intercourse 2-3 times a week about **seven years** to infect another person with HIV! This practically means that it would take the HIV-infected males of 1 million couples 2,739 years of daily unprotected sex to infect all female partners. In the developing world, unprotected sex among heterosexuals can, therefore, not be held responsible for the high number of people who test HIV positive (even if HIV tests were 100 percent reliable, which they are not).

However, the situation is different with regard to infected pregnant women. A baby is directly and constantly exposed to the mother's blood for a period of 9 months. During this period the virus has a 50 percent chance of being passed on to the baby. Retroviruses survive when they reach a new host prenatally (passed from mother to child). This way of passing on a virus is at least 500 times more efficient than through sexual transmission. (Blood transfusion is another obvious way of contracting the virus.)

In contrast to the situation in wealthy nations, HIV in Third World countries is equally distributed between both sexes, which means, it must have been passed on from mother to child for many centuries. Had HIV been a deadly killer virus, the babies of infected mothers would have obviously been born deformed, miscarried, or dead because newly born babies have not yet developed adequate immunity to defend themselves against a killer virus. Even if they somehow managed to survive, they could only last for a maximum of two years - the latency period given to infected babies before developing AIDS. The spreading of the virus would have stopped automatically through the destruction of all new babies that were infected by their mothers.

Due to the low rates of homosexuality in developing countries, the prenatal route of transmission has been their only efficient way (50 percent chance) to pass on HIV to the new generations. Grown female children who become mothers would again have a 50 percent chance of passing the virus to their children. Therefore, in Africa alone, HIV must have been around for many generations before it was able to infect as many as 6-8 million people. The latest argument that the increased condom use in some African nations helped to slow the rate of infection is hardly convincing since the main route of HIV infection in Africa is from mother to child.

Who Gets AIDS?

The situation is much different in the industrialized world where HIV is mostly transmitted through different routes. The most susceptible groups are very active homosexuals, needle-sharing heroin addicts, and hemophiliacs who receive transfusions. They represent the main and easiest routes through which disease-causing microbes can be passed on to others who share one common risk factor: immune deficiency. In other words, the groups in society where HIV is commonly present amongst their members are also the groups with the biggest health risks and, therefore, more likely to produce AIDS symptoms. Still, HIV's most concentrated occurrence among health risk groups cannot be blamed for causing AIDS diseases, just as elevated *cholesterol* levels cannot be held responsible for causing heart disease. These are mere correlations. Another problem is that gay men, drug users, and hemophiliacs who are exposed to semen, drugs, blood transfusions, hepatitis, the Epstein Barr virus, and many other diseases or factors known to cause biological false positives in HIV tests, represent the most unreliable groups in society to demonstrate real presence of HIV.

As prophesied 13 years ago, AIDS has invaded the heterosexual community, or so it appears. Since cervical cancer and other female diseases have more recently been renamed AIDS diseases, AIDS seems to have affected the female population. However, most AIDS patients are still male. Anything and everything that strongly abuses the body and depletes the immune system must be held responsible for causing illness, regardless of whether it is a stroke, cancer, or an AIDS disease. Emotional stress, insufficient nutrition, dehydration, sleep deprivation, alcohol, cigarettes, antibiotics, hard drugs, excessive sexual activity, etc., can all damage the immune system. A dormant piece of viral material such as HIV, on the other hand, can do no harm in a healthy body.

Whoever continuously exposes himself to immune risk factors is also more susceptible to developing the *Acquired Human Immune Deficiency Syndrome*. Someone may argue: "What about an innocent baby who becomes infected with HIV by its parents and dies from pneumonia? Is that not AIDS?" The fact is that at least as many children die from pneumonia with or without HIV, and it doesn't significantly influence the outcome of the disease whether they had a previous encounter with HIV or not. What *can* make a big difference, however, is *how* the pneumonia is treated.

What Really Causes AIDS

Over 35 diseases have now been renamed AIDS diseases, all supposedly caused by one single (inactive) virus. What has been considered normal pneumonia until 10-15 years ago, if linked with HIV, it is now an AIDS disease. The same applies to Candida infection, tuberculosis, *Kaposi's sarcoma,* and cervical cancer. If an African suffers from 'slim disease' and has HIV antibodies in his blood, he is being told that he has AIDS. If he dies from the disease, he obviously must have died from AIDS. This simple logic may sound persuasive to a lay person.

On the other hand, if an African is diagnosed with having 'slim disease' without previous HIV infection and subsequently dies, AIDS is not considered the cause of death. It is worthy to note that there are at least as many cases of slim disease without HIV as there are with HIV, and that the retrovirus HIV has proven to be incapable of causing cell destruction, which is the main characteristic accompanying 'slim disease'.

If the HIV virus cannot be held responsible for causing AIDS diseases, then what *is* the cause of AIDS?

1. Narcotic Drugs

Roughly ten years before the discovery of AIDS, the industrial world experienced a dramatic increase in the use of non-prescribed drugs ranging from hashish, marijuana and psychedelics to LSD, MDA, PCP, heroin, cocaine, amyl and butyl nitrites, amphetamines, barbiturates, ethyl chloride, opium, mushrooms and other 'tailor-made' drugs. By 1974, five million Americans had used the drug cocaine, and only eleven years later, the figure had jumped to over 22 million. In 1990, the American Drug Enforcement Administration had confiscated 100,000 kilograms of cocaine, compared to a mere 500 kilograms in 1980. Within a decade, the number of cocaine overdose victims had increased from 3,000 in 1981 to 80,000 in 1990, an increase of 2,400 percent. Amphetamine use also jumped dramatically. In 1989, the Drug Enforcement Administration seized 97 million doses, up from 2 million doses in 1981. Also, aphrodisiacs became extremely popular during the 1970s. By 1980, five million Americans had become regular users of amyl nitrites, or 'poppers'.

The AIDS epidemic followed a huge jump in drug abuse. Every practicing physician who has seen the severe destruction of body and mind in drug-using patients understands that drugs are capable of doing even more harm to a person than just killing them. Drugs are known for their powerful effect of systematically destroying a person's vital functions, including the immune system. The figures given above can in no way represent the total use of drugs within the population, but they certainly indicate that drug abuse could be playing a major role, if not the biggest role in causing AIDS diseases. Most narcotic drug users have P24 in their blood. An HIV test is likely going to turn them into HIV positive patients that 'need' treatment with expensive and potentially devastating AIDS drugs.

Until recently, drug use was most concentrated among young men aged 25-44 and so AIDS also was most common among this age group. Nine out of every ten AIDS cases were male and 90 percent of all people arrested for possession of hard drugs were male, too. 75 percent of these were aged 25-44 and 72 percent of all AIDS cases among men occurred within exactly the same age group. Could this have been pure coincidence?

Between 1983 and 1987, the death rate among young men of this age group increased by an average of 10,000 per year and so did the number of AIDS deaths within the same period. During the 1980s, deaths from drug overdoses doubled in men of this age group, while deaths from blood poisoning - an indirect result of the injection of drugs into the blood - quadrupled. The same happened to the AIDS sufferers of the same age group during the same period of time.

Now, more females are involved in heavy drug use. Three quarters of all heterosexual AIDS cases and two thirds of all female AIDS cases are injection drug users. Two thirds of all babies born with AIDS have mothers who inject drugs. These figures do *not* include the use of drugs taken orally or in an inhaled form.

The major percentage of AIDS cases, however, is still found among the highly active homosexual men aged 25-44. This group not only abuses large quantities of narcotic drugs, but also antibiotics, antifungals, and antivirals, such as AZT, ddI, ddC, d4T, acyclovir, and gancyclovir, to name a few. A large number of American studies confirmed that over 95 percent of male homosexual AIDS patients typically admitted to popper inhalation and regular use of hard drugs.

AIDS patients suffer from pre-existing immune damage, which in many cases is caused by years of drug abuse. Without an already damaged immune system, AIDS diseases are extremely unlikely to develop. If any of the above risk groups take an AIDS test they are highly likely to test positive, due to the large number of antibodies their bodies have produced to counteract diseases caused by drugs, semen, blood, and viruses, etc.

Why Babies Get AIDS
Babies are strongly affected by the drug abuse of their mothers. Two thirds of all babies with AIDS symptoms, regardless of whether they test HIV-positive or not, have mothers who inject drugs; some large percentage of the rest have mothers who use non-injected drugs. Heroin is one of the most commonly injected drugs. Persistent drug users show symptoms of loss of white blood cells, the main upholder of immunity, as well as lymph node swelling, fever, rapid weight loss, brain dysfunction and dementia, and a marked susceptibility to infections. Heroin addicts often die from pneumonia, tuberculosis, and other opportunistic infections, as well as from wasting syndromes. In all these diseases, the protein P24, generally accepted to be proof of the existence of HIV, is amply present. Although P24 is not unique to HIV but shared with most infectious diseases, they have nevertheless been classified as AIDS diseases.

What is very sad is that babies are defenseless against drug poisoning. Recent research has shown that pregnant women who smoke cigarettes pass cancer-forming chemicals to their babies. It is difficult to imagine what must be taking place in the developing brain of an embryo when it is exposed to heroin injected directly into his mother's blood, which is also his blood.

Many babies born to cocaine-using mothers are born with severe mental retardation and are vulnerable to tuberculosis and lung diseases. The major experimental drugs are so poisonous that regular use can result in dementia, serious bacterial infections, and total destruction of the immune system. The drugs certainly possess a much higher probability of impairing immune functions so typical to AIDS than a simple, inactive virus.

2. Antibiotics

Most of the patients suffering from AIDS also have a long history of taking antibiotics. Antibiotics may be a major co-factor in developing AIDS among the very active homosexual men who depend on them in order to ward off the many venereal diseases and parasites arising from non-hygienic sexual practices. Many gays have received open prescriptions for antibiotics from their doctors who advised them to swallow the drugs before their sexual encounters. Some of them had been on such toxic drugs as *Tetracycline* for as many as 18 years before their immune system succumbed to the devastating side effects they produce. This particular drug causes extreme sensitivity against sunlight. If exposed to sunlight, it can burn one's skin beyond repair. Those affected often suffer from Seasonal Affective Disorder (SAD), a form of depression that arises from lack of exposure to sunlight. The drug is also known to disrupt the body's basic metabolic functions, which may result in virtually any type of disease. It also works as a strong immune suppressant and, perhaps, one of its worst side effects is the destruction of beneficial bacteria in the gut. Eradication of these bacteria makes room for yeast and other infection-causing bacteria, spreading throughout the body and causing continuous flare-ups of disease symptoms

Other commonly used drugs include *flagyl* and *diiodohydroxquin*. Both are used to combat amoeba-caused diarrhea. The drugs can produce severe forms of hallucination and depression.

Corticosteroids, *sulfa drugs*, and *septra* are prescribed for various other conditions, all with serious side effects. They cause severe digestive disturbances, and if worsened by a nutritient-deficient diet so common among active homosexuals, they systematically destroy their bodies' defenses against disease-causing bacteria, viruses and parasites. And so the formerly strong and healthy young men increasingly suffer from opportunistic infections which speed up aging indicators similar to those found only in old and fragile people.

3. Blood Transfusion

All the above mentioned risk factors cause 94 percent of all AIDS cases in the United States, a typical representative for other industrialized nations. But the remaining 6 percent do not seem to fall into any of the risk categories. Over half of this small percentage 'contracted' AIDS through blood transfusions, which to the general population would appear to be a definite indication for HIV to be the cause of AIDS.

However, a closer analysis of the AIDS survival statistics reveals that over half of all blood transfusion recipients die within the first year after transfusion. The same applies to patients who are not HIV-infected. The risk groups for failing blood transfusions are found among the very young and the very old, and those who are severely injured.

Under normal circumstances, healthy people never get a blood transfusion. They are given only to people who have already suffered from long-standing illnesses or after traumatic medical intervention, such as surgery. Anesthesia alone acts as an immune-suppressant, and the same applies to antibiotics administered after surgery to ward off infectious microbes. If a patient undergoes an organ transplant, he will receive steroids and other drugs that prevent his immune system from rejecting the new organ.

Many organ recipients have to take these drugs for the rest of their lives, but since these drugs suppress overall immunity, they often die from 'unrelated' problems within a very short time. The treating doctors rarely attribute these deaths, though, to the side effects of the drugs, and tell the deceased's relatives that they tried everything they could to save their loved ones. If these same problems, however, occur in HIV-positive patients, the cause of death is considered to be AIDS. Accordingly, the victims become part of the 'statistical evidence' that AIDS can be transmitted through blood transfusion.

In the United States, out of the 20,000 hemophiliacs, who rely on regular blood transfusions, few are diagnosed with AIDS despite the fact that over three quarters were infected with HIV through blood supply. Mortality rates for hemophiliacs, in fact, have never been as low as they are today.

It has been proven that blood transfusions can bring up false-positive HIV test results. In a study published in the *Lancet,* patients showed the presence of large quantities of HIV antibodies in their blood immediately after blood transfusion, decreasing thereafter. One healthy volunteer who received six consecutive blood injections at four-day intervals tested HIV-negative after the first injection, but with each subsequent transfusion the HIV-positive antibody response increased. The argument that HIV can be transmitted through blood transfusions may, therefore, only be partially true, if it is true at all. As the above experiment shows, blood transfusions can actually produce human retrovirus material that may be identical or similar to HIV. This certainly doesn't mean that an AIDS disease will automatically develop because of blood transfusion (most hemophiliacs don't develop AIDS). But if the immune system is already severely damaged or low due to other factors, such as drug abuse or surgery, blood transfusions can greatly increase the risk of developing a life-threatening immune deficiency disease or AIDS (see also *Business with Our Blood'* in the following chapter). If blood transfusions can lead to the body producing antibodies against the HIV human retrovirus, as research has shown to be possible, it is misleading to claim HIV-contaminated blood is solely responsible for HIV infection in blood recipients.

4. AIDS - A Metabolic Disorder, not an Infectious Disease

For several years it has been known that AIDS sufferers develop a drastic imbalance of very important amino acids *before* they actually deteriorate. A balanced protein metabolism is the main prerequisite for a healthy immune system. If the concentration of some of the amino acids in the body is too high or too low the immune system can no longer fight acute infections. This is particularly true for AIDS diseases.

The physiological imbalances related to basic protein metabolism in AIDS patients can be caused by any of the above factors, which all have highly stressful effects on the body. To combat such severe stress, the body triggers stress hormones, such as *cortisone,* designed to break down muscle proteins into basic amino acids needed for emergency reuse. This effectively means that the body is feeding off itself. If the stress persists, the amino acid balance can no longer be maintained, which eventually causes the collapse of the immune system so typically found in the AIDS disease.

During the process of destroying its own cells to obtain essential amino acids, the body has to deal with a large amount of cell debris, including the fragments from destroyed cell nucleus. It seems that some of these DNA or RNA fragments are labeled as the retrovirus HIV. Since there are various types of such fragments, there are also several types of HIV, i.e. HIV1, HIV2, etc. as well. This may explain why there are so many people now who are HIV-positive, but never were infected by HIV-contaminated blood or were in contact with HIV-infected people. Research by Dr. Hulda Clark, Canada, showed that babies can test HIV-positive, despite the fact that their parents are HIV-negative.

HIV is much more common than most people think. Many people who go through periods of extreme stress may have a strong presence of HIV in their blood for which their immune systems produce antibodies. Since they are unlikely to test for AIDS, they may never find out that they have encountered this virus. Even if they underwent a reliable AIDS test, they may not test positive for HIV1. However, if the test also searched for presence of antibodies for HIV3 or another of its variations, these individuals may now turn out to be HIV positive. For many years, the testing facilities in most countries could detect only one of the many HIV types. Today, a person's blood may be screened for two types of HIV, which is still not enough to determine whether he is HIV positive or not (considering the high false-positive rates of HIV tests).

Unless the individual's stress reaction continues, he may lead a perfectly healthy life. But if stress-caused cellular destruction becomes a long-term issue, the amino acid balance becomes increasingly disturbed. This in turn may drain the immune system to such an extent that it can no longer defend the body against even the low level infection-causing agents that permanently linger in everyone's body. When the host's immune system fails to neutralize the germs, a simple bacterium can cause a life-threatening infection, as seen among many AIDS patients.

Drug addicts, very active homosexuals, babies born to mothers with an unbalanced amino acid pool, people who are in need of a blood transfusion or have had one, and those who are undernourished, starving, or are otherwise traumatized, all are suffering from an unbalanced amino acid pool and are, therefore, possible candidates for HIV particle generation. Intense stress responses cause the breakdown of cell nucleus, which results in an increased presence of DNA or RNA fragments. The first and natural response by the body is to produce antibodies to these fragments. As mentioned before, Multiple Sclerosis, malaria, hepatitis B and C, tuberculosis, glandular fever, papilloma virus warts, and many other ailments can cause the body to make antibodies for the retrovirus P24. If immunity becomes subdued through any major illness or constant stress, a flood of disease-causing agents begin to invade the body. Wherever the body is most vulnerable and exposed is where the AIDS disease is likely to strike first.

Narcotic Drugs and Rectal Intercourse Can Cause AIDS

Use of intravenous morphine and heroin alters the basic metabolism of the body. The body's own natural morphine compounds, called *endorphins*, are not only capable of reducing pain and producing euphoria, but they also suppress hunger sensation. People who use heroin or morphine tend to lose their appetite and subsequently stop eating and taking enough fluids. The body, while detecting a famine and dehydration, begins the cortisone release mechanisms to try to survive the food and water shortage. When this mechanism reaches a certain level, it will cause an imbalance of the amino acid pool in the blood and lead to an increased breakdown of cell nucleus. The DNA assembly line (double-stranded helix) collapses into its segments of proteins which the body, in turn, uses to restore the amino acid balance to whatever extent possible. These fragments are what tests reveal to be HIV particles. HIV results from a strong imbalance of essential amino acids in the body, which in this case is caused by drug abuse.

This understanding of HIV matches the basic characteristic of HIV being a human retrovirus, and due to its natural design, is not able to kill or harm cells. HIV by itself has no capability of entering a living cell and breaking up the DNA or RNA assembly line, but the body's own *cortisone* can if stress is severe and prolonged enough.

Intravenous drug users who share HIV contaminated needles may test HIV-positive as a result of exposure to the foreign DNA fragments (HIV), but if they die from an AIDS disease it is because of an imbalance in their own amino acid pool. The continued depletion of certain amino acids such as *cystine, cysteine,* or *tryptophan* leads to a suspension of antibody production and, eventually, to a total collapse of the immune system. This is AIDS. All intravenous drug users are at risk of eventually producing HIV particles and developing AIDS diseases.

The same applies to people who have regular rectal intercourse, not because they can infect each other with HIV, but because this unnatural form of sexual practice causes constantly occurring intestinal injury, thus depleting the body's amino acid reserves. As a result of the constant internal injuries, a massive number of cells have to be dismembered, cleared, and replaced continually, which produces a long-term depletion of the body's protein reserves. When one or more amino acids become depleted, DNA or RNA molecules break apart, leaving behind their protein fragments labeled HIV. Therefore HIV is the *effect* of immune deficiency and *not* its cause.

The cells of AIDS patients are consistently short of the amino acid *cysteine* and its precursor *cystine*, which may result from one or several of the causes mentioned before. Laboratory research has demonstrated that when amino acid depleted cells are given back the missing amino acids, these cells stop producing HIV particles because their DNA and RNA molecules are able to sustain their assembly line.

In addition, regular discharge of human semen into the rectum, which has no natural defense lines against the immune-repressive properties of the semen that bathes the sperm, eventually leads to a shutdown of normal repair work and cell replacement. This causes chronic toxicity, which also acts as a constant blow to an already weakened immune system.

Malnutrition, Dehydration, and Starvation Can Also Cause AIDS

As in drug-caused malnutrition, lack of proper nourishment activates the body's stress responses to the point that it starts feeding on itself. This is necessary to keep the amino acid pool balanced. But when too many muscle cells are broken down to release the missing amino acids, large amounts of DNA or RNA fragments are generated which the body tries to neutralize by producing antibodies. The same stress response occurs in cellular dehydration. A severely dehydrated person would, therefore, test HIV-positive.

In the developing world, particularly in Africa, malnutrition, dehydration and starvation have existed for centuries. During a famine, people naturally start feeding on their own bodies. The byproduct of this survival attempt of the body is HIV material, consisting of DNA or RNA fragments. Consequently, the immune system produces antibodies to render these viral particles harmless. Although many of the people in Africa have received inactive HIV from their parents, who at some stage in their lives have gone through a famine, others have produced it themselves from their bodies' natural response to malnutrition.

Wherever the AIDS test is introduced in developing countries, large numbers of the population test HIV positive either because of false-positive HIV tests or because they or their parents once had to endure a famine. The HIV of the latter group is mainly the result of malnutrition or related illnesses, which is clearly demonstrated in the case of the 360,000 HIV-infected and undernourished Haitians. By contrast, the HIV of developed countries results mostly from the above mentioned causes. Although HIV and AIDS are two completely separate issues, they can occur in combination with one another:

1. In developed countries where homosexual intercourse, intravenous drug abuse, and blood transfusions are very common.

2. In Third World countries where wasting disorders such as 'slim disease', tuberculosis, and malaria exist in epidemic proportions.

5. AIDS Drugs Cause AIDS

Christie's story is a sad one. Her two foster-care children, Daniel and Martha, have tested HIV positive. Their birth mother, Christie's niece who is a long-term drug user, was unable to raise the children, so Christie offered to take care of them. Daniel had twice been sent to a Children's Center for HIV-positive children, once soon after he was born, and when he was four years old, and again recently. Her other child had also been taken to the center several months ago and has been kept there since. Christie was accused of being a negligent parent because she refused to give her children the prescribed AIDS drugs.

These children have had a clean bill of health and never showed any sign of illness. But when city health agencies found out the kids weren't on the drugs, they removed them from their guardian and sent them to an AIDS clinic for mandatory treatment, and after that, to the Children's Center. Each day they are forced to take a cocktail of powerful, debilitating and potentially fatal AIDS drugs, such as *AZT*, *Nevirapine*, *Epivir*, *Zerit*, and others. Many of the children there are unable to tolerate so many medications, and so they are drugged through a tube in their stomachs. If a child refuses drugs too many times, they take them away for an operation to feed the drugs directly into the stomach.

And what is the purpose of drugging those healthy HIV positive kids? AIDS research is going to generate the biggest profits from drug sales in the world. There is a whole list of drug studies on children either still running or recently concluded. The research is sponsored by government agencies such as National Institute of Allergy and Infectious Diseases and National Institute of Child Health and Human Development, and huge pharmaceutical companies such as Glaxo, Pfizer, Squibb and Genentech. One of the studies, 'The Effect of Anti-HIV Treatment on Body Characteristics of HIV-Infected Children' seeks to identify the causes of 'Wasting and Lipodystrophy [fat redistribution]' by using drugs known to cause wasting and lipodystrophy. Another study looks at 'The Safety and Effectiveness of Treating Advanced AIDS Patients between the Ages of 4 and 22 with Seven Drugs, Some at Higher than Usual Doses'. Although the seven drugs in the study are all known to cause some of the most severe side effects seen by any drug on the market, they are administered at 'higher than usual doses' in four-year-olds. A third study is using the drug *Stavudine* by itself, or in combination with *Didanosine*. The combined drug cocktail has killed pregnant women.

Then there is the vaccine study involving children of ages 2 months to 8 years. The children are being administered 'live chicken pox virus', despite the fact that live virus vaccine can actually cause chicken pox.

Another study measures 'HIV Levels in Cerebrospinal Fluid'. To obtain cerebrospinal fluid, it has to be gathered from a spinal tap, a dangerous and invasive procedure. And although this may be hard to believe, there is a study on HIV-negative children who were born to HIV-infected mothers that uses an experimental HIV vaccine. The parents or guardians of these legally kidnapped children are rarely ever informed that their kids are subjects or rather, guinea pigs, in these clinical trials. The law prevents them from trying to save their children from the holocaust of human experimentation. The National Institute of Health (NIH) is legally permitted to use HIV-positive children of impoverished, drug-addicted mothers unable to care for them, as test subjects. So far, dozens of trials with AZT and Nevirapine were conducted through the late 90s. And there are 227 studies ongoing or currently completed. The studies are sponsored by NIH subdivisions; many are cosponsored by the pharmaceutical companies that manufacture the drugs being tested. The studies use the standard AIDS drugs: nucleoside analogues, protease inhibitors and Nevirapine. Side effects described on the warning labels of these drugs include:

- Interfering with normal cell division
- Cancer
- Heart Disease

- Preventing formation of new blood
- Bone marrow destruction
- Anemia
- Death in pregnant mothers
- Spontaneous abortion
- Birth defects
- Severe liver damage and liver failure
- Pancreatic failure
- Muscle wasting
- Developmental damage
- Death in children and adults
- Interference with the body's ability to build new proteins
- Bizarre, grotesque physical appearance
- Wasting in the face, arms and legs
- Fatty humps on the back and shoulders
- Distended belly
- Organ failure due to drug toxicity
- Stevens-Johnson Syndrome - a grotesque, violent skin disorder

Despite the fact that these poisonous drugs destroy the human immune system (=AIDS) and have not shown to have any curative effect, they are nevertheless prescribed routinely now. The producers of AIDS drugs protect themselves against liability suits by placing the following notice on the drug labels:

"This drug will not cure your HIV infection. Patients receiving antiretroviral therapy may continue to experience opportunistic infections and other complications of HIV disease. Patients should be advised that the long-term effects are unknown at this time."

The only reason people take these drugs is because they test positive for HIV. Their only (often fatal) mistake is that they don't read or understand the HIV test kit labels and the drug labels. This is especially sad when children are involved.

The Administration for Children's Services (ACS) came down hard on Christie for not drugging her son Daniel. They forced Daniel to go on the 'miracle drug' Nevirapine and within six months, he was on life support due to organ failure. When they put her healthy daughter Martha on a cocktail of AIDS drugs, it completely destroyed her immune system, making her susceptible to constant disease flare-ups she otherwise would never have experienced. The main question is why are doctors permitted and even encouraged to treat AIDS patients with drugs that kill their immune systems? Wouldn't it make more sense to help them build their immunity? These questions will need to be raised again and again if we want to tackle disease in general and AIDS-type illnesses specifically.

Summary: HIV, which consists of human DNA or RNA fragments, cannot be considered to be the cause of AIDS. AIDS, which is an umbrella name for a number of different illnesses that all share a disrupted metabolism and immune system, is caused by one or several major risk factors. If a healthy person *acquires* HIV through an external source, i.e., through contact with HIV-infected blood or through the mother, it is rendered harmless and inactive by the host's immune system. Such a person would have produced antibodies for HIV in his blood just as he would for any other previously encountered viral particles. He is in no greater danger of developing an AIDS disease than any other person without HIV does, as can be seen, for example, in the vast majority of HIV-infected Africans or Asians.

The occurrence of DNA or RNA fragments (HIV) in the blood of a person who actually *produces* abnormal cell destruction, on the other hand, indicates the presence of a serious immune deficiency. Malnutrition, starvation, dehydration, recurring injuries, or cell suffocation from internal congestion results in an imbalance of the body's amino acid pool. To correct such an imbalance the body begins to break down its own cell nuclei in order to obtain the missing amino acids. If there is a shortage of even one amino acid in the body, the percentage composition of all the other amino acids also becomes unbalanced. This can have a simultaneous catastrophic effect on the cells and their nucleus throughout the body. The destruction of cell nucleus results in DNA or RNA fragments; the fragments consist of human proteins called retrovirus. HIV is one the many retroviruses that can be generated in this way. Thus, HIV, which is generated within the body through destruction of cell nucleus, cannot be considered to be the cause of AIDS; it is an unavoidable byproduct of the body's fight for survival. This fight may eventually lead to the destruction of the immune system which is called AIDS.

AIDS - A Process of Awakening

Mankind is rapidly awakening to a new level of understanding that will discriminate between false and correct information. We are living in a time where scandals can no longer be concealed from the public eye. Whatever may be the truth about any subject, it will eventually dominate in collective consciousness. People will simply know from within themselves what is right and what is wrong. The AIDS phenomenon is one of today's great challenges that can urge someone to search for the solutions to his problems within. Andrew, who was my first AIDS patient, made this realization almost instantly.

When I met Andrew five years ago, he was a young homosexual with fully developed AIDS symptoms. He was emotionally unbalanced, depressed and extremely sensitive. He lived in Athens, where, in his opinion, nightlife was the only thing 'worth living for'. First, I motivated him to become a 'day person' again. The Ayurvedic routine, cleansing procedures, improved nutrition, daily meditation, etc. soon improved the multiple lesions on his skin, steadily increased his T-cell counts, and what he felt was most remarkable, improved his appetite and digestion. With all that, his joy of living returned, but the new kind of joy was quite different to what he had ever before experienced. It was the joy of waking up, of appreciating the sun, nature, and day life, rather than clubs, drugs, and nightlife.

When I met Andrew a few years later, he was completely free of all signs of AIDS. He was used to the idea that he was still HIV positive, and with the understanding I was able to provide him with about this virus, it wasn't even important anymore whether he had antibodies against it or not. What he knew was that he had overcome AIDS, which was most essential for his self-esteem and happiness. The stigma of HIV was no longer a matter of disgrace to him. Andrew had changed from being a victim of a disease (that didn't exist) to a person worthy of love, appreciation and recognition. This is what AIDS can do. It can awaken a person to living his life with greater love, dignity, and purpose.

Note: To remove HIV and all disease-causing pathogens, and to restore immune health, please see information about Mineral Miracle Supplement (MMS) and Ojibwa tea in Chapter 7.

CHAPTER 13

Eight Dangerous Myths of Modern Living and How to Shrug Off Each One

1. Antibiotics, Bugs and Why We Attract Them

Are Antibiotics Really Necessary?

Antibiotics have dominated the field of health for nearly 60 years. Known as a 'magic bullet' treatment or 'miracle drug', antibiotics, meaning 'against life', can speedily destroy hordes of disease-causing bacteria. They are the most popular choice of the medical profession for stopping infections and relieving pain. At least one of every six prescriptions written each year is for an antibiotic drug. Antibiotics are so popular with doctors and patients because they provide relief very quickly.

Having grown up in a generation in which antibiotics are frequently prescribed for a stubborn case of cystitis, a sore throat or an itchy skin rash, we may readily accept that the 'magic bullet' prescribed by the doctor is the best option to deal with such bacterial infections. Although every medical student knows that viral infections (including colds and the flu) do not respond to antibiotics, millions of people who are afflicted with these ills still receive antibiotic prescriptions from their doctors. In 1983, more than 32 million Americans visited a doctor for treatment of the common cold and 95 percent of them went home with a prescription drug. More than half of them were unnecessarily given a prescription for an antibiotic. Now 25 years later, this trend has nearly doubled.

Patients are rarely informed that even a single dose of a broad-spectrum antibiotic drug can severely damage the natural flora of the intestinal tract and the blood-forming red bone marrow for as many as four to five years. In the majority of cases, patients do not read the list of side effects written on the drug labels or direction sheets. They simply trust that their doctor knows what's best for them.

It is very disconcerting that many doctors don't even know that penicillin, for example, won't cure a cold or flu. Because of their very design, antibiotics impair the immune system and hence may sow the seeds for problems more serious than a cold in the future. Besides, a cold is not an illness, but rather the body's first and best emergency response to rid itself of toxins. The virus only serves as a trigger for this cleansing response to occur. If you do 'catch' a cold, consider it a blessing rather than a curse, and allow the body to heal itself.

Since most people prefer a quick-fix 'cure' to a time-consuming one, antibiotics have become one of the most preferable forms of treatment today. However, it may take a minimum of 24 hours before infection-causing bacteria can be identified. So the doctor, being pressed for time, tends to use a broad-spectrum drug that can wipe out every microorganism it meets, including those that help *protect* us against disease. This may be justified in the rare event of a life-threatening infection, but certainly not for the vast majority of relatively mild infections. To make matters worse, in a large number of cases specific antibiotics are administered to patients with symptoms of infection even before the lab sample has been analyzed. The chances that they will receive the wrong drug or take a drug for no reason at all are at least 50 percent.

If a man suffering from sinusitis leaves the doctor's office empty-handed and 'merely' receives advice on how to deal with his illness in a more natural way, he may think that his doctor hasn't done his job or is irresponsible. The physician too, facing a viral infection, often prefers the comparatively 'safe' option of an antibiotic to being blamed for not doing enough for the patient, particularly when the patient is a child. Otherwise, the doctor might even risk a lawsuit against him. Even though the probability that a child really requires antibiotics is as low as 1 in 100,000 cases, nearly 95 percent of all children taken to the doctor are given such drugs. In most of these cases, antibiotics are being misused 'to please'" overly worried mothers.

Antibiotics Damage the Immune System

"Antibiotics can hijack the immune system, leaving the body unable to defend itself," says New York-based family physician and natural medicine advocate Fred Pescatore, M.D., author of *Feed Your Kids Well* (Wiley). These anti-life drugs are routinely prescribed for benign or harmless infections. In any case, an infection is not a disease; it represents the body's natural responsiveness to neutralize and remove toxic substances that are generated by such simple events as overeating, dehydration, consumption of junk foods, and previous exposure to antibiotics. The body pays a high price for being exposed to antibiotics. The poison of the drug destroys not only infectious bacteria (pathogens) but also friendly bacteria that help us digest our food, remove toxins, and produce important micro-nutrients such as B vitamins. As these essential, beneficial bacteria become eradicated by the drug, the gut's population of destructive bacteria begins to rapidly grow and dominate the intestinal tract (see section on Candida), turning even nutritious food into strong irritants or poison.

The immune system, of which approximately 75 percent is located in the gastrointestinal tract, tries to neutralize both pathogens and irritants by mobilizing its powerful defense forces. It uses the complex biological response of inflammation to protect the body against these injurious stimuli as well as to initiate the healing process for the affected tissue. Such an inflammatory response may occur anywhere in the body. Swellings of the lymph nodes, fever, skin eruptions, etc., are all indications that the immune system is responding and still intact. This fight can take from 2-6 days or longer, depending on the extent to which a previous course of antibiotics has suppressed the immune system and damaged the natural intestinal flora.

Antibiotic treatment merely succeeds in masking the symptoms of an infection while giving the impression that the patient has conquered the illness, whereas in truth, it has become much worse. Antibiotics actually prepare the ground for chronic disease to develop in the future. Since they stop an acute illness that the body uses to help detoxify itself, the toxins will no longer circulate but are instead deposited in the deeper structures of tissues and organs. Much of the antibiotics remain in the bile ducts of the liver, which in turn alters bile flora and leads to the development of gallstones in the liver bile ducts and gallbladder.

Each new course of antibiotics further disrupts the immune system and intestinal flora, as well as the bile flora, making room for disease-causing microbes to spread throughout the body. With regular intake of antibiotics, the immune system becomes so weak and passive that it is no longer able to defend the body against real life-threatening situations, including those that lead to cancer, heart disease, arthritis diabetes, MS and AIDS. This applies to people everywhere, both in the developed and the underdeveloped world.

For decades, large groups of East Africa's population have been exposed to antibiotics for 'experimental purposes'. Many drugs that are banned in industrialized nations because of their life-endangering side effects are being sold in the drugstores of developing countries. Their powerful immune-suppressive effects may explain the appearance of many new types of diseases that have never occurred in Africa before. Consequently, these immune-suppressive drugs may have actually triggered the recurrence of old infectious diseases, such as tuberculosis.

Biological Warfare

The antibiotic approach to treating infections is costing human society more than anyone could have anticipated. The bugs that were 'successfully' subdued with antibiotics for decades are now taking revenge by producing what is known as 'antibiotic-resistant organisms', i.e. superbugs that defy antibiotic treatment. Some 90,000 Americans suffer potentially deadly infections each year from a drug-resistant 'staph superbug'. According to the U.S. Centers for Disease Control (CDC), more people now die from these superbugs than from AIDS diseases. Recent nationwide outbreaks of infections caused by superbugs killed teenagers in U.S. schools, reflecting the natural consequence of indiscriminate and irresponsible use of antibiotics in this country.

Previously only found in hospital settings, the drug-resistant staph germ is now spreading through prisons, gyms and locker rooms, and poor urban neighborhoods. It can enter the blood, kidneys, liver, lungs and muscles around the heart. Most cases exhibit life-threatening bloodstream infections. However, about 10 percent of the cases involved the so-called flesh-eating disease, according to the study led by researchers at the federal CDC. It is estimated that 18,650 people die annually from this particular superbug, which is about 1,500 more than those who die from AIDS in the U.S. each year.

It is a law of nature that every living organism wants to live and survive for as long as it possibly can. Bacteria that are exposed to regular supplies of the poisonous antibiotic substances will, therefore, try to become immune to the poisons. To survive such assaults, bacteria have their own sophisticated defense strategies, which are in a way similar to ours when we need to defend ourselves against invasive bacteria or viruses. One possible way for bacteria to evade an antibiotic attack is to mutate their genes. As a result, the bacteria become resistant to the active ingredients of a drug, which subsequently renders the drug ineffective.

You may have wondered why so many brands of antibiotics stay on the market for relatively short periods of time. One reason for this is that the bacteria keep outsmarting the antibiotics, and more powerful drugs are then needed kill the newly created strains of bacteria. Another reason for withdrawing brands from the market is the increasingly frequent occurrence of serious side effects that arise from repeatedly giving the drugs to the same patients.

The more we use these drugs, the more resistant the bacteria will become. Top researchers in this field already admit that they are fighting a losing battle. We have overused antibiotics to a degree that every disease-causing bacterium has now developed mutated versions that resist at least one antibiotic.

When an antibiotic attacks a colony of bacteria, *most* of them die. Yet some of the microbes survive because they harbor mutant genes that resist destruction. These mutant bacteria then pass on their resistant genes to other bacteria, and within 24 hours each of them may have left an estimated 16,777,220 offspring, equally resistant to the antibiotic.

The nightmare doesn't stop here. The mutant bacteria begin to share their resistant genes with other unrelated microbes they contact, making all sorts of microorganisms resistant to treatment as well. The well-known microbiologist Stanley Falkow once said that bacteria are 'clever little devils' that can become resistant to drugs they've never met and anticipate confrontations with other ones. In this way, bacteria become supergerms or superbugs, capable of evading any attack by drugs. They lurk particularly in places where antibiotics are most often used, i.e. hospitals and nursing homes. According to recent research findings, five to ten percent of all people checking into hospitals today are going to get infected as a result of antibiotic-resistant bacteria lodging within these buildings.

Except for the sterile environment of surgery theatres, the superbugs can be found riding on dust particles of the heating and air-conditioning systems, in bathrooms and toilets, and even in the food. They account for most of the deaths in hospitals today. The superbugs "choose" those patients whose immune systems have already been impaired through sickness, injury, surgery, and/or previous encounters with antibiotics. In healthy people with a strong immune system, these bugs can live on their skin or in their noses without infecting them. In other words, under normal circumstances, we can live with the bugs without ever getting infected and, even if we did get infected, our body would deal with them effectively while becoming immune to them. However, this natural resistance to the bugs decreases drastically with the first course of antibiotics taken for a simple infection.

Because of the excessive use of antibiotics inside and outside of hospitals, antibiotic-resistant organisms have now become the most common cause of infection. To make matters worse, in many countries people can now acquire antibiotics over the counter. Since precise dosage depends on the individual and the potency of the infection, and since there is no clear time limit to the number of courses a person may require to kill all the germs, antibiotics can never be considered "safe." Interrupted intake or too low a drug dose can encourage the growth of resistant bacteria, which may allow them to be passed on to other people as well. This may increase the risk of infection for those who are near a person who takes antibiotics and may explain why infection is higher in families where they have been used before. However, to become infected, other predisposing factors must be in place, such as poor diet and inadequate personal hygiene.

Indiscriminate use of antibiotics seems to be doing more damage than we can even begin to understand. Antibiotics are among the most powerful immune-suppressants that exist. Most people who are ill and die don't actually die from their diseases. They die from opportunistic bacterial infections that invade while their immune systems are depleted. This applies to cancer, AIDS, and most other so-called "killer diseases." Autopsies revealed that many of the patients who died from an "AIDS" disease had never actually been infected with HIV but were killed by antibiotic-resistant superbugs. These bugs cause similar symptoms to the ones considered AIDS diseases. It is difficult to determine how many millions of AIDS victims are actually victims of antibiotic–resistant bacteria. (Also see chapter 12.)

Antibiotics Can Cause Asthma in Children

Many of you may wonder why so many children develop asthma at a very early age. Now "CHEST." the journal of the *American College of Chest Physicians,* shed some light on this phenomenon. It published a study conducted by researchers at University of Manitoba and McGill University in Montreal, which links childhood asthma to the use of antibiotics. The researchers showed that using antibiotics in the first year of life may double a child's risk of contracting asthma by age 7. They examined a prescription database that included information on 13,116 children and compared incidence of asthma with a variety of risk factors that besides antibiotics included, gender, maternal asthma history, living location, neighborhood income, the presence of pets in the home and the number of siblings at the age of seven.

The higher the number of antibiotic treatments, the higher the incidence of asthma, according to the study. The researchers also found that 87 percent of children who had received antibiotics were treated for respiratory tract infections. However, to be sure the increased incidence of asthma in young children stemmed from the use of antibiotics and not from respiratory ailments, the researchers excluded these cases from the study.

Interestingly, the same study showed that the presence of a dog in the house during the first year of life led to a reduced risk of contracting asthma, even if antibiotics were used. "Dogs bring germs into the home, and it is thought that this exposure is required for the infant's immune system to develop normally. Other research has shown that the presence of a dog in early life protects against the development of asthma," said lead researcher Anita Kozyrskyj.

Losing the Battle with Disease?

The world is not only experiencing a vast number of new man-made epidemics, but old diseases, too, are making a comeback. In 1978, the United Nations adopted a 'Health for All, 2000' resolution, setting goals for eradicating infectious disease by the century's end. But the germs didn't co-operate. Apart from at least 29 previously unknown diseases, 20 well-known ones have re-emerged, including malaria, tuberculosis, pneumonia, cholera, yellow fever and dysentery. The germs causing the diseases are rapidly mutating to forms beyond the reach of today's antibiotics.

Drugs that once cured malaria are being foiled by the mosquito-borne parasite. Its 'changing coat' of mutations baffles scientists. Yesterday's 'super drugs' have become today's weapons of self-destruction. A century of using quinine-based drugs as a prophylactic in people who did not even have malaria has fostered the evolution of new strains of quinine-resistant malaria that defy conventional treatment. The only substance that has shown to cure this type of malaria (within 4 to 8 hours) as well as other similar infections is chlorine dioxide (see Miracle Mineral Supplement (MMS) in chapter 7).

Hemorrhagic dengue, another mosquito fever, has recently struck in India, Africa, and parts of Latin America after an absence of at least half a century. An Asian strain of cholera reached Latin America in 1991 and at least 1.3 million people have been stricken. But it is not just the developing world that is afflicted. The U.S. death rate from infectious diseases rose 58 percent between 1980 and 1992. In 1995, hemorrhagic dengue reached Texas. We seem to be in a battle we cannot win, using the same old symptom-oriented approaches. What is most disconcerting is that those who have used the 'magic bullet' approach to disease in the past have contributed greatly to the new wave of infectious diseases that are sweeping the globe. In a sense, man is now forced to become aware of his mistakes and to employ natural methods of healing instead of using drugs that are designed to kill biological organisms. Tuberculosis (TB) is a typical example of this learning process.

Tuberculosis - Nature Fighting Back

Once the world's premier killer disease, tuberculosis (TB) has now developed resistance to multiple drugs and claims millions of lives each year. The World Health Organization has declared TB a global emergency. In 1990 the disease earned itself the title of the world's number one killer pathogen, responsible for the deaths of nearly three million people worldwide. Fifty years of using antibiotics in the treatment of diseases has made the TB bug so resistant to treatment that, wherever it finds fertile ground, it causes death, especially in developing countries where hygiene is often very poor.

The Western Hemisphere, however, is no longer safe from TB either. The first modern epidemic broke out in New York in 1990 followed by others in several parts of America and Britain. In 2007 an incident involving a TB-infected American man traveling in an airplane sent panic waves through the nation. These superbugs can travel around the world in almost no time. AIDS patients, people regularly treated with antibiotics or those living in poor and unhygienic environments are particularly endangered.

Out of the 40 variations of antibiotics available for the treatment of TB, only one or two still seem to have an effect.

Nobody can foresee the consequences of our collective action in making antibiotics the treatment of preference for infectious diseases. You may remember from chapter 8 that sunlight used to be the preferred and most successful treatment for TB (more about this below). UV-light still is the natural antidote to any germ, including superbugs, yet our obsession with drugs prevents us from even considering the use of a cost-free solution with no side effects. But you and I can make a difference when it comes to creating a healthy world by choosing not to take antibiotics.

Several years ago a major report on drug prescription revealed that 80 percent of all prescribed drugs are of only 'marginal' use, which means that it does not make a difference whether we take them or not, except for the side effects they produce. We are now reaping the consequences of this massive abuse of 'medical' drugs. We have created an entire armory consisting of highly sophisticated antibiotic-resistant weapons - superbugs that defy even the smartest of treatments.

TB took 1,000 million lives within the previous two centuries, but then the deadly disease was nearly eradicated from the earth through a combination of public hygiene measures and antibiotics. One may argue that without the use of antibiotics the disease could never have been brought under control. However, the latest statistical reviews show that TB had decreased *dramatically* through the introduction of new hygiene measures *before* TB-antibiotics were introduced. This clearly demonstrates that antibiotics did not eradicate TB, but improved hygiene measures did.

Today, the situation is not much different. TB strikes where hygiene is poor since dirt is a major source of spreading infectious diseases. Good hygiene, however, does not only include clean fresh water, nutritious food, and proper sanitary conditions, it is also a matter of cleanliness inside our bodies. Modern lifestyle and eating habits have turned our intestines into pools of filth - ideal breeding places for pathogens.

TB and other infectious diseases that defy modern treatment compel man to make major changes for himself and his world. In fact, to live comfortably and without mass epidemics we will have to change nearly everything, from improving our diet to balancing our lifestyle, drastically reducing environmental pollution, regularly exposing the body to the sun, and increasing psychological health. These factors make all the difference with regard to building natural resistance to disease-causing germs of any kind, including TB.

Just one simple adjustment in a person's lifestyle - regular sun exposure - could save millions of lives. Researchers from Queen Mary's School of Medicine and Dentistry, London, and the Wellcome Trust Centre for Research in Clinical Tropical Medicine, Imperial College London, carried out a study at Newham University Hospital and Northwick Park Hospital in London with patients who had been exposed to TB. They found that over 90 percent of TB patients had a vitamin D deficiency. Their findings came from a study that identified an extraordinarily high incidence of vitamin D deficiency amongst those communities in London most at risk from the disease, which kills over two million people each year. In Britain, the amount of sunlight between October and April is usually insufficient to make vitamin D in the skin so much of the population becomes deficient during the winter and spring.

It is a fact that the main source of the body's vitamin D comes from exposing the skin to sunlight. Scientists have shown that a single 2.5 mg dose of vitamin D may be enough to boost the immune system to fight against tuberculosis (TB) and similar bacteria for at least 6 weeks. Of course sunlight is more effective than supplementation. Regular sun exposure, which is a necessity for healthy vital humans, animals and plants, could prevent and eradicate TB for good.

Antibiotic-resistant organisms cannot be eradicated from the surface of the earth, and this may not even be necessary, as we can see from the above research. Although genetically mutated, these and other microbes still require an unclean environment to live and to survive; their population is naturally reduced in size when their food supply becomes limited. Our body's 'ecosystem' is not exempt from this law of nature. The belief that man is powerful enough to bypass the laws of nature and use antibiotic drugs for minor infectious diseases is crushed by a few evasive microbes we cannot even see with our bare eyes. The more people stop 'feeding and fighting' them, the less dangerous they will become for us humans. This is a major lesson for survival on the planet.

Candida - Microbes versus Microbes

An increasing number of Natural Health Care Providers acknowledge that a clean intestinal tract with the proper balance of 'beneficial' and 'destructive' bacteria is one of the most important foundations for achieving a continuous state of optimal health. A healthy intestinal tract is inhabited by over 400 different species of bacteria, of which there are thousands of strains. The delicate balance between the two basic types of bacteria constituting the intestinal flora becomes easily disturbed through the use of antibiotics.

One of the most common side effects of using antibiotics against infection is the overgrowth of *Candida albicans*—a natural and even necessary yeast inhabitant of our gut. A popular misconception is that Candida albicans is a prime enemy of the body and therefore should be eradicated by all means. But nothing could be further from the truth. Candida albicans is one of the essential microorganisms in the body that are termed 'saprophytic', meaning they decompose dead, potentially toxic tissue. Candida only proliferates to help the body prevent a major toxicity crisis. Candida albicans is not out to harm the body. Candida overgrowth problems tend to gradually lessen as the body detoxifies itself.

Candida albicans also helps to break down sugar. When carbohydrate digestion is incomplete or impaired, you can expect a drastic increase of these microbes. Under normal circumstances, Candida bacteria, which reside in most mucus membranes, are kept in check by beneficial, so-called 'probiotic' bacteria, such as *lactobacillus acidophilus* and *bifido*. We have more of these beneficial bacteria in our body than we have cells, and one third of our eliminated fecal matter consists of these tiny helpers. We actually could not survive without them. When excessive amounts of undigested carbohydrates (sugars), harmful waste matter and damaged or dead cells are present in the gut, and the need for the destructive type of bacteria (versus probiotic bacteria) increases. Hence, the proliferation of Candida.

Antibiotics, which target the specific microbes linked to some kind of infection, also kill off the probiotic bacteria in the gut. Subsequently, Candida production goes into overdrive and spreads like mold throughout the intestinal tract. This greatly interferes with the activity of enzymes that break down food, resulting in poor digestion and bloating. If the Candida continues to grow, it develops tentacles that penetrate the bowel walls allowing toxins to enter other parts of the body, including the brain. This can cause an entire range of physical and emotional symptoms. These include sinusitis, ear infections, gastrointestinal dysfunction, weight gain, water retention, hormonal imbalance, mental confusion, depression, insomnia, anxiety, chronic fatigue, vaginitis, increased premenstrual tension, urinary tract infection (cystitis), oral thrush, skin and nail infection, conjunctivitis, constipation, kidney problems, gallstones, and food cravings, particularly for sugar and sweets.

Besides antibiotics, other drugs such as the contraceptive pill and Hormone Replacement Therapy (HRT) have been shown to cause Candida. The latter two increase vaginal glucose by up to 80 percent, which means more food for Candida bacteria. The typical modern junk food diet that is high in fat and sugar contributes to a further spread of Candida. Like most other disorders, Candida too is but a toxicity crisis, and merely one of the body's natural responses to rid itself of accumulated toxins and suffocated, dead cells. Candida spreads wherever toxins need to be 'digested'. Any weakening influence that robs the body of its energy reserves leads to a buildup of toxins and helps to spread Candida further.

Dealing with Candida Infection

A survey of 3,000 patients who had been treated for Candida-related problems revealed that 90 percent of them had reported excessive and prolonged use of broad-spectrum antibiotics before being infected. Antibiotics cannot eradicate Candida bacteria. The more you try to get rid of them with drugs, the more resistant they become and the faster they repopulate.

If you are infected with Candida (yeast), you can starve them by depriving them of the toxins and foods that cause them to multiply. As long as the liver has gallstones, re-infection is almost guaranteed. A series of liver cleanses that releases all stones is one of the most thorough ways to deal with them. Fasting with only water for 3-5 days has also been shown to pacify Candida overgrowth, but fasting this long may be difficult for many people, especially if they are Vata types. Once the food source (toxic waste) is reduced, the yeast bacteria will soon begin to withdraw to their original sites and diminish.

Along with liver flushing, a diet consisting of foods that cause the least amount of digestive trouble and toxicity is able to restore the intestinal flora. Eating fresh salads, freshly cooked vegetables, Basmati rice, millet, beans, lentils, (only if unavoidable), freshly prepared vegetable soups, rice cakes, oatmeal/porridge, and bananas are suitable for most Candida sufferers. Avoid meat, fish, and other cadaver foods or their products. Remember, destructive bacteria target dead cells. Drink plenty of fresh water and herbal teas that have a bitter taste, such as *Chaparral*. Essiac tea (8-herb formula) has shown some of the best results I have seen (see Product Information). Also 2-4 cups of Pau d'Arco (Lapacho) tea a day can help improve the Candida balance. The same applies to green tea and cranberry juice concentrate. The product *Primal Defense* has also proved beneficial for some Candida sufferers, but not for everyone.

Apply the muscle test to all the foods and beverages you normally consume. It is most likely that the following food items will make your arm muscle weak and further the growth of Candida: sugar, yeast or yeast-containing foods such as bread, cakes, biscuits; chocolate and other sweets; tomato ketchup, fruit (except banana), alcohol, Marmite, mushrooms, hard and blue cheeses; fermented products such as vinegar and fermented vegetables; coffee, tea, soft drinks, sports drinks; cigarettes or any other stimulant. You may also need to stop any hormone replacements, including the contraceptive pill and HRT, if applicable.

After a month of dietary restriction, you may be able to reintroduce some previously eaten foods to your diet but, if these cause bloating, they are most likely not part of your natural body-type diet. Candida can be a way to lead you towards a healthier and more fulfilling lifestyle (refer to chapters 6 and 7 for details).

Candida Spit Test: To find out whether you are dealing with a Candida issue, you can apply this simple spit test. After rising in the morning, rinse your mouth and get a glass of fresh water. Work up some saliva and spit into the glass. Observe what happens to the saliva during the next 30-40 minutes, and especially during the first few minutes. If you have a Candida infection, at least one of the following indicators will appear:

1. Strings forming from the floating spit, reaching into the lower parts of the water.
2. Strange-looking saliva at the bottom of the glass.
3. Cloudy specks suspended in the water.

The more quickly the strings and cloudy specks are formed, the more prevalent is the Candida overgrowth. If the above indicators occur right away, the Candida has spread to other parts of the body.

On the other hand, if the spit just floats on top and the water stays perfectly clear, you are unlikely affected by it. If you have extensive overgrowth, this test will show results even if you do it during the day.

If you experience three or more of the following symptoms, you may suffer from Candida overgrowth:

- You feel bloated when you eat or soon after eating.
- You develop gas when you eat.
- You experience acid reflux.
- You suffer from brain fog, drowsiness or headaches.
- You frequently have sinus or ear infections.
- You suffer from fatigue for no reason.
- Your mouth tends to be dry.
- You vision often goes from being blurry to clear, and back to blurry.
- Your blood sugar drops (hypoglycemia), especially in the afternoon.
- You feel shaky if you miss a meal, sleepy after a meal, sweat during sleep.
- You frequently have constipation, diarrhea, or both.
- You are anemic.
- You suffer from skin rashes.
- You have toenail or fingernail fungus.
- You experience repeated vaginal yeast infections or jock itch.

Other symptoms include short-term memory loss, mood swings, dizziness, loss of balance, lack of coordination, ear sensitivity/ringing/itching or fluid in the ears, mucus in stools, postnasal drip, frequent colds, tightness of the chest, white-coated tongue, bad breath, thyroid dysfunction, depression, or sugar craving.

Are Antibiotics Responsible for the Narcotic Drugs Epidemic?

The overuse of antibiotics may have ruined not only individual lives but also entire families. American research shows that the use of narcotic drugs rose by 400 percent within a period of twenty years (1968-1988); the research linked 95 percent of the total increase to the subjects' frequent intake of prescribed medical drugs prior to narcotic drug involvement. Only 5 percent of the total increase during this period was presumably caused by factors such as curiosity, pressure by social groups, drug cartels, etc. This older study remains relevant today, and even more so since the use of prescription drugs has greatly escalated in the past 20 years.

Recent findings in the field of neurophysiology offer some explanations for the way antibiotics may cause substance addiction. Once ingested, antibiotics, as well as painkillers, tranquillizers, and mind-altering drugs, occupy receptor sites on the surface of our cells which trigger the expected responses such as relief of pain, calmness, and lessening of depression. While occupied by these external chemical agents, the cells' receptor sites can no longer receive and respond to the body's own drugs. The body then reduces production of its own drugs like *endorphins, interleukins, serotonin, dopamine*, etc. These natural drugs are related to the experience of satisfaction, happiness and creativity - feelings every person naturally desires.

Endorphins, for example, consist of very strong *morphine* compounds that are needed for the 'happy' and harmonious functioning of the entire mind/body system. We are naturally addicted to them. When they are no longer secreted in sufficient quantities, we begin to look for alternatives. Constant strong cravings for chocolate, alcohol, sugar, tobacco, etc. may already indicate a reduced secretion of these brain drugs. When someone begins to have the feeling that he desperately 'needs' a cola, coffee or drink, he/she is already addicted - a condition that indicates interference with the production of the body's own pleasure drugs. Further interference may even urge the addicted person to look for much stronger *morphine*-type or *morphine*-producing substances which promise to give him the relief or pleasure that his body is no longer able to provide.

The regular use of antibiotics and other medical drugs by young people is certainly not the only interference in the production of the body's own pleasure drugs. Addiction to narcotic drugs is a complex problem that involves unresolved personal conflicts, family issues, social discrimination and a certain amount of karmic discrepancies which all interfere with happiness in life. Narcotic drugs should not be perceived as the real culprit behind the addiction epidemic, just like a gun cannot be blamed for killing someone. The addict's inner void or lack of happiness, and the resulting missing pleasure hormones, makes him/her already 'addicted' long before he/she gets tempted to go on a 'trip'. Only dissatisfied and unhappy people, regardless of age, background or social status, feel the urge for external substitutes for happiness. They all belong to the risk group of substance addicts.

Regular courses of antibiotics given to babies and children may not only impair many of the vital functions in their bodies, including digestion and immunity, but may also deprive them of the sense of internal happiness and satisfaction in life. What's even worse, this treatment could also rob them of the basic right of development. A nine-month survey by the Development Delay Registry of 800 families in the U.S. found that children who had taken more than 20 courses of antibiotics between the ages of 1 and 12 years were 50 percent more likely to suffer from developmental problems, from autism to speech difficulties. Most of the affected children had been developing normally before they were put on antibiotics.

During a medical conference, doctors reported observing children between the ages 1 and 2 regressing, losing their speech, and developing signs of withdrawal and behavioral problems after being administered antibiotics. Children who have taken antibiotics often show signs of restlessness, anxiety, boredom, irritability, and outbursts of anger. Antibiotics may therefore indirectly contribute to substance abuse, whether the substance is tobacco, coffee, alcohol or non-prescribed drugs.

Nature Knows Best - Clearing Infection Naturally

Nature has a cure for every ill. This feature is a built-in necessity to sustain life on the planet. If nature were not able to cure itself from disease, life on Earth would have vanished millions of years ago. All the forms of vegetation, including the trees, flowers, fruits and vegetables, as well as all the animals and insects down to the smallest amoeba and bacteria, are equipped with highly sophisticated defense mechanisms to maintain their own and the planet's existence.

Man's immune system is the most sophisticated among all species and can develop immunity to any invading organism. The power of our healing system, however, depends on our thoughts, feelings, the foods we eat, the quality of the air we inhale, the water we drink, the environment we are in, and the things we choose to do, see and hear. If all or most of these various influences make us feel good, our immune system remains efficient. Even one lingering depressing thought or fearful emotion is sufficient to suppress the immune system, which may make our body susceptible to invading microorganisms.

Recent research found that *toxic* personalities have a much higher risk of becoming ill than *positive* personalities do.

To understand how such simple things as negative thoughts, emotions, or physical experiences can quickly disrupt the energy distribution to the body's muscles, organs, and immune system, apply the muscle test described in chapter 1. It will help you become more selective in what you choose to think, do, see, hear and eat. To support your immune system in its fight against disease or infections, you can use natural remedies known in the traditional forms of medicine.

Ayurvedic Medicine, Chinese Medicine, and Homeopathy, for example, offer excellent remedies for almost every ill. They do not interfere with the mechanism of healing in the body, as is the case with drugs. Instead, their cleansing procedures and immune-stimulating medicines make it easier for the body to rid itself of toxins or deal with pathogens. A major *side benefit* of these natural methods and substances is that they are much more likely to trigger a significant placebo response in the body than drugs.

If you suffer from an infection or any other illness, there is no reason to panic! Your attitude to the disease is the most powerful tool you have to overcome the problem. Fear interferes with your body's healing response. If you ask a friend to test your arm muscle while experiencing this fear, you will find that the energy flow to your muscles is extremely low. Instead of succumbing to this weakening influence, decide to take positive steps to support the body in its healing efforts. Trust that there cannot be a better doctor in the world than your own body because it is equipped with the best pharmacy that could ever exist. It is best to use natural cleansing remedies (that pass the Kinesiology muscle test) before taking antibiotics or other drugs. The latter are useful and necessary *only* in life-threatening situations. And if they are taken, it is good to counterbalance the harmful side effects through a program of cleansing.

For example, coffee enemas, or preferably the liver and gallbladder flush, can help the liver to rid itself from accumulated antibiotic residues and a lot of other toxins as well. Essiac tea, MMS, Chaparral or Lapacho tea can cleanse the liver and the blood from such remnants, too. A kidney cleanse ensures that the toxins which your body releases are actually removed and don't get caught in the kidneys, urinary bladder or skin. The Ayurvedic hot water treatment (drinking hot ionized water) cleanses the tissues. Early bedtimes improve digestion and immune functions. In addition, a nourishing diet according to your body type makes assimilation of food easier and more effective. Exercise serves as a means to bring more oxygen into your cells and helps with the removal of toxic waste from the body. Also don't underestimate the healing powers of sunlight. If properly used, sunlight alone can eliminate many of our ills. And drinking sufficient amounts of fresh water ensures that the body remains hydrated and that detoxification can take place smoothly and efficiently.

Lastly, as shocking as this may sound in today's drugs-for-everything medical world, a new study suggests that doctors of 2,500 years ago knew the secret to stopping a lot of serious infections: bloodletting! Bloodletting is effective against the staphylococcus bacteria, a leading cause of pneumonia and other life-threatening ailments, according to some recent University of Chicago research. The reason for this is quite simple: staph and other germs thrive on iron in the blood. Reducing the amount of blood in the body greatly reduces their food supply (iron) and thereby makes the blood less attractive to them. For the same reason, menstruating women are protected against infection by naturally lowering blood iron before the beginning of their natural bleeding cycle; and pregnant women do the same during the ninth month of pregnancy, thanks to nature's perfect innate wisdom.

2. Business with Your Blood

Are Blood Transfusions Truly Necessary?

Most of us grew up with the distinct impression that donating blood is a highly humanitarian act and helps to save many people's lives. Blood transfusions are currently a standard part of the medical emergency procedure on a patient who has suffered a life-threatening trauma with loss of blood or one who awaits major surgery. However, these transfusions may not be as safe or as necessary as commonly believed. An increasing number of medical experts regard blood transfusions to be an outmoded, unproved, and even dangerous procedure. Yet it is still routinely used as the main method of medical intervention in emergencies - in many cases without any medical justification for its use and without guidelines as to when it should be applied.

Different parts of the blood are used for the medical procedures, including blood albumin, plasma, and whole blood or red blood cells. In its 1989 publication titled 'Blood Technologies, Services and Issues', the Office of Technology Assessment Task Force in the U.S. examined the overuse of the various blood products. It came to the conclusion that as much as 20-25 percent of the red blood cells, 90 percent of the albumin and 95 percent of the fresh-frozen plasma transfused into patients are unnecessary. This situation has not changed since the study was done.

A major Canadian study, which was published in 1998 in the *Journal of the American Medical Association,* revealed that fewer patients died when they were given a restricted amount of transfused blood. During the trial, 52 percent fewer transfusions were given to the restrictive group, and transfusion was avoided altogether in one-third of those patients. The death rate in the control group, which received normal, liberal amounts of blood transfusions, was 24 percent, compared with 18 percent in the restrictive transfusion group. "The bottom line is ; less transfusion is better than more transfusion" said Paul Herbert, the trial's principal investigator. The restrictive transfusion strategy could effectively save one life for every 17 patients transfused.

The most common trigger for authorizing a blood transfusion for hospital patients awaiting surgery is a low *hemoglobin* level (*hemoglobin* in red blood cells is used to transport oxygen to all the other cells in the body; and red blood cells need iron to accomplish that). Women naturally have a lower red blood cell count than men but medics use the same trigger levels for both men and women. "Iron deficiency anemia continues to be among the leading reasons for transfusions, even though it rarely warrants [them]," said the U.S. Office of Technology report in its concluding statement.

The standard hemoglobin trigger-level for justifying a transfusion lies at below ten gram (g) per 100 milliliters (ml) of blood. However, this figure emerged from a misreading by a hematologist during a study of hemoglobin levels in *dogs*! The results of the study, which showed no established links with human physiology, became the main referential guideline for all anesthesiology students thereafter.

Dangers Lurking in the Blood

It is commonly known that diseases can be transmitted by way of blood transfusions. But apart from receiving viruses through foreign blood, patients may develop even more serious complications as a result of a transfusion. Numerous studies show that blood transfusions given to cancer patients can cause depression of their immune system leading to a high rate of recurrence and secondary cancers.

In a controlled study of patients with larynx cancer, the recurrence rate was 14 percent among those who did not receive blood transfusions compared to 65 percent among those who did. More specific research showed that half of the patients who suffered from colonic, rectal, cervical and prostate cancers and received whole blood were reported to have a recurrence compared to a quarter among those who received only red blood cells.

Blood components are routinely irradiated, supposedly to avert rejection of the foreign blood by the recipient's immune system. No studies show that this practice is harmless for the blood cells; it is simply *assumed* that it has no negative consequences. But knowing what we know today about the dangers of radiation, it can be equally assumed that irradiated blood cells could be hazardous to health, especially if they are given to babies and pregnant mothers.

What makes blood transfusion so risky is that there has never been a randomized, double-blind control study to demonstrate its effectiveness and safety. No scientific proof at all is available to justify its use. Like an antibiotic drug, blood transfusion may have its place as a last resort measure to save a person's life. As a standard practice, however, it not only fails to achieve the desired results, it may be doing more harm than good.

A number of studies confirmed that receiving a transfusion during an operation increases the risk of infection fourfold. Considering the high sterility of the objects and environment in operation rooms, having a blood transfusion practically takes a patient back to surgical conditions that existed over two hundred years ago, when precautions against infection didn't exist. The risk of blood infection has practically remained the same and, with the increase in antibiotic resistant organisms, actually worsened.

Genetic blood research has proven that blood, like our fingerprints, is uniquely individual, implying that it cannot be transferred to another person without risking complications. Each person's blood contains a multiplicity of antibodies, antigens, and infectious agents, most of which science has yet to identify. This makes transfusions even more risky because the majority of infectious agents contained in blood have not even been identified and can therefore not be targeted with drugs. But even if a blood-borne infection *is* diagnosed, it is a little too late. In the United States alone there are 230,000 new cases of hepatitis a year that are purely the result of blood transfusions. Just as in the case of the AIDS test, the screening of blood for the hepatitis C virus has turned out to be an equally futile undertaking. Most of the newly developed tests, including Riba-2 and Murex ELISA, proved wrong three-quarters of the time.

Furthermore, a blood transfusion increases a patient's risk of acquiring human T-cell leukemia tenfold when compared with contracting HIV through blood. It may also trigger unforeseeable, life-threatening allergic reactions. In patients undergoing major abdominal surgery, blood transfusion is the dominant contributing factor to organ system failure. It is more and more obvious that neither a blood transfusion nor 'pure' foreign blood is safe.

The Alternatives

Clear evidence has shown that a person's red blood cell count is not as important as his total circulating volume of fluid. With a high volume, your body can speed up the flow of even a low red blood cell count. It is much more problematic if a patient loses a large amount of fluid from the circulatory system, which would coerce the heart into making an enormous effort to send those red blood cells around to all the vital organs. All of the alternative techniques to blood transfusion are based on first stopping the bleeding and second replacing the lost amount of circulating fluids. This can be achieved in a number of ways.

Auto transfusion is a very safe method of supplying patients with their own blood (donated before surgery) after they undergo major surgery, such as coronary bypasses, congenital heart surgery, or surgical removal of cancer.

Hemodilution is a technique that maintains the amount of fluid circulating around the body through artificial volume expanders, either *colloids* (starches or gelatin) or *crystalloids* (sugar or saline solutions). A major study of over 10,000 surgery patients showed that adults can undergo the rapid loss of 1,000 to 2,000 ml blood (about a third of their total volume) and not go into irreversible shock if adequate hemodilution is maintained. Many other studies also demonstrate that adult patients can tolerate seven to ten times lower than normal levels of *hemoglobin* during surgery and still survive. A very large study of 6,000 open-heart surgery patients confirmed that by avoiding blood transfusions altogether and using only volume expanders, patients had improved outcomes, and had to pay less as well. In addition the risk of contracting diseases from other people's blood was eliminated.

Other methods are used to help lower a patient's temperature and blood pressure in order to conserve blood loss and limit excessive bleeding. Drugs are also available that increase red blood cell production. All of these methods have very few or no side effects. Whenever doctors have to conduct surgery on members of the Jehovah's Witnesses, they have no other choice but to use the blood-free procedures (with higher success rates than those obtained by ordinary transfusion). This success has motivated the doctors and some of their colleagues to adopt the procedures for all their patients.

Your Blood is Your Life

Blood holds much more importance than just being a vehicle for the distribution of nutrients and oxygen. Our blood is the most precious thing we have in the body. It carries all our thoughts, emotions, and memories and makes them available to every part of the body. Blood is the creator of life in our body and is different in every person. Each of us has a unique design of blood type, which is co-responsible for the uniqueness of our physical structure and personality. The categorization of blood into a few types ignores this fundamental uniqueness in every human being.

In actuality, only one type of blood exists for each person in the world. Blood carries decoded DNA, which knows what nutrients need to be sent where. It knows of and responds to all our needs, discrepancies, strengths, and weaknesses. The blood is filled with patterns and geometric designs that reorganize themselves according to our state of consciousness. Every new desire, feeling, or intention instantly reprograms the blood and all parts of the body it touches. When you receive another person's blood, you also receive his genetic information and part of his personality. The immune system can easily get depressed when foreign DNA (from one or several donors) suddenly and unexpectedly enters a person's blood through a transfusion. In many cases, the immune system is not able to fight off the many viral particles and toxins that are present in the donor's blood.

The quality of our blood changes according to our thoughts, feelings, and emotions. Negative thoughts create toxic blood whereas happy thoughts make healthy blood. Fearful thoughts, for example fill your blood with *adrenaline*, loving thoughts flood it with *interleukins*. Both literally move your heart but with contrary effects. The 'adrenaline-shot' causes panic to the heart; the 'interleukin-shot' creates emotions of happiness in the heart and protects you against cancer.

Having a blood transfusion may create confusion and chaos within the body and mind. On the other hand, refusing a blood transfusion and not receiving alternative treatments may put your life in danger. If you need a blood transfusion but prefer an alternative and safe method, contact the Blood Transfusion Society in your country. They may be able to put you in touch with a practitioner who is experienced in any of the above transfusion procedures. If you pretend to be a Jehovah's Witness, the hospital will arrange for an alternative approach.

3. Risks of Ultrasound Scans

By the mid-eighties more than 100 million people throughout the world had experienced ultrasound scans before they were born. Today, practically every pregnant woman in Europe and in North America will have at least one ultrasound scan during her pregnancy. Most expectant women receive their first referral for a scan during their first prenatal appointment; only a few of them question whether it is necessary and even fewer know of its potential harm. Most women's magazines, newspapers, and pregnancy books tend to recommend ultrasound scans to ensure the safety and healthy development of the fetus, despite the fact that no study proves that having an ultrasound scan provides more benefits than not having one. In an official statement, the American College of Obstetrics and Gynecology (ACOG) admitted that *no well-controlled study has yet proven that routine scanning of prenatal patients will improve the outcome of pregnancy.*

On the other hand, researchers in New York studied 15,000 pregnant women who received ultrasound scans. They concluded that scanning provided no benefits whatsoever in any of the risk categories such as premature babies, fetal death, multiple births, late-term-pregnancies, etc. In fact, up to this date, ultrasound scans have not revealed any information that is of clinical value. On the contrary, there is more evidence today than ever before that scans can be harmful for both the mother and the unborn child. The Association for Improvements in the Maternity Services (AIMS), England, recorded cases of women who aborted their perfectly fit and healthy babies as a result of misinterpreted scans. It is almost impossible to estimate how many women went through similar ordeals since most cases are not reported.

In 1990 researchers in Finland conducted a large trial study with ultrasound. The ultrasound scans diagnosed 250 women with *placenta previa* in early pregnancy, a condition where the placenta lies low and therefore may prevent the baby from being born vaginally. The mothers were informed that they should expect a *Caesarean* section. But when it came to giving birth, only four women still had *placenta previa*. In almost all cases, the placenta moved out of the way when the womb began to grow. Ironically, the control group, which received no ultrasound scanning also had four women with *placenta previa*; all of them delivered their babies safely.

Human Guinea pigs

Despite the fact that respected medical journals like the *Lancet, The Canadian Medical Association Journal*, and the *New England Journal of Medicine* have all written about the hazardous effects of ultrasound use, mainstream medicine has all but ignored the negative evidence. Even the FDA has commented on the dangers of ultrasound. According to a story by the Associated Press, their position on the technique is this: "Ultrasound is a form of energy, and even at low levels, laboratory studies have shown that it can produce physical effects in tissue, such as jarring vibrations and a rise in temperature... prenatal ultrasounds can't be considered innocuous."

Millions of women around the world, without being aware of the potential health hazards of ultrasounds, are participating in the largest medical experiment of all times. Their babies are the guinea pigs in this experiment. They become vulnerable to external and internal harmful influences when their delicate electromagnetic fields are distorted, misaligned or damaged by highly concentrated doses of ultrasound; exposure to that is neither natural nor suitable for any human being. We cannot solely rely on machines for diagnostic purposes just because machines are considered less likely to make mistakes than doctors. All findings have to be interpreted properly before they can serve as a guide for treatment. As demonstrated in the above study, 98.4 percent of the initial complications during the women's pregnancy cleared on their own simply because the body knows how to handle such problems perfectly well without intervention. Machines don't know that the readings they produce may actually turn out to be a wrong diagnosis.

A false diagnosis is not the only disadvantage that may arise from using ultrasound indiscriminately. In 1993 Australian researchers studied 3,000 women and found that frequent ultrasound scanning between 18 and 38 weeks of pregnancy could produce babies up to a third smaller than normal. Similar studies revealed that babies who had received *Doppler* ultrasound (to scan the baby's blood supply) had a lower birth weight than babies who didn't receive a scan.

If the birth weight of a baby is reduced through ultrasound, what about other functions which are even more important for a baby's growth? One professor in Calgary, Canada, discovered that children developed speech problems twice as often when exposed to ultrasound in the womb. Surgeon James Campbell from Canada found that even one prenatal scan may be sufficient to cause delayed speech. Norwegian studies suggested ultrasound scanning might even lead to mild brain damage in the developing fetus.

One large-scale Swedish study showed a link between ultrasound scanning and left-handedness, which is often the result of slight prenatal brain damage. The study revealed a 32 percent greater chance of left-handedness among the ultrasound group when compared to an un-scanned control group. Needless to say, since 1975, when doctors started aggressive ultrasound scanning late in pregnancy (usually to determine the baby's sex), rates of left-handedness have increased dramatically - especially among male babies.

Ultrasound was approved as a medical tool of diagnosis under a different category than that used to approve drugs. Science has not yet studied the effects of using these different powers of energy. As long as this is the case, ultrasound examinations are under the umbrella of 'legal protection'. The complete lack of scientific research backing up the safety of ultrasound scans should caution both doctors and pregnant women.

Yet the scanning of pregnant woman has become such a routine practice today that not many women want to go without it. Scans give parents the opportunity to get to know their baby long before it is born, although women were able to be in touch with their babies before the invention of ultrasound. Today you can find out whether your baby is male or female, which leaves no room for surprises. You can also get the exact date of delivery although, provided there are no complications, you can calculate the birth date of your child yourself. An ultrasound scan may reveal if a baby suffers from Down's syndrome but it doesn't tell you how serious the condition is. The added information that ultrasound can give makes little or no difference because babies in general cannot be treated before or shortly after birth. After examining all the results from published trials using ultrasound scans, a team of doctors from Switzerland failed to come up with evidence suggesting that the use of ultrasound could improve the condition of the babies.

Furthermore, a large trial study in the United States concluded that receiving an ultrasound scan produced no difference in prenatal mortality rates or in sick babies than not receiving an ultrasound. What is most disconcerting, however, is that the latest ultrasound technology is to be introduced into use without any trials. It consists of a vaginal probe that is covered by a condom and inserted directly into the woman's vagina. With the new technology, doctors will get an even better picture of the fetus but the baby will also get a much higher dose of ultrasound.

Even though an increasing number of health professionals are very concerned about the wholesale use of scans, pregnant women are not informed about the possible harmful consequences that accompany their use. Scans are prescribed routinely but you have the right to refuse one. An ultrasound scan should only be considered if a woman suffers localized pain or complications for which a doctor or midwife cannot find a plausible reason. Such cases though are rare. As for now, ultrasound has been repeatedly shown to make no difference whatsoever to the outcome of a normal pregnancy.

4. Immunization Programs under Scrutiny

Poisonous Vaccines against Harmless Infections

For many decades, leading scientists and doctors have vehemently promoted the idea that immunization of children is necessary to protect them from contracting such diseases as diphtheria, polio, cholera, typhoid, or malaria. Yet evidence is mounting that immunization may not only be unnecessary but even harmful. Pouring deadly chemicals into a lake doesn't make it immune to pollutants. Likewise, injecting the live poisons contained in vaccines into the bloodstream of children hardly gives future generations a chance to lead truly healthy lives. American children often receive some 30 vaccinations within the first 6 years of their lives and children in the U.K. can expect to be vaccinated about 25 times. Within the first 15 months of life, vaccinations including nine or more different antigens are pumped into the immature immune systems of babies. Despite the colossal efforts and large sums of money spent on vaccine research, medicine has never been able to devise a cholera vaccine that works and the drugs for malaria aren't as effective as a single herb. Diphtheria is still combated with toxic immunization programs even though it has almost completely disappeared from the earth. When diphtheria broke out in Chicago in 1969, 11 of the 16 victims were either already immune or had been *immunized* against diphtheria. In another report, 14 out of 23 victims were completely immune. This shows that vaccination makes no difference when it comes to protection against diphtheria; on the contrary, it can even *increase* the chance of being infected.

Immunization against mumps is also highly dubious. Even though it initially reduces the likelihood of becoming infected, the risk for mumps infection increases after immunity subsides. In 1995 a study conducted by the U.K.'s Public Health Laboratory Service and published in the *Lancet* showed that children given the measles/mumps/rubella shot were *three times* more likely to suffer from convulsions than those children who didn't receive it. The study also found that the MMR vaccine increased by five times the number of children suffering a rare blood disorder.

It is interesting to note that the mortality rate for measles declined by 95 percent before the measles vaccine was introduced. In the United Kingdom, despite widespread vaccination among toddlers, cases of measles recently increased by nearly 25 percent. The United States has been suffering from a steadily increasing epidemic of measles, although (or because) the measles vaccine has been in effect since 1957. After a few sudden drops and rises, the cases of measles are now suddenly dropping again. The Centers for Disease Control (CDC) acknowledged that this could be related to an overall decrease in the occurrence of measles in the Western Hemisphere.

In addition to this evidence, many studies show that the measles vaccine isn't effective. For example, as reported in a 1987 *New England Journal of Medicine* article, a 1986 outbreak of measles in Corpus Christi, Texas, found 99 percent of the victims had been vaccinated. In 1987, 60 percent of the cases of measles occurred in children who had been properly vaccinated at the appropriate age. One year later, this figure rose to 80 percent.

Apart from not protecting against measles and possibly even increasing the risk of contracting the disease, the MMR vaccine has been proven to produce numerous adverse effects. Among them are encephalitis, brain complications, convulsions, retardation of mental and physical growth, high fever, pneumonia, meningitis, aseptic meningitis, mumps, atypical measles, blood disorders such as thrombocytopenia, fatal shock, arthritis, SSPE, one-sided paralysis, and death. According to a study published in the *Lancet* in 1985, if children develop 'mild measles' as a result of receiving the vaccine, the accompanying *underdeveloped* rash may be responsible for causing degenerative diseases such as cancer later in life.

In reality, measles is not a dangerous childhood illness at all. The belief that measles can lead to blindness is a myth that finds it roots in an increased sensitivity to light during illness. This problem subsides when the room is dimmed and vanishes completely with recovery. For a long time measles was believed to increase the risk of a brain infection (encephalitis) which is known to occur only among children who live in poverty and suffer from malnutrition. Among upper class children, only 1 out of 100,000 will become infected. Besides, less than half of children given a measles booster are protected against the disease.

In a report issued by German health authorities and published in a 1989 issue of the *Lancet*, the mumps vaccine was revealed to have caused 27 specific neurological reactions, including meningitis, febrile convulsions, encephalitis, and epilepsy. A Yugoslavian study linked 1 per 1,000 cases of mumps encephalitis directly to the vaccine. The *Pediatric Infectious Disease Journal* in the U.S. reported in 1989 that the rate varies from 1 in 405 to 1 in 7,000 shots for mumps.

Although mumps is generally a mild illness and the vaccine's side effects are severe, it is still included in the MMR vaccine. And so is the vaccine for rubella, although it is known to cause arthritis in up to 3 percent of children and in up to 20 percent of the adult women who have received it. In 1994 the Department of Health admitted to doctors that 11 percent of first-time recipients of the rubella vaccine will get arthritis. Symptoms range from mild aches to severe crippling. Other studies show a 30 percent chance of developing arthritis in direct response to the rubella vaccine.

Research confirms that the whooping cough vaccine is only effective in 36 percent of children. A report by Professor Gordon Stewart, which was published in 1994 in *World Medicine*, demonstrated that the risks of the whooping cough vaccine outweighed the benefits. The whooping cough or pertussis vaccine is by far the most dangerous of all the vaccines. DTP, the whooping cough vaccine that was used in the U.S. until 1992, contained the carcinogen formaldehyde, and the highly toxic metals aluminum and mercury. Both this vaccine and its improved' version DTaP have never been tested for safety, only for efficacy.

The new vaccine has proved to be no better than the old one. Both versions cause death, near-death, seizures, developmental delay, and hospitalization. DTaP (formerly DTP) is given to babies as young as six weeks old, although the vaccine has never been tested on this age group. Among the 17 potential health problems caused by the whooping cough vaccine is **sudden infant death syndrome** (SIDS). According to an estimate from the University of California at Los Angeles, 1,000 U.S. infants a year die as a direct result of receiving the vaccine.

These and other vaccines have never been tested for safety on humans; they are only tested on animals. Vaccines cannot be proven safe until they are given to humans, for the first time. Giving vaccines to human turns them into human 'guinea pigs'. It is not possible to predict what reactions they will have. This is the risk all people receiving vaccines have to take. Some will die, others will live but become ill years alter, and many others will live without serious long-term consequences. But since all vaccines are designed to cause the very disease they are to prevent (in order to establish immunity), a truly safe vaccine is one that is not effective.

Children are the most vulnerable because their immune systems are practically defenseless against the poisons in the vaccines. They have a lot against them since their mothers are **not** passing on immunity to them in the breast milk (because they **were** vaccinated and no longer make antibodies). Children die a rate eight times faster than normal after a DPT shot. James R Shannon of NIH understood this when he said: "No vaccination can be proven safe before it is given to children."

Immunization programs against polio have no benefits other than economic ones for vaccine producers. The scientist who eliminated polio now suspects that the handful of polio cases which have occurred in the U.S. since the seventies are caused by the live viruses that were used as vaccines. In Finland and Sweden, where the use of live vaccines for polio is prohibited, there has not been a single case of polio in ten years. If live viruses used as a vaccine can cause polio today when hygiene is generally high, it may well be that the polio epidemics 40 to 50 years ago were also caused by immunization against polio while hygiene, sanitation, housing, and nutritional standards were still very low. In the United States, cases of polio increased by 50 percent between 1957 and 1958, and by 80 percent from 1958 to 1959 *after* the introduction of mass immunization. In five states, cases of polio doubled after the polio vaccine was given to large numbers of the population. As soon as hygiene and sanitation improved, *despite* the immunization programs, the viral disease quickly disappeared. Whatever may have been the reason for polio outbreaks in the past (see section on natural immunization), it is highly questionable today to immunize an entire population against a disease that does not even exist any more. It raises major questions about the motives behind polio vaccination.

Further, the history of some simian virus 40 (SV40) infections in humans is linked to the use of polio vaccines. According to the *American Journal of Medicine*, many studies have reported the presence of SV40 from the polio vaccine in human brain tumors and bone cancers, malignant mesothelioma, and non-Hodgkin's lymphoma. The polio vaccine seems ever more linked to cancers, especially in children. The cancers caused by the use of the polio vaccine in the past still kills 20,000 people a year in the United States. This is quite outrageous given the fact that polio itself hasn't killed anyone for a long time.

Involuntary Vaccinations

The vast majority of vaccinations - for children or adults - are needless. And they cause hundreds of deaths per year from adverse reactions, reactions that wouldn't otherwise occur if mass vaccinations didn't exist. According to a recent announcement (November 14, 2007) by State and County officials in Maryland (USA), parents were threatened with jail if they didnt submit their children to forced vaccinations. State Attorney General Glenn F. Ivey vehemently declared that he would criminalize parents who refuse to bring their children to the courthouse to have them injected, on the spot, with vaccines that contain methyl mercury. A total of 1,600 school children and their parents were ordered to appear in circuit court November 17, 2007 to receive the required shots. Parents now risk losing their children either to autism, brain damage or death caused by this highly toxic chemical, or by having to go to jail for trying to protect them against this medical tyranny of the state.

Along with children, who are helpless against the vaccination assault, soldiers have also been a target of mass immunization. Military troops have to submit to all manner of vaccinations in the name of readiness for warfare. The servicemen and women endure endless injections designed to 'protect' them against bio-toxins like smallpox, anthrax, ricin and others.

Several soldiers have died from the often untested chemicals in the vaccines, and others have been severely sickened by the practice. Not unlike those women involved in involuntary ultrasound studies, soldiers have become guinea pigs in massive drug studies. How else could the pharmaceutical industry legally test poisons on human subjects?

Vaccination of soldiers is mandatory. Those who refuse the shots face court martial and prison time, or at the very least, a dishonorable discharge from the armed forces. Common side effects of the over one million vaccinations so far injected in our soldiers have included joint pain, extreme fatigue, and memory loss. The mandatory anthrax vaccine has even worse effects. A recent report issued by the

General Accounting Office (GAO) confirms that about one to two percent of immunized individuals may end up with severe adverse reactions, including disability, chronic disease and death. Even though this risk seems low, when calculated across the 2.2 million in the service, an estimated 44,000 enlisted could potentially end up in the morgue. That's many times more than war fatalities. A current effort has begun, though, to help soldiers secure their right to refuse vaccination. Let's hope it will be successful.

Prevention of disease through vaccines is rapidly turning into a big business, and the best customer is the U.S. Defense Department. Were it not for the soldiers, drug companies would rather shy away from producing vaccines. They have to be offered at reasonably cheap prices, and also need to be constantly reformulated (which is very costly) to keep up with the constantly mutating killer bugs. During wartime the vaccine industry comes alive and flourishes. Millions of doses of various kinds of vaccines are then finding the perfect market. No liability suits, no major objections from anyone. And no real control for safety. To secure billions of dollars in profits for the drug business, the FDA is declaring even virtually untested vaccines as 'safe'. And so the economy is growing, but it is also becoming sicker. But then we need sickness to keep the economy growing.

Vaccination No longer Makes Any Sense

Or did it ever? The much-acclaimed benefits of the latest vaccine against Hib meningitis also seem to be unfounded. In a pro-vaccine study published in 1993 in the *Journal of the American Medical Association*, the children in the control group who didn't receive the vaccine also experienced a drastic reduction in the cases of Hib infection - from 99.3 to 68.5 per 100,000.

The latest problem arising from the use of vaccines is that they can cause the body to develop viral 'mutants' and even spread the newly created disease to the population at large. Since viral mutants are rarely detected in blood donor screening, they can easily be transmitted through donated blood. This way, the original vaccines may be able to wipe out the strains of virus that are known to cause these various diseases, but in the same stroke they cause other mutant strains of virus to thrive.

Research also showed that a single injection of any kind could increase the risk of paralysis fivefold. Polio, for example, is more common in developing countries where children receive more injections than in developed countries. A study published in 1995 by the *New England Journal of Medicine* showed that injection of the polio vaccine actually caused outbreaks of the disease.

A 1993 report released by the American National Academy of Science Institute of Medicine concluded that virtually all nine vaccines given to children have at some time been proved to cause damage, including such complications as shock, convulsions, or paralysis. The problem is that a child's body is expected to cope with not just one type of poison contained in one vaccine, but with several different ones contained in as many as nine vaccines. Many children have died or become permanently and severely brain damaged within days after immunization. In many cases, however, the adverse effects from vaccination are less devastating but still serious enough to take a good look at the reasons why parents haven't been informed. In many countries parents are actually forced by law to immunize their children.

Unfounded Vaccination Hysteria

It has long been known that, in some illnesses such as measles, chicken pox and scarlet fever, one bout of the illness usually provides lifelong immunity. A second experience with measles or scarlet fever is extremely rare.

The concepts of medicine formulated in the 19th century were partially based on the understanding by the ancient Greek physician Hippocrates, who observed that an illness manifests signs and symptoms that travel from the inner vital organs and blood circulation to the outer surface of the body. These symptoms would often be visible as a rash or as a discharge of blood, mucus or pus. This 'throwing off' of an illness was considered a natural healing response expected to return the body to a state of balance or equilibrium. Hippocrates perceived this labor as a cooking and pepsis of our inner poisons during an inflammatory illness. It was also observed that immunity to or protection from an illness arose when a person had that illness before. Today we consider a disease as being an enemy that we need to battle against.

Contrary to common understanding, an inflammatory-infectious illness does not begin when we become exposed to and are infected with a virus or bacterium, but when our body starts its response. The magnitude of our body's response (severity of illness) is not only influenced by the magnitude of the infection, but also by the stamina and inherent strength in us. The healing force employed by the body depends on multiple factors, such as emotions, spiritual foundation, diet, lifestyle, environment, etc. Our immunity certainly does not depend on whether we have been vaccinated against infectious agents. The crucial factor of strong immunity is due to our immune system's ability to keep the germs at bay or fight them. If the vigor of our immune response is weak, germs are likely to infect us. But normally, the majority of germ 'invasions' occur silently, without ever disturbing us. Symptoms of disease occur only at the time the immune system decides it is necessary to aggressively defend itself against harmful influences.

Louis Pasteur (1822-1895) was the first researcher to postulate that diseases are caused by germs. Pasteur's germ theory proposed that disease germs are after us because they need to prey on us for their own survival while contributing nothing to us in return. He initially believed that infectious/inflammatory diseases are a direct result of germs feasting on us. In microscopic studies of host tissues in such diseases, Pasteur, Koch and their colleagues repeatedly observed that germs proliferated while many host cells were dying. These researchers concluded that germs attack and destroy healthy cells, and thereby start a disease process in the body. Although this assumption turned out to be wrong, it had already made its debut in the world of science, and the erroneous idea that germs cause infections became an undisputed reality. Today, this idea continues to prevail as a fundamental 'scientific truth' in the modern medical system.

Pasteur could have just as easily concluded that bacteria are naturally attracted to the sites of increased cell death, just like they are attracted to decaying organic matter elsewhere in nature. Flies, ants, crows, vultures and, of course, bacteria are drawn towards death. Why would this be different in the body? Weak, damaged or dead cells in the body are just as prone to germ infection as an overripe piece of fruit. Pasteur and all the researchers that followed in his footsteps made the choice of thinking of germs either as predators or scavengers. Had they assumed that cells die for non-apparent biochemical reasons (such as toxicity buildup), our current thinking about illness and health would have been completely different than it is today. We would all have grown up with the knowledge that the occurrence of inflammatory/infectious illnesses can ultimately not be attributed to germs, but must be located in the various human frailties that necessitate the forces of decay and death. Germs only become poisonous to us when confronted with the poisons we create; our body does not battle germs because they are the enemy. An immune system reaction such as high fever or depletion of energy is meant to cleanse the body of harmful substances that otherwise could lead to the eventual demise of the entire body.

In situations of extreme toxicity, the immune system may be so overwhelmed with the poisons it tries to eliminate that it may or may not be able to save the person. In the third scenario, the immune system doesn't respond to the poisons and germs at all, and no acute disease symptoms appear (no fever, inflammations, pain). The result then is chronic, debilitating illness known as allergic or autoimmune disorders.

In the scenario where the immune system has successfully restored the body's functions, the body has acquired immunity to the germs that initiated the rescue mission. Vaccine science has pursued the question of how we can bring about lifelong immunity to an infectious-inflammatory illness without having to experience the illness first. Their assumption is that, by having antibodies in the blood for certain illness-causing germs, you are automatically protected against them. However, no proof has shown whether protection from the germs is due to the presence of antibodies or to a normal healthy immune response. It is actually much more likely that the latter is true, unless vaccine poisons have damaged or even paralyzed the immune system.

Only when the germs' number or rate of growth exceeds a certain threshold are they then recognized by the immune system, resulting in the formation of antibodies specific to the particular provocative bug. A large presence of germs indicates that the cell tissue has become damaged or weak due to the accumulation of acid waste. At that level of infection things get seriously out of control and a tribe of germs proliferates wildly and provokes the full defensive reaction of our immune system. This is what doctors call an 'acute inflammatory response'. Symptoms usually include fever, release of stress hormones by the adrenal glands, increased flow of blood, lymph, and mucus, and a streaming of white blood cells to the inflamed area. The afflicted person feels sick and may experience pain, nausea, vomiting, diarrhea, weakness and chills. The sweating out and throwing off of the illness is a natural response by the body that reflects a healthy immune system. A really sick person would no longer be able to come up with such healing responses.

Once we have successfully passed the challenge of a particular illness, it is less likely that we will experience it again. Somehow the illness and our response to it have made us immune to its recurrence. It is more than doubtful, though, that vaccination can do the same for us by forcing the body to make antibodies for some germs that appear to be causing an infection. It has been shown over and over again that, despite the vaccination of a person against a particular illness, the person may just develop that very illness he is supposed to be protected against, or even more so. The mere presence of specific antibodies cannot protect anyone against any illness, only the cellular immune system can. Although it is true that science knows how to bestow antibodies through vaccination, it mistakenly assumes that it is bestowing the immune strength that can only be developed through the experience of a particular illness. Antibodies alone are not sufficient to produce immunity. It is well known that several diseases such as herpes outbreaks may recur repeatedly despite high antibody levels. Whether or not antibodies are present, immunity to these infectious diseases can only be conferred by our cellular immune system. The theory that exposing the body to disease germs will trigger an immune response similar to the one generated during an actual disease experience is seriously flawed.

Is the Need for Immunization Based on Statistical Errors?

As previously mentioned, the idea of vaccinating our bodies in order to protect them against possible infectious diseases came from the famous Louis Pasteur, who was considered to be the pioneer of immunization. In 1993 historian Gerald L. Geison handed over to the public the 100 private diaries of Pasteur. Surprisingly, his *diary entries* contained especially negative results of experiments with vaccines whereas the *publicized data* had made the experiments look revolutionary. The published results of his most spectacular immunization experiments turned out to be a complete fraud. The authenticity of his research was never questioned until official statistical research revealed that immunization programs directly led to dramatic increases of those diseases they were supposed to eradicate.

Analysis of the official statistics from several countries and their historical occurrences of smallpox, diphtheria, cholera, typhoid, poliomyelitis, tuberculosis, bronchitis, tetanus, etc. revealed astounding findings. For example, diphtheria in France increased to an all-time high with the onset of compulsory immunization and immediately dropped again after the vaccine was withdrawn. The situation was not much different in Germany when compulsory immunization for diphtheria was introduced on a mass scale from 1925 to 1944. During this period the number of diphtheria victims increased from 40,000 to 240,000, with the incidence of infection being higher in immunized patients. In 1945, at the end of World War II, vaccines were no longer available in Germany and, within a few years, the number of diseased dropped below 50,000.

Statistical data shows that most of these diseases were in rapid and continuous decline well before the introduction of immunization programs. The big epidemics began occurring when people from the rural areas moved into the big cities. The streets were used as garbage dumps, contaminating air and water, and becoming the source of infectious diseases. Only major cleanup of the congested cities, and improved sanitation, hygiene, and housing were able to halt the epidemics and lead to drastic improvements in individual and collective health. Vaccination programs had nothing to do with it.

How to Acquire Immunity Naturally

It seems that we humans tend to go from one extreme to the other. Now, the natural balance between immunity and presence of germs is becoming disrupted once again, but this time the cause may be the excessive emphasis on hygiene. Being over-hygienic can inhibit the natural development of immunity to disease-causing agents. The causative agent of poliomyelitis, for instance, is very common among the some native populations in the world; yet to them the virus is completely harmless. They immunize themselves by staying in close contact with nature and also dirt. They rarely wash their hands before taking a meal and whatever else gets into their mouth with the food helps to build their natural resistance to harmful microorganisms.

In the Western Hemisphere, poliomyelitis became a frightening disease only at the beginning of this century, with the onset of the high standard of hygienic living conditions. Regular exposure to dirt and microorganisms kept the people's immune system engaged, strong and naturally immunized. On the other hand, the increased measures of hygiene were necessary in the densely populated areas of big cities where there was little ventilation of air and inadequate sanitation.

Indigenous populations didn't have such needs. If necessary, they boosted their immune systems by injuring each other during rituals or by scarring their skin. They allowed their wounds to suppurate, which we know today is a very efficient way to strengthen one's immunity. For them, bloodletting was a necessary act of survival during times of continuous meat consumption when other types of food were not available; this helped them to keep their blood thin and reduce their body's protein stores, which otherwise could have led to life-endangering diseases (see also chapter 8 on heart disease).

Very often children 'accidentally' injure themselves or even eat dirt because their immune systems are run down and need a major boost to cope with more serious issues of defense. So when you unintentionally cut yourself, try to see it from a holistic perspective. You may have excessive protein in your blood or blood vessels and the bleeding may be just the thing to cause thinning of the blood and to prevent heart problems. This self-regulating mechanism is very powerful and keeps you healthier than any immunization program or mega-doses of vitamin and mineral supplements. This unspecified form of immunization may be necessary from time to time in order to maintain a strong and healthy intestinal flora (two thirds of our immune system is located in the intestinal tract). To remain healthy and immune, we *need* the daily fight with bacteria and viruses.

A recent study conducted at the Institute of Child Health at Bristol University, U.K. observed every aspect of 14,000 children's lives over a period of 7 years. They found that too much hygiene could be damaging children's health, weakening their immune systems and making them prone to illnesses such as asthma. A few decades ago such diseases as asthma, eczema, and hay fever were almost nonexistent. Today, as many as one third of the population suffer from allergies. Scientists now say that our obsession with the latest anti-germ potions and over-reliance on soap and water may explain why the Western world has been hit by a spate of viruses, immune-related diseases, and allergies.

The principle 'what we don't use becomes useless' also applies to our immune system; it needs the regular exposure and adaptation to everyday bugs and germs in order to exercise its ability to recognize what is truly harmful. Rigorous hygiene drastically reduces the number of bacteria and other infectious agents that a developing immune system needs to battle to become stronger and more efficient. Allergies occur when the immune system labels harmless particles (house dust, pollen, etc.) as harmful invaders to which it has rarely been exposed before. To fight them off, the body covers them with poison, which in turn results in inflammation, itching, swelling, and such symptoms as a runny nose. The Bristol study found, for example, that those children who washed their face and hands three or four times a day and bathed once a day suffered a significantly higher incidence of asthma than did the children who used soap and water much less frequently.

Children from larger families are also less likely to suffer from asthma or hay fever. With many children living under one roof, minor infections are constantly brought into the household, which means that the immune system is kept busy and alert almost all the time. If an infection occurs as a result of the body's natural reaction to invading bacteria, the immune system produces 'fighter cells' called antibodies. But if this normal response i.e. an infection, is undermined or prevented by artificial disinfectants or antibiotics, antibodies are no longer made and the immune system is weakened and begins to malfunction. By contrast, letting the infection take its full course strengthens the immune system, making it much more resilient to disease-causing germs afterwards.

Exaggerated cleanliness and fear of infection usually go hand in hand. Many people who fail to employ the natural ways of strengthening the immune system are paranoid about becoming infected; for them, antibiotics and vaccines also remain ineffective.

Vaccination - Attack on Your Body, Brain and Spirit

Vaccines are composed of protein, bacterial and viral material, as well as preservatives, neutralizers, and carrying agents. The vaccine against bacterial meningitis is made from the brains and heart of cows among other highly toxic components. Alarmed by the outbreak of *mad cow disease*, the Italian authorities ordered the seizure of the vaccine in January 1997 for fear it could cause the human version of the disease. By injecting such cocktails of foreign and destructive substances directly into the bloodstream, the human body stands little or no chance of neutralizing the poisons.

Under normal circumstances, all ingested foods, beverages, etc. have to pass through the mucus membranes, the intestinal walls, or the liver before they are permitted into such important areas as the blood, the heart, or the brain. The sudden appearance of a poison in the bloodstream is often met by a counterattack of the immune system that uses an entire arsenal of antibodies to prevent death from poisoning (allergic reaction). This allergic response can lead to a sudden, sometimes fatal, collapse known as anaphylactic shock response. Among the causes of anaphylactic shock are immunizations for diphtheria, tetanus, hepatitis B, and whooping cough. A young person's immune system hasn't typically matured enough to be effective against this type of onslaught

No less dangerous is the Guillain-Barré syndrome which leads to paralysis and is caused by immunizations for measles, diphtheria, influenza, tetanus, and the oral polio vaccine. This is hardly surprising when one considers the high toxicity of the vaccines. It is well known that children whose immune systems are already weak experience more serious complications than those whose constitution and immune system are much stronger. Still, vaccines are given indiscriminately regardless of the children's health status. Many children at infancy don't even get the chance to be healthy later in life because they are pumped full of these poisons against which they are helpless. At this stage of development, a child has not yet acquired full natural immunity and has little ability to protect himself.

Increasing evidence shows that chronic diseases, such as rheumatoid arthritis, encephalitis, multiple sclerosis, leukemia, other forms of cancer and even AIDS diseases are linked to vaccinations administered in the early stages of life. Rheumatoid arthritis is an inflammatory disease of the joints, which had been thought to afflict only the elderly. More recently though, the crippling disease has spread among the young generation and measles and rubella inoculations have been identified as the cause.

Researchers from the American Food and Drug Administration discovered that vaccinations, particularly the hepatitis B shot, could cause hair loss. They estimate that 50,000 Americans suffer hair loss (alopecia) after immunization every year. The report was published by the *Journal of the American Medical Association* in 1997.

It is nearly impossible to estimate the damage and suffering that has been created and will occur in the future as a result of inadequate information about the dangers of modern immunization programs. Parents want to do what is best for their children and they carry a heavy burden of responsibility to keep them healthy and safe. Misinformation can create a strong conflict in parents because they don't want to neglect their children's health or cause them any harm.

Most health authorities are not exactly helpful in supporting parents to choose what is best for their children. In spite of damaging evidence, such as the following, they still support the use of immunizations. For instance, the use of the mercury-based thimerosal as a preservative in vaccines has been associated with autism. Despite the evidence, mercury is still being added to vaccines at completely unsafe levels considering the fact that it is a known neurotoxin. A recent study conducted by the University of Calgary showed that mercury ions alter the cell-membrane of developing neurons in babies and young children, directly contributing to autism.

In the late 1990s, the U.S. Public Health Service and the American Academy of Pediatrics petitioned drug companies to remove thimerosal from vaccines intended for children. Why? Well, in one study that examined CDC statistics, researchers found evidence that children who receive just three vaccines containing thimerosal are 27 times more likely to develop autism, compared to children who get vaccinations containing no thimerosal. That's a 2,700 percent increase. Who needs more proof than that? Apparently, the U.S. government does.

Despite a 2004 campaign promise to the contrary, President Bush promised to veto the HHS-Labor-Education Appropriations Bill, which included a measure to ban childhood flu vaccines that contained thimerosal because of cost concerns. As for now (July 2009), despite the warnings, flu vaccines which contain thimerosal continue to be recommended for all pregnant women, infants and children, even though the Institute of Medicine recommended in 2001 that these population groups not be exposed to thimerosal-containing vaccines. One in every six women of childbearing age has enough mercury in her bloodstream to cause neurological damage to her unborn children, according to the U.S. Environmental Protection Agency.

Is it mere coincidence that rates of autism increased when the Center for Disease Control inserted additions to the recommended vaccination program for infants in 1988? In the 1980s, autism rates were estimated at only six in 10,000 children. Today one in 150 children is autistic, though in some areas autism affects closer to one in 50 children. The U.S. Food and Drug Administration has acknowledged that thimerosal **can** be a neurotoxin (knowing very well that mercury **is** a neurotoxin), and in 2004 stated that thimerosal-containing vaccines were associated with autism. As of 2003, there were 1.5 million autistic U.S. children, adding $90 billion per year to the already skyrocketing health care costs.

According to an ex-vaccine researcher (Dr David) who worked for many years in the laboratories of major pharmaceutical houses and the U.S. government's National Institutes of Health (his true name cannot be mentioned here for obvious reasons), all vaccines are dangerous to health. In an interview he stated that vaccines involve the human immune system in a process that tends to compromise immunity. "They can actually cause the disease they are supposed to prevent. They can cause other diseases than the ones they are supposed to prevent," says this scientist.

While working with different vaccines, this doctor found a number of contaminants in them. In the Rimavex measles vaccine, he found various chicken viruses. In the polio vaccine, he found acanthamoeba, a so-called brain-eating amoeba, and a simian cytomegalovirus. Also discovered was simian foamy virus in the rotavirus vaccine and bird-cancer viruses in the MMR vaccine. Various microorganisms were present in the anthrax vaccine and potentially dangerous enzyme inhibitors were present in several other vaccines. Duck, dog, and rabbit viruses were present in the rubella vaccine, avian leucosis virus in the flu vaccine, and pestivirus in the MMR vaccine.

What most people don't know is that some polio vaccines, adenovirus vaccines, rubella and hepatitis A and measles vaccines have been made with aborted human fetal tissue. Dr. Davis found what he believed were bacterial fragments and poliovirus in these vaccines from time to time which may have come from that fetal tissue. In addition, he also found 'fragments' of human hair and human mucus. Apart from such contamination, it is worth mentioning that standard chemicals like formaldehyde, mercury, and aluminum are purposely put into vaccines. It is left up to your imagination as to what must happen to the health prospects of our future generations when such cocktails of ghastly poisons are directly injected into the bloodstream of a child.

Dr. Davis conceded that no long-term studies have been done on any vaccines, and that long-term follow-up is not done in any careful way. The assumption is made that vaccines do not cause problems, so why should anyone check? Besides, a vaccine reaction is defined so that all negative reactions are said to occur very soon after the shot is given. But a vaccine obviously acts in the body for a long period of time after it is given. A reaction can be very gradual, just as chemical poisoning can occur very gradually. Neurological problems can develop over time. In actual fact, a vaccine that contains mercury may not show any damage for several months. And who is testing or investigating when a child 'becomes' autistic for no apparent reason? Those administering the vaccines claim: "This vaccine is safe." How can they be so sure of this when there is no scientific research to back up that claim, and when no testing procedures are in place to ensure their safety? Quite the opposite is true - plenty of evidence shows that vaccines are not safe.

Questions have recently emerged in the United States and Australia about the effectiveness and possibly dangerous side effects of Gardasil, Merck's newly licensed vaccine for human papillomavirus (HPV). This vaccine is given to young girls to prevent cervical cancer, which kills about 3,700 women each year. On June 9, 2007, *The British Medical Journal* reported that three deaths occurred in the U.S. shortly after immunization with the vaccine; these were among 1,637 adverse reactions reported by Judicial Watch, a public interest watchdog. Judicial Watch obtained the reports from the Food and Drug

Administration using the Freedom of Information Act. The reports were filed through the FDA's vaccine adverse event reporting system.

In Melbourne, Australia, 25 girls at a Catholic high school experienced headache, nausea, and dizziness after receiving their first injection of the vaccine, *The Age* reported.

Merck, the manufacturer of this vaccine, is the same company that made Vioxx, the drug that killed over 60,000 people and that tried to conceal the facts of Vioxx's deadly side effects. Although cervical cancer is easily preventable through non-drug approaches, Merck is trying to make this vaccination mandatory in all U.S. states. The drug-giant is clearly not interested in helping out a relatively few young girls who could be at risk of developing cervical cancer later in their lives; it rather wants to open up the huge potential market for cancer vaccines. Merck's own literature says it is important to realize that Gardasil does not protect women against some 'non-vaccine' HPV types. In other words, even if girls accept the risks and get vaccinated, they can still get HPV.

The Vaccine-Autism Link

Many doctors act as if it is a crime when parents refuse to give vaccines to their children. They equate it with irresponsible parenting. These doctors blindly rely on recommendations made by the Centers for Disease Control (CDC). In October 2004, CDC representatives announced their recommendation that children aged 6 months to 23 months should receive flu shots (which contain thimerosal) as part of the standard schedule of immunizations. Steve Cochi, the acting director of the National Immunization Program, underlined the CDC's official view of the vaccine-autism connection, citing a 'lack of scientific evidence'. This comes at a time when CDC officials were more than once made aware of the large body of scientific evidence that supports the vaccine-autism link. In actual fact, the research used in the study mentioned above was collected from data obtained under the Freedom of Information Act. And, as you may have guessed, the data came from the CDC's own archives. It is still perplexing to me that an institution that was meant to protect people against illnesses gives its blessing and active support to a procedure involving injection of mercury into an 8-, 12- or 16-pound infant.

Statistical research on medical history in the United States covering the years between 1940 and 1970 showed that autistic children were most common among wealthy families. After 1970, autism was equally distributed amongst all income groups. At the end of the sixties, certain immunization programs that only well-off families could previously afford were extended to the poor as well. The same trends were observed in other industrialized nations. Mercury-exposure to children through vaccines has dramatically increased over the past 20 years, while the rate of autism jumped from 1 in 10,000 to 1 in 150 over the same period. If you are a parent, you need to draw your own conclusions. But you certainly should not trust the government's agencies to protect you and your family.

An evidence-based fact analysis provides an irrefutable link between mercury-containing vaccines to autism. According to national statistics, one out of every 200 children in the United States is diagnosed with autism. One reporter wanted to know why Amish children don't suffer the same fate. It is a fact that the Amish don't allow their children to be vaccinated. While checking out one Amish community, the reporter found three children with autism. He discovered that one child was adopted from China and previously vaccinated, another was one of the few Amish children who were vaccinated, and the third had an unclear vaccine history. Although the odds of non-vaccinated Amish children developing autism are slim to none, health officials still pretend they don't know what causes autism in children, while insisting that vaccines are safe and do no harm.

On a different note, the National Institutes of Mental Health recently concluded that it is essential that pregnant women have enough vitamin D to ensure proper development of their fetus's brain. It is equally important for the proper development of a child brain's to have enough vitamin D after it is born. Since the child doesn't get vitamin D from breast milk, the only natural way to obtain it is through sunlight, just as nature intended it. Even moderate sun exposure helps ensure proper brain development. Unfortunately, sun-avoidance has increased dramatically in the last 20 years, ever since the medical community started warning about the dangers of sun exposure. Far fewer parents now expose their babies to the sun, and if they do, the babies are often given sunscreens and even sunglasses to wear. The vitamin D receptors appear in a wide variety of brain tissue early in the development of the baby, and activated vitamin D receptors increase nerve growth in the brain. If you have an autistic child, make sure s/he spends several hours a day outdoors, and if it is warm, without clothes so all the skin can receive this valuable treatment.

If you have an autistic child, you may also want to try out the Emotional Freedom Technique (EFT) by Gary Craig. I have seen great improvements in autistic children whose parents treat them with EFT (the program is available at no cost from www.emofree.com). I have also seen great improvements in autistic children who received a session in Sacred Santémony (see chapter 7).

Other health issues clearly caused by vaccinations include small-scale brain damage, growth inhibition, hyperactivity, learning difficulties, etc. Previously belittled as simple problems of growing up, medical researchers now recognize them as forms of encephalitis (inflammatory disease of the brain). More than 20 percent of the American children - one out of five - suffer from these or related problems. The multi-dose version of the hepatitis B vaccine, which is typically given to newborns before they leave the hospital, still contains thimerosal - the mercury-containing preservative. The central nervous systems of newborns are utterly defenseless against these toxic assaults. It doesn't help that the hepatitis B vaccine has nearly zero benefits for the child.

The hepatitis B vaccine is supposed to protect an adult against hepatitis B infection and liver cancer. Many of these affected individuals also have serious social problems like IV drug abuse, alcoholism and poor nutrition, all of which greatly increase the risk for these diseases. Newborns certainly don't fall into those risk groups and children almost never suffer from a hepatitis B infection or liver cancer. Since the vaccine protects a child only for a few years, by the time he could possibly develop liver cancer, the vaccine would have already stopped providing any benefits. Obviously this extremely poisonous childhood vaccine is absolutely unnecessary.

The documented evidence against the value of immunization is so comprehensive that in 1986 the American Congress passed federal legislation to compensate children for damages arising from vaccination. According to the law, the government is no longer liable for damages, but instead doctors and vaccine producers have to pay millions of dollars for compensation. In the interest of everyone involved, it would be useful to re-examine and re-evaluate the basic theory of Louis Pasteur that immunization is useful or necessary. Could nature have made such a crucial mistake as to make us dependant on injecting foreign, toxic material into our blood when we have an immune system so complex and highly developed that millions of sophisticated computers could not imitate its performance? This is rather unlikely.

How to Stay Immune

The damage that has been caused so far by vaccinations is considerable and surpasses many times the problems that could possibly arise from having no immunization program whatsoever. Many natural ways are available to acquire immunity. All the procedures and natural remedies described in this book can assist you and your family in maintaining natural immunity against disease throughout life. "The best vaccine against common infectious diseases," according to the World Health Organization, is "an adequate diet." Unprocessed, unrefined foods, including plenty of fresh fruits and vegetables, help a child to build up natural immunity and help the adult to maintain it.

The most powerful and all-protective immunization reinforcements a newborn baby can receive are having the doctor wait to cut or clamp the umbilical cord until it stops throbbing[43], and having the mother breastfeed the child. This way, the infant gets all the necessary antibodies to build up a sound system of immunity to effectively deal with any type of infectious agent in the future. Should an illness arise nevertheless, the body will deal with it rapidly and without suffering harm, and in fact will greatly benefit from it.

Breastfeeding should commence during the newborn's first hour of life, according to a 2006 study published in the journal *Pediatrics*. The researchers concluded that this could save 41 percent of newborns who would otherwise die in their first month of life. Breastfeeding right away not only increases the likelihood that infants will continue to breastfeed, but also gives them *colostrum*, a mother's first milk. As research has demonstrated, colostrum is rich in antibodies and essential nutrients, important for building a strong immune system right from the start. Early breastfeeding also helps mothers through improved lactation and less loss of blood. Besides, early breastfeeding helps mother and baby to bond naturally, which is important for the baby's psychological development throughout life. To increase their supply of breast milk, mothers can add fenugreek, a herb/spice, to their food.

For a child's healthy immune system to mature fully and properly in our less-than-perfect environment, it may be necessary to occasionally contract an infectious disease such as the measles, chickenpox, and mumps. We all have to learn to trust nature and our body more than man-made theories and practices. Human DNA has managed to survive millions of years on the planet and it certainly knows how to deal with a few harmless infectious diseases, particularly when they help to strengthen our immune system.

Our immune system shows that it is active and intact by reacting to disease with a normal inflammatory response. This defensive response removes accumulated toxins and the infectious agent from the system through a rash, fever, or cough. The healing process will naturally and profoundly stimulate the immune system so that, when the person recovers from the illness, s/he is equipped with enough immunity to respond to other forms of infection without delay or repeated illness.

Natural Methods of Nursing Children Back to Health

If your child is diagnosed as having chickenpox, mumps, or measles, it may indicate that s/he requires an immunity boost. Most children who have gone through these common childhood illnesses have greatly benefited from them; they are stronger afterwards and even have a growth spurt, either physically or emotionally, or both. Most natural health practitioners see a normal childhood illness as a good opportunity to develop immunity. By nursing a child with natural methods, you can help him to become healthier and more resistant to disease in the long run.

When children become ill with any of these illnesses, the main advice is to encourage their own healing powers. This is first accomplished by letting them get as much rest as possible. Take them out of school, the nursery, etc., and nurse them at home. Drugs such as liquid paracetamol only suppress the body's healing response and lead to many more 'unrelated' physical and emotional problems in the future.

---

[43] See this website for details on how to prevent blood volume loss, autism, anemia, jaundice and many potential illnesses in the life of your baby: http://www.lotusbirth.com.

For a child, the period of illness is often a way to receive additional caring attention from his parents. He may get many extra cuddles, meals in bed, and stories at bedtime, etc. Of course, there may be parents who feel that their child's illness is very inconvenient and show their frustration by being harsh and abrupt with them. Sick children need and deserve special treatment and reassurance, especially when they are frightened or anxious.

A sick child should not be excited or stimulated by exposure to too much radio, television, or even visitors. Quiet activities such as reading to them, drawing, and board games help them to avoid dwelling on their illness too much. Make sure that they get extra sleep with early bedtimes, and daytime naps if they feel tired.

Sick children need to drink plenty of liquid to help remove toxins from the system. Warm water is the best drink for them and should be the first option; herb teas and freshly pressed, diluted fruit juices (except citrus fruit juices if your child has mumps) can also be taken. Avoid giving your child anything cold, such as cold beverages, ice cream, sugar, or sugar-containing foods; milk, yoghurt or other dairy products; meat, chicken, fish or any other form of protein food. As the child's digestive power is weakened during the illness, such foods will only putrefy and acidify the digestive system and further irritate the mucus lining. Sick children, like sick animals, generally do not want or need food. Fasting, while drinking only water, is the best way to encourage the body's healing response. When your child feels hungry, give him freshly cooked vegetable purees, soups, hot cereals like porridge with a little maple syrup, or with good quality honey (which should only be added after the food has cooled down to less than 45 degrees C (115F) but more than body temperature. Children need to know what is happening to them during an illness and that it is going to pass soon. They also want reassurance that you are going to be there for them all the way.

If your child develops a fever, it is a sign of a healthy immune response. A raised temperature shows that the body has taken active charge of the situation and is fighting off an infection. Parents should remember that a high temperature does not necessarily mean that their child is very ill. As has been discovered recently, even a temperature of 41 degrees Celsius, or 106 degrees Fahrenheit, and slightly above is still not considered life-endangering. In 1983, when I lay ill with malaria in India, I refused to take fever-reducing tablets for a temperature of 41.5 degrees Celsius (106.7 Fahrenheit) and after the fever broke at the end of the third attack, I recovered very quickly and have had no relapse of malaria since. The most important thing to remember is that children and babies aged less than six months who are afflicted with fever need to drink plenty of water, as they tend to dehydrate quickly. Sponging them down with tepid water helps to keep the body more comfortable during this phase of healing. Expose and sponge only one part of the body at a time until it feels cool, then move on to the next one. Sponging the child's face and forehead also brings relief.

Another basic rule is to keep a chilly, feverish child warm and covered. This will make him sweat, particularly at night, and help to break the fever, which indicates that the body's 'fight' is nearly over. Hot, feverish children should be kept cool and occasionally be immersed in a bath of tepid water. If your child has accompanying symptoms such as itchy rashes, painful swollen glands, a cough or sore, sticky eyes, he is most likely to recover without any complications. In case he has any unusual symptoms, you may consult a natural practitioner of Ayurveda, Homeopathy, Chinese Medicine, etc., for home treatment remedies. It is better not to give *aspirin* to children during or after an illness as this can interfere with the body's own healing response. If your doctor insists on giving antibiotics to your child when he has one of the above illnesses or symptoms, try to find another doctor to give you a second opinion. In most cases, there is no need for drugs. In one large study published in 1987 in the *British Medical Journal,* 18,000 children received a homeopathic remedy against meningitis. None of the children got infected and not a single adverse effect developed from the treatment.

Elderberry has been used as a folk remedy for flu, colds, and coughs since the time of Hippocrates. And recently, an Israeli scientist discovered exactly why it works so well. In a controlled study that had flu sufferers recovering in record time, she found that elderberry literally 'disarms' viruses. The viruses simply were unable to penetrate the walls of the patients' cells.

As a general precaution, don't take your child to daycare centers or nurseries too early. This can protect him from many childhood diseases. Daycare facilities increase the risk of Hib meningitis, for example, by 24 times. Many of the commercially run centers are frequently 'visited' by all sorts of bugs. The safest environment for a child in the first years of his life is his home.

5. Protection against the Flu?

Protect Yourself Against the Flu Vaccine!

The vaccine industry insists that their vaccines against the flu serve as the key to a healthy winter. Although a serious flu epidemic has not occurred for 38 years, their vaccines are prescribed to millions of people each year. You may wonder why perfectly healthy people are injected with a normally harmless bug whose strains mutate from year to year? Although flu vaccines can never be accurate, employers encourage millions of their employees submit to a flu shot each year, trying to avoid the loss of working days.

Influenza always starts in the Far East, and then spreads to the West in early winter, reaching its peak during February and March. It may come in either of three types, A, B, or C. During the last several years, type A has been the dominant version. What makes vaccination against the flu so unsuccessful is that the strains of the flu virus are different every year and the so-called protection lasts for only six months. So each autumn you require a new vaccination for a different virus. The trouble is, drug companies have no way of knowing in the summer which new strain of the flu virus is going to hit the Western Hemisphere during the winter months.

The vaccine producers grow the vaccines, consisting of live viruses, in hen's eggs. When the vaccine is injected into the body, it can cause side effects such as redness and soreness at the injection site and a mild form of flu. Very serious complications arise in people who are taking immune-suppressing drugs or who have a heart condition. If you are allergic to eggs, having a flu-shot may also endanger your health.

For the average healthy person, coming down with the flu is not serious at all. On the contrary, it can build up natural immunity even against future encounters with new strains of the flu virus. The very reason that nature creates these new forms of virus every year and spreads them with accurate timing is to ensure continued ecological balance and strong immunity in plants, animals, and humans alike. Anyone prone to repeated infections is likely to have a toxic liver with many hundreds of stones accumulated in the liver and gallbladder. Gallstones, which harbor many types of infectious bacteria and viruses, are a constant source of immune suppression. Cleansing the liver of all gallstones is about the best prevention against any type of infection. People who have cleansed their liver in this way have reported that they never catch a cold or the flu anymore.

Flu virus vaccines used until 2002 contained 'live' viruses and produced so many serious, adverse reactions that new vaccines had to be concocted. The new formula for flu vaccines is called the 'subvirion', which basically is a mutilated virus 'blended, spliced and macerated' until just bits and pieces of the original virus are left. This in no way makes the virus less dangerous. In fact, the antigens or foreign proteins in the vaccine, for which the body is forced to produce antibodies, are still as poisonous and harmful as the live virus.

Besides the subvirion, plenty of other substances are added to the flu vaccine, most of which you would never want to consciously ingest. These include:

- *Hemagglutinin antigens* that cause clumping of the red blood cells, leading to cardiovascular disease.
- The enzyme *neuraminidase, which cuts out* neuraminic acid from the cell membrane, weakening all of the trillions of cell membranes in the body.
- A white crystalline substance called *allantoin,* a toxic animal waste product. Due to its high nitrogen content, allantoin is used as fertilizer; it leads to kidney and bladder stones in humans.
- *Gentamicin,* a broad spectrum antibiotic, is added to each embryonated chicken egg to inhibit the growth of bacteria (vaccine is grown in chicken eggs).
- Formaldehyde (carcinogenic), used as a preservative and to inactivate the virus.
- The toxic chemicals, *tri butylphosphate and Polysorbate 80, U.S.P.*
- Resin, to eliminate 'substantial portions'" of tri butylphosphate and Polysorbate 80
- *Thimerosal,* a mercury derivative, to preserve the vaccine cocktail.
- *Polyethylene glycol,* a relative of *ethylene glycol* (antifreeze); often used to poison dogs and other predators of sheep.
- *Isocctylphenyl ether,* a compound of ether; has anesthetic properties; a *teratogen,* causing abnormal prenatal development. It also induces testicular atrophy in animals.

The vaccine producers are unable to guarantee that the vaccine will protect you against the flu. So they carefully tell you that the vaccine "reduces the likelihood of infection; or if you do develop the disease, it will be a milder case." Some express the same uncertainty about their product in this way: "It is known definitely that influenza virus vaccine, as now constituted, is not effective against all possible strains of influenza virus." Perhaps the best lesson of this effect comes from Japan. Compulsory flu vaccination in Japan (1967-1987) revealed no benefit and actually caused more flu- and vaccine-related deaths.

Why would you want to entrust your health to a cocktail of poisonous chemicals when even a somewhat weakened immune system stands a far better chance of protecting you against harm from a bout of influenza. Our body's sophisticated immune system, which has evolved over millions of years, can certainly do a better job of protecting you against the flu than anything made-made. All it needs is some basic caretaking on your part. With each new flu shot, on the other hand, your immune system becomes more depleted and the side effects become more pronounced and severe. And, you may still get the flu anyway. The following list includes the possible consequences you might develop if you choose the road of vaccination:

The most frequent side effects of vaccination:

- Soreness at the site of the vaccination
- Pain or tenderness
- Erythema
- Inflammation
- Skin discoloration
- Induration
- A mass or lump
- Hypersensitivity reactions including puritus and urticaria
- Fever
- Malaise

- Myalgia
- Arthralgia
- Asthenia
- Chills
- Dizziness
- Headache
- Lymphadenopathy
- Rash
- Nausea
- Vomiting

- Diarrhea
- Pharyngitis
- Angiopathy
- Vasculiltis
- Anaphylaxis in asthmatics, with possible death
- Anaphylactic shock, with possible death

Vaccination certainly does not create immunity. You cannot become immune by ingesting poisons that destroy the immune system. Studies by a group of Italian scientists showed that the flu vaccine reduced the occurrence of clinical episodes of influenza by only 6 percent in adults, and effectiveness tended to decrease with age. They concluded that universal immunization wasn't warranted. Stated simply, hand washing and other hygienic and nutritional measures are far superior to the flu vaccine in effectiveness. If you are practicing good hygiene, eating nutritious foods and keeping your intestines and liver clean, influenza will never become a deadly disease. Getting vaccinated against the flu, on the other hand, is a sure way to sow the seeds for new illnesses in the body. All vaccines are poisonous and, as such, act like time bombs that will explode in due time.

Why People Get the Flu

Flu shots lower natural immunity by injecting alien and toxic substances directly into the bloodstream. No other animal in the world chooses such unnatural, superficial and crude means to defend itself against invading viruses. The normal route of contact with a viral particle is via the lungs. The vast majority of the population has a normal, healthy immune system and is perfectly capable of dealing with the invaders without getting sick. But if the body's infection fighters have temporarily gone 'on strike' for reasons other than the lack of a vaccine, the flu virus can gain unrestricted access into the body and cause an infection.

Regular vaccination (of any kind) is one of the major causes of depleted immunity. The yearly-administered flu shots repeatedly burden the immune system and cells of the body with foreign toxic material without giving them a chance to remove them again. The toxic viral particles can remain latent in the cells and gallstones for as long as 20 years; when they emerge, they can cause serious cell damage. With each new vaccination the immune system becomes more and more restricted in its effort to neutralize the live virus that suddenly appears in the blood. It may produce antibodies for the virus (although in many cases the immune system fails to do even that), and thus subdue it, but this encounter leaves the host's immune system unnecessarily tired and weak.

Besides immune damage, vaccines of all kinds produce alterations in genetic material and thereby cause a whole range of malfunctions in the body. Vaccines may even be the cause of the increasing incidence of malignant diseases in children. Mass immunization programs have created such weak immune systems that children are even susceptible to such harmless viruses as the one causing the flu. We may have gone as far as to replace mumps and measles with cancer, leukemia, and Chronic Fatigue Syndrome.

Flu vaccinations are mainly targeted at the older generation and young children. In the United Kingdom, about 10,000 people, most of them of very advanced age, (supposedly) die from flu-related illnesses. It may, therefore, sound reasonable to vaccinate the older people to protect them against the flu virus. But there is no total protection even among those vaccinated. Around 20 percent or more of the elderly people who get the vaccine still get a more virulent strain of flu, and many others get a lighter form of the flu. The same is true for the people in the same age group who haven't been immunized. The weak and elderly people are more likely to die from the flu, *regardless* of whether they have been immunized or not. The bottom line is that there is no real advantage in having a flu shot. And certainly, given the frailty of so many of the oldest members of society, there is absolutely no reliable way of telling whether the flu or something else may have led to their death. The death rate in and out of the flu season is actually about the same. But then, as we have seen with AIDS, statistics can be manipulated in ways that support theories which have only one objective, to keep the medical business going. For instance, when a person who is about to die anyway also catches the flu, he will be listed as a flu victim.

Instead of giving the elderly population vaccines, in the misguided belief that this would take care of them, we could help them much more by improving their general resistance to disease through good diet, social engagements and exercise programs. Many old people don't have adequate nutrition and suffer from depression; both these factors work as powerful immune suppressants. Others don't have a warm home or they live alone. Research has shown that these are the major risk factors for illness and death in the older generation. A series of liver cleanses alone can strengthen natural immunity, improve digestion, retard the aging process, restore health, and enhance mental functions.

In developing countries, where the elderly play an important role in society, general illness is low, provided there is enough food available. In these countries it is more likely that old people die from malnutrition than from a strain of virus.

An increasing number of reports indicate that adults who regularly receive flu shots suffer a worsening of high blood pressure, diabetes, gout, and Parkinson's disease as well as an increase in all kinds of allergic complaints. In 1976 an extensive flu vaccination program in America led to a massive outbreak of Guillain-Barré syndrome, a disease affecting the nervous system. The outbreak, known as the 'Great Swine Flu Fiasco' paralyzed 656 people and 30 elderly persons were found dead within hours after they were vaccinated. Compensation claims were enormous, which slowed down the program but only for a while.

Seniors, of course, are one of the core target groups for the flu vaccine program. So every year we're told how older people are particularly vulnerable to the flu. We're also told that government officials are holding their breath over their fear of a devastating flu pandemic. We're even told that about 36,000 people die of flu-related complications in the United States each year, and most of those deaths are elderly people. The reality of the matter is quite different, though. How many people do you think died of the flu last year? Less than 175, according to Sherri J. Tenpenny, D.O., an internationally known leader in vaccine research! And yet, the official line propagated by media campaigns is to be prepared for another wave of deadly flu epidemic, killing thousands of people each new season.

What about the other high-risk group, young children? Japanese researchers have shown that infants under one year of age fail to even generate a good antibody response following the vaccine. Pumping children full of vaccine poisons is pointless, except to enrich the pharmaceutical companies.

In the Name of Prevention

The pharmaceutical companies producing the vaccines seem to have a more powerful effect on the population than the scientists who invented them. As early as 1980, Dr Albert Sabin, one of the world's leading virologists and a pioneer of the polio vaccine, spoke vehemently against the use of the flu vaccine, claiming that it was unnecessary for over 90 percent of the population. This, however, has not discouraged the vaccination industry to endorse vaccination for *all* in the name of health and protection against disease.

What makes matters worse is that there has never been a properly controlled clinical trial with the flu vaccine. Because we don't know anything about its long-term effects, we may be unknowingly producing generations of people with debilitated immune systems and chronic diseases. Flu vaccination is an unproved and unscientific practice and nothing in the scientific literature can certify or guarantee its safety. The most effective way to fight infections, including the flu, is to prevent it. There is no substitute for a health-increasing regimen. Vaccination, on the other hand, offers no real protection. Injecting the body with foreign and poisonous viral material is counterproductive to improving our well-being. Dr. John Seal from the American National Institute for Allergies and Infectious Diseases warned that we have to assume that every flu vaccination can cause the Guillain-Barré Syndrome. In this sense, prevention is *not* better than cure.

Help From Mother Nature

For those who are concerned about the flu and its possible effects, a remarkable herbal extract called andrographis paniculata is available. It has been used for centuries in Ayurvedic (traditional Indian) therapies and traditional Chinese Medicine to treat everything from isolated cases of the sniffles to full-blown outbreaks of influenza. Apparently, andrographis is believed to have halted the spread of the 1919 Indian flu pandemic.

Scientific evidence supports that theory. Researchers at the Universities of Exeter and Plymouth in the U.K. conducted a survey of medical databases, herbal manufacturer information and World Health Organization reports to select seven studies that met the criteria for double-blind, controlled trials. The combined studies tested the use of andrographis as a treatment for respiratory tract infection in nearly 900 subjects. In all seven of these studies, subjects who took andrographis after the onset of cold symptoms reported faster recovery compared to subjects who took placeboes or medication.

Researchers concluded that andrographis may be effective in treating 'uncomplicated' infection in the upper respiratory tract (throat, sinuses and ears). According to previous laboratory trials, andrographis extract doesn't actually kill the organisms that make you sick - at least not directly. Instead, the herbal compound boosts your immune system and stimulates natural antibodies.

Animal research also showed that andrographis may help inhibit the formation of blood clots, lower blood sugar levels in diabetics, lowered systolic blood pressure, protect the liver against damage and prevent myocardial ischemia (inadequate blood circulation in the heart caused by coronary artery disease).

Kan Jang is a brand of standardized extract of andrographis that has consistently outsold all other cold medications in Scandinavia for 13 years running. The Swedish Herbal Institute, the formulator of Kan Jang, recommends that you take one tablet four times daily to fight colds or the flu. Kan Jang can be purchased at dietary supplement stores and through Internet sites.

COLD-fX is another well-researched panacea for both prevention and treatment of Cold and Flu. It is available over-the-counter from most drugstores. According to credible research of 10 years, COLD-fX regulates both antigen specific acquired and innate immune systems to combat cold and flu viral infection. It will also have effectiveness in the following conditions: travel, work-related fatigue and stress. A 2006 pre-clinical study showed potential benefits in cancer patients. COLD-fX is an extract of American Ginseng.

Warning about cough syrups for children: In 2007, in response to overwhelming evidence about harmful side-effects of cough syrups, the FDA banned the sale of over-the-counter cough and cold medicines for young children. The ban applies to decongestant use in children under 2, and antihistamines in those younger than 6. The products include approximately 800 popular medicines that are sold in the U.S. under names like Toddler's Dimetapp, Triaminic Infant and Little Colds, according to a report in *The New York Times*. It is expected that all infant cough and cold products will eventually be removed from the market. Until then, make sure to avoid any and all cough syrups and decongestants for your children, regardless of the age group. At least 123 children have lost their lives because of them since they became popular in the 1970s.

6. Alcohol - Man's Legal Drug

Much controversy has been generated around alcohol use. Some people say that alcohol can perk you up, reduce tension and inhibitions, and bring more fun into your life. Getting drunk is often seen as a means to 'escape' the burden of personal and interpersonal problems, at least for a while. Alcohol may make you feel euphoric and relaxed but it also has unwanted side effects. You lose control over your mind, your senses, and your body's coordination skills. A hangover demonstrates the powerful toxic effects that alcohol has on the normal functioning of the mind, body, and spirit.

But why do people drink alcoholic beverages? Getting drunk can hardly be considered fun because loss of self-control does not really make a person happy. However, despite the accompanying side effects, many people are drawn repeatedly to having 'another drink'. And why does alcohol make us get drunk in the first place?

The answer to both of these questions may lie in the brain hormone *serotonin*, which is the main chemical equivalent for pleasure and happiness. With the increasing darkness of the night, *serotonin* gets broken down into the hormone melatonin. Alcohol, however, slows down this process and thereby maintains a 'good mood'. However, if *serotonin* is not broken down on time, it reacts with the toxic substance *acetaldehyde,* which the body produces from the ingested alcohol.

The chemical reaction generates an entire group of chemicals that have hallucinating effects; they are known as *tetrahydro-ss-carboline. Salsolinol,* a substance synthesized in the presence of the brain chemical *dopamine,* blocks the breakdown of *serotonin. Dopamine* then begins to form a new chemical called *norlaudanosolin,* a precursor of morphine and 2.000 other types of *alkaloids.* In other words, if you think you are addicted to alcohol, you are wrong. In reality you are addicted to morphine.

However, alcohol consumption does not necessarily turn into an addiction. Genetic predisposition makes some people produce more morphine or opiate from *acetaldehyde* than others. Under normal conditions, the side effects that arise from drunkenness prevent most people from further drinking. So the body rarely gets the chance to make sufficient amounts of such hallucinogenic drugs to cause an addiction. Yet regular consumption of alcohol can eventually increase this chance.

Some people should not risk drinking alcohol at all. Asians in general and Chinese and Koreans in particular lack the enzyme that breaks down the toxic *acetaldehyde* so even small amounts of alcohol lead to a fast pulse, abdominal pain, and a red face. For this reason, alcoholism is rarely existent in Asia; Asians would simply die in large numbers from alcohol poisoning. Also, some people pass out after the first (and only drink) because they have no natural defenses against *acetaldehyde*.

Beer - Hypnotism and a Big Tummy

If you have ever had the chance to smell a hops plant, then you know it has hypnotic effects. Harvesting any of the plants of the hemp family can make you quite sleepy. Cannabis, which is used to produce Hashish and Marijuana, is a close relative of hops. The relaxing effect that beer has on the consumer comes from the hops ingredient *hopein,* among other substances. Hopein is a form of morphine.

With the exception of Muslim countries, beer consumption is legal, yet taking morphine, marijuana, or other hallucinogenic drugs is treated as a criminal act. If a person regularly gets drunk by drinking large quantities of beer, he is not less 'out of himself' or physically and mentally incompetent than he would be under drug-induced hallucination. It would not make a difference whether a hallucinating drug user runs over an innocent pedestrian or a drunk who has had a few bottles of morphine-containing beer. If a person is caught driving while drunk, he will receive punishment by law. If he gets drunk and is not driving, the law cannot touch him. If someone becomes violent under the influence of beer, it is due to reasons similar to a drug user becoming violent under the influence of hallucinogenic drugs.

Apart from their mind-altering effects, hops are known to work as an anti-aphrodisiac, suppressing sexual drive and performance in men. Hops contain the female sex hormones *daidzein* and *genistein,* which are generally used to fatten calves, sheep, and chickens. Contrary to general belief, the body cannot utilize any of the numerous calories contained in whiskey or other alcoholic beverages for producing energy or increasing fat reserves. Beer contains another female hormone, an estrogen, which is also formed in a woman's ovaries. The typical beer belly and breast growth of a beer drinker is caused by these female hormones and has nothing to do with beer calories.

Besides the already mentioned mind-altering chemicals in beer, the malt in beer also has a substance in it that influences the psyche; it is called *hordenin.* Hordenin results from the germination of barley and is related to the well-known stimulants *ephedrine* and *mescaline.* It also has a strong diuretic effect, which causes frequent urination, especially during the night. To process one glass of beer, the body's cells have to supply at least three glasses of water. Hence beer can cause severe dehydration such as is typically found among heavy beer drinkers. When the beer drinker's body signals dehydration, he may be tempted to drink even more beer, which increases dehydration further.

All these factors may result in weight gain, tissue acidification, retention of toxins, and swelling of the body. In addition, if the beer production uses extremely 'hard' water, rich in inorganic (metallic) calcium, the result may be a high incidence of kidney stones and kidney problems among beer drinkers. Also, regular consumption of all alcoholic beverages causes gallstones in the liver and gallbladder. Alcohol is extremely acidic which alters the pH of the alkaline bile to the point of thickening, leading to blockage of bile ducts. Thus, alcohol consumption can become a cause for any illness in the body.

Solving the Red Wine Mystery

Despite what we know today about the destructive effects of alcoholic beverages on liver and brain cells, you may have been advised to drink a glass of red wine or two on a daily basis to benefit your arteries. This advice, however, is misleading. It makes you believe that drinking alcohol is not so bad for you after all, whereas in truth it is not the alcohol in the wine that is beneficial for the heart. A study led by Dr. John Folts of the University of Wisconsin Medical School found that 8 or 10 ounces a day of the purple variety of grape juice has a potent effect on the blood cells called platelets, making them less likely to form clots that can lead to heart attacks.

A group of natural substances found in many kinds of foods, called *flavonoids,* seem to have powerful anti-clotting properties. They are amply present in purple grape juice and, to a lesser extent, also in red wine. Purple grape juice might even be more potent than aspirin, which is widely recommended as a way of warding off heart attacks. The study found that both aspirin and red wine slow the activity of blood platelets by about 45 percent, while purple grape juice dampens them by 75 percent. It is not clear, however, whether the thinning of blood after drinking red wine is caused by flavonoids or by the diuretic effects of the alcohol contained in the wine.

If purple grape juice is turned into wine, it loses some of its flavonoids. To have the benefits advocated for red wine and more, it is better to drink the fresh juice of purple grapes. Plant foods contain about 4,000 flavonoids. Eating a diet rich in fruits and vegetables is one of the best ways to maintain a healthy circulatory system, while alcohol is not. Although the flavonoids contained in red wine may have some beneficial effects on the blood, the alcohol that goes with it, after initially thinning the blood due the alcohol's diuretic effects, makes it thicker than it was before. If you need proof, ask a friend to apply the muscle test from chapter 1 on you while you hold a bottle of red wine or another alcoholic beverage in your hand. If your arm muscle tests weak, it shows that any benefit that may be been left in the red wine from the grape juice has been voided. The alcohol in the wine actually causes the shutdown of energy flow to the muscles.

7. Dirty Business with our Food - Genetically Modified

Genetic engineering of food is rapidly becoming an extremely lucrative business that is likely to place man's global food production in the hands of a few powerful people or governments. Whoever controls global food production will also control the world. In the name of progress and improvement of food production, the plan is to make every nation dependent on using the genetically engineered seeds that the world's leading food industries have produced and for which they own the patent rights. The agricultural products manufacturer Monsanto is doing exactly that. In January 2005, Monsanto announced it will buy the commercial fruit and vegetable seed company Seminis. The deal is said to be worth $1.4 billion. Once the majority of the world is using gene-manipulated seeds to grow their crops, the man-made Frankenstein foods will take their toll on human life. The aim of the wealthiest and most influential group of people in the world is to drastically reduce the size of the world's population. Why? Because a smaller population and the world's natural resources would be a lot easier to control than 8 billion people. Genetically engineered foods play a decisive role in this plan, and unless the rest of humanity wakes up to its responsibility as caretakers of Mother Earth, it is most likely going to succeed.

Monsanto, which also produced the poisonous sweetener aspartame, is inserting genes from plants of unrelated species into the soybean plant to make it resistant to the potent herbicide *Roundup* (glyphosate). The unsuspecting farmers would only welcome such a miracle plant, unless of course they see the risk involved. The Roundup resistant soybean seed can now be heavily sprayed with Roundup to kill weeds, but without causing damage to the soybean. No more problems with weeds suffocating the soybean plants, but bigger problems for the consumer! The new soybean is heavily contaminated with the toxic herbicide, Roundup.

Today, these genetically modified soybean products, which comprise about 80 percent of the beans available, have been found in most baby formulas including Carnation, Similac, Enfamil, Isomil, and Neocare as well as Doritos, Fritos, vegetable oils, soybean oil, margarine, and much more. With soy now being an ingredient of thousands of common food products, the masses are systematically poisoned with harmful herbicides.

One of the genes used in the new soybean is derived from the petunia plant, which is a nightshade variety. This is bad news for people with nightshade-induced arthritis. Suddenly, by inadvertently eating something that contains a soy product, they may end up becoming crippled with arthritis. They may have no problem with soy as such, but soy isn't just soy anymore; it is now also a nightshade, at least on the genetic level.

The method of gene manipulation may even lead to more serious consequences than 'just' a painful joint disorder. When Monsanto inserted the Brazil nut gene into soy, people allergic to Brazil nuts suffered *anaphylaxis* from ingesting a soy product. Anaphylaxis is a serious, life threatening reaction where one is not able to breathe. Monsanto was ordered to remove the gene to avoid further complications of that nature.

The process of genetic engineering of food often involves the use of a live virus, small enough to enter cell nuclei and, thereby, infect other genetic material. Cancer in chickens often results from infection with the *Rous Sarcoma virus*. The chicken cancer virus is used as a carrier to implant the growth hormone gene into farmed fish so they will grow faster. Once the virus has infected the fish, it will likely end up on your dinner plate and also infect you. With the multitudes of genetically modified foods out there, our body will become a host for numerous viruses that normally would never be found in us.

Likewise, Leukemia virus in chicken has been used as a carrier to insert human genes into developing poultry. It gets better, or shall I say, worse. A retrovirus was used to insert human fetal cells in pigs in order to grow aortas for transplantation into humans. When the pig's aorta was transplanted into the human body, it led to infections in humans with the pig's retrovirus.

When these viruses are used as part of genetic engineering, they combine with one another to create new plant and animal diseases. By eating these new foods, foreign genetic material from these viruses can be absorbed through our intestines and become incorporated into our cells. Thanks to genetic research and food production, we are now on the verge of creating new diseases against which we have no natural or unnatural way of defending ourselves.

As more and more foods are grown that include foreign genes to make them resistant to certain pests, pesticides, herbicides or antibiotics, the more of these gene transporters or vectors will end up lodging in our intestinal tract, infecting the bacteria in our gut. The infected gut microbes will not only become antibiotic-resistant, but resistant to any kind of treatment.

Since the U.S. government doesn't require any testing or proof of the safety of genetically engineered foods, the extremely well-paid genetic scientists basically have free and unrestricted reign over designing their sinister programs of gene engineering. As for now, new genes have already been planted in potatoes, corn, sugar beets, tomatoes, and cotton (used to make junk food oil found on roasted nuts given out on airplanes) to make the plants resistant to pesticides. Canola oil is also a genetically engineered product, poisonous for the body.

In 1994, the genetically engineered growth hormone rBGH, designed to increase milk production in cows, was approved for use in the U.S. About a third of U.S. farmers now use it to speed up milk production. The viruses used to make the growth hormone, of course, are in the milk. The prestigious medical journal, *Lancet*, reported in 1998 that breast cancer is seven times higher in women with tiny increases in the growth hormone, Insulin-like Growth Factor (IGF-1), which comes from cows injected with rBGH. Two years before this report, the *International Journal of Health Sciences* stated that IGF-1 concentrations are ten times higher in rBGH milk and *can* be absorbed through our intestines, and increase our risk of cancer among other diseases.

With increasing usage of genetically engineered plants, we will be faced with the following global scenario:

1. Loss of thousands of species of plants
2. All small farmers have to give up their farming businesses
3. Creation of Frankenstein foods that our bodies won't know how to handle
4. Super weeds resistant to all herbicides

5.   Plants resistant to pesticides
6.   New viruses and diseases for which there won't be a cure

Already, 60 percent of processed foods now contain at least one genetically modified food item. Millions of people now consume chips with the firefly gene, potato chips with a chicken gene, or salsa with tomato containing a flounder gene. Cream of broccoli soup can have a bacteria gene in it, and salad dressing is most likely made with canola oil, vegetable oil or soybean oil (all genetically engineered). The tobacco gene is now used in lettuce and cucumbers and the petunia gene is used in soybeans and carrots. If you have celiac disease, you may need to avoid walnuts because they can have the barley gene in them. Even strawberries are not harmless anymore; they can now have 'undisclosed genes' in them, so you will never know what else you are getting when you treat yourself to this delicious fruit. Cheese contains genetically engineered bacterial rennet. Many brands of apple juice contain the silkworm gene, and grapes can contain a virus gene. Trout, salmon, catfish, bass and even shrimp, are also genetically 'enriched'.

Multinational corporations are rapidly changing our food and nobody seems to be able to stop them. They're not accountable to anyone since they do not have to label their foods, and the government (at least in the U.S.) does not require them to do any safety testing.

8. Soy - A Miracle Food or Health Threat?

Soy products have made it into the food industry big time. Soy has been praised as the miracle food that will save the world.   However, in spite of impressive nutritional content, soy products are biologically useless to the body, for reasons explained below. Today, soy is contained in thousands of different food products, which has led to a massive escalation of disease in both developed and underdeveloped countries.

Given the fact that soybeans are grown on farms that use toxic pesticides and herbicides - and many are from genetically engineered plants - increasing evidence suggests soy is a major health hazard. With a few exceptions, such as miso, tempeh and other carefully fermented soy products, soy is not suitable for human consumption. Eating soy, soy milk, and regular tofu increases risks of serious health conditions. In addition, soy is a common food allergen. Numerous studies have found that soy products:

- increase the risk of breast cancer in women, brain damage in both men and women, and abnormalities in infants
- contribute to thyroid disorders, especially in women
- promote kidney stones (because of excessively high levels of oxalates which combine with calcium in the kidneys)
- weaken the immune system
- cause severe, potentially fatal food allergies
- accelerates brain weight loss in aging users

Soy products contain:

- Phytoestrogens (isoflavones) genistein and daidzein, which mimic and sometimes block the hormone estrogen
- Phytic acids, which reduce the absorption of many vitamins and minerals, including calcium, magnesium, iron, and zinc, thereby causing mineral deficiencies

- 'Antinutrients' or enzyme inhibitors that inhibit enzymes needed for protein digestion and amino acid uptake
- Haemaggluttin, which causes red blood cells to clump together and inhibits oxygen uptake and growth
- Trypsin inhibitors that can cause pancreatic enlargement and, eventually, cancer

Phytoestrogens are potent anti-thyroid agents which are present in vast quantities in soy. Infants exclusively fed on a soy-based formula have 13,000 to 22,000 times more estrogen compounds in their blood than babies fed a milk-based formula. This would be the estrogenic equivalent of at least five birth control pills per day. For this reason, premature development of girls (early puberty) has been linked to the use of soy formula, as has the underdevelopment of males. Infant soy formula and soy milk have been linked to autoimmune-thyroid disease, and now also to death.

In 2007, two parents were convicted of murder and given life sentences in prison for starving their 6-week-old baby to death by feeding it with soy milk and apple juice. Now, soy experts are again calling for clear and proper warning labels on all soy milk products - following this and several other babies' hospitalizations or deaths under similar circumstances.

Only properly fermented soy products, such as miso and tempeh, provide soy nutrients that can easily be absorbed. To make soy products nutritious and healthy, they must be carefully fermented - according to the traditional preparation methods used in Japan. Typically, soy must be fermented for at least two summers, ideally for 5-6 years, before it becomes beneficial for the body.

In spite of the documented scientific evidence that shows soy to be carcinogenic and also cause DNA and chromosome damage, the multi-billion dollar soy industry has managed to turn this generally worthless food into one of the most widely used 'nutritious foods' of all times. In a written statement, a spokesman for *Protein Technologies* said that they had "…..teams of lawyers to crush dissenters, could buy scientists to give evidence, owned television channels and newspapers, could divert medical schools and could even influence governments……" We cannot expect that the powerful and wealthy soy industry is going to disappear any time soon, but we can still make the choice to avoid non-fermented soy products or foods that contain soy. Soy acts more like a drug, not a food, upsetting the body's entire hormonal balance. This is enough reason to avoid soy at any cost.

CHAPTER 14

Over 51 Health Myths
Keeping Americans So Sick

1. Vitamin Euphoria - A Shot in the Dark

Vitamins seem to be good for everything. The newborn needs them to grow, women take them to be happy, men use them to maintain or increase potency, athletes ingest them to stay fit, and older people take them to become younger or to avoid the flu. Even foods are categorized into good and bad, depending on how many vitamins they contain. Ever since vitamins were produced synthetically, they were made available in every drugstore or health shop around the world. An estimated 80 million to 160 million people take antioxidants in North America and Europe, about 10 to 20 percent of adults. In 2006, Americans spent $2.3 billion on nutritional supplements and vitamins at grocery stores, drug stores and retail outlets, excluding Wal-Mart, according to Information Resources Inc., which tracks sales.

To stay healthy, you don't have to eat all that vitamin-rich food anymore. Just pop in a couple of those colorful vitamin pills a day and your health is taken care of, or so the ad slogans tell you. But if you don't pay heed to this 'common-sense' advice, doctors tell you that you may become vitamin deficient and put your health at risk.

And so we act obediently, out of fear of risking our lives. If you feel tired or suffer from lack of concentration (which could be due to lack of sleep or overeating), you may be prescribed vitamin B pills. Then there is vitamin C if you catch a cold (which could result from stress, working too hard or eating too much junk food). Vitamin E, you are told, helps you prevent a heart attack (so you may no longer need to watch out for the true risk factors of heart disease, as outlined in chapter 9). Accordingly, we spend billions of dollars on vitamin pills each year to fight off every kind of ill from the common cold to cancer.

Nowadays, artificial vitamins are added to almost every processed food - not because they are so good for you, but because foods that are 'enriched' sell better. Cereals, bread, milk, yoghurt, boiled sweets (hard candy), even dog food with added vitamins leave the supermarket shelves much faster than foods without them. Smokers, meat eaters, sugar addicts and people who drink too much alcohol can now continue enjoying their self-destructing habits without having to fear the dreaded vitamin deficiency, thanks to the blessed food industry. The magic food supplements have become an insurance policy against poor diet, and nobody has to feel guilty anymore over eating junk food. And to top it off, scientific research (financed by the vitamin producers) suggests that taking large doses of supplements may protect you against disease, even though there is no real evidence to support that claim. As seen in the sales figures, the public believes that the more vitamins you take, the healthier you become.

But are vitamins really that good for your health? Despite the massive amounts of vitamins consumed in modern societies, overall health is declining everywhere, except in those countries that still rely mostly on fresh-farmed foods. Could the mass consumption of vitamins be even co-responsible for this trend?

Antioxidant vitamins taken by tens of millions of people around the world at least won't lead to a longer life, according to an analysis of dozens of studies that adds to evidence questioning the value of the popular, largely synthetically produced, supplements. The large review study of separate studies on thousands of people found no long-life benefit from vitamins A, E and C and beta carotene and selenium, according to the Cochrane Hepato-Biliary Group at Copenhagen University Hospital in Denmark. The Cochrane organization is a respected international network of experts that does systematic reviews of scientific evidence on health interventions. For the new report on antioxidants, published in the *Journal of the American Medical Aossociation* in 2007, the researchers first analyzed 68 studies involving 232,606 people and found no significant effect on mortality. When they looked more closely at the most trustworthy studies, they actually found a higher risk of death for people taking vitamins: 4 percent for those taking vitamin E, 7 percent for beta carotene and 16 percent for vitamin A.

Sodium and water are essential to maintain sodium levels and hydrate the body, but too much of either can seriously upset the body's electrolyte balance. Over consumption of vitamin A, for example, can cause loss of hair, double vision, headaches, and vomiting in women, all indications of vitamin poisoning. If a woman is pregnant, the supplement can even harm her unborn baby. As we will see, vitamins can even endanger a person's life.

Vitamin Deficiency - Or Perhaps, Something Else?

In the beginning of the 17th Century, Japan was afflicted with a disease, called *beriberi*, which killed many people. By the year 1860, over one third of Japan's marines had fallen ill with symptoms of weight loss, frequent heart complaints, loss of appetite, irritability, burning sensations in the feet, lack of concentration, and depression. The symptoms quickly disappeared whenever rice, Japan's most important staple food, was replaced with other foods.

Thirty years later the Dutch physician Christiaan Eijkman conducted an experiment feeding chicken white rice. The chicken developed a number of symptoms such as loss of weight, weakness, and signs of nerve infection, which Eijkman interpreted as being *beriberi*. The symptoms disappeared again when the chicken were fed brown rice. Soon after, Eijkman discovered a few, previously unknown substances within the bran of the whole rice; one of them was named B1. This initiated the era of vitamins.

But, as it turned out, beriberi wasn't caused by vitamin B1 deficiency. People no longer suffered from beriberi once they discontinued eating rice altogether. It should have been noticed from the beginning that, with 'no rice - no vitamin B1 - no beriberi', the disease must have had other causes than vitamin deficiency. Japanese marine soldiers died within three days after consuming white rice, yet it takes much longer than that to develop a B1 deficiency. The origin of this mysterious disease was revealed when in 1891 a Japanese researcher discovered that beriberi is caused by the poison *citreoviridine*. Citreoviridine is produced by mold in white rice that is stored in filthy and moist environments.

Yet until today, the vitamin B1-beriberi-hypothesis is still maintained in medical text books around the world. Although it has never been proven that a B1 deficiency causes such symptoms as fatigue, loss of appetite, exhaustion, depression, irritability, and nerve damage, many patients having these symptoms are told that they have a vitamin-B deficiency. During vitamin B1 trial studies, all the participants complained about the highly monotonous diet they were given; they suffered fatigue and loss of appetite, regardless of whether they received B1 in their diet or not. As soon as they returned to their normal diet, even without B1, the symptoms spontaneously disappeared.

Another B-vitamin is *nicotinic acid*, also known as *niacin*. It has become very popular and is now routinely added to many foods. Niacin is supposed to safeguard us against diarrhea, dementia and the skin disease *pellagra*. Pellagra is more widespread among people who eat maize, though not everyone who eats maize gets pellagra. Pellagra was found to be caused by food poisoning through spoiled maize. The poison involved has been identified as *T2-toxine* and is known to disturb niacin metabolism, thus producing pellagra. Besides the great importance given to taking extra *niacin* today, this substance, just like vitamin D, is not really a vitamin at all since it can be produced by the body.

Nobody Knows How Much You Need

Governments and international organizations such as the World Health Organization (WHO) frequently release figures that propose a *Daily Ratio of Allowance* (DRA) for every vitamin that you supposedly need to stay healthy. The nutritional experts in different countries however, have different opinions about how much of each vitamin your body must have. An American, for example, is supposed to take at least 60 mg of vitamin C, whereas a British citizen is considered better off taking only 30 mg. A Frenchman will only remain healthy if he consumes 80 mg of this vitamin, whereas Italians are told they need 45 mg. These figures are 'adjusted' every few years, although our bodies' basic nutritional requirements have not changed over the past several thousand years.

Nobody really knows how many vitamins are good for us because the requirement, physical constitution and absorption rate for vitamins differ from person to person. Vitamins need to be digested before they can be made available to the cells and tissues. If a person's digestive ability (AGNI) has diminished due to congestion of liver bile ducts with intrahepatic stones (see my book The Amazing Liver and Gallbladder Cleanse), for example, foods and also vitamins can no longer be digested properly.

When scientists calculate our vitamin requirements, they usually add a 50 percent 'safety factor' to the original ratios of allowance to make certain that we eat enough of them. And because vitamin extraction from food during the digestive process is so much less than 100 percent, these figures are increased one more time. The official methods of analyzing the amount of vitamins we require are inadequate because we simply *do not know* how much of each vitamin the human body needs. The thin, hyper-metabolic Vata body type, for example, may have a far greater need for vitamin B6 than the heavier-set, hypo-metabolic Kapha type who can never really run out of it.

It is also not known how much of each vitamin is contained in a banana, an apple or a piece of cauliflower. Vitamin contents fluctuate greatly with the size of the fruits, their maturity, the condition of the soil, country of origin, time of harvesting, and the use of pesticides. How many of the vitamins contained in these foods actually end up in our blood depends on our digestive ability and body type. In other words, the amount of any vitamin you take is not necessarily the amount that your body ends up absorbing and ultimately putting to use. Complicating the absorption issue is the fact that your body's ability to absorb nutrients is not necessarily the same from one day to the next. All this makes official nutritional figures highly unreliable and speculative.

The vitamin theories originate in the assumption that the human physiology has stores of vitamins that must always be full in order to saturate the tissues of the body. This assumption, however, has never been proven by scientific research. While calculating human vitamin requirements, nutritional science *assumes* that the body's metabolic processes occur at a top speed, which would require plenty of vitamins. Our bodies, however, are not machines that run at top capacity day and night. Most of us are *not* marathon runners, and even *they* don't run for 24 hours day after day, month after month, and year after year.

It is very questionable whether the saturation of our body tissues with vitamins is even desirable. We need a certain amount of fatty tissue in our body, but this does not mean we should all be excessively filled with fat. Oxygen, too, is considered vital for all our body's functioning, yet if its concentration in the air is too high it can cause serious bodily harm. Why should vitamins be an exception? And anyway, vitamin deficiency is...

...Rarely Caused by Lack of Vitamins

In the majority of cases, a vitamin deficiency does not occur because of insufficient vitamin intake in the diet. A vitamin deficiency is rather caused by a congested capillary network that is unable to diffuse sufficient amounts of the vitamins into the intercellular fluids. This can be due to a number of reasons, of which overeating protein foods is a major one.

A diet rich in protein foods such as meat, fish, pork, cheese, milk, etc. will eventually block the basal membrane (BM) of the small and large blood vessels in the body (see details in Chapter 9 on heart disease). Stress, over-stimulation, and dehydration can exacerbate this effect. The subsequent thickening of the BM and connective tissues makes it increasingly difficult for the basic nutrients, including vitamins, to reach the cells. If trans-fatty acids are consumed, as contained in most processed and refined fats, oils and fried foods, cell membranes become thick and congested, thereby preventing nutrients from reaching the cell interior. All this greatly increases the amount of metabolic waste and toxins in the body, overtaxes the liver, and causes the growth of gallstones. The gallstones inhibit the flow of bile, which subdues AGNI, the digestive power and increasingly hinders the assimilation of basic nutrients, including fats. When fats are no longer properly digested, the fat-soluble vitamins A, D, E, K, which are normally stored in the liver, become deficient. This problem is made worse by eating low fat foods (see section 6 on Light Foods).

If vitamin A becomes deficient, for example, the *epithelial* cells, which form an essential part of all the organs, blood vessels, lymph vessels, etc., in the body, become damaged. This can cause practically any kind of disease known. Vitamin A is also necessary to maintain the cornea of the eye, allow for eyesight in dim light, and reduce the severity of microbial infection. Vitamin A is only absorbed properly from the small intestines when fat absorption is normal. Fat absorption cannot be normal as long as gallstones obstruct the bile flow in the liver and gallbladder. It is, therefore, very reasonable to remove the gallstones and cleanse the digestive system so that the vitamins contained in the foods you eat can actually reach the cells in your body.

Taking extra vitamins can be harmful if the body is unable to make use of them and is left with the additional burden of having to break them down and eliminate them. Because vitamins are strong acids, an overload can lead to vitamin poisoning (vitaminosis) which damages the kidneys, and actually causes the same symptoms that accompany a vitamin deficiency. Instead of filling the body up with large doses of vitamins it cannot even process properly, it would be more healthful and efficient to cleanse the body from accumulated toxins, stored proteins in the blood vessel walls, and impeding gallstones from the liver. Although taking mega doses of vitamins may temporarily increase the pressure of diffusion of these nutrients for a short time and quickly relieve symptoms, any 'benefits' may be short-lived. If digestive functions are impaired, taking extra vitamins may actually endanger your health.

Contrary to popular belief, vitamins do not have isolated functions, but work as a 'team' in the body. If taken in supplemental form instead of deriving them from food, vitamins may be counterproductive, since excess of one vitamin can have a suppressing effect on another. As discussed before, typical vitamin doses in supplements exceed the body's true requirements. When isolated and extracted from foods, vitamins tend to arouse your nervous system, should you take them. Feeling stimulated, and therefore energized, you naturally assume these vitamins must be doing you good. But stimulants never give you extra energy; to the contrary, they force the body to spend and give up energy.

The best source of healthy vitamins is fresh fruit, vegetables, grains, legumes, nuts, seeds, etc. Fruits and vegetables also contain important health-essential nutrients known as *phytochemicals* - nature's food coloring agents. They give fruits and vegetables their color. And to obtain vitamin D, the best and cheapest source is sunlight. B12 basically consists of microbes living in your mouth and gut. There is no need to look for other sources of vitamins.

Hidden Perils of Vitamin Pills

Vitamins D and A

Calciferol, known as **vitamin D**, is not a vitamin in the real sense since the body is capable of producing it itself. With the help of UV light from the sun, the body synthesizes it from cholesterol (7-dehydrocholesterol) in the human skin. Vitamin D, which acts rather like a hormone than a vitamin, facilitates the absorption and utilization of calcium and phosphorus, necessary for maintaining strong bones and teeth. Although vitamin D levels cannot be influenced through diet, the official nutritional textbooks speak of 2.5 µg daily requirement for adults. Babies and breast milk are supposed to have the biggest deficiencies in vitamin D, implying that nature made a crucial mistake when it invented breast milk. Mothers are warned that, without taking extra amounts of this important vitamin, their babies could risk rickets or bone deformation.

Yet mothers are rarely informed about the risks they take when they overuse vitamin D. Vitamin D poisoning leads to something very similar to rickets. Professor Ernst Lindner from the University of Giessen in Germany has warned that if large amounts of vitamin D are given to a person, calcium is removed from the bones; and this can cause bone deformation. He also states that it is very risky to add vitamin D to food.

Bone deformation is more likely to occur in babies who are *not* breast-fed. Until the expensive vitamin D pill came on the market, rickets was effectively treated with breast milk, and I might add, for thousands of years.

Nature deemed it necessary to supply mother's milk with only very little vitamin D. As studies have shown, the amount of vitamin D in mother's milk does not increase when the mother takes vitamin D supplements. This proves that a mother's body filters out vitamin D to protect the baby from being poisoned (by the vitamin). A baby's body easily synthesizes vitamin D from sunlight once it is exposed to it. Since being exposed to natural sunlight is one of the most natural needs humans are born with, it is, therefore, unnecessary to have this vitamin present in the mother's milk. Just like plants need sunlight to grow, humans need sunlight as well. The major cause of vitamin D deficiency among babies is keeping them in dark rooms with little or no natural light. But even with less than adequate sun exposure, they are still capable of absorbing sufficient amounts of calcium from the blood necessary for the building of healthy bones. While being breast-fed, an infant receives plenty of milk sugar and phospho-caseins, both excellent transporting agents for calcium. If there is anything that could cause rickets in babies, it is lack of mothers' milk and underexposure to sunlight.

Adults are not as well protected against vitamin D ingestion as breastfed infants are. One report issued by the University of Tromso in Norway showed that the long-term intake of vitamin D at the dosage of just slightly above the 400 IU recommended amount (many people take as much as 4,000 to 5,000 IU per day!) may trigger a heart attack and cause degenerative joint disease and arthritis. Another finding emerged from the New York University Goldwater Memorial Hospital, which suggests that large doses of vitamin D can cause magnesium deficiency in the heart tissue and cause heart attacks.

Pregnant women are particularly at risk. Dietary intake of vitamin D has led to kidney calcification and severe mental retardation in their offspring. Children born to mothers, who take extra vitamin D in their diet, may develop a certain type of congenital heart disease called *supravalvular aortic stenosis* and show extreme deformations of facial bones.

Taking vitamin D supplements can also contribute to arteriosclerosis and even be fatal. In 1991, several Americans died from vitamin D in cow's milk. The supplement was added during the production process, but the measurement was faulty. Dairy inspection revealed that the instrument used to measure vitamin concentrate was broken, implicating the unmeasured addition of vitamin D to the milk as the cause of the excess fortification. In a different incidence, the milk wasn't blended properly.

Now this is where it gets complicated. Milk enhances the potency of vitamin D by up to ten times, a fact that is routinely ignored by milk producers. Milk that has been enriched by 90 units of vitamin D is poisonous and can kill an adult person. But milk with added vitamin D just sells better. If you feel you need more vitamin D, then it is best to sunbathe regularly or go for regular walks. But avoid using sunscreens.

It is also a well known fact that too much vitamin A causes deformity in unborn children. For this reason, there is a law preventing the use of this vitamin in food. Yet this law does not apply to animal feeds even though it is well known that vitamin A is accumulating in the liver of farm animals. Pregnant women are warned not to consume liver to avoid damaging their babies. If taking extra vitamin A is considered poisonous for pregnant women or unborn babies, it cannot be considered safe for the rest of the population either.

B-vitamins

Pyridoxine or **vitamin B6** is a combination of six substances. Since most parts of this vitamin occur in bound form, analytic methods fail to determine how much of it is contained in food. It is also not possible to make any reliable statements about how much of it we require. Still the nutritional textbooks suggest a 1-2 µg daily intake, which is pure guesswork. What *is* known, though, are its side effects.

Vitamin B6 is often used as a drug. Its use is indicated for depression, premenstrual tension, schizophrenia, and child asthma. It was considered safe until 1983 when scientists discovered a syndrome accompanied by strong circulatory problems in the hands and feet of a number of patients who were given large doses of vitamin B6. The patients developed symptoms similar to the ones caused by the drug *thalidomide* (which recently has been reintroduced for specific disorders). Mothers who had taken large amounts of B6 during their pregnancy also reported deformities in their children's bodies. It took a long time before the nerve damage was linked to vitamin poisoning. As it turned out, many patients, who had been diagnosed with *multiple sclerosis*, were poisoned by vitamin B6. There are many unsuspecting people taking vitamin B6 today without the faintest idea that they are slowly injuring their bodies from the inside out.

The statement that *Cobalamins* or **B12 vitamins** can only be found in animal foods, such as meat, fish, eggs, cheese, etc., is plain false. B12 has been detected in fermented plant foods and algae. A deficiency of this vitamin is thought to cause pernicious anemia and degeneration of nerve fibers of the spinal cord. The argument that people who don't consume any animal foods must have a B12 deficiency and endanger their health is unscientific, unfounded and misleading. Apart from producing vitamins K, B1 and B2, as well as energy-providing short-chain fatty acids, the billions of beneficial bacteria residing our intestines and mouth produce more than enough B12. The amount of vitamin B12 a healthy person will require throughout his lifetime is about the size of half a pinky nail.

In addition, the liver can store B12 for many years and knows how to recycle this vitamin. This may explain why *vegans* (those who don't eat any type of animal product) eating a balanced diet almost never suffer from B12 deficiencies (contrary to public opinion). I can personally attest to that. Before I started eating purely vegan 35 years ago, I suffered from a severe chronic anemia. It vanished two months after I stopped eating meat, poultry, eggs, fish, cheese and milk.

If the body for any reason required more of this vitamin, it would instinctively desire foods (versus craving them) that would meet the increased demand. However, if the liver and intestines are congested, a B12 deficiency may eventually develop, *regardless* of whether a person is a meat-eater, a vegetarian, or vegan. In addition taking antibiotics and other medical drugs destroy the beneficial bacteria in our mouths and intestines, which is the most common cause of B12 deficiency.

Niacin is one of the most popular B-vitamins. Added to a large number of manufactured foods, including breakfast cereals, niacin also is not without risks. After large doses of niacin (3 g) were given to patients suffering from psychiatric diseases, these patients developed hepatitis and other liver problems. Among other symptoms of niacin-poisoning are hot flushes, itching skin, arrhythmia, and nervousness. Illegal use of niacin in minced meat and hamburgers has repeatedly led to similar symptoms. The main reason for adding niacin to meat is to color it red and give it the appearance of being fresh. If you turn bright red, like a tomato, and get an itch right after eating meat, then you are likely to have been poisoned with niacin.

The **B-vitamin** *Folic acid* is also a common food additive, and potentially one of the most harmful ones. After researchers first discovered that people in malaria regions suffered from folic acid deficiency, they gave them this B vitamin in the belief that it would make their immune systems more resistant to the malaria bug. The children who were given this vitamin felt worse after the treatment and were found to have much higher concentrations of malaria-causing agents in their blood than before.

The explanation for this phenomenon lies in the understanding that the malaria bugs themselves require large amounts of folic acid to spread. People who have a deficiency in this vitamin are naturally protected from malaria infection. A British doctor in Kenya discovered that children who took folic acid developed malaria. He gave folic acid to one group of monkeys and compared them with another group monkeys who were folic acid deficient. All the monkeys with 'normal' levels of this vitamin were infected with malaria whereas the ones with 'abnormally low' levels stayed healthy.

Over 40 percent of the world's population is threatened by malaria today and it is no longer restricted to developing countries. Malaria is rapidly becoming the leading cause of death in the world. It is impossible to imagine the disastrous consequences that may have arisen from giving millions of healthy people vitamins to help their assumed vitamin deficiency. A vitamin deficiency in one person may actually be a life-saving response for another person. It is sad to know that many people have to pay with their lives because we so crudely interfere in the self-regulating mechanisms of nature and human physiology that protect us against disease.

Vitamin C

The most popular of all vitamins is *Ascorbic acid* or **vitamin C,** a deficiency of which is believed to cause multiple hemorrhages, slow wound healing, anemia and scurvy (damage of blood vessels). It is in fact very easy to cure scurvy with red peppers, citrus fruits, or cranberries, all containing high concentrations of this vitamin. Since the Hungarian scientist Szent Gyoerkyi identified vitamin C in oranges to be an effective substance, it became common knowledge that vitamin C and orange juice must have the same benefits. But as it turned out, scurvy cannot be cured by vitamin C alone. Regardless how large a dosage of vitamin C you use, the blood vessels will remain damaged. By contrast, eating a few oranges or red peppers cures scurvy quickly, without a trace of damage left.

Vitamin C-rich fruits contain at least one other vitamin ingredient which is known as vitamin C2. Scurvy can only be cured if vitamin C and vitamin C2 are taken together. When Gyoerkyi studied vitamin C, he included both compounds of vitamin C. But as the years passed, the scientific community began omitting C2, and today nobody talks about it anymore.

When vitamins became popular in the United States, there was a sudden jump in the number of newly born babies developing scurvy. It was thought that scurvy was a disease eradicated a long time ago. As the mysterious development was investigated, it was discovered that the mothers of the affected babies had taken extra vitamin C preparations (without C2) in the belief that it was good for their babies. Dosed with the vitamin, the mothers' bodies started eliminating more of it than they ingested. When the babies were born they also continued removing whatever vitamin C they had received from the mother, because this is what they had learned to do while in the womb. Since their baby food did not consist of large amounts of vitamin C, they soon developed the dangerous baby scurvy.

The body of an adult, who consumes vitamin C regularly, may eventually produce a similar response. He may even develop scurvy because the body becomes programmed to eliminate vitamin C faster and in larger quantities than it is ingested or can be absorbed. Adults are known to develop further complications when, after using this vitamin regularly, they suddenly stop taking it altogether. It is also known that large doses of vitamin C can destroy another vitamin, that is, vitamin B12. There is too little research to tell what further damage large amounts of vitamins can do to us but experimenting with these powerful substances on the human body is similar to handling an explosive device.

A friend of mine developed a dangerous swelling of his kidneys after taking 2 g of Vitamin C a day for several weeks. By taking him off the vitamins and giving him tea made from the herb Pau d'Arco helped remove the excessive vitamin from the kidneys and restore them to their normal size and efficiency. Added to the current uncertainty and confusion about taking vitamins, there is still no conclusive proof that vitamin C protects you from infection, which is one of the main reasons people use it.

Even if vitamin C were able to stop an infection, in many instances this could turn out to be disastrous for the body. To prevent a cold from reaching its climax interferes with the body's efforts of removing accumulated toxins, and thus may become the first stage in a series of future illnesses. If the body is 'toxic' because of an unhealthy lifestyle, diet and stress, its most important primary response is to initiate a toxicity crisis that permits the body to cleanse itself. A cold is not a disease, and it should not be treated as one. It is very ill advised to stop the body from eliminating toxins and purifying itself.

Handing out vitamin C as a preventive measure against colds is a practice that may also be counterproductive. Although small doses of vitamin C may successfully trigger a cleansing response in the body, large amounts of vitamin C can interfere with an ongoing, and possibly life-saving, cleansing process. The often-cited argument that all water-soluble vitamins, such as vitamin C and B, are harmless because the body can easily eliminate excessive amounts without a problem is pseudo-science and misleading. *Cyanide* is also water-soluble, but it can kill a person.

The 2004 November issue of the *American Journal of Clinical Nutrition* reported that according to new research older women with diabetes who take high doses of vitamin C for the sake of their hearts may be doing themselves more harm than good. The study, which followed nearly 2,000 postmenopausal women with diabetes for 15 years, found that those who took heavy doses of vitamin C supplements - 300 milligrams (mg) a day or more - were nearly twice as likely to die of heart disease or stroke compared with women who took no supplemental C. Interestingly, high intakes of vitamin C from food were not related to a greater risk of death from cardiovascular causes.

The researchers of the study suggest that taking supplements to correct the lower blood levels of vitamin C commonly seen in diabetes is not necessarily the right choice. And although the research focused on older women, the findings may apply to men as well, according to the study's senior author. "Our results, if confirmed by other research, would suggest that diabetics should be more cautious than others about taking supplements," Dr. David R. Jacobs Jr., of the University of Minnesota in Minneapolis, told Reuters Health.

The current recommended dietary intake for vitamin C is 90 mg per day for men and 75 mg per day for women. While vitamin C is clearly necessary for good health, studies have garnered conflicting results on whether supplements help lower the risk of heart disease and stroke. According to Jacobs, vitamin C has been shown, in the test tube, to damage cell proteins in the same manner that high blood sugar harms diabetics' body cells. Jacobs also pointed to the complexity of the 'antioxidant defense system'. When antioxidants interact with free radicals, he explained, they become 'pro-oxidants' that must be detoxified by other antioxidants. "It's possible," Jacobs speculated, "that this detox process happens more slowly in diabetics - both women and men - and that under certain circumstances, the altered vitamin C molecules are able to harm body cells." Jacobs said he and his colleagues favor getting vitamin C, along with the full complement of nutrients, from food rather than supplements. One ounce of chia seeds, for example, can supply you with six times the amount of vitamin C that several oranges can give you.

Whereas antioxidants in food may be 'balanced bio-chemically', Jacobs and his team write, any vitamin pill would lack such balance. Taking high doses of a single antioxidant, they speculate, may 'perturb' the body's balance of antioxidants and pro-oxidants. These findings support other research, showing that high daily doses of another antioxidant, vitamin E, may not extend life, and instead may slightly raise the risk of dying earlier.

It is important to understand that the body cannot live without free radicals. It uses the chain reaction of the free radicals to turn air and food into chemical energy. Free radicals also play an essential role in every immune response, attacking and destroying foreign invaders and bacteria. Using antioxidants, such as vitamin C, to eliminate or reduce free radicals, might actually cause more serious harm than having too many of them in the body. A study published in the August 10, 2007 issue of the journal *Cell* reveals that an overload of antioxidants could actually lead to heart failure.

As has happened so many times before, both medical and nutritional science continue to underestimate the innate wisdom of the body. Their isolationistic approaches to understanding and treating the human body are based on a little knowledge of how the body works, while dismissing its innate wisdom and thereby endangering its life. Provided you supply the body with wholesome, natural foods and avoid or significantly reduce your intake of processed foods, which are loaded with artificial chemicals, it will automatically self-regulate free radical activity and all other processes. To avoid imbalance in one way or the other, you should obtain your antioxidants only from one source - food, including, fruits, vegetables, grains, legumes, nuts, seeds, herbs, spices, teas, etc.

It is not entirely clear, whether natural forms of vitamin E are harmful. I strongly suspect that the harmful side effects from vitamin E are due to taking it in synthetic form. There are numerous people who claim to have greatly benefited from vitamin E. The problem is that the general population is not made aware of this important distinction. In fact, most people use the synthetic form, which can risk their health.

On a different note, you may be surprised to know that China is actually one of the largest exporters of many drugs and vitamins. About 90 percent of all Vitamin C sold in the United States is from China.

China also produces 50 percent of the world's aspirin and 35 percent of all Tylenol. The same is true for the majority of Vitamins A, B12 and E. Since there are no safety regulations and only minimal inspections for these products, you can never quite know what you will get. The pet food and toy scandals and reported instances of toxic food and toothpaste from China have shown that we need to be cautious about foods and supplements that originate from places we know nothing about.

Conclusion:

The vitamin euphoria has hit the world's population at a time when there are no reliable methods to determine if and when someone suffers from a vitamin deficiency. Reviewing the harmful effects caused by vitamin intake, it is likely that a deficiency, if it really exists, is either caused by an overtaxed digestive system and subsequent congestion of the capillary network or by overdosing the body with vitamins. Blood vessel wall congestion and intestinal trouble prevents vitamins from reaching the cells, tissues, organs and systems in the body. Taking extra vitamins in such a situation can actually trigger a defense mechanism that empties the body's vitamin reserves.

Furthermore, it is not known how much of each vitamin each particular body-type requires to be vital and healthy, and it also not possible to find out how much of each vitamin the body is able to extract from the foods consumed. What's more, it is erroneous to assume that by taking extra vitamins the body will automatically make use of them. We simply don't know how much of the vitamins will leave the stomach unharmed, in what amounts they are going to be digested and how much of these are likely to be absorbed by the blood and the body cells. What is known, though, is that synthetically produced multi-vitamin pills have an intestinal absorption rate of no more than 3 to 5 percent; the rest ends up in your toilet, if you are lucky. There are no people on the planet with exactly the same vitamin requirements and absorption rates. What may be normal for one person may not be normal for another, which makes the 'standardized vitamin requirements for all' questionable, if not potentially harmful.

The argument that our foods today are so depleted of vitamins that we need to take additional helpings of synthetically derived vitamins is only partially correct. *Most* of the foods consumed by *most* people in modern countries are highly acid-forming, which means that they damage blood vessels and deplete the body's vitamins and minerals. The foods that have the most acidifying effects in the body include milk, dairy products, meat and its products, tinned or frozen foods, white bread, pasta and pastry made from bleached and refined flour, refined sugar, alcoholic beverages, diet beverages, soft drinks, sports drinks, packaged fruit juices, preserved foods, processed breakfast cereals, chocolates, ready-made cakes, potato chips (crisps), hydrogenated oils and fats, and most fast/junk foods. The exaggerated ratio of daily-required vitamins may apply only to the severely undernourished person. Fresh fruits, vegetables, legumes and grain foods, ideally of organic origin, still contain more than enough vitamins to supply the body many times over.

Taking vitamin pills, which don't contain much *Life Force Energy,* (also known as *Chi* or *Prana*), does not substitute regular intake of healthy, fresh food. Vitamins that have been removed from their natural environment, i.e. fruits, vegetables, etc. can in fact upset both AGNI and the delicate balance of minerals and vitamins in the body. This especially applies to multivitamin preparations. Although there are conditions when taking extra vitamins may be beneficial, for example, before and after removing amalgam fillings from the teeth, they ought not to be taken in large doses and for more than 10-14 days at a time. This is best done under supervision of a health practitioner who is aware of the side effects that vitamins can have. In any case, synthetic vitamins should be avoided at all cost.

A large study testing the potential benefits of antioxidants such as Vitamin C, Vitamin E and beta carotene for the heart in women found no benefits whatsoever. The study was reported on CNN August

14, 2007. You will need to determine whether it is worthwhile to spend a lot of money on supplements that don't work, but could possibly affect you negatively.

What about Taking Extra Minerals?

Mineral salts found in the earth's soil and rocks are classified as inorganic, and must be incorporated within the structure of plants in order to be usable by your body. Most mineral supplements are inorganic, and their consumption causes serious problems, as they commonly end up deposited in your various tissues. This can result in serious health problems including arthritis, Alzheimer's, and arteriosclerosis. Calcium supplements are notorious for this. Your best source of all usable organic minerals is fresh vegetables, with fruit providing your second best source. Some nuts and seeds are also abundant with minerals, such as in the case of sesame seeds, which supply a whopping 1160 milligrams of calcium per 100 grams. The super-grain, Chia seeds, is packed with numerous minerals. (It is widely available on the Internet, such as this web site: www.chiaforhealth.com.)

Unlike vitamins, minerals cannot be synthesized by plants. Plants take up mineral salts (inorganic compounds) from the soil and convert them into colloidal minerals (organic compounds). The inorganic minerals, also called metallic minerals, are very difficult to be absorbed by a healthy digestive system, and even more so if the small intestine is impacted with toxic waste material. In the case of a very healthy adult, the absorption rate for metallic minerals is 3 to 5 percent; the rest merely passes through the body system without benefit, but often not without causing harm. Although these minerals now come in chelated form, i.e. amino acids or protein are wrapped around them to improve assimilation, they are still inorganic and of very little use to the cells of the body. Ionic minerals, on the other hand, have an absorption rate of 98 percent, which indicates that only minerals in its organic (angstrom size) form are meant to be used by the human physiology.

If the soil is not replenished with minerals after harvesting, it becomes increasingly mineral deficient. Modern methods of agriculture don't include putting minerals back into the soil. Before the era of continuous soil depletion, the topsoil consisted of as many as 90-100 different minerals. The great rivers such as the Nile in Egypt and the Ganges in India caused extensive flooding every year, bringing new minerals from the glaciers and mountains to the land, automatically fertilizing it. The people living in these areas were generally in perfect health and lived on average 120-140 years. The situation changed with the erosion of forests and building of dams. Today, there are merely 12-20 minerals found in plant foods.

Whatever is contained in modern chemical fertilizers (nitrogen, phosphorus, and potassium) may be sufficient to raise normal-looking crops; yet the healthy-looking plant foods are short of minerals, which is reflected in their poor taste. This may cause some mineral deficiencies in the body. We are consistently missing out on the majority of minerals. And if the digestive system does not function efficiently, a health crisis may arise. Almost every disease today is linked with or caused by a deficiency of one or several minerals or trace minerals.

Taking supplements consisting of metallic minerals is not only inefficient because of their relatively low absorption rate but also because of their non-physiological value. Large quantities of metallic minerals can even be toxic to the body, as seen in people who, for example, take iron tablets. The iron may make them sick, a natural response by the stomach against the toxic metal. Iron oxide is nothing other than 'rust'. New research has shown that taking extra iron can triple one's risk for heart attacks.

Taking calcium tablets may weaken the bones by causing zinc deficiency. High dosed mineral supplements consisting of metallic minerals can block the absorption of other bio-usable minerals, which can upset the body's entire biochemical balance. Most of the metallic minerals are derived from oyster shell, limestone, soil, clay, calcium carbonate, and sea salts. In fact, taking metallic minerals can lead to serious mineral deficiencies.

It may be beneficial, on the other hand, to take extra ionic liquid minerals. Plant derived minerals are water-soluble, ionic and enzymatically active which makes it very easy for the body to digest and utilize them. The iron, contained in Lapacho tea, for example, is of ionic form and has an immediate positive effect.

Plant-derived minerals rarely have negative side effects, even if you overdose on them. If you feel that you need extra minerals, check out Eniva® or Kornax (see *Product Information*) for their ionic liquid minerals. But as is the case with vitamins, most serious mineral deficiencies occur because of inadequate nutrition, too many acid-forming foods and beverages, overstimulation, dehydration, stress, etc. There is not much point in taking extra minerals when they are removed right away or destroyed by one or more of these factors. So before you spend a lot of money on mineral supplements, try to eliminate the causes of the deficiency first.

3. Breakfast Cereals and Junk Foods - Poison for our Children

'Super Food' of the Century

Breakfast cereals have never been more popular than they are today. Packed with vitamins and minerals, they promise power, health and vitality, especially to the young generation. There is hardly a commercial breakfast cereal in the world that does not seem to contain everything a child needs to receive the 'perfectly balanced' dietary nutrition. However, despite this 'valuable' contribution to family health, a frightening number of children show signs of ill health and lacking immunity. The vitamins that are added to the cereals supposedly protect the child against the vitamin-destroying sugar, but it seems that this guarantee is no longer guaranteed.

Besides cornflakes, which still top the list of American and European breakfast cereals, the sales of new 'tasty and healthy' breakfast foods soar as never before. The main marketing targets for these 'healthy' breakfast foods are children. Research suggests that as many as 79 percent of all households use ready-made breakfast cereals to start the day. Children are usually very keen to try the latest cereal model, which contains essentially the same ingredients as all the other types but comes in a different shape and color. The well designed packaging depicting a healthy-looking family or natural scenery promises the parents that the contents are of pure and natural origin, often organically grown, and good for the entire family. The kids love the happy friendly figures on the cardboard. "If Mickey Mouse, Donald Duck, Bugs Bunny, or the strong Dinosaurs like the cereal then it must be good for me, too," some children might argue.

Packaging has a powerful manipulative influence on children. Researchers at Packard Children's Hospital in California asked 63 children, ages three and five, to taste-test servings of hamburger, French fries, chicken nuggets, baby carrots and milk. Some of the servings were wrapped in containers with a McDonald's logo, and some were wrapped in containers with no logo. As expected, most of the kids thought the food in the McDonald's containers tasted better than the identical food with no logo.

It doesn't take much to convince an unsuspecting mother that the beautifully packaged foods are actually good for her children. The mother, who naturally wants to secure the best possible nutrition for her child, finds her mind put at ease when she learns about the high nutritional value of the product in the food table. It convincingly states that the cereal has the balanced amounts of carbohydrates, protein and fats, and is most importantly enriched with all the essential dietary supplements. If the right amount of milk (mostly pasteurized and homogenized) is added to the super food, the child would have the best possible start of the day that nature could provide, or so she may believe.

Shocking Revelations

Yet the reality of the matter is quite the opposite. An American team of researchers decided to prove to the world once and for all that factory-made breakfast cereals are "truly" man's super-food. So they fed the common breakfast cereals enriched with the most important vitamins and minerals to young, healthy laboratory rats. The researchers divided a total of 240 rats into two groups; one group received cereal and water and the other one normal food and water. The experiment lasted for 45 days. The result was totally unexpected and devastating. The rats that were fed with cereals, which according to common nutritional sense and advertising should have turned them into strong and vital grown-up rats, were close to death. They suffered from fatty livers, anemia and high blood pressure. In a separate experiment, rats were fed with cornflakes, which consisted of *useless* cornstarch and white sugar. In this group some of the animals died.

The researchers had expected that the animals would grow faster with cereals, yet they did not grow at all, and some of them even lost weight. Especially the rats which received cereals with high sugar content (sugar is thought to be fattening), had the least growth rates. This is a summary of the results:

> The products that contained the least amounts of fat significantly increased the *cholesterol* levels of the rats. Some products were able to lower the rats' *cholesterol* levels but also caused fatty livers.

> Those rats that were fed with cereals containing only small amounts of salt increased their blood pressure whereas the ones that received cereals with higher salt contents lowered their blood pressure.

> Some of the products were enriched with iron, which should have raised *hemoglobin* concentrations in the blood of anemic animals. However, the results took the researchers by surprise: **1)** There was no connection between higher intake of iron and *hemoglobin* levels. The rats stayed anemic despite ingesting large amounts of iron. **2)** Those rats that had little iron in their blood deposited excessively large amounts of iron in their liver, which led to worsening of anemia (for a similar reason it is very questionable to give extra iron to people who suffer from anemia).

Poison that Tastes and Looks like Food

The main conclusion we can draw from this experiment is that the purely theoretical approach to diet and nutrition (using food tables and daily nutritional recommendations) has not only been insufficient to raise the standard of health in the population but has in fact caused more harm and confusion than is currently assessable. Sanctified by theories of nutrition, which in actuality contradict the body's natural responses to food, the food industry has been given the green light to produce anything that fulfills the official nutritional requirements, even if the 'foods' have a poisoning effect and create havoc in the body. There is no legislation to test man-made foods on animals before giving them to millions of human beings. The average consumer takes it for granted that the food produced by a reputable company must be safe for human consumption, even if it contains plastic. (Using animals to find out whether these foods are poisonous or not is cruel and I don't advocate animal testing. I have reasons to believe that all man-made foods have harmful effects on the human body, and I therefore recommend that you avoid eating them.)

Not all governments support this disconcerting trend. According to an August 2004 issue of the Guardian, some few health-conscious governments in Europe that are less dominated by the food industry and big pharmaceutical companies, are beginning to protect their people from obvious harmful practices.

Health officials in Denmark recently banned the addition of vitamins and minerals to 18 varieties of breakfast foods and cereals produced by Kellogg Co. The reasons given include increasing evidence that eating those products regularly can ruin the health of children and pregnant women. Cereal is one of the first solid foods introduced to babies, and pediatricians typically encourage parents to start feeding cereal to their babies from between 4 and 6 months. Their advice grossly contradicts findings from a study that cereals introduced in the diets of babies increased the risk of insulin-dependent diabetes in the children.

Kellogg had hoped to add iron, calcium, folic acid and vitamin B6 to some cereals and cereal bars, as it is so common in other countries. However, Danish health officials believe that these toxic additives in the cereals can seriously harm the livers and kidneys of children as well as unborn fetuses in pregnant women. A government laboratory delivered the ban after examining the ingredient lists provided by Kellogg.

Resolving the Whole Grain Mystery

Recently, the largest U.S. food producer *General Mills* announced it will start using whole grains in some of the popular cereal products for kids. Processed flour will be replaced by whole grain flour. Whole grain is fashionable now, so the change seems timely and healthy.

The problem is that the whole grain actually does not qualify as genuine whole grain. It is made of flour that is processed with a newly developed milling method that grinds the whole grain into particles of uniform size. *U.S.A Today* states that General Mills executives would not discuss the new technology behind the development of their new type of whole grain. So what's the big secret? They're asking us to accept their word that it's healthier, but they're not giving us specific details. The second biggest food company, *ConAgra*, now uses *Ultragrain*, similar to General Mill's 'Whole Grain'. It has the look, texture and flavor of processed grain.

The question concerning this new trend in food production is: how did they manage to make a completely different whole grain that's just as healthy as whole grain? To have a long shelf life, which whole grain products certainly don't have, they must have done something to the grain to preserve it and make it last as long as refined grains, an absolute necessity in packaged cereals.

Even if real whole grains were added to these super foods feeding our nation at breakfast time, this certainly wouldn't turn them into health foods. Consider what's in a cup of Trix, for example. The nearly iridescent colors of the popular cereal show that it is saturated with artificial coloring agents. To keep it fresh, it has to have preservatives which 'preserve' (prevent) it from being digested properly. Trix also contains plenty of trans fatty acids (as found in canola and rice bran oil) that clog up the cell membranes and damage blood vessels. Not to mention the 13 grams of bleached, refined sugar per cup, leaching minerals from the muscles and bones, and leading to the beginning stages of insulin resistance. The entire concept of manufacturing a packaged cereal that is healthy is an absolute impossibility.

The food industry is entitled to use a large variety of solvents and chemicals to improve the taste, color, and texture of its products. Food producers have free reign over food production, and there is nobody out there that is going to make sure our children don't get fed with another sweet tasting poison.

But the common practice of producing food *synthetically* and making it 'healthier' by adding *synthetically* derived vitamins and minerals is at the root of many health problems afflicting both children and adults in the developed world.

To determine whether a cereal is healthful or harmful for you and your family, try using the simple muscle test described in chapter 1. Take your children to the grocery store and let them test out different products. This will teach them to trust their body and its responses and reactions and make them aware that not everything that *looks* healthy actually *is* healthy. Synthetically derived 'nutrients' are foreign matter to both animals and humans alike. Making laboratory foods palatable and attractive does not mean they are harmless. The muscle test is a fairly reliable tool you can use to protect yourself and your family from the harm caused by such non-foods.

Hot breakfast cereals, which were in common use before the era of cold, ready-made cereals, include cream of wheat, steel cut oats, the old fashioned porridge oats, rye flakes, millet, corn meal, cream of rice, etc. Although they take more time to prepare than the ready-made cereals, at least you know what's in them. Also check with your body-type food list.

Note: Most muesli mixtures or cereals with nuts and fruits in them contain the fruit preservative sulphur dioxide (E220), which can spark asthmatic attacks and is blacklisted by the Hyperactive Children Support Group in England. The cracked nuts react with oxygen and turn rancid, a common source of allergies. The dried fruits in cereals develop molds, which can interfere with vitamin and mineral absorption and suppress immunity. Crunchy or roasted oats contain lots of refined sugar and inferior oils loaded with trans fatty acids.

Hyperactivity in Kids Caused by Food Additives

Food is wreaking havoc on kids. Artificial food colorings and benzoate preservatives increase hyperactive behavior in preschool children, according to a new report in the June 2004 Archives of Disease in Childhood.

Dr. John O. Warner from Southampton General Hospital, U.K., and colleagues studied the impact of artificial food colorings and benzoate preservatives on the behavior of 277 preschool children. At the start, 36 children had hyperactivity and allergies, 75 were only hyperactive, 79 had only allergies, and 87 did not have either condition.

The result of the study: Parents' ratings of their children's hyperactivity fell after withdrawal of food additives from the children's diets. And there was an increase in hyperactivity when food additives were re-introduced. Parental hyperactivity ratings increased significantly when children were exposed to food additives regardless of their hyperactivity status or the presence of allergies at the start of the study. "Additives do have an effect on overactive behavior independent of baseline allergic and behavioral status," Warner told Reuters Health.

If you or your children suffer from 'hyperkinetic disorder' or 'attention deficit and hyperactivity disorder' (ADHD), make certain to avoid junk foods. Choose to have healthier menus, using organic foods, and transition to organic ingredients (no pesticides, antibiotics, hormones, irradiation or genetically engineered ingredients). Read the food labels and look out especially for the following chemicals:

- Sunset yellow (E110 or FD&C Yellow 6) is a dye used in, among other foods, orange jellies and squashes, apricot jam and packet soups. It's also in Smarties, and at least one variety of Lucozade (a popular British and now also American sports drink).

- Tartrazine (E102 or FD&C Yellow 5), one of the more controversial coloring additives used in the U.K., is another yellow dye used in fizzy drinks, ice cream, sweets and jams.
- Carmoisine (E122 or Red 3), a red dye, is used in jellies, sweets, blancmanges, marzipan and cheesecake mixes. You'll also find it in novelty cakes.
- Ponceau 4R (E124 or Red 7), also red, is used in European tinned fruit, jellies and salamis. Smarties and Simpson's cakes also contain it.

In addition to the devastating effects of additives in children (and adults), the excessive consumption of sugar by children has highly destructive effects on their development. It sows the seeds for many illnesses, including diabetes and obesity. A 1998 study published in the *Journal of the American Dietetic Association* showed that children get 20% of their daily calories from sugar. Kids consume on average 29 teaspoons of added refined sugar each day. Every year, teenagers eat 93 pounds of refined sugar on average. I'm afraid this amount has only continued to grow since these figures were researched. Sugar consists, however, of 'empty' calories that have no nutritional value for the body whatsoever. Sugar robs the body of precious minerals and makes the immune system vulnerable to pathogens. It has led to the enormous obesity problem among children today.

The High Fiber Trap

Official health reports advise us to pack large amounts of whole grain and bran-enriched cereals into our diet. Studies have shown that those who follow this advice have a significantly lower fat intake compared with those who don't. They also want to eat fewer calories at lunchtime, which seems desirable. A high fiber cereal for breakfast subdues AGNI, the digestive fire for many hours, which might tempt you to even skip lunch (for lack of proper appetite). But by the evening, the body, sensing a 'famine', wants to eat twice as much to make up for the lack of nutrient supplies during the day. By then AGNI is too low to handle large quantities of food, which results in the accumulation of toxic fecal matter in the intestines. Consequently you *put* on weight, *despite* your good 'health habits'.

The commonly held belief that indigestible fiber cannot be digested and leaves our body unaltered applies *only* to the small intestine. But when it reaches the large intestine, the fiber is attacked and broken down by large numbers of residential bacteria. This causes fermentation and the common flatulence, headaches, heart pressure, irritability, tiredness, sleeping problems, etc. Fiber is a plant's skeleton, and can only be found within plants. It is vital to the health of your digestive system as it stimulates the waves of muscular contraction that coerces food through your intestinal tract. If your diet is low in vegetable fiber, your intestinal musculature becomes weak, resulting in the sluggish transit of foods. This can cause many problems: including intestinal gas, constipation and irritable bowel syndrome. The vegetable fiber helps you to feel full, and reduces the likelihood of you overeating. It also assists in the evacuation of any excess cholesterol from your system. Your body is designed to process the soluble fiber found in fruits: not the insoluble fiber found within grains (bran), which is sharp and can leave microscopic lacerations on the wall of your intestines.

Doctors at the South Manchester University Hospital, England, studying Irritable Bowel Syndrome (IBS) have discovered that after eating bran - the one time cure-all food for IBS - more than half of their patients felt much worse. Today over 20 percent of the British population suffers from IBS, and it is even more so in the United States. High fiber cereals cause loose stools, a major reason why people with constipation choose bran or bran-enriched foods as a method of producing regular bowel movements. Added bran, however, leaches minerals from the colon cells, weakens peristalsis, and causes chronic colon problems. If intake of bran is discontinued, constipation results.

Many health-conscious people follow a low fat diet - so highly recommended by nutritional experts. Yet if cereals don't contain enough fat, they miss out on the 'fuel' required to properly digest and absorb their carbohydrates. The result is that they pass through the small intestine far too quickly. The colon bacteria then act on the undigested food, producing many unpleasant side effects, including flatulence, bad-smelling gases, constipation or diarrhea, and weight gain.

The high fiber theory definitely has its good sides, though. Another major factor of intestinal obstruction is small feces. A diet rich in natural, soft vegetable fiber produces larger feces that retain a lot more water than a diet consisting of refined and processed foods. The average British meal takes about 83 hours to pass through the intestinal tract with an average stool weight of only 104 g. By contrast, British vegetarians take about 41 hours and produce 208 g of stools - whereas the average meal of a Ugandan villager, consisting of low protein high-fiber diet, takes only 36 hours and generates 470 g of stools a day. Ugandans rarely suffer from constipation, and they *don't* add bran to their foods.

It is much better for the body to obtain fiber from fresh fruit, salads, cooked grains, beans and vegetables. Cooked vegetables in particular contain plenty of fiber, which helps the digestive process but does not overwhelm the colon in the same way as added bran does. Also, the high water content of cooked foods and fruits generally make the passage through the intestinal tract much easier. This brings us to the next subject: Is eating raw and unprepared food better than eating cooked and prepared food?

The belief that regular bowel movement is important for health is very ancient. But the present theory is based on Dr. Dennis Burkitt's discovery that relatively few rural black Africans suffer from cancer of the colon. He attributed this to their relatively crude diet. The theory was that, as fiber made food travel through the gut faster, it allowed less time for cancer-inducing agents to form. This, of course, presupposed that food became carcinogenic in the gut.

3. Raw Whole Foods

There was no evidence that the above presumption is true. Neither was there any evidence that moving food through the intestine at a faster rate decreases the risk of colon cancer. Moreover, the rural African's lifestyle was far from that of the Western city dweller: their diet is different, but also they were not exposed to so many pollutants, toxins or mental stresses. Indeed, there were many factors that could have been responsible for a difference in disease patterns. Other communities - the Mormons of Utah, for example - also enjoyed a low incidence of colon cancer although they ate a low-fiber diet.

So Dr. Burkitt's theory was unsubstantiated at the time and it was to be disproved in practice later as the rural Africans moved into towns and adopted a Western style low fiber diet. Their incidence of colon cancer has remained low and this has continued with the second generation. Nevertheless, these later findings were never publicized. Burkitt's theories caught the attention of the media. Always ready to exploit a good story, they expanded what was at best a very weak hypothesis into a treatment dogma that today teaches that fiber is a panacea for all manner of illnesses.

Commercial interests were quick to see the potential in the recommendation and jump on the bran wagon. Burkitt's recommendation was based on vegetable fiber. Bran (cereal fiber), on the other hand, has a far higher fiber content. A practically worthless byproduct of the milling process, until then, bran had been thrown away. Almost overnight, it became a highly priced profit maker. Although totally inedible, backed by Burkitt's fiber hypothesis, bran could now be promoted as a valuable food. But Dr. Hugh Trowell, Burkitt's partner and another strong advocate of dietary fiber, stated in 1974:

"A serious confusion of thought is produced by referring to the dietary fiber hypothesis as the bran hypothesis, for many Africans do not consume cereal or bran."

Fiber-caused Diseases on the Rise

There is no evidence to suggest adding extra fiber to your diet has the effect of curing or preventing diseases. Although bran has been a popular way to manage Irritable Bowel Syndrome (IBS) for about thirty years, there is no placebo-controlled study of bran in IBS that has shown any convincing beneficial effect. A study, published in 1994, found that while fruit fiber was helpful in IBS, bran only made the situation worse. Far from being a cure for IBS, the researchers found that it was the bran that was actually causing it! Bran also led to bowel disturbances, abdominal distension and pain. There is also a growing skepticism in the U.S. that lack of fiber causes cancer; some studies even suggest that a fiber-enhanced diet *increases* the risk of colon cancer.

Other Adverse Effects of Added Fiber

While fruit and vegetable fiber is quite harmless for the body, bran fiber from grain foods should be avoided as it poses a considerable health risk. Research conducted on the supposed benefits of dietary fiber shows that eating fiber-enriched foods can upset basic physiological processes. Food absorption through the gut wall should neither be slowed nor be rushed. However, fiber abnormally speeds up food transportation through the gut, which leads to decreased nutrient absorption. Eating fiber-enriched foods or foods containing rough fiber can significantly inhibit the absorption of iron, calcium, phosphorus, magnesium, sugars, proteins, fats and vitamins A, D, E and K. Phytates found in cereal fiber (bran), for example, bind with calcium, iron and zinc making them indigestible, which in turn causes poor absorption.

In one study comparing the body's ability to utilize nutrients from whole wheat bread and white bread, subjects actually absorbed more iron from white bread than from whole wheat bread. Remarkably, although the whole wheat bread contained fifty percent more iron than the white bread, the body wasn't able to extract it. In addition, bran has also been shown to cause fecal loss of calcium, iron, zinc, phosphorus, nitrogen, fats, fatty acids and sterols, thus depleting the body of these materials.

These findings are of particular concern to people suffering from conditions related to nutrient deficiencies. The *get-your-daily-fiber-mania* can put several sections of the population at considerable health risk from eating too much fiber in their diet. The following are some of the risks:

- The incidence of osteoporosis (brittle bone disease) is rapidly increasing and now affects one in two post-menopausal women. Osteoporosis is also now a leading cause of death among men. Osteoporosis is a metabolic disorder caused by many factors, including poor calcium absorption due to bile duct blockage in the liver and gallbladder; milk, cheese, meat, and other acid-forming foods and beverages; and bran. Bran both inhibits the absorption of calcium from food and depletes the body of the calcium it has. Bran also depletes zinc the body requires to restore bone health.
- Sufferers of Alzheimer's disease (senile dementia) are found to have abnormal amounts of aluminum in their brains. Tests on the people of Guam and parts of New Guinea and Japan, who get Alzheimer's disease at a much younger age, suggest that it is a lack of calcium - causing a hormonal imbalance - that permits the aluminum to penetrate the brain.
- Infants may suffer brain damage when fed with soy-based baby formula. Soy is rich in phytates, which inhibit the absorption of zinc. Zinc is essential for proper brain development.

- Vitamin deficiency diseases such as rickets are on the rise again. This bone-deforming disease nearly disappeared in Britain until huge advertising campaigns led to steep increases in the consumption of dairy products and meat.
- The intake of 'anti-nutrients' such as dietary fiber is greatly increasing the risk of iron deficiency anemia.
- Depression, anorexia, low birth weight, slow growth, mental retardation, and amenorrhea are associated with deficiencies of zinc and, with the exception of amenorrhea, iron.
- Excess fiber consumption affects the onset of menstruation, retards uterine growth and, is associated with menstrual dysfunction.

Because of phytates, Dr. David Southgate, considered the world's leading authority on the effects of fiber, concludes that infants, children, young adolescents and pregnant women whose mineral needs are greater should avoid excessive consumption of fiber.

Writing of the **colon cancer** risk, Drs. H. S. Wasan and R. A. Goodlad of the Imperial Cancer Research Fund stated in 1996:

"Until individual constituents of fiber have been shown to have, at the very least, a non-detrimental effect in prospective human trials, we urge that restraint should be shown in adding fiber supplements to foods, and that unsubstantiated health claims be restricted."…"Specific dietary fiber supplements, embraced as nutriceuticals or functional foods, are an unknown and potentially damaging way to influence modern dietary habits of the general population."

In January 1999 the results of the largest trial into the effects on fiber on colon cancer ever conducted were released to the public. After studying 88,757 women for sixteen years, doctors at the Brigham and Women's Hospital and Harvard Medical School state: "No significant association between fiber intake and the risk of colorectal adenoma was found." … "Our data do not support the existence of an important protective effect of dietary fiber against colorectal cancer or adenoma." Surprisingly, the women who ate the most fiber - nearly 25 grams per day - were just as likely to develop colon cancer and pre-cancerous tumors as those who ate the least (about 10 grams per day).

There are close to 30 published studies which all confirm that fiber intake has not only no beneficial effects, but is indicated in multiple complications of the gastrointestinal tract. For example, in one study published in 2000, researchers randomly assigned 1,429 men and women with a history of colon polyps (a pre-cancerous condition) to eat either a high-fiber or low-fiber wheat-bran supplement in addition to their ordinary diet. After three years, researchers found at least one polyp in about 50 percent of the participants in each group.

Chocolate - Facts and Fiction

The recent desperate attempt of the food industry to boost sluggish sales of their products, after the dampening effects of the low carb craze, has caused it to heavily invest in serious 'scientific' research to prove that their unhealthy products are not just safe, but even good for you. Although hard to believe, chocolate is now being pushed as a health food. Add chocolate to your healthy diet, and your heart health will improve. At least, this is what they are now trying to make you believe.

Apparently, there is a new study that suggests eating chocolate can improve your blood vessel functions. This clearly shows how much the food industry, similar to the pharmaceutical industry, wants you to buy more of their products, with utter disregard to your health.

According to the editors of the *Journal of the American College of Nutrition* (JACN), flavonoid-rich dark chocolate may improve artery flexibility while increasing an antioxidant that may help prevent blood clots. Whereas this is likely, and may be true, the problem with the study is that it didn't include a control (placebo) group. So there was no one to compare to. Besides, the common chocolate you buy in stores doesn't improve artery flexibility - it's the flavonoids in dark chocolate and raw cocoa beans that have this effect. These same flavonoids are also found in apples, grapes, broccoli, onions, berries, and dozens of other foods, some of which the subjects of the study most likely consumed besides the chocolate. Of course, the study was sponsored by a chocolate producer, Mars Candy Company, which was so generous to also supply the chocolates for the 'study'. If the study has any real value, why didn't the researchers announce that flavonoids, as found in most plant foods, such as broccoli and fruits, grape juice and, yes, also chocolate, are beneficial for your arteries? But no, they were obliged by their sponsors to announce that 'chocolate is beneficial for your arteries'. All this is in total disregard to all the other things that are contained in chocolate, that is, lots of sugar, milk, preservatives, coloring agents, artificial flavorings, etc.

The American Dietetic Association (ADA) which is supported by a grant from Mars Inc. has a section on their website titled 'Chocolate: Facts and Fiction'. Although dietary sugar intake is a big factor for the millions of people who have Type 2 diabetes or peripatetic conditions, the ADA advices, "If you have diabetes, ask your health professional how to incorporate chocolate into your eating plan." This sounds like 'sound' medical advice. I would stay away from any of the ADA's dietary advice. You never know what kind of sickness you may develop because of it.

The truth of the matter is that real chocolate consists of largely fermented, roasted chocolate beans that are packed with nutrients. The word 'chocolate' comes from the Aztecs of Mexico who called it 'bitter water'. They associated chocolate with the goddess of fertility. It was always used as a beverage, never as a solid food. Its numerous benefits were known to them.

Today's largely 'fake' chocolate consists mostly of cocoa butter, milk or milk powder, sugar, and other ingredients such as emulsifiers that improve smoothness and flavor. The finest plain dark chocolate contains at least 70% cocoa (solids and butter), whereas the most expensive milk chocolate usually contains about 50% cocoa. High-quality white chocolate contains around 30% cocoa. Most mass-produced chocolate contains as little as 7 percent cocoa and fats other than cocoa butter. These 'chocolate' products have little to do with chocolate because of the low or virtually non-existent cocoa content.

The chocolate that most people consume is relatively inexpensive. Production costs can be decreased by reducing cocoa solid content or by substituting cocoa butter with a non-cocoa fat. The announcement by Mars and other candy producers that 'chocolate is good for your heart' applies only to a tiny fraction of the chocolates sold, and therefore is misleading. The health claims made are part of a clever marketing campaign to sell more chocolate of any kind, knowing well that most people buy the cheapest chocolate available. The proclaimed health benefits of chocolate can, however, only be applied to fermented, roasted cocoa beans and the more expensive dark chocolate with mostly natural and healthy ingredients.

Dark chocolate, which has a strong bitter taste, has shown the same blood-thinning benefits as aspirin, but without the harmful side effects and increased risk of heart attack and stroke. Regular chocolate has never shown any health benefits, but lots of harmful side effects, including weight gain and obesity.

4. Raw Versus Cooked Foods

The Pros and Cons

The arguments in favor of a raw food diet sound very convincing: Food should be left whole and unprepared. Only then can we benefit from its natural goodness and vitality. With the plenty of vitamins, minerals and trace elements contained in raw food we will never suffer any deficiencies. We should live like all the other animals in nature; they don't prepare their food, cook their vegetables, or bake bread - the reason why they are so healthy and strong. On the other hand, we destroy most of the essential and health-promoting nutrients through methods of cooking, preparing, and baking, causing all the vitamin and mineral deficiencies prevalent today.

The promoters of raw food diets propose that if the general population ate more of the untreated whole foods, many diseases could be prevented. This could save billions of dollars in treatment costs. Many chronically ill patients have found sudden relief and improvement, thanks to raw vegetables and soaked grains.

The initial and sometimes lasting benefits of a raw whole food diet can be so promising that a person may decide to continue eating solely raw foods, although he may not like their taste. But is it possible that raw and whole foods, except fruits, which are already 'cooked' or ripened by the sun, can actually be harmful to some of us if eaten on a continual basis? And why does 98 percent of the world's population favor prepared and warm foods to raw and cold foods? Have we all forsaken our natural instincts?

Karl Pirlet, Professor of Medicine at the University of Frankfurt, Germany, claims that he has a nearly endless collection of cases where health was restored to patients after they stopped eating a raw whole food diet. He found that most of these patients suffered a physical breakdown after several years (in some cases after 10-20 years) of eating raw whole foods. The effects were varied but were all marked by the occurrence of sudden aging as seen in a deterioration of joints and arteries. Most patients looked fragile, felt low in energy, and had excessively bloated stomachs. Their bodies could no longer cope with breaking down hard grains and raw vegetables; they were literally starving themselves.

So does this mean that raw foods are not good for us? This depends on each person's constitution and condition. Young Pitta types with a strong AGNI and plenty of exercise can cope with such a diet for many years without harmful side effects. But eventually even their digestive system may become exhausted because of trying to breakdown raw whole grains and raw vegetables.

Many people who start on a raw whole food diet have already suffered from health problems and a weak AGNI. Unable to break down the high food fiber, the intestinal bacteria start taking over that job instead. This results in fermentation and putrefaction of the food. The poison, which the bacteria produce during the fermenting process, greatly stimulates the immune system and helps the body to dispose of it. This strong cleansing reaction initially helps clear the intestines from impacted fecal matter, stops constipation, and through the intense immune activity releases plenty of energy. The relief from congestion and constipation and the increased energy and vitality are very noticeable to the person and strikes him/her as very 'positive' signs. This response can even lead to a spontaneous remission of cancer or the relief of arthritic pains. But eventually the intestines may begin to bloat up like a balloon, unable to deal with the toxic gases and poisonous compounds. Healthy Pitta types on mostly raw foods may never get to this stage, but Vata types and Kapha types may suffer ill-effects within days or weeks.

Many nutritionists and dieticians may then give the advice to eat even more fiber because only fiber can absorb such toxic substances as ammonia, which is very caustic, and protect the intestinal walls against injury. But it is highly unlikely that a fermenting and putrefying mass of undigested fiber, which produces ammonia, *reabsorbs* it in the same 'breath'. Nutritional science assumes that the nutritional ingredients of food alone determine whether they have physiological value for us or not. Such an approach, however, is incomplete and misleading unless we include the common-sense understanding that we need a well functioning digestive system to digest, absorb and metabolize these nutrient components in order to benefit from them. A weak digestive system can even make poison out of nectar. The saying "You are what you eat" is therefore only partially correct. You rather are the food you are able to digest and metabolize. In other words, a long-term raw food diet is only good for you as long as you are able to digest it properly. You are the ultimate judge whether raw food works for you or not.

What makes Plants so Poisonous?

Every microbe, insect, plant, animal, and human being on this planet wants to survive. But there are potential dangers out there that can lead to their destruction. For this reason, all living things, including plants, have developed a sophisticated defense apparatus to ward off anyone or anything that wants to eat or harm them.

It is only natural for the species of any life form to create difficulties for the invading or devouring predators; otherwise ecological balance would be impossible. Despite innumerable numbers of lice, pests, beetles and locusts, plants have managed to survive and keep the planet green and oxygenated. This is due to their highly advanced 'healthcare system'. Similar to our bodies, plants have immune systems to ensure their own survival and health. They use prickly thorns, poison as in the case of the deadly nightshades, or they envelop themselves in a wax-covering that is impenetrable for microbes and insects such as lice, beetles, etc. If any of these predatoros somehow manage to enter the plant's interior, inborn defense mechanisms attempt to destroy the invaders, not dissimilar to our own defense responses.

Most destructive microbes that are present in the air, food and water never reach the inside of our bodies. They are promptly neutralized by enzymes located in our noses, lungs, saliva, and stomach juices. The rest of them are taken care of by our immune systems with a sophisticated arsenal of antigens and immune cells, including the macrophages and T-cells.

Plants, however, have to do more to protect themselves since locusts and animals such as cows, mice, or man, can eat them altogether. For this reason, they produce antibodies of which 20,000 kinds are known to date, still only a fraction of what they are capable of producing. These antibodies, when ingested by animals or humans (now considered antigens) can make them sick, which stops them from eating the plants, or at least not eat up all of them.

Another potential sensitivity, that protects plant species from becoming extinct, is a reaction to toxic *salicylates* - natural preservatives stored in the bark, leaves, roots and seeds of plants and found in many foods. In vegetables, they're mostly concentrated in the peels and rinds or the outer leaves. The salicylate content in fruit is highest when the fruit is not fully ripened yet, and decreases during the ripening process. Properly sun-ripened fruits (cooked by the sun), versus those ripened after they are harvested, have great beneficial effects on the body. In general, raw foods, dried foods and juices contain higher concentrations of salicylates than cooked food. To avoid the natural poisons contained in many raw foods, all major ancient civilizations traditionally prepared their foods.

Why Prepare Foods?

The populations of the High Andes were the first ones to introduce the potato to their cultures. But the potatoes had to undergo vigorous cleansing procedures before they were considered edible. First, they were spread on the ground to freeze them overnight. This ensured that the cells burst open. Then the men and women trampled on the potatoes to destroy their skins. Still frozen, the potatoes were then placed into a well base for several weeks to surround them with water. This removed 97 percent of the *alkaloids* and turned the green pulps into a snow-white color. After pressing the potatoes, they exposed them to the hot sun. You may ask: "But what about the so-important vitamins and minerals?" The Andes populations with their high standards of health and stamina obviously preferred taste to nutritional values. They knew that most bitter substances are poisonous and they trusted their taste buds more than any theories of nutrition.

Ayurveda, the most ancient health science in the world, categorizes foods only according to their tastes and after effects. It emphasizes that if the body receives all the six tastes, i.e. sweet, sour, salty, pungent, astringent, and bitter, it will be stimulated to produce many of the important nutrients itself and thus remain balanced. The sense of taste is our body's supreme judge to know whether certain foods are right for us or not. Situated in the taste buds of the tongue and in coordination with the constantly changing requirements of the body, the sense of taste controls our natural instinct and desire for healthy food.

The taste buds for bitter taste are very developed and can detect even the slightest trace of bitter-tasting substances. We have this facility because bitter foods may contain alkaloids and can be poisonous. If toxins build up in the blood the body requires a bitter-tasting antidote or medicine that purifies it and restores its balance. Blood-cleansing herbs or teas generally taste very bitter. The human body accepts chocolate, coffee, tea, and beers, which are of predominantly bitter taste, only after our persuasive mind or added sugar manages to override the taste barrier. Such foods or beverages become desirable quite quickly because they contain morphine-type compounds. This may lead to a substance addiction. There are many types of food that have a slightly bitter taste to them, including lettuce, broccoli, and leafy green vegetables. Yet the bitterness of these foods is well balanced by their natural sweet taste, caused by the sugar-composed carbohydrates. Hence these foods have a cleansing effect but do not poison you.

The natural Indian populations of South America eat potatoes only if there is a scarcity of food. But when they eat them they mix them with clay from the Earth which is known to absorb any toxins that may be left in the potatoes and remove them from the system. This practice also removes vitamins and minerals, which seems to make no difference to their health. Clay is used by many types of folk medicine around the world to absorb the toxins generated by bacteria during diarrhea.

The Aboriginals who live in the wilderness prepare their food similarly to our cooking procedures. Each plant, seed, or root requires a separate process of preparation to make it edible. Certain roots, for instance, are peeled, soaked for half a day, and then baked for thirty minutes. The sometimes-elaborate preparation of their food serves a very important purpose, that is, the removal of natural food poisons or plant antibodies, which the body treats as antigens.

Even animals 'prepare' their food. Cows, for example, bring up their food and chew it again after it has been 'cooked' in the stomach. In fact they have 12 stomachs to make certain that the blood does not absorb the ingredients of flowers, grains or grass before they are thoroughly detoxified. Birds are equipped with goiters to soak (ferment) the grains before their muscle stomachs 'chew' them up. Rabbits have their own way of dealing with the potentially dangerous food; they eat part of their own feces, which is an alternative to chewing the same food twice.

Low Nutrient Foods - A Key to Survival

The time-tested methods of food preparation may weaken the theory that we are supposed to eat our food in the state nature has given it to us, with all the nutrients retained. But how could the original inhabitants of our planet have survived for so many thousands of years without having sufficient vitamins and minerals in their diet? They made certain that only very few toxins could enter their digestive systems. With so little toxicity to deal with, the small amounts of nutrients contained in their foods were almost sufficient to keep up the healthy functioning of their physiology. Their bodies produced the rest.

It is known, for example, that the human body has eight different ways to make calcium, using bicarbonate of soda (a product of our digestive system), other minerals and certain enzymes. The body is its own factory. It can make many minerals and even vitamins. Whatever it cannot produce itself, the trillions of friendly bacteria residing in the gut produce for it. Whatever the body requires in terms of nutrient complexes it is capable of producing them from even the simplest of foods. This may explain why certain North Mexican tribes can live on eating only corn (mainly starch) and some beans and be more healthy and fit than the healthiest and fittest individuals in the 'well-fed' world. Out of necessity, their digestive systems are so sophisticated and efficient that they can produce everything their body needs from corn (and beans). In comparison, most of our 'well-fed' bodies are so inefficient that they have even 'forgotten' how to make essential vitamins and amino acids.

Raw whole foods supply us with plenty of vitamins and if the soil is naturally fertile also with many minerals. But this doesn't necessarily mean that we need them all and that we can use them in such large quantities. The initial boost in energy and vitality after going on a raw food diet is not due to the vitamins; it is rather caused by the sudden mobilization of the immune system which tries to counteract the massive influx of enzyme inhibitors and antibodies contained in the food. In time, the digestive system becomes increasingly dependent on large supplies of vitamins and minerals. And when suddenly there are not enough of them in the food we eat, the body begins to suffer from what is generally called a vitamin or mineral deficiency, which is just another word for weak digestion. Our time is characterized by lazy digestive systems. We have cultivated our own dependency on large quantities of external supplies of these basic nutrients.

We can easily afford to eat a fresh salad with our meal today because we have 'cultivated away' the natural antibodies of the plants and vegetables. This makes them less 'poisonous' for us but at the same time also more vulnerable to all kinds of attacks by insects, lice, bugs, beetles, locusts, fungus, and harsh climatic conditions. To make them resistant against the bewildering number of possible enemies we give the plants synthetically derived poisons (insecticides, pesticides, and other fertilizers) to make up for the missing antibodies. We have effectively impaired the plants' immune systems, and without our chemical assistance, most cultivated plant foods would never reach the ripening stage.

By contrast, the wild-growing herbs have retained their immunity and know very well how to survive. They contain potent medicinal substances, which are nothing other than the plants' antibodies. If they are cultivated, too, removed from their natural environment and climatic conditions, their medicinal properties become less potent; thus, they are less effective as a medicine. Many of them no longer have medicinal values and they are now merely used in cooking to flavor the food.

The Grain Food Mystery

If you give pigs too much grain in their feed, their growth rate is retarded. By contrast, the same grains fed to cattle ferment in their stomachs without a problem. Grains contain several substances that can reduce our ability and that of other animals to absorb minerals, trace elements, and even vitamin B1. They also can block our digestive enzymes and render proteins indigestible. Wheat in particular contains material components that interfere with the digestion of fats by blocking such enzymes as the *lipase* of the pancreas. Our ancestors have traditionally used plenty of lard or oil when preparing dishes made from grain, often at the ratio of 1:1. This may explain why people who eat too little fat with their bread and other wheat products often develop excessive weight; they suffer from a disturbed fat metabolism.

Each type of grain has specific antibodies and enzyme inhibitors that can disrupt digestion and slow normal cell growth in both children and adults. These natural poisons are found in the most 'precious' parts of the grain, the wheat germ, and in the layer directly under the husk. The husk itself is wooden, enhanced by stored silicate, and contains *tannins* which bond with proteins. The putrefaction of these proteins produces bad-smelling gases, ammonia, and toxins. If eaten as raw grain muesli it can virtually 'burst' one's intestines.

But even whole grain bread has become difficult to digest for most people since the old baking procedures have been 'modernized', saving time and money. For thousands of years, man has imitated the fermentation process that grains undergo in the cow's stomach system. The dough used to be left alone for as long as twenty hours. This helped to pre-digest the grains and break down some of the most notorious antibodies or *alkaloids*, freeing the otherwise useless nutrients. The initial stages of baking also increased the process of fermentation, which got rid of the rest of the poisons.

Today's time-saving baking methods use a mixture of chemicals that reduce the need for long fermentation but fail to break down the toxic contents of the grain. The use of yeast completely inhibits their destruction. The result is that the bread, though tasting delicious, is difficult to digest and causes bloating. However, it may work very well as a laxative. Most people who eat uncooked whole grains, commercial whole grain bread, or even just added wheat bran, find that their bowel movements begin to be 'normalized'. To be relieved from constipation is certainly a great advantage over being all blocked up. Still, the main reason for the sudden 'improvement' is the body's desperate attempt to remove the toxic antibodies in the wheat products as quickly as it can. This should not be confused with a voluntary healthy bowel movement; it simply is a normal immune response. But if the situation continues, the constant irritation can lead to Irritable Bowel Syndrome, diarrhea, Crohn's disease, or cancer of the colon.

Another immediate advantage of properly fermenting bread dough is the production of various types of natural antibiotics, which help to ward off mold-producing microbes. This protects the intestinal lining against possible irritation. Commercial whole-wheat bread and wheat flakes in breakfast cereals have therefore no natural defenses against mold attack, which makes them 'risky' foods. Allergies are a common result.

In most cultures of the world, white bread has been the dominating wheat product for thousands of years. This shows that the older generations knew more about the potential dangers of whole wheat than we do. The Ancient Egyptians sifted the flour again after milling. Even Hippocrates declared 2,500 years ago that white bread was more nourishing and the ancient Romans favored white flour too. Too much of it, however, is constipating. French baking is known to have avoided wheat bran for hundreds of years. Rye, on the other hand, has never been refined which gives rye bread its darker color. Barley is usually eaten in roasted form. Oats are normally heat-treated; otherwise they would taste bitter. Cooked as oatmeal/porridge, preferably soaked overnight, they are good for an irritated stomach. Rice obviously is edible only in cooked form.

Warning: Most commercially made flour is bleached and conditioned, which increases its shelf life and makes it better for baking. Some added ingredients are relatively harmless, while others are outright dangerous and can cause cancer, heart disease and diabetes. Processed and altered flour and its products should be avoided, just like white sugar.

Making your Own Cultures

If you enjoy cultured breads, you may make and use your own culture. Just take a small amount of any type of organic wheat flour and mix it with some distilled water, put a few layers of cheesecloth over the jar, and let it sit in or on a screened patio where it is above room temperature. After 3 to 6 days check if it smells like bread or beer. If it does, it is ready for use to make your own bread. (Use a sourdough recipe.)

Alternatively, you may use organic raisins. Soak them in water, covered with 2-3 layers of cheesecloth (follow the same instructions as above). Keep container in the fresh air and wait a few days up to a week. Use the water as a natural culture, once it turns or smells fermented.

Conclusion:

Nutrients are not the only components of our food. Natural food also contains toxic plant antibodies (antigens once ingested), a fact that should be considered by all those who live on unaltered whole foods. Ayurveda knew of these dangers even 6,000 years ago and recommends that we prepare and cook a considerable portion of our foods. Mankind has used fire for food preparation for over one million years to make food digestible and to remove any toxic components. A mixed diet, consisting of raw and possibly organically grown salad foods, fruit, cooked vegetables, cooked staple foods such as rice, wheat, and other grain foods, as well as legumes, offers a large selection of natural foods that can accommodate every body-type.

As mentioned, balanced Pittas, with their naturally strong AGNI or digestive fire, can eat relatively more raw foods than the other two major body types, particularly in the summer season. Vata and Kapha types benefit more from eating mostly warm and cooked foods, as their bodies tend to be cool by nature. A Kapha's AGNI may easily get 'subdued' by a lot of raw food, and a Vata, whose AGNI is 'changeable' can become constipated, nervous, and depressed if he eats too much of it. But, whatever body-type you are, start trusting your intuition and listening to the signals from your body each and every moment of the day. One day you may have eaten a particular food such as a bar of chocolate and the next day you suffer a headache. If you ate a salad or fruit for supper, you may feel sluggish and irritable the next morning, because it has fermented in your intestines during the night. Nobody knows your body better than you do.

If you feel inclined to only eating raw, unprepared foods, it means that your body may require cleansing. Still, keep listening to your body's signals of comfort and discomfort. If one day you get an aversion to these foods, return to a mixed diet immediately because your body is telling you that it has had enough and can no longer cope with so many toxic and irritating antigens. A cleanse consisting of raw vegetables or their juices has saved many people's lives by triggering a strong immune response. This helped remove toxic waste that may have lingered in the intestinal tract for many years. The body usually sends a clear message of discomfort when the antibodies begin to damage the intestines, which is the time to stop the cleansing.

Your physical needs, emotional state, behavior, digestive ability, environmental factors, geographic conditions, and many other influences determine what kind of food, of what quality and how much of it your body requires each new day. You are not a machine that runs with one specific fuel oil; you are a living organism that is changing every moment according to uncountable influences. By increasingly relying on the body's wisdom and natural instinct regarding the choice of food we can break out of the man-made, restrictive rules of nutrition and discover what we really need to nourish ourselves.

5. The Milk Controversy

Is Cow's Milk Suitable for Human Consumption?

Dairy milk has become a major target of criticism over the past few years due to its long lists of negative side effects. More and more health practitioners report that patients are allergic to dairy products or suffer from food intolerance to milk-containing foods. Eczema, asthma, migraine, constipation, hay fever, arthritis, stomach trouble, lymph edema, heart disease and testicular cancer are all linked with high consumption of dairy products.

One such case was Tim who just turned 11 years old when his parents brought him to see me. He had developed asthma when he was five months old. The former treatment consisted of three different types of drugs, including *cortisone* and an inhaler. The boy's condition worsened steadily and he developed herpes and other symptoms of high toxicity. Six months before his visit to me, Tim had caught a cold, which was treated with antibiotics. Since then his lungs showed strong signs of congestion. He complained about being tired all the time and unable to run or play with his friends. Kinesiology muscle testing revealed that Tim was highly allergic to milk or milk products. His parents confirmed that by the age of five months he was no longer breastfed but was instead given infant milk formula.

Tim's asthma was caused by his body's inability to break down the protein of cow's milk. The fragments of undigested protein caused a strong immune response aggravating the entire mucus lining from the anus to the lungs. His condition was chronic because he consumed large quantities of animal protein, including milk and dairy products throughout his young life. After two weeks of abstinence from these foods, his asthma and herpes subsided and have never recurred since.

Could it be that cow's milk is meant only for calves just as cat's milk is meant only for kittens? Would we consider feeding our babies with, for example, dog's milk instead of human breast milk? The ratio of nutrients contained in dog's milk does not suit human requirements. Yet the same applies to cow's milk. Cow's milk contains three times as much protein, and almost four times as much calcium as human mother's milk. These amounts are unsuitable for the human physiology at any age.

Cow's milk is designed to contain the exact amount of calcium and protein necessary to feed a calf that will end up being at least 3-4 times larger than the human body is. If we gave human breast milk to a calf, it would not grow strong enough even to survive. By contrast, human babies require more carbohydrates in the beginning stages of their lives than calves do. For this reason, in comparison to human mother's milk, cow's milk contains only half the amount of carbohydrates. Calves on the other hand require much more salt than human babies do; naturally, salt content in cow's milk is three times higher than in human milk. It is for a good reason that most of the original populations living in Asia, Africa, Australia, and South America don't regard cow's milk as a food fit for human consumption.

Once weaned, mammals no longer look for milk to satisfy their hunger or thirst. If human babies, who have been breastfed for 14-18 months, were given the option of choosing from various types of natural and suitable foods, two out of three would no longer want breast milk as a food, according to classic study. Babies who are fed with cow's milk tend to look puffy, bloated and fat. It is not uncommon for 1-year olds to have gallstones in the liver as a result of drinking, and not digesting, cow's milk. Many of them suffer from colic, gas, and bloating, which makes them cry and develop sleeping disorders. Other problems include tonsillitis, ear-infections, breathing difficulties, excessive mucus discharge and drooling from the mouth.

Michael Klaper, M.D., and author of Vegan Nutrition: Pure & Simple, summarized the milk controversy as follows: "The human body has no more need for cows' milk than it does for dogs' milk, horses' milk, or giraffes' milk."

Milk-caused Osteoporosis

Since milk intolerance is becoming increasingly common among all age groups in the Western world, nutritionists and doctors are starting to suspect that cow's milk may not be such a natural food for humans after all.

Milk is a highly mucus-forming food that can cause irritation and congestion throughout the gastrointestinal tract. If regularly consumed, milk can leave an increasingly hardening and almost impermeable coating on the inside of the intestinal membranes. This restricts absorption of nutrients, including the calcium, magnesium and zinc needed to form bones. It is virtually impossible to successfully treat people with natural medicines as long as they continue to clog up their digestive systems with milk or dairy foods; the medicines are not able to penetrate the hardened layer of mucus in the intestines.

Most people wouldn't drink milk if they weren't so influenced by the myth that milk is essential for the bones. If you are prone to osteoporosis, or osteoarthritis, then consider the following facts:

- Cow's milk may be very rich in calcium but its high calcium to magnesium ratio can make it difficult to absorb. In certain people or body types, the calcium may be deposited in places where it is not required, hence, the development of calcification of bones and other parts of the body.

- Most of the calcium contained in cow's milk is bound by the milk chemical *casein*, which makes it far too crude for proper absorption by the human intestinal membranes. Cow's milk contains 300 times more *casein* than human milk. You can get more absorbable calcium out of 6-8 almonds or a teaspoon of molasses than you can get from one liter of cow's milk.

- There is quantitatively more phosphorus in cow's milk than there is calcium. To metabolize that much phosphorus, the body requires extra amounts of calcium, which it extracts from the bones, teeth and muscles. This leads to calcium deficiency in these parts of the body. To compensate the sudden loss of calcium, the body tries to mobilize more of it. As mentioned before, the body has several methods to manufacture the much-needed mineral. If the body depended totally on external supplies of calcium, 80 percent of today's population would have lost at least one third of their bone mass by the age of 30. Because of this self-regulating mechanism, we are able to survive even extremely poor diets with very little calcium intake. We can even fast on distilled water for several weeks without developing a calcium deficiency (distilled water removes calcium from the body). Yet if the consumption of dairy foods continues for a long time, the calcium reserves get depleted faster than they can be replenished, leading to damage of the bone tissue.

- Milk proteins contain about three times the amount of sulphur-containing amino acids than proteins from vegetable origin. Regular consumption of milk and dairy products would turn the blood acidic and kill it if the body didn't mobilize large amounts of minerals to save itself from acid death. Yet, in the long term, this emergency measure leads to demineralization of the tissues and organs, and subsequent acidosis.

- Storage of excessive amounts of milk protein in the connective tissues and basal membranes of the capillaries reduces the diffusion of essential minerals and vitamins to the tissues of the body. This causes a depletion of nutrients in the tissues, especially of those that form the bones and joints.

Cows maintain strong and hardy bones and teeth throughout their lives and get most of their calcium from the greens they eat. Gorillas, elephants and other strong animals also don't suffer from osteoporosis. Occasionally they lick on limestone, but this is certainly not enough to supply the large quantities of calcium they require to build and rebuild their heavy skeletons. If milk were the most useful and important source of calcium for grown animals then nature would certainly have designed ways of supplying them with milk throughout their lives. But as it turns out, they have access to milk only at the beginning stages of their lives.

The human body requires large amounts of bile to digest whole milk. Drinking whole milk regularly can eventually exhaust the liver's bile-producing capacity. Drinking low fat milk makes matters worse. Low fat milk requires less bile to digest the fat contained in the milk, yet milk protein cannot be digested without the naturally high concentrations of milk fat. Added to that, without sufficient bile, calcium cannot be properly digested or absorbed either. The large amounts of undigested milk protein increase acidity in the body and the unused crude milk calcium can cause calcification of joints, arteries and kidneys. This can make protein foods with lowered fat-content hazardous to health.

Leafy green vegetables contain four times more calcium than whole milk. There is also plenty of calcium in almonds, black molasses, sesame seeds, broccoli, Brazil nuts, millet, oats and citrus fruits. The calcium contained in these foods is readily absorbed by the human digestive system, provided the digestive system functions efficiently. Osteoporosis and osteoarthritis are basically metabolic disorders that are caused by severe congestion and an unbalanced diet/lifestyle, and almost never by insufficient calcium intake. Osteoporosis is virtually unknown in such places as Africa where people eat far fewer proteins than those living in developed countries.

Milk Consumption Linked to Diabetes and Allergies

Initial studies on diabetes revealed that the frequency of *insulin dependent diabetes* is linked to breast-feeding. The longer children were breastfed by their mothers, the less was their risk of developing diabetes later in life. The interpretation of this finding was revised, however, after it was found that children who are fed with cow's milk formula rather than with mother's milk were the most likely candidates for diabetes. More precise studies revealed that diabetics have a striking number of antibodies against a particular protein in their blood. Diabetes is considered an 'autoimmune disease' which means that the body supposedly directs its defenses against itself. The particular protein that the body tries to combat here comes from the whey of cow's milk. If the milk protein becomes lodged in the body's connective tissues, it is only natural for the body's immune cells (white cells) to attack and remove it. The fact that this response by the immune system inflames the cells surrounding these tissues (which is essential for healing) should not be misconstrued to be an autoimmune disease.

Ever since cow's milk has been used to make cheese, whey, which is a waste product of cheese production, has been fed to pigs. This practice continued even after scientists attributed great nutritional value to whey. Since nobody really liked drinking this 'precious' ingredient of milk it was mixed in with foods. This 'coincided' with a dramatic increase in allergies in the developed world. Scientists have discovered that the *beta-casein* (a particular protein) in cow's milk can trigger an immune response that may, in turn, cross-react with an antigen to cause an allergic reaction. An allergy is the body's response to fight a substance that it considers dangerous to its health and survival.

Today, millions of people in the Western Hemisphere are suffering from allergies caused by milk or products that contain milk powder or whey. Perhaps this is the reason most populations in the world avoid drinking cow's milk. The current 'allergy epidemic' in developed countries may have well been caused by the 'miracle food' whey which is added to so many food products, including children's foods, fresh cheese, ready-made soups, diet foods, etc. We are practically infested by this milk protein unless we live off purely natural foods.

Watch out for the Milk Hormone

Bovine somatotrophin (BST) is a hormone which, when fed to cows, can increase their milk yield by 20-30 percent. In the United States, BST was licensed by the American Food and Drug Administration (FDA) in 1994. This effectively gave farmers the legal permission to treat their herds with the controversial hormone. The license was accompanied with a new labeling policy, previously unheard of in the United States. Traditional dairy farmers are prohibited from labeling their milk as 'hormone free' - while those using the hormone are not required to say that they use BST. Because uncontrolled hormone intake is linked to a number of serious health problems, there has been great concern among farmers who use BST that people would prefer the natural milk to the hormone treated one. Their pressure ensured the above legislation.

The granting of a license to increase milk production through hormones comes at a time when milk production is already much higher than is milk consumption. Most industrialized nations destroy enormous quantities of milk and butter to manipulate the prices with no regard to the cows' health. Cows are naturally made to produce a certain amount of milk according to the demand from their offspring. The hormone-induced artificial increase of milk yield causes a number of cow's diseases that are met by administering large quantities of antibiotics. The drug's poisons seep into the milk and its products. How much a cow must be suffering when its udder is being extended to beyond it natural capacity is not even considered an issue.

Is Milk Bad for Everyone?

Cow's milk is the food used to raise cows. Drinking the milk from another species is less than ideal. Under normal circumstances, you will not find young animals going around and begging other animals to give them some of their milk. Any adverse reactions to partaking of the milk of another species are to be expected. However, if milk causes allergies or other diseases why doesn't everyone who regularly consumes cow's milk suffer from the same problems? One reason may be that they don't remove the fat from the milk. Left unaltered, cows milk is completely balanced regarding its natural ingredients. By removing one essential part of the milk, that is, fat, the milk protein can no longer be digested completely, hence there will be a 'leftover' of undigested and irritating proteins that the body's immune system begins to combat and get rid of.

In my practice I have found that persons who are of Vata constitution seem to digest and metabolize milk much better than Kapha types, provided it is fresh, whole fat, and boiled before consumption (Pasteurizing of milk differs from boiling it in that is uses an extremely high temperature, namely, 285 degrees F (141 degrees C). Vata types often suffer from dryness, lightness and coldness. The mucus-producing effect of milk may help lubricate their intestinal lining, which has the tendency to be dry. The milk's heavy and warming qualities may pacify Vata and thereby outweigh some negative effects that milk may have for other body types. Healthy Vata types and, to a certain extent, healthy Pitta types seem to produce more of the specific digestive enzymes, which are used to break down milk proteins, than Kapha types.

In Kapha types, milk protein remains undigested and can trigger allergic reactions with intense mucus irritation and sinus congestion. The Kapha's blood vessel walls tend to clog up quickly with excessive proteins as a result of overeating dairy foods or meat. This may explain why this particular body type is more prone to obesity and congestive heart failure than the Vata type.

Once milk is pasteurized, i.e. ultra heat-treated, its natural enzyme population is destroyed. Yet the enzymes are needed to make the milk nutrients available to the body cells. Newly born calves die within six months when fed with pasteurized cow's milk. One can only imagine the turmoil that must be going on in the tiny intestinal tract of a baby who is fed with pasteurized milk or sterilized milk formula. As mentioned before, such babies usually develop colic, become bloated and chubby, discharge mucus, catch colds frequently, are restless, and cry a lot. The best advise is to breastfeed as long as is possible, avoid dairy-based formulas altogether, use alternatives such as coconut milk (the closest to human milk) as well as some almond milk, hemp milk or rice milk; and give freshly mashed fruits, vegetables and rice when the baby is ready to eat solids.

Boiling fresh, non-pasteurized milk before consumption seems to have a beneficial effect. Milk protein begins to break down into amino acids during boiling, which makes it easier to digest and absorb. This may be one of the reasons why Indians always boil their milk before use. They also know that milk has adverse effects when its fat is removed. For some reason, milk protein, unlike egg or meat protein doesn't coagulate when heated. In addition, many of the milk's enzymes survive. To preserve milk and to kill any existing germs Indians simply put a silver coin or a silver spoon in the milk. Silver is strongly anti-bacterial. And to avoid mucus congestion, they put 2-3 pinches of either turmeric or dry ginger into the milk before boiling it. Whereas boiling the milk helps to reduce some its irritating effect in Vata and Pitta types, pasteurizing it upsets all the three *doshas*. Kapha types don't do well with milk at all; they develop mucus congestion almost right away.

Cold milk is very difficult to digest. As the cold milk touches the warm stomach lining, the nerve endings of the stomach become "numb" or insensitive, and its cells tighten or shrink. This inhibits the secretion of gastric juices, which is required to digest milk protein. The cold condition of the milk may even be responsible for leaving those proteins undigested that are known to cause allergic reactions. Enzymes require a specific temperature to be able act on the food; if the temperature is too low the proteins will be broken down properly, hence the intense irritation of the mucus lining. Vata types who are very sensitive to cold are rarely attracted to taking milk in cold form (from the refrigerator). Pittas often have an excessively high temperature in their stomach, which gets lowered only slightly by cold milk. Consequently Pittas are still able to secret a good amount of gastric juices to digest some of the milk proteins. But if they take milk cold on a regular basis, their AGNI or digestive power also begins to be affected.

If you have access to fresh, full-fat, and non-pasteurized milk and if you are a Vata or Pitta type with no Kapha imbalance (signs of excessive mucus in chest, nose or sinuses), you may use milk in moderation by applying the above procedures of preparation. If milk still causes you mucus, then it is simply a 'no-food' for you. I personally have not yet met a person who hasn't shown signs of congestion and irritation as a result of milk consumption, especially in the United States. In all the U.S. with the exception of California, Washington and Georgia, it is illegal to sell whole, raw milk, despite the fact that raw milk contains far less potentially harmful bacteria than pasteurized, homogenized milk. Pasteurized, homogenized milk does not qualify as food per se. The homogenization process breaks up an enzyme (xanthine oxidase), which in its altered (smaller) state can enter the bloodstream and react against arterial walls, causing the body to protect the area with a layer of cholesterol.

The demand for raw, non-pasteurized milk is booming. According to Sally Fallon, president for the Weston A. Price Foundation, the number of raw milk drinkers is now at about half a million people across the United States - many of them willingly breaking the law, purchasing their milk from 'underground black markets' and other creative setups. Raw milk comes with its own risks. Even if the cows grow up on organic farms, their milk bladders are constantly filled and extended, day after day, month after month, year after year. A continuous process of milk production (lactation) is unnatural for any animal. The resulting repeated injuries of the bladder wall leads to infections and inflammation, and a lot of dead cells (pus). Millions of units of pus are found in every quart of milk, especially in older cows. It is irrelevant whether the milk is raw or pasteurized; the dead cells remain in the milk. However, since bacteria are attracted to dead cells, and raw milk is not pasteurized, the latter is more susceptible to bacterial contamination.

In July 2007, the U.S. Department of Agriculture tested raw milk from 861 farms in 21 states. According to their report, nearly a quarter of the samples contained illness-causing bacteria, including five percent with listeria, three percent with salmonella, and four percent with less dangerous types of E. coli. Regardless of the real figures of contamination, either type of milk comes with its own risks. Again, if you are not sure about milk's health benefits for you, apply the muscle test and your body may give you some good clues about it. Or take a look at your tongue in the morning after consuming milk or cheese the day before. If it is coated white, you should avoid them. A white coating on the tongue indicates mucus aggravation in the gut, which in turn reflects turmoil in the digestive system. In my own case, eating lots of raw whole milk and cheese led to years of painful juvenile rheumatoid arthritis, constipation, lymphatic congestion, heart disease, anemia and a lot of gallstones in the liver and gallbladder. Soon after I quit eating foods derived from animals, my health returned to normal.

As in every respect, vegans appear to enjoy equal or better health
in comparison to both vegetarians and non-vegetarians.
~T. Colin Campbell, Ph.D. Professor of Nutrition, Cornell University

6. Aspartame and Other Sweet Killer Drugs

Aspartame is the sweetener in Diet Coke, Diet Pepsi and thousands of 'diet' foods. Donald Rumsfeld, who once was the CEO of a major drug company, managed to bring this poisonous food/drug to market during the Reagan administration. He used his political influence to quash an FDA toxicologist's report naming aspartame as a cause of not only cancer, but brain tumors as well. In 1996 the Food and Drug Administration published a list of 92 adverse aspartame reactions that included seizures, blindness, obesity; testicular, mammary and brain tumors; sex dysfunction, and death, acquired from 10,000 consumer complaints.

Through clever advertising campaigns the world population was made to believe that aspartame and all the other artificial sweeteners are just simple, harmless, food additives that give you the sweet taste, but help you keep slim, or even shed some extra pounds. However, the sweeteners are actually patented for 'appetite enhancement'. And these drugs really do what they promise - they make you crave carbohydrates, and thereby make you fat.

And now, the aspartame drug has even been patented to treat sickle cell anemia, one of the many diseases it is responsible for causing. Researcher Carl Manion found that a single dose of aspartame lowered the sickle cell count in the blood. Aspartame metabolizes into formic acid, a blister poison that transfers from cell to cell killing all them and leaving a blister of dead tissue.

Aspartame is a synergistic methanol poison. Methanol is known to cause serious birth defects and major developmental disorders such as autism and attention deficit in the offspring of aspartame users. Ever since the 1950s when Aspartame, MSG, and fluoride were being pushed into our youth, along with the harmful immunization programs, the IQ of the average high school graduate has fallen 10 percent.

Sweetness at a Price

Aspartame, Sucralose (in Splenda®) and *saccharin* are the most commonly used artificial sweeteners and have gained huge popularity among people who are concerned about their weight. In the belief that they are doing something good for themselves, they are thrilled to have found the 'ideal' sweetener that satisfies their sweet tooth yet doesn't make them fat. However, mounting evidence shows that artificial sweeteners are a major health risk, causing brain damage and other problems of the nervous system.

The use of artificial sweeteners in Britain alone has rocketed from a total of 615,000 tons in 1988 to 1,801,000 tons in 1993, an increase of 370 percent for *aspartame* and 250 percent for *saccharin* in five years. The situation is even worse in the United States. The sharp increase in the use of artificial sweeteners is very significant in relation to their sweetening potency. *Saccharin* is more than 400 times as sweet as regular sugar and *aspartame* 200 times as sweet, with Splenda® in between the two. The recently approved sweetener, *neotame*, appears to have super strength sweetness, hence it is named 'super aspartame'.

Considered non-toxic and safe by the British government, both *saccharin* and *aspartame* have found their way into the food chain. Both sweeteners are not only found in beverages but also in children's jellies, lollies and numerous other types of candies, puddings, as well as beans, and even tinned pasta. *Aspartame,* which is sold under the names NutraSweet®, Hermesetas, Gold Choice, and Canderel, has been included in some 14,000 foods in America and hundreds of products in Great Britain and other European countries. The products include fruit juices, diet soda, frozen lollies, a sugar substitute for tea or coffee, instant breakfasts, chewing gum, cocoa and other instant beverages, medical drugs, food supplements, and even yoghurt.

The British government has issued a call for clear warning labels (why warn people if it is so safe?), but only a few manufacturers have complied, claiming that it would 'clutter up' their labels and confuse consumers. Yet it is more confusing to the consumer to not know whether a food product contains *aspartame* or *saccharin* than to know it.

A survey conducted by BBC2's *Money Program* revealed that up to 40 percent of the public do not expect to find artificial sweeteners in their fruit juices and drinks, not to mention in their foods. But there is hardly any drink on the market that does not contain an artificial sweetener, even if the drink is labeled 'sugar free'. The most popular brands give the impression that they are totally natural whereas in truth they contain synthetically derived sweeteners. The European Union has urged producers to label these beverages 'with sweetener', but surveys have shown that up to 50 percent of consumers would then no longer buy these products.

The same applies to sucralose, the sweetener behind Splenda®. Disguised by its lovely sweet taste, it is yet another Frankenstein food additive of the industry. It is produced by chlorinating sugar molecules. Chlorinated molecules actually accumulate in body fat and can come back to haunt a body many, many years later. Splenda is synthetic and, having a chlorinated base like DDT, it can cause autoimmune disease (the body's natural reaction to attack and neutralize such poisons). Sucralose or Splenda is not safe. In the original research Splenda was shown to cause many health problems.

Sucralose as used in Splenda is not yet approved for use in most European countries, where it is still under review. Few human studies of safety have been published on sucralose. One small study of diabetic patients using the sweetener showed a statistically significant increase in glycosylated hemoglobin (HgbA1c), which is a marker of long-term blood glucose levels. According to the FDA, increases in glycosylation in hemoglobin reduces control of diabetes.

Research with animals has shown that sucralose can cause many problems in rats, mice, and rabbits, such as:

- Shrunken thymus glands (up to 40 percent shrinkage)
- Enlarged liver and kidneys.
- Atrophy of lymph follicles in the spleen and thymus
- Increased cecal weight
- Reduced growth rate
- Decreased red blood cell count
- Hyperplasia of the pelvis
- Extension of the pregnancy period
- Aborted pregnancy
- Decreased fetal body weight and placental weight
- Diarrhea

Many European countries have discontinued the use of artificial sweeteners for good reason. Tests on animals have revealed that *saccharin* can cause cancer of the bladder. And a recent study on aspartame conducted by the Ramazzini Foundation shows that aspartame causes a dose-dependent increase in all sorts of cancers (lymphomas, leukemias and breast cancers) when consumed at levels comparable to those ingested by humans in diet soft drinks. The study was published in the peer-reviewed journal *Environmental Health Perspectives* (EHP), the most widely-read environmental science journal in the world. It confirms the results of a previous study by the Ramazzini Foundation documenting the cancer-causing effects of aspartame in animals.

The European Food Commission is particularly concerned about the overconsumption of sweeteners by children. In the mid 1990s, the British government announced that 2.5 mg/kg of body weight was the acceptable (safe) daily intake (ADI) of *saccharin*. Today, the average person consumes about 14 mg/kg of body weight per day. Diabetics consume even of it. Since not every person uses saccharin or eats foods that contain it, many people must therefore be consuming as much as 20 mg/kg/day or more. Through repeated intake of the sweeteners, many children and adults 'expect' that a variety of foods and drinks taste very sweet, a characteristic most of them never have in their natural form. The masking of the natural taste of these products has consequences - there is a price to be paid for falling into the 'sweet' trap.

Check out the ingredients in artificial sweeteners nowadays. NutraSweet®, for example, contains Formaldehyde, L-Phenylalanine, Acetaldehyde, Benzaldhyde, Methane, Dimethoxy, Propanone, Ethane, Propane, Benezene, Paraformaldehyde, L-Phenylalanine, L-Aspartic acid, Oxazolidinecarboxylic acid, and many more deadly chemicals. Even if you don't know any of these poisons, the next time you eat or drink anything that contains neotame, aspartame or sucralose, remember that there is nothing natural about them at all. None of these chemicals are suitable for human consumption. Formaldehyde alone is a powerful cancer-causing agent.

Politics versus Ethics

Fortunately, a resistance movement is growing to prevent further damage from these harmful products. On April 6th, 2004, lawsuits were filed in three separate California courts against twelve companies that either produce or use the artificial sweetener aspartame as a sugar substitute in their products. The suits were filed in Shasta, Sonoma and Butte Counties in California. The suits allege that the food companies committed fraud and breach of warranty by marketing products to the public such as Diet Coke, Diet Pepsi, sugar-free gum, Flintstone's vitamins, yogurt and children's aspirin with the full knowledge that aspartame, the sweetener in them, is neurotoxic. Although such lawsuits can last many years, they bring an increased awareness about the fraudulent practices of the pharma-medical and food industries to the unsuspecting population.

Aspartame is a drug masquerading as an additive. It interacts with other drugs, has a synergistic and additive effect with MSG, and is a chemical hyper-sensitization agent. As far back as 1970, studies on aspartic acid, which makes up 40 percent of aspartame, showed that it caused lesions in the brains of mice. It was also shown to lead to behavioral and psychiatric problems triggered by aspartame-caused depletion of serotonin.

Aspartame consumption can cause headache, memory loss, obesity; testicular, mammary and brain tumors; seizures, vision loss, coma and cancer. It worsens or mimics the symptoms of such diseases and conditions as Fibromyalgia, MS, lupus, ADD, diabetes, Alzheimer's, chronic fatigue and depression.

The effects of aspartame are documented by the FDA's own data. In 1995 the agency was forced, under the Freedom of Information Act, to release a list of ninety-two aspartame symptoms reported by thousands of victims. In 1996 the FDA stopped taking complaints and now denies the existence of the report. On Sept 30, 1980 the Board of Inquiry of the FDA concurred and denied the petition for approval of aspartame as a food additive. In 1981, the newly appointed FDA Commissioner, Arthur Hull Hayes, ignored the negative ruling and approved aspartame for dry goods. As recorded in the Congressional Record of 1985, then CEO of Searle Laboratories Donald Rumsfeld said that he would call in his markers to get aspartame approved. Rumsfeld was on President Reagan's transition team and, a day after taking office, Reagan appointed Hayes. No FDA Commissioner in the previous sixteen years had allowed aspartame on the market.

In 1983, aspartame was approved for use in carbonated beverages. Today it is found in over 5,000 foods, drinks and medicines.

Why Sweeteners Make You Fat

A major American controlled study on 80,000 women showed that those who regularly use artificial sweeteners put on more weight per year than those who do not use them. What is even more surprising is the finding that, with the widespread use of sweeteners, the consumption of ordinary sugar and sugary foods has increased, too. In other words, the more artificial sweeteners you consume, the more food urges you have, thereby fulfilling their patent as an 'appetite enhancement'.

There is overwhelming proof that these food poisons are making us fat. Research conducted at Purdue University shows that a group of test subjects fed artificial sweeteners subsequently consumed three times the calories of those given regular sugar. According to the study, it is far less fattening to eat sugar than artificial sweeteners, although eating this much regular sugar isn't good for anyone either.

Most mainstream doctors recommend that their overweight patients consume diet soda, Sweet-N-Low, etc. for weight loss, but in actual fact their advice causes the patients to crave calories and binge on unhealthy carbohydrates. The obesity epidemic is spreading like wildfire ever since diet foods and beverages gained popularity. The following explanation resolves this mystery.

The body has a self-regulating mechanism, a kind of thermostat that measures the amount of energy (or calories) it can obtain from a particular meal. When your body has received enough energy from the food you have eaten, then your mouth, stomach, intestines, and liver send messages to the brain that all energy requirements have been met. Subsequently, your nervous system secretes hormones that stop your desire for more food. This point of saturation is essential for your wellbeing, for without it you would continuously want to eat and never feel satisfied. If, for instance, during one particular meal, you eat foods that contain only very little energy or at least not enough to fulfill your energy requirements, then your body will tempt you to eat more during the next meal. This way, the body makes up for the loss of energy during the previous meal. The same happens when your AGNI or digestive power is low and you are not deriving sufficient energy from the food you eat

On the other hand, when you eat food during one meal that has a higher content of calories than your body really requires at this moment, it will signal for less energy during the next meal. Your body will strive to keep your individual 'set point' or energy distribution point as balanced and normal as possible. Whenever you deprive yourself of eating enough and are unable to meet the energy needs of your body, you will look for more food the next day, the day after, and so on. This leads to chronic overeating which packs plenty of low-energy food into your intestinal tract. Since your body is incapable of digesting and absorbing low-energy food properly, it turns this food into fat and waste, and clogs up your lymphatic, digestive, and circulatory systems.

This is the time when your body signals 'famine'. You start craving foods, particularly refined carbohydrates such as ordinary sugar, chocolate, sweet beverages, coffee, etc. which all give you an instant boost of energy. But they also contain only 'empty' energy and just raise the sugar level in your blood for a short time. After a little while the sugar levels drops below normal, which may cause depression, moodiness, and exhaustion.

If you are overweight and believe that you can reduce weight by restricting your daily intake of calories, you will be very disappointed. Within a few days, your body will run out of energy and want to eat, hence the increased appetite or craving. If you still don't eat enough, you will fall into a depression, which may cause you to binge on food ravenously. Your body thinks that periodic famines are going on and tries to convert some of the food into fat deposits to prepare for the next one. After each 'voluntary famine' or 'weight reducing' diet, your body will put on weight much faster than it did before. This is known as the yo-yo effect.

Under normal circumstances, the body converts calories into heat, which then simply evaporates. Well-circulated brown fat tissue, which is located near the large arteries and in the underarms, is the main source of this energy. New research suggests that in some obese people this mechanism may be disturbed and that the best dietary rules would be of no avail. Abusing the body's digestive system through frequent strict dieting may be the main cause of this problem.

Because artificial sweeteners are low-energy foods and non-physiological, the body deals with them in the same way as described above. It recognizes their complete absence of potential energy and signals 'low energy'. As a result, it stimulates the desire for more food. This principle is a well-known and commonly applied practice, both in the food industry and in animal feeding. Animal feeds contain highly concentrated *saccharin* to stimulate the animal's appetite so that they eat more frequently and grow fat faster. The same mechanism applies to the human body, including children.

Children eating diet foods in lieu of the full-calorie versions may lead to overeating and obesity when they grow up, according to a 2007 report from the University of Alberta, Canada. Lead researcher Professor David Pierce stated: "Based on what we've learned, it is better for children to eat healthy, well-balanced diets with sufficient calories for their daily activities rather than low-calorie snacks or meals."

Deceiving the Body

For both humans and animals, *aspartame, sucralose, saccharin and other sweeteners* belong to the category of 'sweet' food. The sweetness of natural foods is caused by sugar. Because sugar can move straight through the stomach walls, it will appear in the bloodstream within 3-5 minutes. However, the body has to keep the blood sugar level in check since too little or too much sugar can be dangerous. The body regulates sugar levels automatically through simple reflex mechanisms. When sugar touches the taste buds for the sweet taste on the tongue, the pancreas is given the instruction to secrete *insulin*, which is required to make it (the sugar) available to the cells.

If you eat artificial sweeteners, the body naturally responds to their sweet taste by secreting *insulin*. Rather than receiving sugar in the blood as expected, however, it receives a combination of protein compounds. Doing its normal job, the pancreas has already prepared a portion of *insulin* that now floats about in the bloodstream searching for the expected sugar. Since it isn't found there, the insulin removes some of the blood sugar instead. This effectively lowers your sugar levels. However, since this situation can be life endangering, your body quickly signals 'hunger' which becomes a sudden, strong 'craving'. Since foods with artificial sweeteners are not able to meet the demand for an increase in blood sugar, you begin to look for sugary foods.

Instead of saving the calories that are contained in ordinary sugar, you have artificially increased your need and appetite for more sweet food. If you try to satisfy this desire by eating more foods containing artificial sweeteners (without calories), the urge to eat will become even stronger than before and you will start *overeating*. Researchers have found that the urge to eat more food after ingesting artificial sweeteners in a drink can last up to 90 minutes, even when all blood tests show normal values.

A more serious situation arises when the body is given artificial sweeteners on an ongoing basis. Since the sweeteners repeatedly stimulate the taste buds responsible for detecting sugar, the brain maintains an almost continuous urge to eat. At the same time, the liver is instructed by the brain to store sugar supplies rather than to release them, which causes chronic fatigue. The pancreas, which had wrongly assumed that real sugar was entering the bloodstream, eventually realizes that it has been cheated. Hence it reduces its secretion of *insulin*. One might think that this solves the problem but the body reacts with depression.

Sweeteners Cause Obesity, Depression, Brain Damage

Sugar is known to 'improve' moods for relatively short periods of time. With the help of *insulin*, sugar increases the secretion of *serotonin* in the brain. *Serotonin* is the neurotransmitter of happiness. If *insulin* secretion fails to occur, happiness remains low. The only way to get out of this situation, it seems, is to eat sugar so that the body can secrete *insulin* again.

You may believe that the fewer calories you eat, the more weight you will lose. But food manufactures know that the more artificially sweetened foods and beverages you consume, the more you will want their normal sugar-containing foods and beverages as well. Diet foods and diet beverages have not only contributed to a massive increase in sugar consumption and obesity but also led to an epidemic of depression. I have seen numerous depressed people over the years, a large percentage of whom regularly used artificial sweeteners. By cutting out diet foods and 'light' products, they have returned to their normal moods, *and* they have lost excess weight, too.

Apart from causing obesity and depression, sweeteners have been linked to insomnia, headaches, giddiness, loss of memory, nausea, pre-menstrual syndrome, panic attacks, epileptic fits, and even overstimulation of breast glands leading to breast cancer. *Aspartame* in particular may cause extensive damage to the central nervous system. Once it has entered the intestinal tract, *aspartame* is converted into two highly excitatory neurotransmitter amino acids, *aspartic acid* and *phenylalinine*, as well as into *methyl alcohol* (wood-grain alcohol) and *formaldehyde (embalming fluid)*.

Wood alcohol is one of the most dangerous substances that result from eating artificial sweeteners. It may directly enter the bloodstream and move through the brain barrier into the central nervous system where it can influence the neurotransmitters, alter brain function, and cause brain damage. Wood alcohol can cause blindness and formaldehyde can cause cancer. In some cases *aspartame* may suppress appetite and 'kill' AGNI, the digestive fire, altogether. Both can lead to quick, excessive weight gain. According to *Consumer Reports*, aspartame has a shelf life of between two and three months. After that it begins to break down and pose an increasing danger to the consumer. The same occurs when aspartame or an aspartame-containing food is heated.

Aspartame accounts for more than 75 percent of the total adverse reactions to food reported to the U.S. Federal Drug Administration. Hundreds of airline pilots have reported symptoms of memory loss and confusion, headaches, seizures, visual disturbances and gastrointestinal reactions as a result of consuming sweeteners. If pregnant women consume large quantities of diet sodas to avoid weight gain, their placenta may accumulate methyl alcohol, causing mental retardation in the fetus. They also risk maternal malnutrition because of the gastrointestinal problems and diarrhea associated with sweeteners.

Other sweeteners besides aspartame have similar effects. Added to soft drinks, they are now even linked with testicular damage and other key areas of the body. Stimulating the brain of a child with these 'pleasure-enhancing' chemicals in beverages will, in some cases, program their senses to look for and use stronger addictive substances such as hard drugs or large amounts of alcohol later in life. The latest sweetener, *acesulfame K*, may also be carcinogenic, i.e. cause cancer, according a report published in the *British Medical Journal* in 1996. To avoid serious health problems, it is best to stick to foods and beverages that come from purely natural sources.

A sugar called *tagatose* is one of the next sweeteners that will be appearing on products labeled under the pseudo-hygienic appellations of 'Light', 'Lite', 'Low Calorie', 'Sugar Free', 'Sugarless', 'Low Fat', or 'Low Sodium' etc. Hyperuricemia is an unhealthy and unacceptable result from ingesting tagatose. Some researchers believe hyperuricemia is a risk factor for ischemic heart disease, and it has been associated with lipid abnormalities, hypertension, stroke, and preeclampsia. It is an especially hazardous effect with regards to diabetes because hyperuricemia is damaging to the pancreas as well as possibly causing major harm to other organs and systems in the body. Having too much uric acid in the blood predisposes you to developing gout, a painful joint condition. If you wish to protect yourself and your family from the dreadful consequences of universal deceit and actually benefit from the foods you eat, start with fruit, vegetables, grains, nuts, seeds, and legumes. And be sure to prepare your foods from scratch.

7. Light Food - A Weight Booster

'Foolproof' Slimming Diets

Most dietary approaches in the past were based on the simple mathematical concept that, because 1 kg of body fat contains 7,000 calories, taking in 1,000 calories less each day would cause a person to lose 1 kg of body fat a week. Since this equation sounded so logical and convincing, many people tried to shed the undesirable weight by controlling their daily intake of calories. However, this theory is erroneous. Actually, the more people reduced their calorie intake, the faster they put on weight.

When you analyze the results of all the prominent slimming techniques and dietary plans, you face the following facts. Most people who go on a diet give up before completing it. Of those who continue, only a few lose weight and most of those people put the weight back on again. The biggest craze on the slimming market concerns the consumption of 'light' food. As the name suggests, the new products promise to make you lighter. You can eat as much as you like and will not put on weight because the products contain few or no fattening substances at all. With these, you supposedly don't have to restrict yourself or curb your appetite any longer, and at the same time you become slim.

For these or similar reasons 'light food' has become extremely popular in the industrialized nations. At last, food manufacturers have complied with the demands made by nutritional scientists and dieticians to produce foods with fewer calories. Consumers feel relieved that the new food is fat-free and without sugar, and instead contains fat substitutes, water and artificial sweeteners. This saves massive amounts of calories. And by adding artificial flavors to the food and using other forms of chemical manipulation, the taste buds believe that it is the real thing. Man seems to have finally succeeded in creating the ideal food for man; at least this is what the majority of consumers have started to believe.

However, the theory that eating low fat or fat-free food is healthy turned out to be one big fat lie. An eight-year study of 48,835 women published in February 2006 by the *Journal of the American Medical Association* found that the study participants failed to lose a measurable amount of weight on the low-fat diet. To the contrary, most of them remained overweight which put them at an even greater risk for cardiovascular disease despite following their low-fat regimen. In addition, the study showed that low-fat diets had zero health benefits in regard to avoiding the risk of getting cancer and heart disease. The study cost the American taxpayers $415 million, but this money seems to have been wasted. The mass media, medical industry and food manufacturers have not taken much notice of this important finding. In the meanwhile, the low-fat hysteria continues to escalate.

"Light Fats" and their "Amazing" Effects

Take for instance 'light-butter' or half-fat butter, which has been heralded as one of the greatest 'achievements' of food technology so far. In this high-tech product, at least half of the fat content of butter is replaced with water. It tastes like butter, it spreads like butter and it melts like butter in the mouth, but in reality it is mostly water. To turn water into butter, you have to mix it with a thickening agent like gelatin, an emulsifier that permits mixing fat with water, and then add artificial coloring, aromas, and preservatives. It is difficult, though, for a layperson to detect from the labels whether a product has been manipulated in this way. Still there is one way to find out. Place the light butter or light margarine in your frying pan and see what happens. The artificial fats quickly disintegrate and turn into what they really are - mostly water.

However, not all food imitations can be enriched with water. Fat-free salad dressings contain modified starch as a fat substitute. Principally being very dry by nature, starch (mostly cornstarch) is treated with hydrochloric acid and enzymes derived from mold. The end product leaves you with the feeling of cream in the mouth. The same can be achieved by using cheap protein and other carbohydrates. The products have fancy names such as 'Trailblazer' and Nutrifat PC and have already been on the U.S. market for several years.

'*Olestra*' is the name of a pseudo-fat that has been approved for sale on the U.S. market to fill the gap for zero-cholesterol fat. The pseudo-fat mimics the properties of ordinary fats, with a similar 'mouth-feel' and taste. Fat-free chips, diet-friendly crisps, and cholesterol-lowering tortillas can now be staples in the otherwise fatty American diet. It seems wonderful to be able to have all these 'naughty' foods and not become fat or risk heart disease. The only problem with this non-physiological food is its side effects.

The pseudo-fat can actually cause substantial anal leakage and diarrhea. It is as indigestible as plastic, which means it comes out completely unaltered. To prevent the product from becoming unpopular, the manufacturers have now added an 'anti-anal leakage agent', a mixture that slows the elimination of the oil from the large intestine.

One of the more serious side effects of such products is that they are capable of removing the fat-soluble vitamins A, D, E, and K from the body as they pass through the intestinal tract. For this reason, U.S. food manufacturers are required to fortify their olestra-containing products with all these vitamins; this gives the false impression that these foods are now safe for human consumption. But uncontrolled intake of vitamin K can endanger the lives of hemophiliacs; and a pregnant mother may risk her baby's life by taking too much vitamin A. Apart from removing vitamins from the body (and thoroughly confusing the body), olestra also reduces the absorption of *carotenoids* that help us to prevent cancer, heart disease and stroke. Pseudo-fats cannot fool even animals. When the fat replacement olestra was fed to dogs for 20 months, their weight did not decrease but actually increased.

Olestra is the first food additive with negative nutritional value. It is hard to conceive how much damage this 'plastic' food will cause if it remains in our food chain for several decades and, what makes things worse, it will be extremely difficult to trace any health damage to the use of olestra. It is very unlikely that there will be any further research done on the side effects of olestra or similar foods. Hence it is up to each one of us to take more responsibility for our health and that of our families. If we desist from buying such synthetic foods, they will disappear from the market as fast as they appeared.

Beware of the latest diet drug *Orlistat*, marketed under the name *Alli* and sanctioned by the FDA. This new wonder drug is actually a lower-dosage version of the old prescription drug *Xenical*, which has never shown to have any effects on fat reduction. Alli is the first drug of its kind sold without a prescription, and it is selling like hotcakes. But instead of enjoying a real hotcake, you may experience extremely unpleasant and embarrassing side effects, including gas with oily spotting, loose stools and abdominal pain. The drug's official website states that if you take the drug, "I''s probably a smart idea to wear dark pants, and bring a change of clothes with you to work."

The manufacturer, GlaxoSmithKline, has predicted that 5 million to 6 million Americans a year will buy the drug, which may be true, given the 70 million Americans who resolve to lose weight by going on a diet program. The drug blocks the absorption of about 25 percent of consumed fat. That would eliminate about 225 calories from a 3,000 calorie per day diet, in exchange for loose stools and gas with an oily discharge.

The combined sales of all the diet products advertised and sold by the weight-loss industry earns $58 billion a year from consumers desperately searching for a solution to their weight challenges. In order to lower weight, Olistat is designed to block the absorption of dietary fat. Since this interferes with the absorption of vital fat-soluble vitamins A, D, E, K and beta carotene, users are instructed to take a daily multivitamin. Alli's official website, MyAlli.com, admits that weight loss cannot be achieved with Orlistat alone, stressing the importance of a good balanced diet and regular exercise - the typical disclaimer found on any weight loss product that doesn't work.

High Protein Foods Make You Fat and Low Energy Foods Deplete Energy

Not such good news for the Atkins diet friends. The results of a four-nation study involving more than 4,000 men and women ages 40 to 59 produced a stunning conclusion in our Atkins diet-fueled society: the thinnest people on Earth eat the most carbohydrates. What is even more alarming, the people who ate the most protein in their diet were actually the heaviest.

"Without exception, a high-complex-carbohydrate, high-vegetable-protein diet is associated with low body mass," study leader Linda Van Horn of Northwestern University said in a news conference reported by Reuters. "High-protein diets were associated with higher body weight."

Of course, this does not mean that your favorite doughnut, French fries, pasta and white bread are going to make you slim. These refined carbohydrates don't offer you the complex sugars that your body needs as a primary source of energy. Only complex carbohydrates found in grains, fruits, vegetables, nuts, seeds and beans are suitable to fill the body's energy requirements. Most notable is this finding: the more animal protein a person consumed, the higher his weight was.

Why Light Foods Make You Feel So Heavy

Many people wonder why they have put on so much weight since consuming light foods. Or, they may ask, why don't light foods seem to contribute to slimming? The answers to this question are quite simple. Low-energy foods deplete your energy and, thereby, slow down your metabolism, making it more and more difficult to metabolize even the light foods and lose any extra weight. In addition, after eating light foods a couple of times, your body begins to realize that it is deprived of energy. Consequently, it sends you urgent messages to consume energy-containing foods. Since carbohydrates are the foods that keep your serotonin and beta-endorphin levels normal, not eating them makes you cranky, restless and moody. To overcome the discomfort, you eat more of these same low-energy foods than you normally would. Much of it, though, gets converted into fat and waste matter. This natural response occurs in everyone, even in children.

Children are generally more in touch with their natural instincts and have not yet been influenced by theories about diets, calories, and light foods. When researchers tested the eating habits of children, they wanted to find out whether children extract fewer calories from their food and lose weight if they consume light products. The scientists were surprised to discover that those children whose diet included light foods (low calorie) had actually *increased* their appetites and started eating more to balance the loss of energy caused by the light foods.

The body is constantly aware of how much energy is required to conduct all its activities and subsequently sends the appropriate signals of how much we should eat in order to satisfy its needs. The requirements, of course, change as the day goes on. A theoretical system of how much you should eat at each meal and how many calories you can use up without becoming fat is therefore useless, if not harmful. It strongly interferes with the body's natural and uniquely programmed weight control mechanisms. The accompanied anxiety of eating too much or eating the wrong type of food may even shut down the digestive functions, which means you are converting much of the ingested food into undigested toxic waste. This clogs up the system even more and adds extra weight to the body.

The body always knows when it has reached a point of satiety. This was shown in another experiment during which a group of children were given the permission to eat as much as they wanted and whatever they wanted for six consecutive days. They were even allowed sweets, cakes, and other kinds of 'unhealthy' foods. Parents were not permitted to influence their children in any way.

The researchers carefully recorded what and how much of each food a child ate during each meal, throughout the six 24-hour periods. Some children ate only minute amounts during some meals but then greatly increased the amounts at other meal(s). The children's calorie intake fluctuated substantially from meal to meal; yet, when calculated for an entire day, calorie consumption remained the same.

Gaining 'Waste-weight'

Many studies show that light foods encourage appetite and overeating and do **not** reduce weight. The more enzymatic energy contained in food, the faster we feel satisfied. But not only light foods are energy depleted and dissatisfying. Refined, processed, chemically treated foods contain no *Prana* or life energy, which is the type of energy the body needs to help digest food.

There may be plenty of calories in the highly refined white flour products but the body is not able use this form of 'dead' energy. Our digestive system is naturally programmed to extract energy from *live foods* or complex staple foods, which contain plenty of *Prana*. The body regards such lifeless foods as meat, cornflakes or light foods to be indigestible and tries to 'dump' them as quickly as possible. All they do is to congest the intestines where they ferment and putrefy. This is the first location in the body where waste, meaning extra weight, starts to accumulate and, when the intestinal 'vessel' is full, it begins distributing the waste to other areas of the body as well.

This increase of waste-weight may tempt you to go on a restrictive diet for a while. But the more often you go on a diet, the less successful it becomes. Each new diet requires a different type of metabolism. The continual abuse of your natural weight regulation reduces AGNI, the digestive fire, to a point when almost no foods, even fresh, healthy foods, can be tolerated and utilized by the body. At such a stage, obese people complain that they are putting on weight although they are hardly eating anything.

The producers of light foods know all that. Since light foods have become available in the supermarkets, the sales of normal foods have increased too. If light food had the effect of curbing appetites and reducing the consumption of ordinary foods, you can take it for granted that light products would have never made it into the food market. These man-made foods have certainly not been made available to create a healthier population.

The Calorie-plan Fiasco

What is most discouraging in the confusion around food today is that our generation is perhaps the first one in the entire history of mankind to lose its natural instinct to know which foods are good for us and which ones are not. We have left it to experts or nutritional scientists to make certain that we are being nourished in the best possible way. Food is no longer considered to be God's gift to man but a mere collection of chemical components, including calories or joules, vitamins, fats, proteins and their various amino acid components, carbohydrates, trace elements, etc. If the figures of nutritional daily requirements were correct, no one in the world could ever be healthy because everyone would miss out on one vitamin, mineral, trace element, or the other. For example, we would have to eat massive amounts of liver and herring, to avoid vitamin D deficiency. Yet those who have never eaten fish or liver in their entire lives have no less vitamin D in their bodies than those who eat it regularly.

Actually, the official figures for nutritional requirements are unreliable and misleading. In a major study at the University Hospital in Vienna, researchers first calculated the nutritional values of the patients' diet according to the official nutritional figures and then analyzed the same food items in the laboratory for their true nutritional contents. The experiment lasted for 38 days and the results were astounding. The calculated figures for calories were 1/3 higher than were actually found through chemical analysis. The difference with regard to carbohydrates was 44 percent, with regard to protein 50 percent, and with regard to fats 60 percent! The conclusion of the study was that no process reliably shows what is contained in food. Besides, foods such as tomatoes, potatoes, fruits, and vegetables change their nutritional contents according to seasons, preparation, and storage and have different constituents in different countries due to varied climatic, soil, and geographical conditions.

In addition, the information that indigestible fiber contained in whole foods doesn't release calories is incorrect. It is true that *our body* has no enzymes to digest fiber but we have plenty of *bacteria* in our intestinal tract that can do this job even better than enzymes do. All fiber reaches the colon in undigested form. Just as the bacteria in nature easily break down food fiber, so do the bacteria of the intestinal flora digest the fiber that passes through the intestines. This may result in undesirable gases caused by fermentation and release various fatty acids that are absorbed by the large intestines to serve as a source of energy, which means they provide calories. Pectin, for example, is a fiber found in apples and can provide 283 calories per 100 g, as much as in a 100 g of ice cream!

The dilemma that arises from eating according to a calorie plan is that nobody can tell you for sure how many calories are locked in a particular food, nor is it known how many calories are being utilized by each individual. A Kapha type, for instance, has a slow metabolic rate and uses up less energy than a Vata type who has a very fast metabolic rate. Vatas may eat three times as many calories and still put on no extra weight whereas Kaphas may just 'look' at food and put on weight. If a healthy Pitta type eats excess amounts of calories, let's assume 2,000 instead of the recommended 1,000, he simply converts the unused calories into heat and becomes slightly more 'energetic' than before. His body weight will remain unchanged, unless he overeats regularly. Research has documented that the average overweight person does not consume more calories than a slim person does.

If excessive consumption of calories always led to weight gain, then most people in the world would be obese by now. According to the calorie theory, a person who eats two extra pieces of chocolate a day (50 calories) should put on 25kg of body fat within a period of ten years. Imagine how this person would look if he ate that much chocolate for sixty years, according to the theory.

Fortunately, the body is not a machine that counts calories. A strong digestive fire (AGNI) can make use of more calories than a weak one. If AGNI is weak, then most calories are not used which means that plenty of unused and undigested food is left. Consequently, the energy requirements of the body are no longer met. This lowers the metabolic rate and general circulation, and the resulting accumulation of toxic waste congests vital areas of tissues and organs in the body. The lymphatic system becomes severely blocked and retains large amounts of lymph, hence the swelling that accompanies weight gain.

Weight Regulation is Natural

Weight loss occurs spontaneously when the natural weight regulation mechanisms are restored. Excessive body weight is a symptom of disturbed digestion and metabolism. In addition, it is a sign of chronic toxicity in the body. Trying to remove the symptom (excessive weight) can turn out to be very harmful and disappointing if the accumulated toxins are not removed first.

The body has a natural resistance to losing excessive weight quickly because sudden weight loss could release a flood of trapped toxins into the circulation and even have fatal side effects (collapse of liver functions, kidney failure, and heart attack). The body never behaves in an irrational way. Weight regulation has to begin by removing the root causes behind the metabolic problems responsible for weight gain.

Boston researchers discovered that people whose pancreas secretes high concentrations of insulin have more difficulties losing weight than those who produce smaller amounts of insulin. This, however, has very little to do with genes, as some doctors may tell you. The reason 200 million Americans are overweight or cannot shed excess weight is not because of genetic flaws. It is well known that overweight people secrete more insulin. However, over-secretion of insulin is an effect of weight gain, not its cause. The reason 200 million are overweight is because they have become insulin resistant (see chapter 11 about the causes of insulin resistance). When the insulin receptors of the cells block out insulin, blood sugar begins to rise. To deal with the increase in blood sugar, the pancreas makes more insulin to help remove it from the blood. One way to deal with this dangerous situation is to have the body convert the excessive amounts of sugar into fat. The more fat a person has accumulated, the less likely he is to move the body and exercise.

Insulin also inhibits the body's fat-burning hormone, 'hormone-sensitive lipase'. This hormone is responsible for releasing fat into your bloodstream to be used as fuel. Once this hormone is deactivated, the body can no longer burn fat for energy. Instead, it must use amino acids and complex sugars stored in the muscles as fuel. This in turn will make the person weak and excessively hungry (as in cravings), which creates an endless cycle of increased insulin secretion and fat generation. To escape this vicious cycle, one must keep the body's insulin secretions low. Low levels of insulin allow your body to produce large amounts of hormone-sensitive lipase, thus burning fat as needed. This keeps your weight naturally regulated. Processed, refined and otherwise manufactured foods all increase insulin levels, and thereby diminish the body's energy reserves. The following list includes other factors responsible for weight gain.

People who put on extra weight may have been weakened by the following factors:

- Junk food (now the typical American diet)
- Overworking
- Lack of exercise
- Overstimulation of senses
- Strenous lifestyle and exhaustion
- Sleep deprivation (especially the two hours of sleep before midnight) increases hunger
- Irregular eating habits
- Heavy evening meals and frequent snacking
- Overeating to compensate for intake of non-nutritious and low-energy foods
- Stimulants such as coffee, tea, and cigarettes
- Pesticides and other chemicals in foods change hormonal activity, which can boost body fat
- Air conditioning and heating prevent sweating and shivering, so we don't burn as many calories
- Antidepressants and diabetes drugs have weight gain as a potential side effect
- Most other medications cause weight gain; they tend to suppress digestive functions
- Soft drinks and sports drinks (high in fructose corn syrup and salt)
- Less than adequate amounts of water drunk each day
- Negative responses to stress
- Alcohol consumption
- Unresolved conflicts (impairing digestion)
- Fear and other emotional upsets
- Any other weakening influence.

Sleep Well - Lose Weight

By some estimates, Americans average about six hours of sleep per night. That may be enough for some, but not for the majority of people, especially for those concerned about their weight. According to a study from Columbia University, presented at the annual scientific meeting of the North American Association for the Study of Obesity (NAASO), people need to get a lot more than six hours of sleep each night to stay healthy and fit. Researchers used almost 10 years of data collected on nearly 18,000 subjects who took part in the National Health and Nutrition Examination Survey (NHANES). The study gathered information on general dietary and health habits. After accounting for other factors that are known to contribute to obesity, the Columbia team reported these estimates:

- Less than four hours of sleep per night increases obesity risk by 73 percent, compared to subjects who slept seven to nine hours each night
- An average of five hours of sleep per night increases obesity risk by 50 percent
- An average of six hours of sleep per night increases obesity risk by 23 percent

The researchers believe that the link between sleep deprivation and obesity is altered body chemistry. According to the research, a lack of sleep increases *grehlin*, a hormone that sends a hunger signal to the brain. The usual foods of choice are ready-to-eat carbohydrate snacks. At the same time, the level of a protein called *leptin* drops. Leptin helps suppress appetite, so when the level is low, appetite increases. This causes you to look for something to eat. Combine too much grehlin and too little leptin, and you've set the stage for the ingestion of extra food that your body neither needs nor can digest properly. The inevitable result is intestinal congestion and weight gain.

If you have children who are putting on more weight than is normal, the reason for that may be that they are not getting enough sleep. A recent study (November 2007) announced by major television networks showed that, for every extra hour of sleep a 3rd-grader gets, s/he has a 40 percent reduced risk of becoming obese by grade 6. Younger children seem to need at least nine hours of sleep, whereas teenagers actually need 10 to 12 hours of sleep to remain slim and healthy, according to the research.

On a different note, independent research published in November 2007 shows that lack of sleep also causes brain disorders.

Physical Cleansing

The body needs to be cleared of toxins before it can restore its natural weight. Cleansing it also ensures that weight loss takes place smoothly and without causing adverse effects. The most powerful and thorough of all the cleansing procedures described in this book is the *Liver and Gallbladder Flush*. Its most important effect is to restore AGNI, the digestive fire. When AGNI is stronger, food is digested more efficiently and less waste becomes deposited in the intestines. This, however, can happen only if you also clean out your colon through colonic irrigation or similar colon cleansing methods. A kidney cleanse ensures that any toxins released by the body don't get caught in the kidneys. The main principle here is that weight loss will take place naturally and without harm if the eliminative organs are first cleared of any accumulated waste deposits.

All this will effectively restore the body's health and natural weight. One liver cleanse, however, will not be sufficient to restore AGNI on a permanent basis. You need as many such cleanses as it takes to remove all the gallstones. After each cleanse, there may be an increase in energy, the abdomen may feel tighter, and you may lose several pounds. Yet within less than a week, some of the old sluggishness may return and previous food cravings may re-emerge. This shows that gallstones from the rear parts of the liver have traveled forward and clogged up the major bile ducts again, thereby reducing AGNI once more. By the time your liver is completely clean, your body weight should be ideal and your energy boundless, provided your diet and lifestyle are healthful and balanced, too.

A Healthy Body - Normal Weight

Only a healthy body can be of normal weight. Theories of how much each person should weigh (calculated according to gender, height, etc.) ignore each person's unique constitutional requirements. Healthy body weight varies according to individual body types. A healthy Vata type will always be very slim, and a healthy Kapha type will always be corpulent and muscular. The bones of Vatas are light and thinly built, whereas Kaphas have very heavy, dense and compact bones. Both body types have very different, if not completely contradictory, requirements regarding, food, exercise and living conditions. Pitta types, who have more heat in their body, have entirely dissimilar energy requirements to the other body types.

Weight loss for the right reasons, i.e. to improve your health, is easy. Trying to shed weight without removing the accumulated toxins first goes against the body's principles of survival and is therefore difficult to achieve. The body merely protects itself against acid death by keeping the toxins in a neutralized state inside fat cells and bodily fluids. Your health will improve automatically once you remove the toxic waste products and keep the eliminative organs and systems open and clean. The focus needs to be on moving toward good health, rather than on fighting ill health. Once you have learned the lessons of creating health, you can easily turn your body into a finely tuned instrument that helps you fulfill your desires and lead a life filled with happiness, vitality, abundance and wisdom.

8. MSG - The Obesity Factor

As a nation we are becoming increasingly dependent on processed foods, and each year the FDA approves more and more chemicals as additives in food production. While some of these chemicals increase shelf life of foods, others kill bacteria, improve taste, and replace fats and carbohydrates, enhance flavor and color of foods, and much more. Although adding chemicals to natural foods is not really necessary, it certainly increases profits many times. The unsuspecting consumer has no clue that some of the chemicals they ingest in their delicious meals are neurotoxic and/or carcinogenic (cancer-causing). One of the most dangerous poisons is *MSG* (processed free glutamic acid).

In a 1968 study conducted at Washington University Medical School, laboratory mice that were fed MSG subsequently developed retinal damage and became grotesquely obese. The mice had lesions in the hypothalamus of the brain - the part that is prominently involved with the functions of the autonomic nervous system and endocrine system. Hormonal imbalances often lead to obesity.

As of May 13, 2004 more than 150 studies confirmed this earlier piece of research. There are now more studies on the effects of MSG on the hypothalamus leading to obesity than on the effects of aspartic acid. During animal studies neuroscientists found that glutamic acid and aspartic acid (40 percent of aspartame) load on the same receptors in the brain, and cause identical brain lesions and neuro-endocrine disorders. The victims usually develop compulsive eating habits.

MSG can easily pass through the blood-brain barrier in newborns and young children. A fetus is almost completely unprotected against toxic compounds. Many diseases, aging, and overuse of medical drugs, regular ingestion of food additives, such as aspartame and MSG, can all damage the blood-brain barrier and the brain itself. Since most of the processed foods contain MSG, as do many personal care items, supplements and pharmaceuticals, it is almost impossible for an expectant mother to protect her baby from being affected.

Following birth, an infant is exposed to MSG and, possibly, aspartic acid through childhood vaccinations. All infant formulas contain some free glutamic acid and free aspartic acid. An infant on a hypoallergenic soy-based formula will ingest more excitotoxic amino acids (glutamic acid, aspartic acid, and L-cysteine) per day than is contained in any serving of food found on grocery store shelves.

MSG is most often added to common foods under names that give consumers no clue to its presence. (Refer to the list of other names following.) Both MSG and aspartame cause lesions in the hypothalamus, the portion of the brain that is recognized to affect weight. If you are concerned about your weight and that of your children, I suggest you start identifying the sources of MSG in your grocery shopping cart, before taking them home.

Dietary supplements, processed food used by vegetarians, and products labeled 'organic' are some of the industry's favorite places for hiding MSG. California proposes legislation to allow more crops to be sprayed with MSG. Like so many other live virus vaccines, the nasal spray flu vaccine called FluMist contains MSG in the form of monosodium glutamate. Monosodium glutamate is described as a '*mutagen* and *reproductive effector*' by the Centers for Disease Control in their *Registry of Toxic Effects of Chemical Substances*.

More and more personal care products that are labeled 'organic' actually contain free glutamic acid (MSG). Soon soaps, shampoos, and other body care products will have glutamate surfactants in them, as well as products that contain hydrolyzed proteins. Much of that MSG will enter your body through the skin.

The following is a list of some common names that MSG hides behind:

- Monosodium Glutamate
- Monopotassium Glutamate
- Hydrolyzed Protein
- Hydrolyzed Vegetable Protein (vegetable and animal)
- Plant Protein Extract
- Textured Protein
- Hydrolyzed Corn Gluten
- Yeast Extract
- Autolyzed Yeast
- Yeast Nutrient
- Yeast Food
- High Flavored Yeast
- Calcium Caseinate
- Sodium Caseinate
- Textured Soy Protein
- Malt Extract
- Malt Flavoring
- Bouillon
- Broth
- Stock
- Flavoring
- Natural Flavoring
- Seasoning
- Accent
- Textured Soy Protein
- Soybean Extract
- Hydrolyzed Oat Flour
- Glutamic Acid
- Gelatin (which includes Jell-O)

On a final note, the common myth as to whether 'bad genes' are responsible for obesity was dispelled by a group of scientists in New Zealand. In what is referred to as a breakthrough discovery, scientists from Auckland University's Liggins Institute discovered that genetic predisposition to obesity, which is caused by poor dietary habits of the mother, can be reversed through good nutrition in early childhood. If genes were responsible for causing obesity, it would not be possible to reverse it.

9. Microwave Oven - Death in the Heat

Did you ever wonder what microwaves can do to water, food and your body? Russian researchers have found decreased nutritional value, cancer-making compounds and brain-damaging radiolytics in virtually all microwave-prepared foods. Eating microwave-prepared meals can also cause loss of memory, concentration, emotional instability and a decline in intelligence, according to the research. The Russian scientists also found decreased nutritional value - or significant dimming of their 'vital energy field' - in up to 90 percent of all microwave-prepared foods.

In addition, the B complex, C and E vitamins linked with stress-reduction and the prevention of cancer and heart disease, as well as the essential trace minerals needed for optimum brain and body functioning, were all rendered useless by microwaves, even at short cooking durations. Microwave-cooked food is basically reduced to the nutritional equivalent of cardboard. If you don't want to develop nutrient deficiencies, you may be better off throwing this appliance out of your kitchen. The radiation has been found to accumulate in the kitchen furniture, becoming a constant source of radiation in itself.

Microwave usage in the preparation of food has been found to lead to lymphatic disorders and an inability to protect the body against certain cancers. The research found increased rates of cancer cell formation in the blood of people eating microwave-cooked meals. The Russians also reported increased rates of stomach and intestinal cancers, as well as digestive and excretive disorders, plus a higher percentage of cell tumors, including sarcoma.

Microwaves rip apart the molecular bonds that make food to be 'food'. Microwave ovens hurl high-frequency microwaves that boil the moisture within food and its packaging by whipsawing water molecules dizzyingly back-and-forth at more than a billion reversals per second. This frantic friction fractures food molecules, rearranging their chemical composition into weird new configurations unrecognizable as food by human bodies. By destroying the molecular structures of food, the body cannot help but turn the food into waste, but not harmless waste, rather, 'nuclear waste'.

Other side effects of microwaves than just making food useless and 'wasteful' include:

- High blood pressure
- Migraine
- Dizziness
- Stomach pain
- Anxiety
- Hair loss
- Appendicitis
- Cataracts
- Reproductive disorders
- Adrenal exhaustion
- Heart disease
- Memory loss
- Attention disorders
- Increased crankiness
- Depression,
- Disconnected thoughts
- Sleep disturbance
- Brain damage

Eating microwave-damaged foods can lead to a considerable stress response in the body, and thereby, alter the blood chemistry. While eating organic vegetables zapped by microwaves, you will send your cholesterol soaring. According to Swiss scientist Hertel. "Blood cholesterol levels are less influenced by cholesterol content of the food than by stress factors." The Russian government had banned microwave ovens for over 50 years, but they were recently introduced to the Russian market (for 'economic' reasons). Microwave ovens have taken over the cooking chores in nine out of ten American homes, and American and Chinese microwave manufacturers hope that the same will happen in Russia.

Reporting for the Forensic Research Document of AREC Research, William P. Kopp now states: "The effects of microwaved food byproducts are long-term, permanent within the human body. Minerals, vitamins, and nutrients of all microwaved food is reduced or altered so that the human body gets little or no benefit, or the human body absorbs altered compounds that cannot be broken down."

In a classical experiment 2,000 cats were given only food and water that were previously placed in the microwave oven, even for just one minute. The foods selected were the most nutritious and natural ones available. Within six weeks, all cats mysteriously died. While investigating the surprising result of the test, it was discovered that, although the cats looked well fed, the cells in their bodies virtually contained no trace of nutrient-components. The cats literally starved to death, despite all the nutritious foods. Microwaves turned their food into deadly poison. Seeing the unprecedented sickness epidemic in the U.S. and other countries that largely rely on microwaves to cook their foods, it may be wise if we followed the example of some countries where healthy cooking methods are still mainstream, such as Russia, Greece, Italy and France, as well as most developing countries.

TV-caused Autism

If you have children under three years old and are concerned about their health and wellbeing, you ought to take this good advice from the British publication the *Guardian Unlimited* on April 24, 2007. It reported new research linking autism in young children to the harmful effects that watching television can have on their physical and mental wellbeing. According to the research, allowing children under 3 to watch television can impair their linguistic and social development, and also increase their risk of health problems including attention-deficit disorder, autism and obesity.

Before the age of 3, children's brains go through rapid development and are being physically shaped in response to whatever they are exposed to, says the report. It further points out that exposing children to fast-moving images for sustained periods at this time in their lives can inhibit their ability to sustain attention, and hinder their development of social skills.

Other research suggests that television can also cause irregular sleep patterns for infants and toddlers, and decrease their resting metabolic rate, which compounds the physiological problems that come with lack of exercise. Furthermore, there are several studies suggesting early exposure to TV can be a trigger for autism.

CHAPTER 15

What Doctors Should Be Telling You –
37 Health Threats To Avoid

1. Potential Dangers of Medical Diagnosis

What do you think is the leading cause of death in the United States? You may say, it must be a disease, such as cancer or heart disease. Whereas it is true that most deaths have something to do with disease, it is actually not the disease itself that kills most people, but the medical treatments administered or prescribed by doctors. In 1995, the *Journal of the American Medical Association* (JAMA) admitted that doctors are the third leading cause of death (iatrogenic acts), causing 250,000 deaths each year. This disturbing trend has now worsened. Today (as of 2007), doctors are, in fact, the leading cause of death in the United States; or to clarify, it is the many unnecessary procedures and drugs they prescribe, as well as the mishaps and false diagnoses they make. Based on reviews of thousands of published studies and statistics (collected and published by Gary Null, Ph.D., Carolyn Dean, M.D., N.D., Martin Feldman, M.D., Debora Rasio, M.D., Dorothy Smith, Ph.D.), the annual doctor-caused death rate averaged 783,986 in 2007. By comparison, heart disease kills 699,697 annually, and cancer kills 553,251 annually. Since only 5 to 20 percent of all iatrogenic acts are ever reported, the annual rate of doctor-caused deaths may actually be over one million. Surprisingly, the most dangerous method applied by the current medical system is the *diagnosis* of disease.

The categorization of disease begins with its diagnosis. Depending on the particular symptom of discomfort or pain a person may be experiencing, a visit to the doctor will most likely result in the diagnosis of a disease, which the physician knows by its name and description. However, before you are given the certainty of diagnosis, you may have to undergo a series of routine examinations. There is the stethoscope, which has become a symbol of the healing profession; a measuring device to take the blood pressure; counting of the heart beat through feeling of the pulse; blood and urine tests; perhaps x-rays, EEG, EKG and more... In total, there are over 1,400 test procedures available that the modern doctor can use today to monitor and measure virtually every bit of your body.

Although in some cases, the use of these methods of diagnosis is justified and can save a person's life, in the vast majority of cases it is unjustified, misleading and potentially harmful. In theory, high tech diagnostic tools seem to be impartial and yield correct results, but in reality, they are grossly unreliable and can be as dangerous to health as some of the riskiest drugs and surgical procedures. It is therefore important that they are not applied routinely, but much more selectively and, if possible, only during emergency situations. The following are some of the most commonly used methods of diagnosis and their discrepancies.

ECG and EEG - Machines *Can* Lie

One of the instruments most frequently used to monitor heart activity is the *Electrocardiogram* or ECG/EKG. Repeatedly conducted tests have shown that at least 20 percent of diagnoses made by ECG/EKG experts were false. In addition, 20 percent of all ECG/EKG readings turned out to be different when the same person was tested a second time. When ECG/EKG measurements were taken on people who had suffered a heart attack, the machine detected an abnormal heart function in only one-quarter of the patients, no sign of a heart attack in the second quarter, and indecisive results in the remaining half. A sudden 'abnormal' curve in the ECG/EKG reading, caused by a jet flying over the hospital, can put a person into the group of those 'at risk' for suffering a possible heart attack.

One 1992 report published in the *New England Journal of Medicine* proved that ECG/EKGs could not be trusted. When these tests were performed on a group of perfectly healthy people, over 50 percent of them showed an extremely abnormal heart condition. In other words, if a healthy child or adult goes through a highly recommended health check-up and is diagnosed by an ECG/EKG expert as having an abnormally behaving heart that requires urgent treatment, the chance that this diagnosis is a false-positive is an astounding fifty/fifty. To avoid being treated unnecessarily with potentially harmful drugs, it is necessary that additional methods of diagnosis be employed to verify the correctness of the ECG/EKG readings. Having a second or third ECG/EKG reading at another hospital is also highly recommended, just to be on the safe side.

The *Electroencephalogram* (EEG), which is used to measure brain activity and detect brain tumors and epilepsy, often gives highly unreliable diagnostic results, too. Twenty percent of people who suffer from epileptic seizures produce normal readings. What is even worse, 15-20 percent of healthy people produce an abnormal EEG. To show how unreliable the EEG machine can be, when it was once connected to the head of a doll, it showed that the doll was *alive.* In order to avoid costly and potentially risky treatment programs, one should not rely solely on the diagnosis produced by the EEG.

X-rays - Handle with Care!

One of the riskiest of all diagnostic tools is the x-ray machine. Most people who visit a doctor will experience at least one exposure to these high-frequency waves of ionizing radiation (x-rays). These are the facts that have been discovered *so far* about the adverse effects of x-rays:

- If children are exposed to x-rays while in the mother's womb (in utero), their risk of all cancers increases by 40 percent, of tumors of the nervous system by 50 percent, and of leukemias by 70 percent.
- Today there are thousands of people with damaged thyroid glands, many of them with cancer, who were radiated with x-rays on the head, neck, shoulder, or upper chest 20-30 years ago.
- Ten x-ray shots at the dentist's are sufficient to produce cancer of the thyroid.
- Multiple x-rays have been linked with multiple myeloma - a form of bone marrow cancer.
- Scientists have told the American Congress that X-radiation of the lower abdominal region puts a person at risk for developing genetic damage that can be passed on to the next generation. They also linked the 'typical diseases of aging' such as diabetes, high blood pressure, coronary heart disease, strokes and cataracts with previous exposure to x-rays.
- It is estimated that at least 4,000 Americans die each year from x-ray related illnesses.
- In the U.K., one fifth to one half of all x-rays given to patients are without real necessity. In the

U.S., the FDA reports that a third of all radiation is unnecessary.
- In the U.K., x-rays ordered by doctors account for over 90 percent of the total radiation exposure of the population (Cambridge University Press, 1993).
- In Canada, almost everyone gets an annual x-ray of one sort or another.
- Old X-ray equipment still used in many hospitals gives off 20 to 30 times as high a dose of radiation as is necessary for diagnostic purposes.

Unless it is for an emergency situation, x-rays should be avoided because their harmful side effects may pose a greater health risk than does the original problem. As a patient you have the right to refuse x-ray diagnosis. By discussing your specific health problem with your physician, you can find out whether exposure to x-rays is really necessary or not. Many physicians today share this concern with their patients and try to find other ways to determine their exact condition. [To reduce radiation poisoning, see Chapter 7s section on metal tooth fillings and uses of magnetic clay.]

Mammography - Yes or No?

A recent study showed that mammography - a diagnostic tool that uses x-rays to detect breast cancer in women - is highly inaccurate. Only 1 to 10 out of 100 'positive' mammography tests are truly positive, which means that there is a 90 to 99 percent chance of a woman being diagnosed with breast cancer who doesn't have it. Since these tests are not taken only once in a lifetime, the chances of becoming a victim of false diagnosis for breast cancer are very high.

In Great Britain, about 100,000 women per year receive a false diagnosis for breast cancer (not excluding other forms of diagnoses). The women undergo many unnecessary biopsies and an unknown number of mastectomies (breast amputations). Many of the women suffer unnecessarily from depression, desperation, and fear of dying as a result of the diagnosis. In the United States, mastectomies have skyrocketed since mammography became the most popular 'preventive' method for diagnosing breast cancer.

The medical establishment is very nervous that the truth about the mammogram technology is finally beginning to surface. After all, it is a huge moneymaker. Peter Gotzsche, M.D. - a researcher at the Nordic Cochrane Center in Denmark - and his associates recently published a peer-reviewed study that found major fault with the results of a large trial that reported a 31 percent reduction in breast cancer mortality as a result of mammogram screening. After carefully reviewing the data, Dr. Gotzsche's team discovered that a large number of breast cancer deaths in the original data had 'somehow' been left out of the final report. The Gotzsche study was originally published last in an online edition of the European Journal of Cancer (EJC). Three weeks later, the study vanished from their web site. Apparently, EJC editors removed his study because they received complaints from pro-mammogram doctors.

To suggest mammography to be a diagnostic tool for detecting pre-symptomatic stages of cancer is deceptive and dubious. In most cases of breast cancer, it is irrelevant whether breast cancer is detected at an early or late stage. It is rather the type of cancer and whether it tends to metastasize ('spread to', which in reality means 'develop in' other parts of the body as well) at an early stage, that determines the outcome of the disease. Contrary to common belief, early detection has not shown to lower mortality rates for these types of cancer. Also by having many mammograms performed, a woman may put herself at risk for developing the very disease mammography is supposed to prevent, or worsen it if it is already present. Mammograms certainly aren't the 'magic bullet' for breast cancer prevention/detection that everyone seems to think they are. For one thing, mammograms are of very limited effectiveness because they seem only to be able to detect tumors of a size that is large enough to signify a rather advanced stage of cancer.

What is most disturbing about this diagnostic method is the excessive compression of the breast that is required during a routine mammogram. To produce good pictures and to avoid being sued for missing a tumor, the technician squeezes the breast extra hard. Squeezing can rupture internal tissue, including tumor tissue. If there is a tumor in the breast, performing a mammogram can actually break apart cancerous cell masses, spill the deadly poisons they contain and cause the disease to develop in other organs. New research shows that small tumors are especially prone to such potentially fatal damage.

Forcible flattening of a breast during a mammogram cannot be considered an acceptable risk, especially when the test is so ineffective anyway. A large body of research suggests that mammograms may be only marginally more effective (if at all) than physical exams in detecting breast cancer. So why use a method that can exacerbate a disease unnecessarily? Mammography is a major-league moneymaker for hospitals, doctors and cancer clinics nationwide. The unsuspecting women believe that the screening reduces their risk of death from breast cancer by 50-75 percent! In truth, according to research conducted by the U.S. Preventive Services Task Force, it would be necessary to screen over 1,200 women aged 40-74 every year for 14 years to prevent even one death from breast cancer.

Fortunately for women, the massive increase in lawsuits as a result of missed tumors is contributing to an increasing reluctance among doctors and clinics that once offered mammography to continue doing so.

A 1997 report by the American National Cancer Institute stated that mammograms showed no mortality benefit unless women in their 40s had been followed for 10 years. Other studies have shown that women who have mammograms suffer about the same rates of death due to breast cancer as women who do not have mammograms. Despite the fact that over 90 percent of the abnormalities discovered by mammography have been benign (not cancerous), 63 percent of U.S. women in their 40s keep having a mammogram every one or two years. This poses a great risk on healthy women who wish to prevent developing breast cancer in the future. Given the powerful cancer-inducing effects of mammograms, there is little if any benefit having a yearly mammogram.

Prevention of breast cancer does not begin with having a mammogram; it starts with taking active responsibility for one's body and mind. It can be said that most natural foods have a cancer preventive effect, and this includes food. Commenting on a recently released study on the prevention of cancer, John Pezzuto, leader of a food research group at the University of Illinois in Chicago, U.S.A, said, "...the study does show that a diet loaded with fruits and vegetables is a good defense against cancer." Research has identified a substance in grapes called *resveratol* that keeps cells from turning cancerous and inhibits the spread of cells that are malignant already. Most other natural foods contain similar or even more powerful cancer-fighting substances.

Women don't need to rely on *mammography* to feel safeguarded against breast cancer, especially since it is highly unreliable as a diagnostic tool. A series of liver, kidney and colon cleanses are often enough to prevent, stop and regress any type of cancer.

Hair dyes (highlights are okay), make-up (women who use make-up on a daily basis can absorb up to 5 pounds of chemicals into their bodies each year, many of them carcinogens), deodorants, toothpaste, commercial synthetic shampoos, moisturizing creams, hand lotion and other such substances, all release large amounts of chemical toxins into the lymph ducts of the breasts, causing lymphatic congestion and high levels of toxicity there.

A Note on the Risks of Wearing Bras

Wearing bras regularly also impairs proper lymph flow and may greatly increase the chance of developing breast cancer. Researcher David Moth has conducted an experiment where he measured the actual pressure exerted by bras. He says, *"The results suggest that the lightest possible bras will still exert pressures in excess of that found within the lymphatic vessels."*

There are studies which confirm the link between bra wearing and breast cancer. In 1991 Hsieh & Trichopoulos studied breast size and left/right handedness as risk factors, and noted in the findings that premenopausal women who do not wear bras had less than half the risk of breast cancer compared with bra wearers. The study was published in the European Journal of Cancer, 1991;27(2):131-5.

Another more recent study (2000), published in *Chronobiology International* (the journal of biological and medical rhythm research), found that wearing a bra decreased melatonin production and increased the core body temperature. Melatonin is a powerful antioxidant and hormone that promotes good sleep, fights aging, boosts immune system, and slows the growth of certain types of cancer, including breast cancer.

The most comprehensive studies on this subject were performed by medical researcher Sydney Singer. Singers found that the Maoris of New Zealand who integrated into white culture had the same rate of breast cancer, while the marginalized aboriginals of Australia had practically no breast cancer. The same was true for 'Westernized' Japanese, Fijians and other bra-converted cultures.

In the early 1990s Singers studied 4,500 women in 5 cities across the U.S. about their bra-wearing habits. He found that 3 out of 4 women who wore their bras 24 hours per day developed breast cancer. Furthermore, 1 out of 7 women who wore bras more than 12 hour per day but not to bed developed breast cancer. By comparison, merely 1 out of 152 women who wore their bras less than 12 hours per day had breast cancer, and only 1 out of 168 women who wore bras rarely or never developed breast cancer. In other words, the difference between 24 hour wearing of a bra and not at all was 125-fold.

A Note on the Dangers of Breast Implants

Over 300,000 women a year get breast implants. Having breast implants and undergoing mammograms can endanger your health. I have received many letters from women who have or had silicone breast implants that ruptured. One woman had this to say: "… I have had them for 23 years with no problems. Then they started to leak. The way I knew was I had pain in my chest and numbness and tingling down my arms. I got them out as quickly as possible and did not replace them. The doctor told me that it was a bad rupture and I had silicone in my lymph nodes and chest, and he could only clean up so much of it because it is like glue." There are many other ingredients in the implants (listed below); heavy metals such as aluminum and platinum are used as catalysts to turn the liquid to silicone gel. Silica is used as a filler; it is deadly if it gets into the lungs.

- cyclobexanone
- isopropyl alcohol
- denatured alcohol
- acetone
- urethane
- polyvinyl chloride
- lacquer thinner

- ethyl acetate
- epoxy resin
- epoxy hardener
- amine
- printing ink
- toluene
- freon

- silicone
- flux
- solder
- metal cleaning acid
- formaldehyde
- talcum powder
- color pigments

- oakite (cleaning solvent)
- cyanoacyrylates
- ethylene oxide
- carbob black
- xylene

- hexone
- hexone 2
- thixon-OSN-2
- rubber
- acid atrearic

- zinc oxide
- naptha (rubber solvent)
- phenol
- methylene chloride
- benzene

If you are concerned about getting breast cancer, it is best to avoid anything that is as unnatural as the above substances/chemicals. Women can actively contribute to a carefree future by taking care of their bodies' daily needs and requirements. (Also see *'Cancer - Who Makes It?'* Chapter 10).

What about Saline Implants? Saline implants aren't much better than silicone implants. Plastic surgeons like Susan Kolb, M.D., Atlanta, have seen the implants turn black, darkened by a fungus. The fungus can easily migrate into the blood causing severe symptoms of illness, including suicidal tendencies. The risks are real and serious, and the complication rate is extraordinarily high. And it makes sense why this danger exists. The labels on 1-quart bottles of saline IV solution recommend storage at 77 degrees and include a discard date of about 18 months. With implants, the saline is stored in the body at 98.6 degrees Fahrenheit degrees for years, which naturally makes it a perfect medium for fungi and other microbes to grow. Many women have had their saline implants for 10 or more years, and are suffering from unexplained symptoms of illness and sub-clinical infections. Women with saline implants complain about the same autoimmune problems that those with silicone-gel sacs experience.

Can You Trust Medical Laboratories?

Some of the weakest points in the field of medical diagnosis concern the bacteriological tests conducted in medical laboratories. In 1975, the Center for Disease Control (CDC) in the United States released the findings of an investigation of medical laboratories throughout the country and published the following results:

- 10-15 percent of the bacteriological tests were insufficient.
- 30-35 percent of the simplest clinical tests turned out to be false.
- 12-18 percent of tests to determine the correct blood groups and blood types, and 20-30 percent of tests to determine the blood serum and hemoglobin levels were incorrect.
- Over one-quarter of all tests showed faulty results.
- 31 percent of the laboratories were not even capable of detecting a simple form of anemia.
- Other laboratories falsely found infectious mononucleosis (glandular fever) in one out of every three tested persons. Between 10 and 20 percent of the laboratories detected leukemia (blood cancer) in samples that were free of it.

Another countrywide American study showed that over 50 percent of the laboratories with 'high standards' and permission to conduct all different types of medical tests did not fulfill national requirements. The worst results surfaced during a study when 197 out of 200 tested persons with abnormal test results turned out to be completely healthy after they were tested a second time! It may be added that the CDC study investigated only the best laboratories, which make up less than ten percent of the total number of medical labs in the United States.

In 1989, an editorial in the *Lancet* bluntly announced that many routine laboratory diagnostic tests are a waste of time and money. One study showed that the diseases of only six out of 630 patients were diagnosed from routine blood and urine tests. In another major study involving 1,000 patients, only 1 percent benefited from routine blood and urine tests.

Sarah is in her late 30s and has been having some gastrological problems. Her doctor referred her to a specialist, whom he described as 'widely recommended'. The specialist examined her and ran some tests, including the fecal occult blood test (FOBT). Surprised when one of the tests came back positive, this doctor recommended a colonoscopy. He also assured Sarah there was no risk to the procedure.

In recent years, colonoscopy has become the standard procedure for detecting cancer or precancerous polyps in the colon. Colonoscopy is an invasive procedure, requiring sedation while a flexible, tubular instrument is inserted into the colon.

When Sarah asked her doctor whether the original test result could be flawed, he told her that there can be a number of reasons an FOBT sometimes brings back false positive results. In order to get a second opinion and clear her doubts about possibly having a colonoscopy unnecessarily, Sarah asked her doctor to refer her to another gastroenterologist. After scheduling a new FOBT, her doctor handed her a list of things she needed to avoid for three to five days before the test in order to prevent a false positive result. These included:

- Eating red meat, fish, broccoli, potatoes, mushrooms, cantaloupe, grapefruit, carrots, cabbage, cauliflower, radishes, Jerusalem artichokes and turnips
- Eating iron-rich foods or taking iron supplements
- Taking acetaminophen or nonsteroidal anti-inflammatory drugs (NSAIDs), such as aspirin or ibuprofen
- Supplements of 200 mg or more of vitamin C

As it turned out, Sarah had eaten some of the foods on the list, in addition to taking Vitamin C at six times the dosage permitted for this test.

The main question that arises from this case is: "How many people undergoing FOBT tests are not receiving this list from their doctor, and subsequently end up having a false positive test result which makes them a candidate for colonoscopy?" I speculate that this applies to many or most patients.

On different note, a Canadian study reported in the *Journal of the American Medical Association* (Volume 295, page 2366) confirms that a 10-year interval between colonoscopy screenings may be appropriate for those who have had one negative procedure, meaning no cancer was found. Ten-year screenings have long been recommended for detecting possible colon cancer, but the new research shows that repeat screenings even after the ten years bear few or no benefits. Researchers studying cancer risks at the University of Manitoba looked at records for nearly 36,000 patients who had negative screenings for colon cancer between 1989 and 2003. They compared the incidence of colorectal cancer in this group with that in the provincial population. The research team found that the risk of developing colon cancer within less than 10 years of a negative colonoscopy was very low and remained lower beyond that time. In fact, at 10 years, the risk of developing colon cancer was 72% lower. So much for the hype of making colonoscopy every ten years a standard test for everyone.

Hypertension Produced in the Doctor's Office?

If your visit to the doctor is accompanied by the fear of anticipating a serious physical problem, your anxiety may trigger a stress response and raise your blood pressure. This phenomenon is known as 'white-coat hypertension'. While the doctor is measuring your blood pressure (using the old system of measurement), the pressure of the inflating cuff against your blood vessels and the accompanying nerves raises it even more. By the time the pressure in the cuff is lowered to read the pulsation level, you inevitably have an artificially raised blood pressure. Both factors, the anxiety and the taking of the blood pressure, may be sufficient to 'make' a person hypertensive.

A healthy blood pressure can vary tremendously - as much as 30 mm Hg - over the course of any day. To be really certain that you are hypertensive, the doctor would either have to take several readings each day over a period of six months (as recommended by the WHO) or give you a portable electronic device to do the same. Another complication lies in the fact that the systolic blood pressure may vary between each arm by as much as 8 mm Hg. In some cases the difference can be up to 20 mm Hg.

There is also the question of whether the doctor or health care worker takes the blood pressure while the person is lying down, then sitting, and then standing. If the person is asked to stand, how long does the doctor wait before taking the blood pressure? Furthermore, is he also checking the person's heart rate in the three different positions? Just taking a blood pressure measurement when the person is sitting will not tell him much about what happens when he is standing for any amount of time. But how rare is the patient who asks his doctor to do such detailed testing? The general mode of behavior in a doctor's office is to let the doctor do his job without questioning him. A recent study revealed that more than 70 percent of health care workers failed to use the proper arm position established by the American Heart Association. This position calls for the elbow to be slightly flexed and held at heart level.

In a study from the University of California, San Diego, 100 subjects' blood pressure was taken in six different positions. The researchers found that when the subjects were seated with the arm perpendicular to the body, hypertension was recorded in 22 percent. However, when the same subjects held the arm parallel to the body, 41 percent had readings that indicated high blood pressure. This raises a very important question: "How many people leave the doctor's office or hospital with a blood pressure prescription in hand who 'suffer' from high blood pressure because the doctor or nurse didn't follow the proper measurement guidelines?" My conservative estimate is, hundreds of thousands of them.

With regard to testing the blood pressure of pregnant women, no consensus exists as to which of the several available tests are truly reliable.

Furthermore, high blood pressure often is a temporary stress-related phenomenon and returns to normal levels after things calm down. In the case of white-coat hypertension, your blood pressure may drop to normal levels soon after you leave the doctor's office. But whether your blood pressure is chronically elevated or not, you may be asked to take anti-hypertensive drugs that have little or no effect on your real condition. In addition, they may produce severe side effects including headaches, lethargy, nausea, sleepiness and impotence. Anti-hypertensive drugs are popular because patients believe that swallowing a pill a day can prevent a possible heart attack. Research published in 1997 by the *Journal of the American Medical Association* found that drugs for high blood pressure may be overprescribed, especially if blood pressure measurements are taken by the doctor instead of by the portable device used for ambulatory monitoring.

Breeding Hypertensive Patients

What is more disturbing is that the medical system is trying to create a problem where none actually exists. What is considered 'normal' blood pressure has been modified nearly a dozen times in the past 35 years. The American Medical Association's recommendations now cite anything over 115/70 mm Hg as 'high'. Just 10 years ago, that number was 140/90 mm Hg, which is actually still quite low. Perhaps, soon everyone with 100/60 mm Hg may be considered at risk. How far do they want to take this deception before everyone is considered to be in the high risk group for hypertension and heart disease?

We are certainly heading in the wrong direction with our medication policies in the U.S. and other countries. We have indiscriminately turned huge portions of the population into hypertensive patients when, in fact, these people are not sick at all. According to a recent Reuters online article, a Ben Gurion University study with 500 subjects showed that patients over 70 years old with mild hypertension (by today's standards) actually thought more clearly and creatively than those with lower blood pressure. Both men and women in the study whose blood pressure was deemed high enough to warrant treatment with prescription drugs - and also those with clinically uncontrolled (untreated) hypertension - performed significantly better on tests of cognitive function, memory, concentration and visual retention. Surprisingly, those with 'normal' blood pressure, lowered with medication, showed the worst performance among all three groups in the study. The research clearly implies that senior citizens are overmedicated, and not just for blood pressure. Just as we have seen with blood cholesterol levels, a normal blood pressure among the elderly population is naturally higher than it is for the younger population. Lowering their blood pressure with medications that have harmful side effects is not only harmful to their brain cells and other parts of the body, but it is highly unethical, too.

While research has established that mortality rates remain uninfluenced by hypertension drugs, their side effects are often severe and include the collapse of the lungs and heart attacks. In contrast, many controlled studies have shown that relaxation therapies and a change of diet and lifestyle can lower a person's blood pressure faster and more consistently than medication can. Going on a balanced vegetarian diet alone can normalize blood pressure on a permanent basis. The *water therapy* described earlier is also a natural and quick method to restore normal blood pressure. Furthermore, the daily full body oil massage (especially with sesame oil) greatly benefits blood pressure. If taken internally as a cooking oil or salad dressing, sesame oil also helps to reduce high blood pressure and lessens one's dependence on medication. According to a recent study, participants (with an average age of 58) who consumed 35 grams of sesame oil a day for 60 days lowered their blood pressure from an average of 166/101 mm Hg to 134/84 mm Hg.

All of the other cleansing methods described in this book can significantly improve blood pressure, too. In most cases, a series of liver cleanses and a kidney cleanse are sufficient to eliminate hypertension altogether.

Conclusion:

I have used the examples of several diagnostic techniques to highlight the potential disadvantages and dangers of *just having a test*. There are many other tests that are as equally risky as the ones mentioned above, including angiography, bone scans, CAT scans, MRIs, various types of oscopies (such as colonoscopy) the AFP tumor marker test, and, of course, pap smear tests. (Whereas a pap smear test by itself is harmless, a positive test result for cancer may prompt you to choose cancer-suppressing treatments, instead healing it at the causal level, as explained in Chapter 10. The high percentage of false positive readings with these 'objective' methods of diagnosis shows that the diagnosis of disease is not as clear cut and obvious as it may seem to a layperson.

Today's methods of clinical diagnosis for chronic problems are mostly symptom-oriented and, therefore, leave the causes of the symptoms concealed and untreated. The cause-oriented diagnostic skills of an experienced practitioner of natural medicine, on the other hand, may be able to reveal the true nature of the imbalance prevalent in the body of a chronically ill patient. The health practitioner would incorporate in his treatment plan, the elimination of the four major risk factors of disease as outlined in chapter 3.

However, in the case of an accident, an injury, severe burns, or a number of other acute health problems, there can hardly be a better option than to place one's life in the hands of an experienced practitioner of conventional medicine.

2. Medical Treatment is Rarely Safe

"If all the medicine in the world were thrown into the sea, it would be bad for the fish and good for humanity." ~ *Oliver Wenddll Holmes, (Professor of Medicine, Harvard University)*. In conventional medicine, the treatment of disease is a highly controversial issue. On the one hand, many lives are *saved* through the procedures and drugs used during medical intervention. On the other hand, harmful side effects that arise from the treatment can *take* lives.

When you visit a doctor and receive a prescription for a drug or procedure aimed at a specific complaint you have, you (and your doctor) are most likely to presume that what he recommends has been proved by extensive testing and scientific reviews. Yet it is a well-documented and published fact that 85-90 percent of all the medical treatments we generally trust and accept to be 'scientifically verified' and 'proven effective', have actually been adopted and widely used without a single scientific study backing up their claims.

Drugs Should be the Exception, not the Rule

In a 2004 article, *The Times* talked about the 'Pharmaceutical Man'. I sincerely doubt that being as drug-dependent as we are now, it could be considered an evolutionary step of the Homo Sapiens! Rather it should be seen as a sign of the dissolution of life.

The illusion that there is a successful treatment for every disease has led to the escalation of increasingly complex forms of illness and increasingly prohibitive health care costs. Many patients who are released from hospitals leave with the conviction that they are healed from whatever was wrong with them. They believe that since the problem has been 'fixed' they can *just get on with their lives again*. Drugs, surgery, and other medical treatments deceive in this way.

When penicillin came on the market, it was considered a wonder drug that could bring dying patients back to life within a few days. In fact, penicillin did save many lives, although simple methods of cleansing and supporting the body in its efforts to throw off poisonous substances could have achieved the same. Today, penicillin causes the very problems for which it is often prescribed. Side effects include skin eruptions, diarrhea, fever, vomiting, mononucleosis, allergic shock, fainting, heart collapse, arrhythmia and low blood pressure.

Whatever applies to penicillin also applies to most other drugs. Their side effects frequently outweigh their benefits, and patients should be aware of the complications they may generate before they agree to take them. The signs of this 'evolution' abound. Nexium, Prevacid, Lipitor, aspirin, Celebrex, Crestor and other such drugs have become household words. Neighbors, friends and relatives are all taking at least one pill, and more often, several pills, each day for months and even years. Television, radio and print media are full of praise for their 'life enhancing' benefits. Newspapers go even one step further. Not a day passes without an article or two heralding the latest study 'demonstrating' the supposed benefits of the wonder drugs.

In 2003 Americans spent $163 billion dollars on pharmaceutical drugs, which is more than we spend on fruits and vegetables, all dairy products and all bakery products combined. So naturally, there are many more pharmacies around than grocery stores! To sustain our health, we now rely more on pharmaceutical products than on food. The pharmaceutical man has become a living reality.

There are now pills for every acute as well as every chronic illness. As pleasing this should be to those selling these pills, those who take them do not reach a higher level of health or happiness. This, of course, does not stop drug companies from designing and manufacturing billions and billions of additional pills, supposedly to make your life easier and more comfortable.

There are pills for when you or your child's attention wanders from time to time. You can buy pills to reduce or end pre- or post-menstrual aches and pains (which often occur in woman with endometriosis). If you have an unwanted pregnancy, there are pills to induce an abortion. If you cannot curb your appetite, you can suppress it just by popping a pill. If you complain to your doctor about not having an appetite, he can prescribe a pill that can increase it for you. There are pills for allergies and to attract the opposite sex (based on pheromones). Mood-enhancing and anti-stress pills also abound. Eventually, your dependency on pills will make you depressed. But, of course pills exist for that condition, too. Taking antidepressants doesn't really resolve depression, though; in fact, the use of such drugs can drive you to take your own life.

If you search for it long enough (just use Google search on the Internet), you can find a pill for every physical and emotional difficulty you can think of.

Pill-Popper Drama Unfolding

"Medical practice has neither philosophy nor common sense to recommend it. In sickness the body is already loaded with impurities. By taking drug-medicines more impurities are added, thereby the case is further embarrassed and harder to cure." ~ *Elmer Lee, M.D., Past Vice President, Academy of Medicine.*

The famous physician, Dr. William Osler, expressed the dilemma of taking medicinal drugs in just a few simple words: "The person who takes medicine must recover twice, once from the disease and once from the medicine." Be careful to check for the side effects of any prescription medicine you may be considering; they are always listed on the instruction list accompanying the drug. But also be aware that many potential side effects are not listed, including death. Only when serious side effects get reported frequently by practicing physicians, may the FDA sometimes (when under public pressure) actually order the withdrawal of a drug.

A frequent side effect of medical drugs that is hardly ever mentioned is the development of an addiction to them. The best-selling author of *Confessions of a Medical Heretic,* Dr. Robert Mendelsohn, said this: "We are prone to thinking of drug abuse in terms of the male population and illicit drugs such as heroin, cocaine, and marijuana. It may surprise you to learn that a greater problem exists with millions of men and women dependent on legal prescription drugs." Just because prescription medicine is legally available and given to you by your doctor, does not mean it is any less addictive than hallucinogenic drugs.

Senior citizens in particular should be cautious when taking medicines prescribed by their doctors. A new study from Duke University reveals disturbing evidence that more than 20 percent of all seniors who are prescribed drugs are receiving medications that are known to be harmful to older patients. Another study published in the *Lancet Neurology* (May 1, 2007) showed that seniors who regularly take regular aspirin and warfarin to prevent strokes could instead actually be increasing their risk. Especially in healthy older people over 75, aspirin may very well be doing more harm than good. The number of strokes associated with these drugs increased by a factor of seven. The researchers concluded that the increasing use of these drugs means that they may soon overtake high blood pressure as the leading cause of intracerebral hemorrhagic stroke in those over 75.

Drugs can greatly interfere with the absorption of nutrients in everyone, and especially in seniors. For instance, acid blockers (such as Prilosec and Nexium) have been shown to significantly decrease absorption of vitamin B12, which is one of the primary vitamins needed to prevent anemia.

Other medications related to nutrient-depletion are among the most frequently prescribed drugs on the market. They include antibiotics, anti-depressants, anti-inflammatory drugs, blood pressure medications, cholesterol-lowering drugs, estrogen, and tranquilizers. Any of these drugs can strip valuable vitamins and minerals from the body. When two or more of these drugs are combined, especially in an older patient, the risk of developing anemia rises almost exponentially. Anemia is a serious condition that can dramatically increase mortality risk for patients with chronic health problems, such as heart disease and cancer.

Many doctors and patients underestimate the risks associated with anemia. Anemia is a deficiency in the oxygen-carrying capacity of the blood. Hemoglobin (Hb) is the protein in red blood cells that picks up and transports oxygen throughout the body. When this function of the blood becomes disturbed, symptoms of weakness, fatigue, trouble concentrating, sexual dysfunction, shortness of breath, dizziness and paleness of the skin are likely to develop.

Anemia can exacerbate the symptoms of underlying heart disease and may be a risk factor for frailty. If you have been diagnosed with anemia, your doctor may have told you that you suffer from iron deficiency and need to take iron supplements. The truth is, however, that the liver will limit the uptake of iron from food to a level below normal only if there is an underlying condition that requires blood iron to be low. For example, if the liver bile ducts are blocked and excessive iron cannot escape from the liver, the blood iron levels could reach toxic concentrations and cause hemochromatosis, a condition that can destroy the pancreas and liver. To prevent death, the body will try to absorb as little iron from the food as possible. Another cause of iron-deficiency absorption would be the loss of red blood cells during chronic, low-level gastrointestinal bleeding. Internal bleeding can result from prolonged aspirin or nonsteroidal anti-inflammatory drug use, colon polyps, stomach ulcers, and gastrointestinal cancer. The most natural blood iron loss (caused by the liver) occurs just before a woman's menstrual period or during the last few weeks before a mother gives birth to a baby. Since iron is a favorite food for destructive bacteria, by keeping blood iron low, the body makes the blood (which is exposed to the air during the menstrual period and the birthing process) unattractive to air-borne bacteria, thus preventing a possibly fatal blood infection. Since medical approaches are not based on the knowledge and understanding of how the body responds to internal and external challenges, most doctors settle for fixing the symptoms, totally disregarding their underlying cause or wisdom, for that matter. In the case of anemia, prescribing iron tablets can actually risk a patient's life.

Anemia may also be caused by chronic inflammation, chronic infection, rheumatoid arthritis and kidney disorders. Once again, treating these illnesses as separate diseases and applying suppressive drugs instead of seeing the illness as the body's appropriate response to an underlying threat, can have serious consequences. As a society, we are now sicker than we have ever been before. We may live a little longer, but with a lower quality of life.

The medical and pharmaceutical industries have managed to persuade the older generation that it needs to take more drugs to stay alive and healthy. Accordingly, the average senior citizen now receives 25 prescriptions annually! But the wider variety of drug intake increases the chances of serious drug interactions, while further robbing the patients of the very nutrients they need most when fighting an illness. According to a recent study, this situation has escalated into a very serious problem: 20 percent of all emergency room visits are made by senior citizens suffering drug-related side effects or interactions. Another problem is overdosing on the medications. One 2002 study identified 2.2 million cases of seniors taking more than the recommended dosages of their medications. The only solution to this problem is assisting the elderly to deal with the root causes of their health problems, rather than encouraging them to suppress the symptoms of their ailments.

Doctor-Caused Diseases Surging

Iatrogenesis (illness caused by the doctor) is one of the most rapidly spreading epidemics of our time. Behind heart disease and cancer, medical doctors are the third-leading cause of death in the U.S. The famous physician Charles E. Page, M.D., once stated: "The cause of most disease is in the poisonous drugs physicians superstitiously give in order to affect a cure." Medical intervention used for some of the most benign conditions has created even life-threatening situations for many patients. Therefore, the question arises: which is more dangerous to your health, the disease or the treatment for the disease? The following statistics released by the U.S. Department of Health & Human Services may provide the answer.

In the United States there are 700,000 physicians. Accidental deaths caused by physicians are 120,000 per year. The risk at dying at the hand of your doctor is therefore substantial. In a recent Harvard University study, researchers found that 'long-shift' doctors committed five times as many diagnostic errors as their shorter-shift counterparts. These weren't just errors in diagnosis. In one instance, a long-shifter ordered 10 times the correct dose of a powerful blood-pressure drug. Another error caused a patient's lung to collapse when a sleepy intern botched inserting a tube into a nearby artery.

In yet another instance, a tranquilizer overdose caused one patient to suffer a dangerously low heartbeat and blood pressure. Hospitals have a tight strategy for keeping costs down and making more profits. So rather than paying additional doctors, they double-up the shifts of the least experienced staffer they have. (The study's report cites an average 80-hour work week for interns.)

Death Lurking in Prescription and Over-the-Counter Drugs

In addition to accidental death caused by physicians, patients also face the risk of dying from the side effects of prescription and over-the-counter (OTC) drugs. According to a January 2005 report, the dangerous arthritis drug Vioxx apparently has killed over 135,000 people. Then consider the hundreds of OTCs, such as aspirin. This 'harmless' drug increases the risk of potentially lethal internal bleeding; it also makes blood more likely to clot, not less!

And did you know that taking ibuprofen (Advil, Motrin) in combination with aspirin actually doubles your risk of death from heart-related causes! According to a study of over 7,000 patients' medical records spanning eight years, if you take ibuprofen for any reason - say, arthritis pain relief - while engaged in aspirin therapy for heart disease, you are twice as likely to die from a heart attack or stroke because of the way these two powerful drugs interact. The study, which was conducted by Britain's Medical Research Council and published in *The Lancet*, was confirmed by another study published in the journal, *Annals of the Rheumatic Diseases*, on April 5, 2007. This proves the point that over-the-counter drugs can be lethal in the stomach of an unsuspecting patient. In fact, because of complications, some 56,000 users of OTCs in the United States end up in the emergency room every year. Just because some 5 billion over-the-counter medications are sold in the United States annually does not mean you should believe they are safe.

Take for example, acetaminophen, also known as Tylenol. Besides causing cardiovascular problems, Tylenol is actually the most common cause of liver failure, not hepatitis C, as you might believe. Tylenol 3, which is given to women for postnatal pain, can produce deadly concentrations of morphine in their breast milk. A lawsuit over the death of Toronto newborn Tariq Jamieson, who died as a result of opiate toxicity in his mother's breast milk, is shedding new light on the dangers of prescribing such drugs as Tylenol 3 to breastfeeding mothers. Tariq died after 11 days of breastfeeding, according to *National Review of Medicine,* June 15, 2007. He was found to have high blood levels of acetaminophen and a blood concentration of morphine 6 times higher than is considered safe in a neonate. Tylenol 3 contains both acetaminophen and codeine (the most widely used narcotic in medical treatment in the world). Codeine is metabolized to morphine in the body.

Mothers cannot expect doctors to protect them and their babies from the dangers of prescription and over-the-counter drugs. The doctors didn't make these drugs and often have no clue about what's in them. Most doctors never even look at the list of side effects. Patients need to inform themselves about the side effects of the drugs they take. It makes little sense to replace one relatively minor symptom of discomfort with some or all of the following potential consequences of taking Tylenol: nausea, vomiting, constipation, lightheadedness, dizziness, drowsiness, flushing, vision changes, mental/mood changes, slow/irregular breathing, slow/irregular heartbeat, change in the amount of urine, dark urine, yellowing eyes or skin, stomach pain, extreme fatigue, possibly fatal liver disease and allergic reactions.

To stress the seriousness of the situation, a survey conducted by the National Consumers League found that 44 percent of adults knowingly exceeded the recommended dose of OTC pain relievers - while only 16 percent had even read the warning label! Federal officials estimate that over 150,000 Americans each year end up in the emergency department of hospitals because of complications from OTC pain-relievers. These 'harmless' medicines, as most doctors and patients consider them, kill 16,000 Americans outright every year.

Furthermore, while you may believe that aspirin is good for getting rid of a headache, a new study reveals that certain heart patients may actually be at greater risk for heart attacks if they use aspirin, as reported in the July 2004 issue of the *American Heart Journal.* The lead researcher of the study, Dr. John G. F. Cleland, University of Hull, England, stated that any theoretical benefit of using aspirin after a heart attack "is outweighed by real evidence of harm." Discontinuing the treatment once it has been started is also problematic. A French study showed how severe angina and fatal heart attacks might be prompted by the sudden halt of regular aspirin intake. The researchers even stated that aspirin therapy "cannot be safely stopped in any case."

In stark contrast to drug therapy, a 15-month study of almost 2,000 subjects showed how those whose diets included the highest fruit intake had more than a 70 percent reduced risk of heart attack and other cardiac problems compared with those who ate the least amount of fruit. Vegetable intake produced a similar effect. Subjects who consumed vegetables three or more times each week had an approximately 70 percent lower heart attack risk than those who ate no vegetables at all.

Antibiotics may have their place if someone is dying and could be saved by the drugs. But it is very risky, for instance, to give children who are infected with the flu virus H, the antibiotic *chloramphenicol.* The drug is known to destroy bone marrow, which requires subsequent blood transfusions and many other therapies that cannot guarantee a recovery at all. Chloramphenicol preparations are still prescribed even for such minor problems as a sore throat.

According to studies cited by the American magazine *Newsweek,* seven out of ten Americans who seek treatment for the common cold receive antibiotics - even though it is a fact that antibiotics are useless against viral infections such as colds or the flu. When these powerful yet ineffective drugs are administered to patients with such relatively mild illnesses, neither patient nor doctor seems to be aware of the chaos the drugs can create in the body of an infected person. After killing most of the invading germs and substantial numbers of friendly bacteria in the host's intestines, the body's immune system is left with the nearly impossible task of removing their rotting carcasses. Since the good bacteria have been destroyed, too, there is 'nobody' left to clear up this toxic mess, which consists mostly of putrefying protein. Some of the protein, though, does end up in the connective tissues and is packed into the basal membranes of the capillaries and arteries. In time, the increased congestion in the circulatory system may lead to heart attacks, stroke, or congestive heart failure.

Nearly every day, drugs are removed from the market because they have been shown to produce such strong side effects that their use is "no longer" justified. Somehow, drug makers and the FDA omit to emphasize the fact all drugs are potentially dangerous because the poison they contain is 'anti-body' oriented, which means that they are also destroying parts of the body.

The heart drug *nifedipine,* a calcium-channel blocker used to treat high blood pressure, has been linked with serious, and sometimes fatal, side effects, including heart attacks and other cardiac abnormalities. Although the *Journal of the American Medical Association* argues that because of its severe side effects, the drug should be abandoned, it is still prescribed world-wide in certain hypertensive emergencies. The U.S. National Heart, Lung and Blood Institute has warned doctors to use nifedipine only with great caution, if at all. One study published in 1995 in the *Lancet* found that patients who received calcium-channel blockers were 60 percent more likely to suffer a heart attack than those put on either diuretics or beta-blockers. Nifedipine turned out to be the most dangerous of all calcium-channel blockers.

Beta-blockers are hazardous, too. In 1998, the *Journal of the American Medical Association* reported that apart from being ineffective, the elderly are more likely to suffer a sudden and fatal heart attack while taking these drugs. New analysis of 10 trials from a Medline search revealed that beta-blockers, which have been used for over 30 years to treat high blood pressure, are no more effective than a sugar pill.

The American drug *reserpin,* which is also used to lower elevated blood pressure, has been shown to increase the risk of breast cancer by *300 percent,* but it is still given to patients with high blood pressure. Several other classes of drugs - including diuretics and anti-hypertensives (for lowering blood pressure) - are suspected to cause cancer of the kidneys. The beta-blocker *atenol* also became suspect after it was discovered that cancer was twice as common in hypertensive sufferers taking the therapy. Both British and U.S. studies have shown that only a fifth to a third of patients on drugs managed to reach the blood pressure targets set by their doctors. Even placebos are able to achieve that. This makes the so urgently-advised treatment of high blood pressure all the more questionable.

Another major side effect of hypertensive drugs is *hypotension* - or a sudden drop in blood pressure when one stands up. Thus, these drugs can be considered a major risk of dizziness and falling, and therefore, bone and hip fractures among senior citizens. In 1994, the *British Medical Journal* published a study showing that diuretics (drugs used to lower blood pressure) cause an 11-fold increase in diabetes. As reported in the *Journal of the American Medical Association* in 1993, *ACE* inhibitors (a group of pharmaceuticals that are used primarily in treatment of hypertension and congestive heart failure) can cause potentially fatal kidney damage and even death, if they are given too soon after a heart attack.

Even the highly praised 'miracle' drug insulin, which is injected into diabetics, has now been proven to cause diabetic blindness. Another drug, the anti-malaria medication *plaquenil,* which is supposed to be useful against lupus, rheumatoid arthritis, and skin problems, is often prescribed. Its sale is legal in the U.K, where authorities have no objections to recommending the drug for children provided the daily dosage does not exceed 6.5 mg per kg of body weight. In the U.S., any doctor who prescribes plaquenil to a child faces the risk of a lawsuit because a number of fatalities have been reported among children who have taken doses as low as 0.75 g. Not only children risk their health and possibly their lives by using this drug. Those suffering eye problems, psoriasis or liver problems, and also alcoholics and pregnant women could find their condition worsening. Side effects of the drug include irritability, nervousness, nightmares, convulsions, nerve deafness, blurred vision, edema, bleaching of the hair, alopecia (loss of scalp hair) aplastic anemia, anorexia and nausea.

A whole range of drugs also exists that were designed to cut down your stomach acid production. If you want to avoid developing pneumonia, among other serious health problems, you had better stay away from antacids and instead deal with the true causes of acid reflux. Subduing the secretion of stomach acid, no matter what approach you choose, is a serious intervention with long-term consequences, if pursued over time. Undermining the stomach's ability to commence a normal digestive process becomes the genesis of an entire host of disorders.

According to a 2004 Dutch study published the *Journal of the American Medical Association*, several popular heartburn medications may sharply increase the risk of pneumonia. The drugs involved are the proton pump inhibitors: Nexium, Prilosec, Prevacid, Protonix and Aciphex, as well as the H2 receptor antagonists: Pepcid, Zantac, Tagamet, Rotane and Axid.

There are also a large number of drugs that, in turn, cause heartburn because of acid reflux. Take for example, ibuprofen, a non-steroidal anti-inflammatory drug (NSAID). Originally marketed as Nurofen, it is also known under the names Act-3, Advil, Brufen, Dorival, Herron Blue, Panafen, Motrin, Nuprin, Ipren, Ibumetin, Ibuprom, IbuHEXAL, Moment, Ibux, Íbúfen and Ibalgin, depending on the country in which it is sold. Mostly it is used for symptoms of arthritis, primary dysmenorrhoea, fever and as an analgesic, especially where there is an inflammatory component. Popping the occasional Advil can lead to years of agonizing stomach distress. This and other anti-inflammatory drugs cause stomach tissue to tighten (but not esophagus tissue), thereby widening the esophagus passage and allowing stomach acid to pass through. Before anti-inflammatory drugs such as Advil became widely available, heartburn was rare and was almost always related to diet. Today, up to 70 percent of all acid reflux cases may be linked to the prolonged use of anti-inflammatory drugs. Since their introduction a few decades ago, acid reflux disease experienced an enormous jump. This example shows once again that taking anti-inflammatory drugs versus dealing with the causes of the health condition, is not a solution at all, but leads instead to even bigger problems than those that existed before.

Consider the anti-cancer drugs that cause cancer. Tamoxifen, for example, is a common drug prescribed to high-risk women to prevent breast cancer, and it is usually taken for five years. However, research conducted in Israel found that Tamoxifen can cause cancer instead. According to a study published in the *International Journal of Gynecological Cancer*, the treatment of breast cancer with tamoxifen results in an increased risk of uterine cancer incidence and mortality. Merely substituting one cancer for another is not a treatment option that should be offered to cancer patients.

Prozac Scandal Revealed; Antidepressants

The most favored antidepressant drug to make people 'happy' is *Prozac* (fluoxetine). In the U.S., it is now used by millions of people to cope with stressful living conditions. This may lead people to believe that the drug is safe. The first studies on *Prozac*, however, show that the drug is not harmless after all. Researchers from the University of California made the discovery that women who take *Prozac* while pregnant are more than twice as likely to give birth to babies with defects. If the drug is still being taken during the third trimester, the baby is nearly five times as likely to be born prematurely and twice as likely to need the help of special-care nurseries. The baby also faces nine times the risk of having breathing difficulties, cyanosis (lack of oxygen) during feeding and jitteriness. Other published side effects of Prozac include the following: anxiety, significant weight loss, cardiac arrhythmia, visual disturbances, tremors, nausea, diarrhea, asthma, arthritis, osteoporosis, stomach bleeding, loss of sex drive and impotence.

And it gets worse. On January 2, 2005, CNN reported that an internal document purportedly from Eli Lilly and Co. revealed that the drug maker had data more than 15 years ago showing that patients on its antidepressant, Prozac, were far more likely to attempt suicide and show hostility than were patients on other antidepressants. For obvious reasons, the company attempted to minimize public awareness of the drug's side effects.

The document was provided to CNN by the office of Rep. Maurice Hinchey, D-New York, who has called for tightening FDA regulations on drug safety. "The case demonstrates the need for Congress to mandate the complete disclosure of all clinical studies for FDA-approved drugs so that patients and their doctors, not the drug companies, decide whether the benefits of taking a certain medicine outweigh the risks," he said.

This would certainly be a step in the right direction, but it is simply not the way in which the FDA is moving. In a bold move designed to sell even more prescription drugs, the FDA has announced its intention to bypass doctors and allow pharmacists to prescribe certain drugs directly to consumers. The move would subject patients to prescription-strength pharmaceuticals, even though they had not been examined, diagnosed with any condition or given a non-drug alternative treatment plan by the person prescribing the drugs. It is a 'drugs only' approach that moves the U.S. medical system another step closer to being the world largest legalized, drug-pushing cartel.

This is how the FDA justifies its recent move, as stated in a Federal Registry notice: *"Some groups have asserted that pharmacist interaction with the consumer could ensure safe and effective use of a drug product that otherwise might require a prescription. Because pharmacists have the training and knowledge to provide certain interventions, they may be able to ensure that patients meet the conditions for use and educate patients on appropriate use of the drug product."* Why do we need doctors then, you might ask? Who are the 'some groups'? Will this move by the FDA do anything to reduce the number of doctor-caused diseases and fatalities? Isn't it likely that drug dispensaries will increase their profits by this move? And who is going to suffer most from this from of legalized drug pushing? Unfortunately, drugs like Prozac are already considered harmless recreational drugs. By making drug acquisition even easier, this disturbing trend will only continue.

The 1988 Eli Lilly document indicated that 3.7 percent of patients attempted suicide while on Prozac, a rate more than 12 times that cited for any of four other commonly used antidepressants. The document, which cited clinical trials of 14,198 patients on fluoxetine, the generic name for Prozac, also stated that 2.3 percent of users suffered psychotic depression while on the drug. This was more than double the next-highest rate for patients using another antidepressant. In addition, the paper noted that 1.6 percent of patients reported incidents of hostility, more than double the number that patients on any of four other commonly used antidepressants reported. Finally, the trials reviewed in the document said that 0.8 percent of users of Prozac reported causing an intentional injury - eight times the rate associated with any of the other antidepressants.

In the paper titled 'Activation and Sedation in Fluoxetine Clinical Trials', the authors said that the drug may produce nervousness, anxiety, agitation or insomnia in 19 percent of patients, and sedation in 13 percent of patients.

The *British Medical Journal* reported that the documents disappeared in 1994, during the case of Joseph Wesbecker, a printing press operator who had killed eight people at his Louisville, Kentucky, workplace five years before, while taking fluoxetine. He then shot and killed himself.

The FDA has recently warned that antidepressants can cause side effects such as agitation, panic attacks, insomnia and aggressiveness. This is truly bad news for people in Great Britain where Prozac is being taken in such large quantities that it can now be found in Britain's drinking water. Environmentalists are calling for an urgent investigation into the revelations, describing the buildup of this antidepressant as 'hidden mass medication'. The Environment Agency has revealed that Prozac is building up both in river systems and the groundwater used for drinking supplies.

Meanwhile, in the U.S., Prozac has been in major waterways for months already. A Baylor University toxicologist (Brooks) discovered traces of Prozac's active ingredient (fluoxetine) in the tissues of blue gill fish in a lake in Dallas, Texas. Brooks speculated that the fluoxetine made its way from the urine of Prozac users through a water treatment plant and into the lake.

Researchers from the University of Toronto recently published a study in the *Lancet*, showing that all classes of antidepressants are dangerous for the elderly (aged 66 and over) to take, and will greatly increase their risk of falling and fracturing a hip.

In recent years, the herb Saint John's Wort, or Hypericum perforatum, has been recommended by numerous psychiatrists for their patients suffering depression. The herb, which is often taken in pill form, is at least as effective as Prozac and other antidepressants, and has few or no side effects.

A staggering 4 million children a day line up at their school nurse's office for their daily afternoon doses of Ritalin. Starting millions of small children on a prescription drug for attention deficit disorder without ever taking a moment to seek out the root cause of the problem being treated is a true form of 'medical negligence'. While taking Ritalin or a similar medication will bear results practically overnight, it could take several weeks or months to figure out the root causes behind the behavior. In so many cases, it is sugar, insulin resistance, and poor nutrition that are causing the mental irritation, poor concentration and nervousness. Giving the child more loving attention is often enough to make him feel safe and secure and to help restore his emotional and physical balance.

Steroids, Arthritis Drugs, and NSAIDs

A medical investigation in the United States has shown that three times more people die from legal prescription drugs than from illegal narcotic drugs, such as heroin and cocaine. This study does not account for the contra-indications of the drugs, which kill at least 30,000 a year in the U.S. These are people who take medications, but have conditions (including drug allergies) that would cause these drugs to be dangerous for them. It is nearly impossible to determine how many people are being hospitalized because of contra-indications from drugs, but careful official estimates indicate that they make up about 5 percent of all lying in American and British hospitals today. *Steroids* belong to another group of drugs that were formerly used only for extreme, life-threatening conditions. Today, they are used for minor problems such as sunburn, skin eruptions, acne and glandular fever. Patients are rarely aware of the dangers that may arise from taking these drugs. Side effects include high blood pressure, stomach ulcers with possible perforation of the stomach wall (this is how my father died), cramps and dizziness, inhibited growth in children within six weeks of taken the drugs, irregular menstruation, weakening of muscular strength, slowed healing of wounds, vision problems, skin atrophy, allergic shock, loss of libido, decrease in bone density, manic depression, and the emergence of latent diabetes. Steroids are now handed out, even for babies, at the first sign of inflammation of any kind. But these drugs cannot cure a single condition; all they do is stop the body from responding to an abnormal condition. The new diseases caused by such drugs may require further treatment using even stronger drugs, thus adding more side effects to the ones that have already occurred.

The latest 'breakthrough' drugs for arthritis produce such strong side effects that it might be better to live with arthritis than to risk one's life. The manufacturer of one popular brand known as *Butazolidin alka* was obliged to warn the consumer that this particular drug was very strong and had led to cases of leukemia (cancer of the blood) even after short term use. Additionally, the drug can have 92 side effects including hepatitis, high blood pressure, dizziness and unconsciousness, as well as headaches. The manufacturer advises the attending physician to enlighten his patients about the possible dangers that can arise from taking the drug, particularly if they are over 40 years old, and to use the smallest possible, but still effective, dosage. The manufacturers admit that the drug can cause serious and life-threatening reactions while having no effect on improving the condition of the disease!

NSAID's, the common name for over a dozen or more non-steroidal anti-inflammatory drugs (including aspirin, ibuprofen and acetaminophen), are used to treat rheumatoid and osteoarthritis[44]. However, for the past few years, these drugs have been given to people for such simple complaints as recurring headaches or inflammation. In return for the pain relief, however, the patient may die as a result of gastric bleeding caused by the extreme toxicity of the drugs. A warning placed on each NSAID prescription says: "Serious gastrointestinal toxicity such as bleeding, ulceration, and perforation can occur at any time, with or without warning symptoms, in patients treated chronically with NSAID therapy." If this doesn't sound like *Russian Roulette* to you, the death toll from taking these drugs may convince you otherwise. In the U.K., 4,000 people die each year from taking NSAIDS. In the U.S., the fatality figure is up to five times as high as it is in the U.K. Each year, hundreds of thousands of people are hospitalized due to gastric bleeding caused directly by taking NSAIDs. Other side effects include perforation of the colon, colitis, Crohn's disease, blurred vision, Parkinson's disease, liver and kidney damage, hepatitis and hypertension.

A 20-year-old acne medicine that millions of American teens are, no doubt, taking every day has been linked to a stunning array of negative psychiatric conditions including suicide, depression, psychosis, violent and aggressive behaviors, mood swings, emotional instability, paranoia and changes in personality. This makes one wonder if any drug, no matter how commonly prescribed, is even remotely safe.

With the enormous variety of drugs available today, many doctors no longer have the time to study the side effects of each drug they prescribe, and most patients never read the list of side effects that accompanies the drug. Also, few patients read the small printed contraindications or ask their doctor about the possible dangers of the drugs. Doctors don't seem to have the time to warn their patients about possible side effects either. One report on a survey published in a 1996 issue of the *British Medical Journal* found that less than two-thirds of patients recalled receiving any advice from their doctors on potential side effects. Although the doctor has a moral as well as a legal obligation to inform the patient about the risks of treatment, in most cases this important step is omitted. The drug company is legally protected as long as the side effects and contra-indications are listed. This leaves it up to the patient to decide whether to take a drug.

Read Side-Effect Labels to Save Your Life

Side effects arising from the use of common pharmaceutical drugs can develop into some of the most grotesque symptoms imaginable. The Stevens-Johnson Syndrome (SJS), which can progress into a complication called TENS (toxic epidermal necrolysis), is caused by adverse drug reactions. Before you start taking common prescription drugs, you may need to inform yourself about this often-fatal reaction. The list of drugs that may be problematic includes antiepileptic and anticonvulsant drugs, sulfonamides, ampicillin, allopurinol and nonsteroidal anti-inflammatory agents (NSAIDs), as well as some vaccinations (such as anthrax).

The frightening fact about these drugs is that the body's reaction to them is completely unpredictable. For instance, you may have taken ibuprofen, a popular NSAID, a hundred times, but you can never

---

[44] A new study by the Tel Aviv University in Israel and a second one by the University of Miami concluded that ginger extract (255 mg per day for 6 or more weeks) may be optimal for the treatment of osteoarthritis.

know for sure whether or when the body will suddenly become hypersensitive to the drug. When your body starts fighting the drug, it will go into an extreme inflammatory response that causes your skin to die and literally burn away. This side effect can occur with any age group, from infants and teens to the elderly. The mortality rate ranges from 25-80 percent. Those who survive the ordeal are scarred for life, often to a point of total disfigurement. As the number of people taking these drugs rises, the number of victims increases.

There is no real need to take any of these drugs. Suppression of symptoms jeopardizes the body's own healing efforts and only makes matters worse. If you do opt to take a prescription that puts you at risk for SJS or TENS, watch for any signs of an allergic reaction, such as a rash, blisters, a scalding sensation or fever, and discontinue the medication immediately. Don't wait for your doctor to take you off the medication because your life may be at stake.

Demented Dirt

There is more dispiriting news to come. As I have mentioned before, Americans over 60 are the drug companies' best customers. They are also the most likely group to be prescribed a class of mind-regulating drugs called atypical antipsychotics, not to be confused with antidepressants. Conventional doctors consider these drugs to be among the best courses of treatment for mild to moderate levels of the dementia associated with Alzheimer's disease. However, in recent months, four major medical organizations have issued simultaneous warnings about the significant risks many of today's atypical antipsychotic drugs carry with them. The harmful side effects they cause include obesity, blood lipid imbalances and adult-onset (Type 2) diabetes. All of these conditions clearly increase the chance of developing heart disease or lead to a greater risk of suffering a heart attack or stroke.

In a recent issue of *Diabetes Care*, The American Diabetes Association, The American Psychiatric Association, The American Association of Clinical Endocrinologists, and some other associations all joined forces to warn about this class of drugs. The reason for this unprecedented move is that the companies which produce these drugs have refused to list their side effects on package labels out of fear that no one will be willing to take the drugs. In 2003 the FDA ordered these companies to do so, but to date, they have not complied.

Scandalous Drug Business

Naprosyn is a common drug of American origin used for treating arthritis. Even though the FDA discovered that the drug company had forged the documents which reported its drug testing on animals with regard to tumor formation and mortality, it is not in the power of the government to prohibit the sale of this drug.

Similar scandals are occurring in the treatment of hyperactive or tense children. Over one million American children, whose behavior is considered aberrant, receive *psycho-pharmaceutical drugs*, although not a single diagnostic technique exists to determine whether a child suffers from one of the nearly two dozen symptoms related to emotional tension. Yet the children are treated as 'slightly brain damaged'. The side effects of the drugs are often severe. The children show signs of retarded growth, develop high blood pressure, nervousness, sleeplessness and turn excessively passive and lethargic. They become depressed and apathetic, a common symptom among those who took the drugs. Making changes in their diets, such as eliminating stimulating foods like sugar, chocolate and other unnatural sweets, chips, breakfast cereals and basically all junk food, can help most of these children. Many children are highly allergic to artificial colorings and preservatives, soft drinks, packaged fruit juices, and foremost of all, artificial sweeteners that may cause brain damage. As discussed previously, artificial sweeteners are found in most unnatural, sweet-tasting foods and drinks.

Most clinical tests on new drugs are financed by the pharmaceutical industry, and nearly all information supplied to doctors about the products' effects and benefits comes from the drug companies. An investigation conducted by respected scientists, including four Nobel Laureates, found that clinical tests on new drugs are highly scandalous. When the FDA made spot checks on these tests, it discovered that 20 percent of the involved researchers used highly irregular practices, such as applying the wrong doses of drugs and/or forging documents. In one-third of the examined 'clinical tests', there were no tests done at all, and another one-third did not comply with the standard requirements for conducting such tests. The *Journal of the American Medical Association* reported on November 3, 1975, that the results of *only one-third* of all clinical tests could be considered reliable.

Therefore, at a time when most drugs are entering the market without scientific backing and justification, both physicians and patients ought to be vigilant and cautious about their use of drugs. Since there are no long term studies to prove that a certain drug a patient is using today will not cause him cancer, diabetes, or heart disease 15-20 years from now, he can never be sure that they won't. As long as one's life is not in real danger, it would be better to avoid drugs, especially if they are combined with other drugs, which amplifies their side effects by 2, 3, 4 or more times. If you want to know more about a drug, read the list of side effects accompanying the drug or consult the drug advisory board in your area (if available). Most medical doctors can only pass on the information they receive from the drug manufacturers.

The whole drug side effect issue is complicated by the fact that drug reactions are only rarely reported by general practitioners. The *British Journal of Clinical Pharmacology* reported in 1997 that "most prescription drugs are more dangerous than they appear because doctors rarely report side effects to the appropriate authorities." This tragic situation was confirmed by French researchers, who discovered massive underreporting of adverse reactions to prescription drugs. The French research revealed that only one out of 24,433 adverse reactions is reported to the various drug monitoring agencies. All drugs are poisonous, and even if they happen to have a few beneficial side effects, in the majority of cases these do not warrant their use.

Doctors are not innocent in this regard. Three out of four physicians fail to tell their patients about the toxic side effects of the prescription drugs they recommend. Many of the doctors claim that they just don't have the time to explain the risks involved to their patients. However, they obviously have the time to treat them during repeat visits for the diseases that result from the side effects of their prescriptions. Patients need to draw their own conclusions on this. Perhaps the following facts will help to make it easier.

- Over the last 10 years, the FDA has approved 12 drugs that have deadly side effects, including Vioxx, Celebrex, and Aleve, among others.
- The *Journal of the American Medical Association* reported several years ago that an estimated 125,000 Americans die each year from the side effects of FDA approved drugs. Since the new drug scandals that occurred in 2004-05, this figure is quite likely to be 10 times as high.
- The FDA approved the sale of the statin drug Baycol to lower cholesterol. One severe adverse reaction, discovered later, was the potentially fatal condition known as rhabdomyolysis, in which destruction of muscle tissue occurs. Despite such a severe adverse reaction, the FDA continues to approve the use of other statin drugs that are also associated with this deadly side effect.

- The FDA has aggressively suppressed natural alternatives to drugs. Red yeast rice, for example, known to be a safe and effective alternative to cholesterol-lowering drugs, was banned by the FDA in 2001.
- One in five patients is completely misdiagnosed by his doctor, who writes prescriptions for health problems the patient does not have.
- Up to 20 percent of all prescriptions given in hospitals could be just plain wrong, causing severe side effects, for which treatment is required with more prescriptions.

The Contraceptive Pill: Catastrophic Risks...

In the United States alone, about 15 million women are taking the contraceptive pill. The Pill seems to be the easiest method of preventing an unwanted pregnancy, but it is also one of the most risky ones. Although natural methods of contraception have at least the same success rate and are a fraction of the cost or free, they are rarely publicized. Despite warnings by an increasing number of health officials about the strong side effects of the drug, it is still regarded as the 'best and safest' method of contraception.

Women who continually use contraceptive pills are more likely to develop circulatory problems, liver tumors, headaches, depression and cancer than those who don't use them. The risk increases with age. Women taking the Pill who are between 30 and 40 have a three times higher risk of dying from a heart attack than women of the same age group who are non-users. Women who are over 40 and still using the contraceptive pill have a six times higher risk of developing high blood pressure, a four times higher risk of having a stroke, and a five times higher risk of developing thrombosis and embolism, a condition where a blood clot may form and then lodge in an artery close to the heart. The risk of suffering thrombosis is greatest among short-term users.

In August, 1996 newspapers were awash with the shocking story that the Pill has a 'time bomb' effect in causing breast cancer. A four-year study of the Pill, carried out by the Imperial Cancer Research Fund in Oxford, England, reanalyzed epidemiological evidence on the Pill from more than 150,000 women. The results show that *all* users face an increased risk of breast cancer, even for up to 10 years after they stop taking it.

According to the study, published in 1996 in the *Lancet*, women on the Pill faced a 25 percent increase in the risk of breast cancer, and that risk was still 16 percent for up to five years after the medication was discontinued. Another large study conducted at the Netherlands Cancer Institute, also published in the *Lancet*, showed that girls who started taking the Pill before the age of 20 were three and a half times more likely to get breast cancer. Among women over 36 who took the Pill for less than 4 years, the risk of developing breast cancer increased by 40 percent. What is very disturbing is that 97 percent of the women younger than 36, who had contracted breast cancer, had taken the Pill at some point in their lives, even for a short period of time. This raises a lot of questions, such as: "Is taking the Pill by a large portion of the female population responsible for the continuous breast cancer epidemic?"

Klim McPherson, arguably the most experienced British epidemiologist on HRT and the Pill, estimates that up to one in four long-term Pill users, who start on it early in life, will wind up with breast cancer. More studies are surfacing almost every other month. Another major Pill study, which concluded in September, 1996, determined that women who have taken the Pill at any time have a 60 percent increased risk of cervical cancer[45]. The repeatedly used medical argument that the risk of developing

---

[45] If you have a teenage daughter and are concerned about vaccinating her to protect her against cervical cancer, consider the following finding by the *New England Journal of Medicine*, Vol. 356, 19 May 2007. New information about the human

breast cancer with the Pill is outweighed by its benefits of protecting women against endometrial and ovarian cancer is no longer valid. In any event, risking one type of fatal cancer to prevent another type of fatal cancer is a very questionable conclusion. Because the Pill causes breast cancer and other diseases, it is outright dangerous and should not be sold to unsuspecting women.

The *intrauterine device* (IUD), also known as coil or loop, is not a safe method of contraception either. The IUD has been associated with a number of debilitating side effects. A 1974 report by the *Lancet* showed that women who have an IUD fitted and become pregnant nevertheless are 50 percent more likely to have a miscarriage as opposed to a 17 percent rate of miscarriage for those using any other kind of contraceptive. Pelvic inflammatory disease is also common among users. Other problems include cramping, backaches, the risk of an ectopic pregnancy, perforation of the uterus, a greater incidence of tubal infertility, skin rashes, and increased susceptibility to infection.

If you consider a potential pregnancy, which is not a dangerous illness, to be less of a disadvantage than risking your life by developing breast cancer, cervical cancer, a stroke or thrombosis, you are better off avoiding the Pill or any of the other highly invasive contraceptive methods such as *Inject-and-go contraception* and IUDs. I personally recommend mental birth control, the most ancient method of conception choice, as the preferable method for avoiding an unwanted pregnancy. It is very effective, cost-free, and without any side effects. The method can be learned within a few minutes from the little book *Mental Birth Control* by Mildred Jackson (costs less than $1). There are other approaches teaching mental birth control, such as a self-hypnosis (tape) by Barrie Konicov. (Do a Google search for mental birth control)

Other methods include 'Fertility Testers' which can determine the days of the month in which a woman is fertile. All that is required is a drop of her saliva. 'Persona' is another new method of contraception. Through simple urine testing, a small, computerized device informs a woman of the days she is at risk for becoming pregnant. 'Persona' is 93-95 percent reliable when used according to the instructions, which makes it as dependable as the condom. It is readily available at all 'Boots stores' in the U.K. In any case, the condom remains an option as well.

Caution about the new birth control pill: Lybrel recently launched Wyeth Pharmaceuticals' new birth control pill that eliminates women's periods. Women on the new pills do not menstruate, unlike those on the original oral contraceptives, which include a week of placebo pills at the end of the cycle to bring on menstruation. Since the drug has only been tested for one year (I wonder why), there is no way of knowing what the long-term side effects will be. Considering the serious side effects that have resulted from the use of traditional oral contraceptives, the new drug will most likely cause the same harm as the old ones, if not more.

Women who menstruate shed the thick lining of the uterus that builds up during the cycle. Although those on the new pill may not produce such a thick lining of the uterus, eventually, not discarding the thinner lining can lead to uterine diseases. In addition, menstruating women naturally remove excessive iron and protein from their blood, which greatly reduces their risk of cancer and heart disease. Not having this opportunity increases their chances of serious illness in the future. As always, a short-term gain may actually turn out to be a long-term loss. Being able to interfere with the body's natural design

---

papillomavirus (HPV) cervical cancer vaccine Gardasil has raised serious questions about its effectiveness. Although Gardasil blocked almost 100 percent of infections by two strains of HPV, it only reduced the incidence of cervical cancer precursors by 17 percent. Gardasil may, by blocking only specific strains, allow other varieties of HPV to flourish. The vaccine's manufacturer, Merck, has said that the vaccine reduces the number of pre-cancerous lesions caused by HPV. But some have pointed out that Merck's study was not long enough to demonstrate the vaccine's effectiveness; it only lasted three years, although it was examining a disease that can take decades to develop. The U.S. state of Ohio is now considering making this vaccine mandatory.

in such a drastic way is not an indication of scientific advancement but of poor judgment and shortsightedness that will once again (mis)lead millions of people into the abyss of sickness and suffering. For Wyeth Pharmaceuticals it will mean a $250 million profit for the first year and many more to come.

3. Menopause - Disease or Natural Transformation?

The Folly of Hormone Replacement Therapy (HRT)

One of the most commonly treated 'diseases' among women today is the appearance of menopausal symptoms - indications that a woman's body may be going through major changes in her life. Doctors believe that these changes (and the symptoms) are caused by a decrease in the production of the female hormones, estrogens and progestogens, which the body uses to conduct the monthly cycles, pregnancy, and birth, among other rhythms. To postpone the onset of the dreaded illness 'menopause', which is often seen as a sign of rapid aging, and to reduce or eliminate the accompanying symptoms, doctors commonly prescribe a combination of hormones known as *Hormone Replacement Therapy* (HRT) (Or at least they used to until the recent media scare). The drugs are also supposed to prevent major illnesses that have been linked with diminished hormone production, including osteoporosis, heart disease, stroke and senile dementia.

Influenced by medical authorities and media reports, many menopausal women feel that they are suffering from a serious hormone deficiency, which may endanger their health. Consequently, they become convinced that Hormone Replacement Therapy (HRT) can help them lead a more comfortable and carefree life during and after menopause.

Yet it turns out that HRT is everything but preventive medicine, and the risks involved are serious. Taking extra hormones can even endanger a woman's life. According to research conducted at the Boston University Medical Center, U.S.A., the risks of suffering a thrombosis increase by 3.6 times with a 'normal' dose of hormones and by nearly 7 times if a woman is taking as much as 1.25 mg or more a day. As with the contraceptive Pill, the researchers found the risk to be greatest during the first year of usage.

In the United States, five million menopausal women are presently using hormone replacements. Numerous studies show that the longer a woman takes HRT, the greater is her risk of cancer. Specifically, breast cancer risk increases by three times and the risk of endometrial cancer by four times. An analysis of 16 studies on women who had been taking HRT for 15 years revealed that taking *estrogen* alone increased the risk of uterine and cervical cancers by 20 times and the combined HRT (estrogen and progestogen) increased the risk by up to 30 times. A Swedish study which looked at 23,000 women, showed that women who used only estrogen increased their risk of developing breast cancer by 80 percent over a control group. When progestogen was added, these women actually quadrupled their risk of cancer after four years! The most comprehensive combined analysis of studies (thirty-seven in number) of breast cancer risk found that long-term estrogen use increases a woman's risk of breast cancer by 60 percent. The results of the very large *Nurses' Health Study*, published in 1995 by the *New England Journal of Medicine*, found that for HRT-using women over 60, the risk of breast cancer was 71 percent. This is a severe blow to those doctors who recommend that women take HRT forever, or for at least for ten years after the onset of menopause. In addition, one study by the American Cancer Society involving 200,000 menopausal women found that those who stay on HRT for more than 10 years show a 70 percent increase in ovarian cancer over those who use HRT for a shorter period of time.

According to another study by Smith JS, Green J, 'Cervical Cancer and Use of Hormonal Contraceptives: A Systematic Review', The Lancet, 2003 Apr 5, cervical cancer is closely linked to oral contraceptives.

Apart from increasing one's risk of developing cancer, excessive estrogen causes salt and fluid retention, increases body fat, impairs blood-sugar control, interferes with the thyroid hormone, causes excessive hairiness and loss of scalp hair, increases blood clotting, causes depression and headaches, diminishes libido, reduces oxygen levels in all cells, causes a decline of zinc and the retention of copper, and gives rise to a cystitis-like syndrome. Over 70 per cent of women on estrogen or progestogen experience such strong side effects that half of them stop taking the drug after 6 months. In 1992, the *British Medical Journal* listed some of the side effects of HRT, which are very similar to the PMT-like symptoms these hormones are supposed to treat. They include: monthly period-like withdrawal bleeding and eventual breakthrough bleeding, abdominal cramps, bloating, breast tenderness, irritability, depression and anxiety.

Progestogens can also cause abnormally high calcium levels in the blood, alter its sugar and insulin concentrations, increase the severity of migraines, and lead to gallbladder disease, liver cancer and urinary tract infections.

Yet many doctors still prescribe HRT routinely as a preventive to avoid discomfort during menopause, wrongly assuming that every menopausal woman will also suffer from discomfort. Hormones are even sold as rejuvenatory drugs and prescribed for circulatory problems. They are recommended to middle-aged women who develop signs of depression, although depression can occur at any age and may be caused by numerous other factors than a drop in hormone levels.

In America, doctors use a highly detailed manual called the *Physician's Desk Reference*. By law, the drug manufacturers are required to list all the risks of their drugs in this manual. The entry for Hormone Replacement Therapy includes: *womb cancer; breast tenderness/enlargement; undesirable weight gain/loss; elevated blood pressure; mental depression; reduced carbohydrate and glucose tolerance; hair loss; vaginal candidacies (thrush); jaundice; abdominal cramps; vomiting; cystitis-like syndrome.* Menopausal symptoms may begin to seem mild when compared with any of these side effects.

HRT Fails to Prevent Bone Loss

Many older women take HRT to prevent osteoporosis - a disease characterized by a loss of minerals from bone tissue. A large number of them have been warned by their doctors that their bones will crumble if they don't take it. The latest results from an ongoing study of 670 women in Framingham, Massachusetts, published in the *New England Journal of Medicine*, October, 1993 shows, however, that HRT fails to protect women from *osteoporosis* - therefore eliminating one of the main reasons for its use. Only those women who were on HRT for longer than 7-10 years, far longer than most women stay on the drug, had higher bone mineral density. However, even those on HRT for 10 years were still not protected from osteoporosis. As soon as they stopped taking HRT, bone mineral density declined rapidly, so that by age 75 it was only 3.2 per cent higher than it was in women who had never taken the hormones.

Increased bone mineral density has always been considered a positive effect of the long-term use of estrogen and progestogens contained in HRT and the contraceptive pill. But researchers from the University of Pittsburgh, U.S.A., found that women whose bone mineral density increased as a result of taking extra hormones also have a far greater chance of developing breast cancer. The indicator for breast cancer risk is therefore not, as previously assumed, bone mineral density but hormone supplementation.

Since most women begin menopause in their fifties, and the greatest risk of fractures is when they are in their eighties, HRT offers no benefits, unless they take it for 30 years or longer. In such a case, the risk of developing cancer and other health problems is so high that the use of these drugs is rarely warranted.

In 1992, the *New England Journal of Medicine* provided clear evidence that *lack of estrogen does not cause osteoporosis*. In fact, some evidence suggests that estrogens actually contribute to osteoporosis. Women experience significant bone loss during the 10 to 15 years before menopause, despite an ample supply of estrogen. During this time there is an almost total decline of *progesterone*, another female hormone. Synthetic progesterone, called *progestins,* is now given, combined with estrogen, but the combined drug has no less serious side effects than estrogen does alone. On the other hand, natural *progesterone*, as contained in wild yam, for example, has no negative side effects. If it is applied topically in the form of a cream, it can drastically reduce menopausal symptoms and rebuild bone. Natural progesterone affects the bone-building cells whereas estrogen affects the cells in control of bone reabsorption. For this reason, HRT can only temporarily reduce the rate of bone density loss; it cannot stimulate the body's bone-building cells to produce more bone material.

The body is extremely reluctant to utilize synthetic drugs. It knows what it natural and what is fake. Hence the difference in the effects of natural and synthetic progesterone. The main reason for poor progesterone production in the body is congestion in the liver, reproductive organs, and other organs of elimination, as well as an unbalanced diet and lifestyle.

What Really Causes Brittle Bones?

An increasing number of health practitioners and women recognize that meat, milk and cheese, instant soups and puddings, carbonated beverages, sugar, and other stimulants such as caffeine and tobacco, alcohol and chocolate can remove calcium and other minerals from the bones faster than they can be absorbed or synthesized by the body. Consuming such foods contributes to *osteoporosis* more than a decrease in hormones does (if the hormonal decreases affect done density at all). The rate of urinary calcium excretion, for example, increases significantly after the consumption of a high protein meal, that is, one consisting of meat. According to a 1988 study of 1600 women, published in the *American Journal of Clinical Nutrition*, vegetarians have more bone density than age-matched meat eaters. Another safe way to increase bone mineral density is exercise. Research, published in 1996 in the *Lancet*, shows that weight-bearing (as opposed to aerobic) exercise can substantially increase bone mineral density by between 14 and 37 percent.

Calcium absorption is directly linked with the hormonal form of vitamin D, which is synthesized through sunlight. Lack of exposure to sunlight alone can lead to bone density loss. Also, excessive exercise and activity (anything that causes exhaustion) deplete the body's calcium stores. One of the main reasons for decreased availability of calcium in the body is diminished bile secretion in the liver due to the accumulation of gallstones in its bile ducts. Without enough bile, calcium cannot be absorbed properly. To meet all the calcium requirements of the bones the body has to rely on its own abilities to produce this mineral. For example, the enzyme *alkaline phosphatase* works with magnesium to produce calcium-crystals in the bone. Women on HRT have the lowest levels of alkaline phosphatase and are therefore not able to produce enough new bone tissue. (HRT only prevents the loss of old bone)

The body's original design does not include the premature destruction of its own skeleton. If it becomes weak or is destroyed, this is due to factors other than hormone deficiency, such as gallstone accumulation in the liver, a highly acidic diet and lack of simple weight-bearing exercise. Menopause is a natural phenomenon for which the body is well prepared, provided its basic metabolic functions have not been interfered with.

Can HRT Prevent Heart Disease?

Claims that HRT protects against coronary heart diseases are highly spurious. Why should we believe that while *estrogen* in the contraceptive pill is known to increase the risk of cardiovascular disease, in HRT it prevents this very condition? To achieve clarify in the midst of so much confusion, a group of Dutch scientists analyzed 18 major HRT studies. They found that women on HRT were healthier than non-users, not because they were taking HRT, but because they represented a segment of society that could afford regular medical care and would be likely to have lower rates of all illnesses (*British Medical Journal*, May 1994).

Being in a low risk group for illness, however, is no guarantee for preventing the side effects of HRT. The extensive 1991 *Nurses' Health Study* showed a 46 percent increase in ischemic stroke risk among nurses using HRT, despite the fact that this group is comprised of women with less diabetes, less cigarette smoking, and less adiposity than those not using *estrogen*. Six years earlier, the Framingham, Massachusetts study suggested that the risk of heart disease actually increased with the use of HRT. Similar results were reported by the *Journal of the American Medical Association* in 1995. One of the first placebo-controlled trials studying the relationship between HRT and heart disease showed more cases of heart disease among those taking HRT than those given a placebo. In 2004, one of several Women's Health Initiative (WHI) studies on HRT was shut down because using these hormones endangered the lives of too many women. This eight-year study of 11,000 women was stopped in its 7th year when it was determined that estrogen therapy may increase the risk of stroke.

Claims that HRT can prevent Alzheimer's disease are also unfounded. There is not a shred of evidence that indicates HRT can keep the brain clear and sharp. A 15-year study published in 1993 by the *Journal of the American Medical Association* has shown that estrogen intake does not slow any reduction in cognitive functions among women. Furthermore, a 2003 study showed that combined HRT actually increased the risk of developing Alzheimer's disease and other forms of dementia. The FDA now requires a warning about this on all HRT drug labeling.

Furthermore, a University of Rochester study reported that women who took HRT suffered from impaired hearing. If all of this does not deter a woman from using HRT, a recent study from Brigham and Women's Hospital in Boston, Massachusetts, showed a sharply increased risk of asthma for women taking either estrogen alone or combined HRT. Arguably, none of these health problems is as significant as the 2002 revelation that HRT increases the risk of heart disease, the one disease that kills more women than any other.

As I have shown, this risk was known years before 2002, but was purposely concealed from millions of unsuspecting women who are now suffering the long-term consequences of a treatment program that was pushed by relentlessly greedy drug producers. Their policies are calculating and manipulative. Drug makers conduct trials in preparation for an FDA review and then withhold the studies that could be damaging - submitting only the research that encourages regulatory approval. Obviously, by withholding the negative studies' results, doctor are encouraged to prescribe a drug without knowing about some of the associated problems. Fortunately, the scandalous practices surrounding HRT research were discovered and announced by the mass media.

Menopause - Not a Disease

There exists only a *correlation*, not a *causal* relationship, between low female hormones and frequent headaches, heavy bloating, hot flashes, and depression that some women experience as they enter menopause. If a woman's body were genetically programmed to develop a true hormone deficiency which would affect her vital functions, every woman in the world reaching a certain age should be suffering from these or similar symptoms. Yet, only a fraction of women worldwide encounter menopausal symptoms. Most of those who do live in developed countries. To understand menopause and the unpleasant and, often, unbearable symptoms that sometimes accompany this change in a woman's life, we need to separate these two issues and see them for what they truly are.

Beginning of a New Phase of Life

Women who view menopause negatively - as a sign of mental and physical decline - can experience adverse psychological consequences with the onset of menopause (Gannon, 1985). By contrast, in countries where women achieve higher status in middle age, like Sweden, Finland, India and China, few, if any signs of menopause are reported (Varpa, 1970). These findings point out the importance of cultural attitudes. In other words, what women expect or feel about the midlife phase in their life determines what they will actually experience.

Menopause is one of the most important time periods in a woman's life - a time when major transformations occur on the physical, mental and spiritual levels. It is a time for re-evaluating life and entering a new phase of maturity, wisdom and success. With a greater sense of maturity and wisdom, a woman can more easily revise some of her outdated beliefs and habits, improve her diet and lifestyle, and begin to focus on the deeper issues of life. Sometimes, changes in one's marital relationship, children growing up and leaving home, caring for ailing parents or employment-related issues may coincide with hormonal changes and produce a physical/emotional crisis.

The inner transformation that the menopausal woman goes through can use up a lot of energy, as well as tax her immune system and emotional strength. This is likely to bring to light any hidden anxieties or physical imbalances that may have been suppressed or left unnoticed for a long time. If a woman was able to live an unhealthy lifestyle or have a poor diet without developing major health problems before menopause, she won't be able to afford doing the same during and after this transition. Her 'new purpose' in life, whatever that may be, requires a pure and well-functioning physiology.

The ovaries of a woman entering menopause *purposely* reduce their production of estrogen. Menopause is not a sign of becoming old or the body becoming useless; it simply prevents a woman from conceiving children so that she can devote the rest of her time and energy to the process of developing and maturing new, formerly untapped skills and capabilities. During midlife and advanced age, a healthy woman's adrenal glands and fat cells begin to take over the role of producing enough female hormones to keep her body vital and efficient. Since she cannot reproduce any longer, it would actually be harmful if she did maintain the old levels of hormones. (High estrogen levels are responsible for breast cancer.) So menopause, as such, does not cause hormone deficiencies at all. The story, however, is very different if a woman hasn't been healthy before the onset of menopause.

It's Not the Lack of Hormones…But…

Hormones are made from the food we eat. The body's ability to produce the right amount of hormones is mostly determined by the quality of food we eat, the body's digestive ability and the condition of the liver. Women who suffer from severe menopausal symptoms do not experience this upset because of a sudden drop in hormone production, but rather because a long-standing digestive weakness is now becoming more apparent. During a woman's midlife transition, dietary imbalances and stress generally cause more chaos and confusion in the body and mind than they did before. As a direct result of this now-amplified interference in the balanced performance of mind and body, the woman's ovaries may receive fewer nutrients. This, in turn, will lower her hormone production. For similar reasons, the adrenal glands and fat cells may also be unable to maintain their normal output of these hormones.

Stress, alone, can greatly affect the endocrine system that controls blood sugar levels (which affect mood swings), energy levels, calcium balance, weight, and sex hormones. Stimulants have the same effect as stress. Regular consumption of alcohol, coffee, sugar, chocolate, soft drinks, sports drinks, diet drinks and foods containing sweeteners like aspartame, and cigarettes strongly interferes with hormone production and is, therefore, sufficient to trigger strong menopausal symptoms. Cigarette smoking by itself accelerates the destruction of estrogen. During menopause a woman's ovaries naturally reduce hormone production. The above stimulants can trigger powerful and regular stress responses in the body that eventually lead to hormone deficiency. A middle-aged woman simply has no hormone reserves that she can afford to waste. It is incorrect to attribute the occurrence of menopausal symptoms to the natural decrease in ovarian hormones. If menopause is a 'hormone-deficiency disease', it is certainly not caused by a lack of hormones.

How to Make the Best of Menopause

A balanced diet and lifestyle according to body type (see chapters 4-7) can make a woman's transition into the next phase of her life much smoother and more comfortable. A well-balanced vegetarian, low or no dairy diet that is rich in natural fiber often works wonders. Foods that are processed, refined, preserved, microwave heated, frozen or reheated may still contain enough nutrients but are all deprived of their natural life force (Chi, Ki or Prana). Without life force, these foods may reach the bloodstream but are unable to enter the cells where they need to be in order to keep the body healthy. This basic physiological principle was demonstrated in a classic experiment involving 6,000 healthy cats (as mentioned earlier). The cats were given highly nutritious food that was warmed in a microwave oven prior to feeding them. All 6,000 cats died from cell starvation within six weeks.

Freshly prepared meals composed of salads, cooked vegetables, grains and legumes serve the menopausal woman best. Fresh fruits eaten in between meals (mid-morning or mid-afternoon) provide her with extra nourishment and life force. Bile secretions and other digestive juices peak at midday, which makes it easier to digest a heavier meal at this time than one eaten in the evening. Heavy meals eaten in the evening, especially after 7:00 p.m., tend to putrefy and ferment in the gastrointestinal tract during the night.

Hot flashes are not necessarily a sign of estrogen deficiency. However, they often, but not always, indicate that bile and toxins from undigested food are back flowing from the intestinal tract into the stomach, chest and head areas. The afflicted person is unable to digest food properly, causing food intolerance and food allergies. **Note:** To test for food allergies, take your pulse; then place a small piece of the food under your tongue and take your pulse again; if it is higher than before, you may be allergic to that particular food.

Hot flashes may also indicate excessive concentration of food protein in the blood and protein storage in the walls of the capillaries and arteries. This may raise one's blood protein values - *Hemocrit* and *hemoglobin* - which give the appearance of redness and heat in the face and chest. Eating a high-protein diet also means that calcium is constantly being leached from the bones, furthering the risk of osteoporosis. The thickening of the blood and connective tissues reduces the nutrient supply to cells, including the *estrogen-producing* ovarian cells and fat cells. The resultant lack of adequate estrogen, in turn, disrupts hormonal balance and may also bring about a disturbance of proper fluid maintenance, also known as water retention. A weakening of eliminative functions, which causes nervous disorders, including headaches, irritability and depression may also occur.

Menopausal symptoms, however, can just as often have a spiritual basis. Hot flashes, for example, may be triggered by an awakening of the spiritual energy *Kundalini*. The heat waves can 'strike' like lightening during mealtimes, while resting and even during sleep. As this intense energy rushes upward from the base of the spine or uterus toward the head, it can cause tremendous heat in the body along with severe sweating. Following the hot flash, the body may experience a cold spell.

Treat Your Body Kindly

Energy boosting therapies such as yoga, shiatsu, reflexology, meditation and relaxation exercises, and brisk walking may make you more comfortable during menopause. In fact, this time period may even become one of the most rewarding stages in a woman's life. Although in some cases, hormone replacements can give almost instant relief of symptoms, they unwittingly allow toxins to build up to the point of saturation. This becomes the cause of more serious illness later, such as cancer or thrombosis. HRT does not correct metabolic imbalances in the body. On the contrary, it interferes with the body's own synthesis of hormones, upsets basic digestive and metabolic functions, and causes strong withdrawal symptoms once it is discontinued.

Some of the most effective herbal compounds to regulate menstruation, ease menopausal symptoms and maintain proper hormone production by the pituitary gland include *black cohosh, agnus castus* and *false unicorn root*, best utilized when taken together. *Agnus castus* is known for safely removing fibroids, cysts and endometriosis. Taking 25-35 drops of *agnus castus* tincture with water each day for three months can normalize and stabilize female hormone production. Another effective natural alternative to HRT is *pfaffia. Wild yam root*, applied topically, may relieve hot flashes almost immediately. *Evening primrose oil* also helps the ovaries maximize their output of estrogen during the early stages of menopause. For those who still don't find relief, *maca root* may be the answer - it jogs the pituitary and hypothalamus and balances hormones in the body. Maca root has helped to reduce hot flashes by 80 percent. Start taking two teaspoons per day, one in the morning and one in the late afternoon. Since maca has an energizing effect, you should avoid it too close to bedtime. When symptoms die down, reduce your intake to a ¾ teaspoon twice daily. Mix it with juice or take it in capsule form, as its taste is somewhat unpleasant.

Still, the best preventive action for reducing or avoiding menopausal symptoms is cleansing the liver, colon and kidneys. Removing the hundreds or thousands of gallstones that are typically found in the liver bile ducts of almost every middle-aged American woman today not only helps to make the menopausal experience smoother and more comfortable, but it also greatly reduces the risk of the following ailments: *bowel cancer, ovarian, uterine and breast cancer, cardiovascular disease, osteoporosis, breast cysts and breast tenderness, polycystic ovary syndrome, endometriosis, heavy menstrual bleeding, fibroid symptoms, constipation, varicose veins, gallstones, and premenstrual symptoms*. For details, see my book *The Amazing Liver and Gallbladder Flush*.

Menopausal problems can be an opportunity for a woman to put her life in order on all levels. Menopause brings to the surface whatever issues a woman may not have dealt with successfully while she was busy taking care of her family or career. The midlife phase doesn't need to be a midlife crisis.

Instead, it can be a woman's greatest opportunity to deal with any unresolved issues in her life, thereby freeing her from all kinds of limitations - physical, emotional and spiritual. The first and most important step in that direction is to know that menopause isn't a disease and that the body isn't doing anything wrong. Supporting it and treating it with kindness and respect during this important time in a woman's life can make all the difference.

4. What Makes Medical Drugs so Expensive?

Thanks to *Judicial Reform Investigations* (JRI) we now know why pharmaceutical drugs are so expensive. Some companies claim the active ingredients of the drugs cost a lot, which leads to the high prices. Many drugs sell for more than $2 per tablet. JRI did some investigating and located the offshore chemical synthesizers that supply the FDA-approved active ingredients to the drug manufacturers. JRI collected the data and pricing for the active ingredients and the consumer markup price for the most popular drugs in the U.S. For example, the popular drug Xanax sells for $136. At a cost price of 0.02 for its active ingredients, the markup for Xanax is a staggering 683,950 percent. Norvask sells for $188.29 but costs $0.14 to make; its markup is 134,493 percent. Zolofts's markup is 11,821 percent. Prozac is among the biggest money makers of all times, with a 224,973 percent markup. Lipitor is one of the most expensive drugs to produce ($5.80), but it sells for $272.37; its markup is 4,696 percent. Some generic drugs were marked up as much as 3,000 percent or more.

CBS's famous *Sixty Minutes* national TV show, aired 1st April, 2007, revealed the biggest ever health scandal, which so far cost the American public nearly $1.5 trillion. The scam is orchestrated by the pharmaceutical companies, which through powerful lobbying in the American Congress, helped pass a prescription drug bill that prevents Medicare from buying prescription drugs at a discounted rate for their members. Other institutions, such as the U.S. Department of Veterans Affairs (VA), negotiate the price for prescription drugs directly with the pharmaceutical companies and pay merely 10 percent of the amount that Medicare has to pay for the top 10 prescription drugs. Since this bill was passed over three years ago, Medicare has been legally required to pay an average of 60 percent more than the VA pays for the same prescription drugs. Most other countries in the world, which receive their prescription drugs from the same source as Medicare, also pay the lower rates. The Medicare drug plan, devised by the pharmaceutical industry and approved by lawmakers benefiting from it, will earn the pharmaceutical companies over 1.5 trillion dollars over the next 10 years, all paid for by the taxpayers who finance the Medicare program. In other words, all U.S. taxpayers directly contribute to the already astronomical profits of the pharmaceutical industry.

Just consider the enormous profiteering taking place in the cancer industry. The newer anticancer drugs are very expensive, especially when they are used in combination. The price of drugs for eight weeks of treatment can be $10,000 or more. If other drugs are added, this raises the cost of the medication alone to $20,000-$30,000. According to Johns Hopkins University *Health Alert:* "When these therapies improve survival by only a few months, this presents troubling issues for cancer patients, their doctors, insurers, and society as a whole." Considering that the production costs for these drugs are a tiny fraction of their selling price and that nearly one in every two people in the U.S. will develop cancer at some stage in his or her life, you can readily understand why the cancer industry makes no real attempt to find a true cure for cancer. Instead, it tries everything in its power to keep this most profitable business in the world growing.

David Walker, who was the nation's top accountant - the Comptroller General of the United States - from 1998 to 2008, said the following about the new Medicare plan: "The prescription drug bill was probably the most fiscally irresponsible piece of legislation since the 1960s." He perceives it as the most powerful force driving the United States toward bankruptcy. With one stroke of the pen, Walker says, the federal government increased existing Medicare obligations nearly 40 percent over the next 75 years. "We'd have to have eight trillion dollars today, invested in treasury rates, to deliver on that promise," Walker explains. Asked how much we actually have, Walker says, "Zip." In addition to the financial fiasco, the plan forces millions of older Americans to accept inferior drug coverage. All the government does is to borrow money to pay for what it cannot afford to pay. The main beneficiaries are the drug companies and those politicians who are paid handsomely to close their eyes to the fraud at hand.

The drug companies (and politicians) are not the only ones making a fortune from these drugs. The pharmacies also take a big cut. For example, if you want to buy a brand name drug that costs $100 for 100 pills, but your pharmacists offers you a generic version of the same drug for $80; you may think you are getting a great deal. This is not the case. The pharmacy gets the 100 pills for $10 and sells them to you for $80! That's why the pharmacy business is doing so well, as evidenced by the abundance of pharmacies everywhere.

5. Surgery is Rarely Necessary

Several years ago a committee of the American Congress investigating procedures of surgery in the United States came to the conclusion that 2.4 million operations are performed unnecessarily each year. The cost of these unneeded surgical procedures is 12,000 lives and 4 billion U.S. dollars. The latest figures show that some six million unnecessary surgeries are now performed each year.

A major study found that most people who underwent surgery did not actually need it, and half of them did not even require medical treatment. Many were children suffering tonsil infections. Parents rarely object to the removal of their children's tonsils, especially since not many side effects are recorded for this type of surgery. The death rate from tonsil operations amounts to only 1 in 3,000 or even less, statistically insignificant, unless the one child happens to be yours.

Only a few parents know that tonsils are an important part of the immune system and are needed to keep the head area free from toxins, bacteria and viruses. It has been shown that many children become depressed, pessimistic, fearful, insecure and shy after surgery, 'character traits' that may stay with them for the rest of their lives. Natural methods can support the body in overcoming an infection of the tonsils without the need for surgery. (See *Natural Methods of Nursing* in chapter 10.) What applies to small operations applies equally to more serious ones. The need for surgical intervention is indicated only in certain extreme situations.

Most people believe that removing an inflamed appendix is a necessity, and that diagnosing appendicitis is routine and reliable. But surgeons get it wrong up to 45 percent of the time, even when they perform an exploratory *laporotomy* in order to come up with a diagnosis. False-negatives - claiming there isn't a problem when there is one - also run high, at around 33 percent. One in five patients with appendicitis leaves the hospital without a correct diagnosis ever being made, and one in five appendixes removed by surgery is found to be normal. In the U.S. this amounts to 20,000 healthy appendixes mistakenly removed every year.

One of the most common operations performed today is coronary bypass surgery. A seven-year controlled study has demonstrated that except for very rare cases where the left aorta is affected, coronary bypass surgery does nothing to improve the heart's condition. In addition, the mortality rate among patients with low risk heart disease who undergo a bypass operation is higher than it is among those with a high risk. A 1998 study, published by the *New England Journal of Medicine*, showed that patients who suffer a mild heart attack and are given a bypass or balloon angioplasty are more likely to die as a result of the surgery. Another study that involved researchers from 14 major heart hospitals around the world, found that up to one-third of all bypass operations were not only unnecessary, but actually hastened the death of the patient.

Angioplasty, a relatively new procedure used to open arteries, offers an even lower survival rate than bypass surgery. Several research studies confirm that patients who have undergone these types of surgery are as likely to suffer a heart attack as those who haven't. The relief of chest pain (angina) that patients may experience after a bypass operation cannot always be attributed to an actual improvement of the condition. Oftentimes the perceived improvement is due to the cutting of nerve strands during the procedure, to the secretion of endorphins, which are the body's natural painkillers, and/or to the placebo response.

In the case of a bypass operation, the newly inserted pieces of coronary arteries can block up easily again if the cause of arteriosclerosis is not removed. The U.S. National Institute of Health estimated that 90 percent of America's bypass surgery patients receive no benefits. Major lasting improvements were attributed to an improved diet and lifestyle, stress reduction, smoking cessation and regular exercise. (See also chapter 9)

All artery-opening methods, like bypass surgery and stents, the widely used wire cages that hold plaque against an artery wall, can alleviate crushing chest pain for a certain period of time. Stents can also rescue someone in the midst of a heart attack by obliterating an obstruction and keeping the closed artery open, at least for a while.

But as it turns out, the vast majority of heart attacks do not originate with obstructions that narrow arteries. "There has been a culture in cardiology that the narrowings were the problem and that if you fix them, the patient does better," said Dr. David Waters, a cardiologist at the University of California at San Francisco.

Heart researchers now know that most heart attacks do not occur because an artery is narrowed by plaque. Instead, they say, heart attacks occur when an area of plaque bursts, a clot forms over the area and blood flow is abruptly blocked. They assert that in 75 to 80 percent of cases, the plaque that erupts was not obstructing an artery and would not have been stented or bypassed. Because the plaque which is attached to the artery walls is soft and fragile, it produces no symptoms and would not be seen as an obstruction to blood flow. This makes heart attacks very unpredictable. True blockages in an artery would make themselves known as severe chest pain and breathing difficulties.

Since heart patients may have hundreds of vulnerable plaques, surgeons cannot go after all of them. In fact, coronary artery surgery does nothing to the soft plaque, which is the real time bomb ticking in the coronaries of heart disease patients.

Other dangers lurk in a hospital's operating room. According to a *New England Journal of Medicine* report, 1,500 patients a year in the U.S. leave the operating table with some of the hospital's equipment still inside them. Wayward clamps, sponges, electrodes, retractors and various other instruments take up permanent residence in the chest, abdomen, hips and body cavities like the vagina. According to these findings, the chances of having such items planted in your body are higher if you happen to be overweight.

Complications from these blunders can lead to internal bleeding, infection and sometimes death. In quite a few patients, though, these missing items are not discovered until the person undergoes another procedure or has an X-ray or ultrasound.

Fear-Motivated Operations

In the United States alone *nearly one million women a year* sacrifice their uterus to the scalpel. This means that more than half of all American women will have had a *hysterectomy* by the time they reach the age of 65. Many of these women will suffer from post-operative syndromes such as depression, anxiety and increased susceptibility to stress. I have seen in my own practice that most women who have had a hysterectomy developed ovary problems, breast lumps, digestive disorders or breast cancer 1-5 years after the operation.

An investigation carried out in six New York hospitals found *that 43 percent of all uterus operations were unjustified*. Other research shows that only 10 percent of hysterectomies are warranted. 15 percent of hysterectomies are carried out to remove cancerous tumors, and are thus considered necessary. The other 85 percent are due to uterine fibroids, endometriosis, or other causes of pelvic pain and excessive bleeding. Thousands of women every year have a *full* hysterectomy (including the removal of the ovaries), but have not given their consent prior to the surgery. Only a few of them make use of the law to seek compensation, but money cannot return a woman's uterus, which is symbolic of womanhood.

Even from a surgical perspective, a woman has less invasive and traumatic options. First, there is the less invasive *nryomectomy*, which preserves fertility by removing just the fibroid, but keeps the rest of the reproductive system intact. However, nryomectomy can be just as traumatic as having a hysterectomy. A second new procedure is called a uterine artery embolization (UAE) and is performed by an interventional iadiologist. Of course, there are also a number of natural methods, like the ones explained in this book that can be used to prevent and remove fibroids and other reproductive disorders. Balancing estrogen levels through liver cleansing and dietary changes is very important for any woman suffering from female disorders. It is a well-known fact that fibroids tend to shrink and disappear after menopause when estrogen levels decrease. The liver is in charge of breaking down estrogen, but is prevented from doing so properly when it is congested with intrahepatic gallstones.

Most fibroids develop when congestion of the cisterna chyli vessels (a group of sac-like lymph vessels located in the middle of the abdomen) prevents the proper drainage of metabolic waste products and dead, turned-over cells from the female reproductive organs. In most cases, there is also a history of constipation. By addressing the underlying causes of fibroids, the reproductive organs can resume their full functions. Having a hysterectomy, on the other hand, is not without risks. The mortality rate is 1 in 1,000 procedures, and serious complications occur 15 times more frequently than that. Side effects can occur in more than 40 percent of operations; they include urinary retention or incontinence, significant reduction in sexual response, early ovarian failure, risk of a fatal blood clot and bowel problems.

Induction, Cutting and Caesarean Section

Pregnant women are generally treated with respect and special care, but the methods of delivery used today can have an adverse effect on mother and baby alike. Before the era of hospital deliveries, the responsibility for handling deliveries was given to competent women. Home was considered the best place for all involved. This had been a common practice around the world for thousands of years. Provided that the appropriate hygienic measures were taken, very few birth complications occurred. Today, however, with most deliveries being handled by male doctors and taking place in the sterile environment of a hospital room, we have the highest rates of complications at birth. Research from Britain, Switzerland and Holland, published by the *British Medical Journal* in 1996, found that planned home births were the safest of all options, including hospital deliveries.

In hospitals, delivering mothers are watched over by a number of electronic instruments and machines that monitor every possible change and that signal the need for an operation just in case something goes wrong. One of the most common types of surgery during delivery is known as an episiotomy or 'cutting'. The procedure helps to widen the vagina so that the baby's head and shoulders come out more easily. This routine operation is supposed to prevent tearing of the vagina. Yet if the mother were not induced and/or made numb by drugs and were properly prepared for the delivery, she would know perfectly well how and when and when not to push to release the child from the birth canal at the right time. The pain would tell her exactly what to do during the birth process. This would naturally prevent tearing of the vagina. Even if it did tear, the injury would heal much faster than a cut inflicted by a surgical knife. Because it severs important nerves, 'cutting' also lowers the mother's sexual sensitivity, something that doesn't happen with 'natural' tearing.

The second most unnecessary but most commonly applied operation during delivery is the *Caesarean section*. If the monitoring electronic instruments indicate a sign of irregularity in the heartbeat of the baby, the mother is often cut open and the baby is pulled from her womb. It is well known that the baby's heartbeat can react to a sudden loud noise made in the proximity of the mother, something that is more likely to occur in a hospital or operation room than it would at home. An unborn child may increase his heartbeat because of irritating lights shining on the mother's stomach or strong electromagnetic fields caused by nearby electronic appliances such as monitors. Controlled birth studies have shown that a Caesarean section is performed 3-4 times more frequently if electronic devices were used to monitor the birth rather than a simple stethoscope.

Mothers in the midst of labor often consent to a Caesarean section when they see intensified signals of their baby's heartbeat flashing on the monitor in front of them. It is quite likely that a baby's heart activity produces erratic changes when cold electrodes are attached to its head while it is squeezed through the narrow tube of the mother's womb. The procedure of connecting electrodes to the head of the baby before it is born is itself an invasion that may have serious consequences. A controlled study revealed that 65 percent of all children whose birth had been controlled electronically were at risk for developing growth and behavioral problems later in their lives.

The very setup of a delivery room in the hospital, which looks much like an operation theater, can induce a fear and stress response in a sensitive mother. The sudden release of anxiety-provoking stress hormones by the mother may also affect the fetus and make him fearful. The mother's worries become his worries, and her fears become his. Recent studies have shown that within a fraction of a second after fear has caused the racing of a mother's heart, a fetus's heart begins pounding at double its normal rate. Fear can paralyze many important functions in the body, including those needed for delivering a baby.

Often it is no longer in the hands of the mother to 'decide' the time of delivering her baby. Unlike a wild animal, the human mother may be forced to give birth when the doctor tells her it is the 'correct' time, even though, as it has been shown, his calculations can be wrong by several days or even weeks. Artificially induced delivery is considered more practical than natural delivery and also fits the doctor's schedule more conveniently. Induced birth, however, causes nearly three times as much pain to the mother as natural birth does. To deal with the pain she is given strong medications, all with strong side effects. It is a lesser-known fact that many of these mothers and their newly born babies end up in intensive care units.

In October 2007, the British Medical Journal published a major study of more than 94,000 births which found that women who have a planned (elective) caesarean section put themselves, and their babies, at increased risk of serious complications and death.

Over half of all Caesarean operations have serious complications. The mortality rate for mothers who have a Caesarean is *twenty six* times higher than among mothers who give birth naturally. Since 75-80 percent of them are performed unnecessarily due to excessive use of the new electronic monitoring devices, a change of policy could drastically reduce mortality rates among Caesarean mothers. Risk of requiring a hysterectomy after a caesarian was four times higher than after vaginal birth.

In addition to the harm done to mothers, babies who are delivered by Caesarean section are exposed to the danger of developing serious lung damage, which causes a shortage of breath previously found only in prematurely born babies. In naturally born babies (which includes not clamping the umbilical cord before it stops throbbing; see lotusbirth.com), the uterine contractions press out all the accumulated secretions in the baby's chest and lungs and eliminate them through its mouth. Caesarean deliveries account for more than 25 percent of all births today, of which only a few of these are justified. There are indicators when there is a *real* emergency, and the doctor normally knows well in advance when a Caesarean delivery will be necessary.

Fewer Surgeons and Medical Interventions - Fewer Deaths

The American College of Surgeons conceded that the U.S. population would require only about 50 percent of its current number of surgeons to secure America's needs for surgery during the next fifty years. In 1976, Los Angeles County registered a sudden reduction of its death rate by *eighteen* percent when many medical doctors went on strike against the increase of health insurance premiums for malpractice. In a study by Dr. Milton Roemer from the University of California, Los Angeles, 17 of the largest hospitals in the county showed a total of *60 percent* fewer operations during the period of the strike. When the doctors resumed work and medical activities went back to normal, death rates also returned to pre-strike levels.

A similar event took place in Israel in 1973. Doctors staged a one-month strike and reduced their daily number of patients from 65,000 to 7,000. For the entire month, mortality rates in Israel were down 50 percent. This seems to happen whenever doctors go on strike. A two-month work stoppage by doctors in the Columbian capital of Bogotá led to a 35 percent decline in deaths. This practically makes the medical profession, together with hospitals, the leading cause of death.

6. Hospitals - A Major Health Threat

In 1995, a report in the *Journal of the American Medical Association* (JAMA) said: "Over a million patients are injured in U.S. hospitals each year, and approximately 280,000 die annually as a result of these injuries. Therefore, the iatrogenic death rate dwarfs the annual automobile accident mortality rate of 45,000 and accounts for more deaths than all other accidents combined." These statistics have become a lot worse since 1995. Unless you require an emergency treatment, it is better to avoid hospitals altogether. Many hospitals today may pose a major risk to your health for the following reasons:

- They are filled with infection-causing bacteria that cannot be found anywhere else. Hospitals, which often house very large numbers of sick people, are the ideal breeding environment for the sometimes deadly bugs. Hospital patients generally have a lower level of immunity and offer little or no resistance to them. Many of the microbes are passed on to the patients through the cooling towers, air conditioning and heating systems in hospitals. The hospital staff, due to constant exposure to the bugs, is fairly immune to them, but may pass them on to patients by touching them or their food, bedding, clothing, or medications.
- Contrary to common belief, hospitals are among the most contaminated places in the world. In fact, it is virtually impossible to keep hospitals spotlessly clean, and it does not take much dirt to become a breeding place for billions of deadly infectious bacteria.
- Doctors can be the worst transmitters of disease in hospitals. Most doctors do not wash their hands except before an operation, when they wear sterilized gloves and gowns anyway. They may sometimes touch many dozens of patients within several hours, one after the other, without

washing their hands even once. Even the doctor's white gown is not as clean as it looks. It is only clean if it is washed every single day, which rarely happens. When it is washed, it comes into contact with the dirty laundry from the operating room, bed covers, pillowcases, etc. Many extremely harmful bugs survive the washing machine and dryer.

- Bed sheets may be clean, but mattresses and pillows are not. The chance of being infected by bugs living in them is 1 in 20.
- Fifty percent of all infections in hospitals occur because of the patient's contact with non-sterile medical instruments such as catheters and intravenous infusion installations. Before they were in common use, such infections occurred only very rarely.
- In the United States, over 90,000 people a year die from hospital-acquired infections. This figure does not account for those who are considered to be dying, or are already weakened by an operation. Yet they too are killed by a hospital-acquired infection.
- A 1,500-page report of a 3-year study on the causes of death in American hospitals revealed that a further '300,000 Americans die each year in hospitals as a result of medical negligence'.
- The most dangerous place in a hospital is the maternity ward because infants have not gained immunity against any disease-causing agents. The most vulnerable babies are these who are deprived of the antibodies contained in breast milk.
- A hospital patient may receive up to 12 different kinds of medication, all of which produce side effects that can lead to serious complications and even death.
- Many studies have shown that between 25 and 50 percent of the long-term patients staying in U.S. and U.K. hospitals are suffering from malnutrition due to a poor hospital diet. Malnutrition was found to be the major cause of death among older people in hospitals. An undernourished body is hardly able to defend itself against any type of illness. Add the toxic side effects of the drugs, the presence of deadly bugs, as well as the stress and anxiety that accompany an illness and a stay in a hospital, and a poorly nourished elderly person has very little chance of surviving.
- A spot check of 105 U.S. hospitals conducted by the American government showed that 69 of them had violated basic laws and rules. The commission in charge of granting licenses to hospitals (JCAH), however, refused to close them down.
- Most deliveries today take place in the operation theaters of hospitals, which when compared with home deliveries, increases the infant's risk of injury during delivery by six times, of getting stuck in the mother's birth canal by eight times, of requiring resuscitation techniques by four times, of becoming infected by four times, and of developing chronic physical problems by thirty times. In addition, a mother is three times as likely to hemorrhage if she gives birth in a hospital.
- More than 3,000 hospital patients in the U.S. undergo wrong-side surgery each year.

Given these and other major health risks linked with a stay in the hospital, it can be said that hospitals are among the most dangerous places in the world. I, therefore, advise you to do everything necessary to prevent illness from arising in the first place so that you can avoid hospitals altogether, unless of course, it is for an emergency like an accident.

Conclusion

This book may challenge many of our most ardently held beliefs about the nature of disease manifestation, and the practices and theories of modern medicine and nutritional science. Our currently held world views no longer seem sufficient to provide for a prosperous and healthy future. In fact, they may even superimpose upon us the frightening premonition that the future of life on Earth is at stake. Yet the new world is just beginning. The abolishment of outdated principles of living that have kept mankind limited and fearful for centuries leaves behind a mess of scattered pieces of knowledge that no longer make any sense. The views, which I have presented in these last few chapters, are certainly not the final answer to the puzzle of health and illness. As a matter of fact, any viewpoint is a limitation, whereas our true potential is unlimited.

It is not correct to say that the drug AZT used to treat AIDS, or the chemotherapy drugs, radiation or surgery applied to a malignant tumor are all useless or harmful. Conversely, it is also not right to claim that all natural treatments are useful or harmless. Considering the power that the placebo effect can have in any one person, it becomes clear that even poison like AZT may turn into nectar if a patient is convinced that it will cure his AIDS. Both disease and medicine are illusory projections of ourselves that can turn into 'reality' when we begin to identify with them or 'energize' them in one way or another. It may well be that a hopeful person receiving radiation therapy for cancer experiences no negative side effects at all and has a spontaneous remission. On the other hand, a depressed person who swallows a placebo pill to combat a headache may suffer a stroke. There are instances where people become so enraged that they suddenly suffer a fatal heart attack, even though their blood vessels are perfectly clean. By contrast, a person with 100 percent blocked arteries may create his own bypass and suffer no physical problems at all.

The deep conviction that a particular medicine can help you overcome an illness may be just as powerful as the pessimistic view that a certain illness like cancer can terminate your life. Deep trust, however, is rarely present in a person who has AIDS, MS or cancer diseases that are mainly caused by low self-worth and repressed emotions. As a recent study has found, distrust, anger and doubt are more common among people who are ill. Happy people with 'non-toxic' personalities rarely fall ill.

Health and disease are accurate projections of ourselves, and they mirror back to us everything we are or who we are. If a person wants to 'uproot' his cancer, which may be a manifestation of repressed anger and frustration, through x-rays, chemotherapy or radical surgery instead of learning to use the same energy to regain his peace of mind, the projection of his anger will sabotage any long-term benefits a given therapy may have. The basic message here is that *we can change the projection by changing ourselves*. This book suggests that you take responsibility for everything that happens to you. With it comes the power to make the appropriate changes that will unerringly lead you to the discovery that **you carry the key to the timeless secrets of health and rejuvenation within you.**

*"The natural force within each one of us
is the greatest healer of disease."*

~ Hippocrates

Product Information

To order books, Ener-chi Art pictures, and Ionized Stones
please contact:

Ener-Chi Wellness Center, LLC
Web Site: http://www.ener-chi.com
E-mail: andmor@ener-chi.com

Toll free (1-866) 258-4006 (U.S.A)
709-570-7401 (Canada)

See Product List below for products mentioned in this book

Ionic Water-Soluble Minerals

ENIVA Corporation
P.O. Box 49755
Minneapolis, MN 55449
U.S.A.
Toll Free: 1-866-999-9191
Tel: 1-763-398-0005
Fax: 1-763-795-8890
Web Site: http://www.eniva.com
Note: To order any products from Eniva,
you require a sponsor name and ID. You may use
the name and ID of the author,
Andreas Moritz, #13462.

Kornax Enterprises, L.L.C. (for the WaterOZ
products)
P.O. Box 783
Lyons, CO 80540
U.S.A.
Toll-free:1-877-328-1744 (U.S. & Canada)
Tel. 303-823-5813
Fax: 303-823-6780
Web Site: http://www.kornax.com

Unrefined Sea Salt

Redmond Minerals, Inc.
P.O. Box 219
Redmond, UT 84652
U.S.A.
Toll Free: 1-800-367-7258
Tel: 1-435-529-7402
Fax: 1-435-529-7486
E-mail: mail@redmondminerals.com
Web Site: http://www.realsalt.com

The Grain and Salt Society
273 Fairway Drive
Asheville, NC 28805
U.S.A.
Toll Free: 1-800-TOP-SALT (1-800-867-7258)
Fax: 1-828-299-1640
E-mail: topsalt@aol.com
Web Site: http://www.celtic-seasalt.com

Colema Board &
Colon Cleanse Equipments

Colema Boards of California, Inc
3660 Main St Suite C
Cottonwood, CA 96022
Tel (800) 745-2446
Web site: www.colema.com

Or for home colonics:
http://www.homecolonics.com/

Amen Health Products
P.O. Box 1635
Cottonwood, CA 96022
U.S.A.
Contact at: info@amenhealth.com
Toll-free 1-888-387-2636 Web site:
http://www.amenhealth.com

Free Colema Board Video Demonstration:
Web Site: http://www.colema.com/videodemo.htm

**Home and Professional Colon Hydrotherapy
Equipment:** Web Site: http://thecolonet.com

Herbs for the Kidney Cleanse

The Present Moment
3546 Grand Avenue
Minneapolis, Minnesota
U.S.A.
Mail Order: 800-378-3245
        612-824-3157
Fax : 612-824-2031
E-mail: herbshop@presentmoment.com
Web Site: http://www.presentmoment.com

Metallic Clay Bath Kits

www.magneticclay.com

www.magneticclaybaths.com,
Toll Free: 800-257-3315 (USA)

www.relfe.com

Therapeutic Living Clay
www.globallight.net

Ojibwa (8-herb Essiac) Tea

**Contact Daryl Toll Free: 866-840-338
(USA)**

http://www.premium-essiac-tea-4less.com
(best value)

An alternative web page with ratio/breakdown of
herbs: http://www.biznet1.com/p2699.htm

Or see Michael Miller formula according to Renee
Caisse below:

Burdock Root 60.5% - Sheep Sorrel 19.5% -
Rhubarb Root 4.8% - Slippery Elm bark 4.8%
Kelp 4.8% - Blessed Thistle 2.4% - Red
Clover 2.4% - Watercress 0.3%

Virgin Coconut Oil

Wilderness Family Naturals
Ken and Annette Fischer
Box 538
Finland, MN 55603
U.S.A.
Toll Free: 800-945-3801
Tel: 866-936-6457
E-mail: info@wildernessfamilynaturals.com
Web Site: http://wildernessfamilynaturals.com

Products for the Alternative Versions of the Liver and Gallbladder Flush

Prime Health Products
15 Belfield Road, Unit C
Toronto, Ontario, Canada M9W
Tel: 1-416-248-2930 or 1-416-248-0415
E-mail: jchang@sensiblehealth.com
Fax: 1- 416-248-0415 or 1-416-233-5347
Web Site: http://sensiblehealth.com

- Gold Coin Grass
- Chinese Gentian and Bupleurum

BulkFoods.com
http://www.bulkfoods.com
(419) 537-1713 USA
Presque Isle Wine Cellars
94440 W Main Rd
North East, PA 16428
U.S.A.
Tel: 1-814-725-1314
Web Site: http://www.piwine.com

- Malic Acid Powder, Food Grade

The Family Health News
9845 N.E 2nd Avenue
Miami Shores, FL 33138
U.S.A.
Tel. 1-800-284-6263
1-305-759-9500
Web Site: http://www.familyhealthnews.com

- Colosan

Ashaninka
Web Site: http://www.ashaninka.com

- Chanca Piedra Extract

Water Treatments/Filtration

Puritec
9811 W. Charleston Blvd., Suite 2-836,
Las Vegas, NV 89117
Email: info@puritec.com
Phone Numbers:
Toll Free: 888-491-4100 (USA)
Local: 702-562-8802 (USA)

Prill Beads
www.globallight.net
Toll Free: 888-236-2108 (USA)
Local: 210-651-0505 (USA)

Water Ionisers
Jupiterionizers
2120 Las Palmas Drive. Suite E
Carlsbad, CA 92011, USA
Phone: (800) 578 5939 or (800) 699 3475
Local: (760) 431 8047
Fax: (760) 431 0126
Web site: www.jupiterionizers.com

Beeswax Candles

Gift Winds, Inc
531 Prospect Ave
Little Silver, NJ 07739
U.S.A.
E-mail: giftwinds@giftwinds.com
Web site: http://www.giftwinds.com

Sunshine Bay Trading Company
Call Toll Free: 800-558-7292
Fax Toll Free: 800-765-7145
email: info@sunshinebay.com
Web site: http://www.sunshinebay.com

Beneficial Sugars

Global Sweet.Com
125 Tremont Street
Rehoboth, MA 02769
U.S.A.
Telephone:
800-601-0688 (in U.S.A)
508-252-5294
Fax:800-778-2357 (in U.S.A)
508-252-5888
Website: http://www.globalsweet.com

- **Xylitol and D-Mannose**

Web Vitamins
920 River St.
Suite E
Windsor, CT 06095, U.S.A.
Phone 800-919-9122
Web Site http://www.webvitamins.com

- **FOS Supplement**

Aloe Vera in Powder Form

Good Cause Wellness
http://www.goodcausewellness.com
Tel. 520-870-2484
Email: alan@goodcausewellness.com

Soladey Toothbrushes

Ener-Chi Wellness Center
Tel 866-258-4006
709-570-7401 (Canada)
www.ener-chi.com/soladey.htm

Waterless Cookware

Web site: http://www.NorthAmericanSales.com

Web site: http://www.fitsmybudget.com

Web site: http://www.100cookwares.com
Tel: 866-265-4875
Web site: http://www.overstock.com

Chia Seeds (Super Grain)

Chia for Health (Nature's Emporium)
20825 Highway 410 East #322
Bonney Lake, WA 98391, USA
Tel 253-826-0510
Web Site: www.chiaforhealth.com

Squatting Toilet Platform

Nature's Platform
186 Westside Drive
Boone, NC 28607, U.S.A
828-297-7561
http://www.naturesplatform.com

Anti Warts / Skin Cancer Herbs

Risingsun Health Alternatives
1106 W. Park #199
Livingston, Montana 59047, USA
Tel: 406-222-9257
Web Site: http://www.bloodrootproducts.com

- Bloodroot Paste

McDaniel Life-Line LLC
Voice 580-426-2481 Toll Free: 866-393-5540
Web Site www.lifelinwater.com
E-mail sales@lifelinewater.com

- Indian Herb

Blemish Free: http://www.blemish-free.com

Miracle Mineral Supplement (MMS)	**Detoxified Iodine**
Ener-Chi Wellness Center Toll Free 866-258-4006 Local 709-570-7401 (Canada) **More Information on MMS** www.miraclemineralsupplement.bravenet.com www.miraclemineral.org (free Ebook)	Magnascent www.mnwp.org Atomic Iodine, www.baar.com Atomidine, http://edgarcayceproducts.com

Botanical Names *Kidney Cleanse Herbs* (Follow the directions given in Chapter 7)	*Botanical Names* *For Liver Herbs* (Follow the directions given in the Amazing Liver and Gallbladder Flush)
Marjoram [Origanum majorana] Cat's Claw [Uncaria tomentosa] Comfrey Root [Symphytum officinale] Fennel Seed [Foeniculum vulgare] Chicory Herb [Chichorium intybus] Uva Ursi or Bearberry [Arctostaphylos] Hydrangea Root [Hydrangea arborescens] Gravel Root [Eupatorium purpureum] Marshmallow Root [Althaea officinalis] Golden Rod Herb [Solidago virgaurea]	Dandelion root [Taraxacum officinale] Comfrey root [Symphytum officinale] Licorice root [Glycyrrhiza glabra] Agrimony [Agrimonia Eupatoria] Wild yam root [Dioscorea Villosa] Barberry bark [Berberis vulgaris] Bearsfoot [Polymnia uvedalia] Tanners oak bark [Quercus robur] Milk thistle herb [Silybum marianum]

Other Books and Services by the Author

The Amazing Liver & Gallbladder Flush
A Powerful Do-It-Yourself Tool to Optimize your Health and Wellbeing

In this revised edition of his best selling book, *The Amazing Liver Cleanse,* Andreas Moritz addresses the most common but rarely recognized cause of illness - gallstones congesting the liver. Twenty million Americans suffer from attacks of gallstones every year. In many cases, treatment merely consists of removing the gallbladder, at the cost of $5 billion a year. But this purely symptom-oriented approach does not eliminate the cause of the illness, and in many cases, sets the stage for even more serious conditions. Most adults living in the industrialized world, and especially those suffering a chronic illness such as heart disease, arthritis, MS, cancer, or diabetes, have hundreds if not thousands of gallstones (mainly clumps of hardened bile) blocking the bile ducts of their liver.

This book provides a thorough understanding of what causes gallstones in the liver and gallbladder and why these stones can be held responsible for the most common diseases so prevalent in the world today. It provides the reader with the knowledge needed to recognize the stones and gives the necessary, do-it-yourself instructions to painlessly remove them in the comfort of one's home. It also gives practical guidelines on how to prevent new gallstones from being formed. The widespread success of *The Amazing Liver & Gallbladder Flush* is a testimony to the power and effectiveness of the cleanse itself. The liver cleanse has led to extraordinary improvements in health and wellness among thousands of people who have already given themselves the precious gift of a strong, clean, revitalized liver.

Lifting the Veil of Duality -
Your Guide to Living without Judgment

"Do you know that there is a place inside you - hidden beneath the appearance of thoughts, feelings, and emotions - that does not know the difference between good and evil, right and wrong, light and dark? From that place you embrace the opposite values of life as *One.* In this sacred place you are at peace with yourself and at peace with your world." ~ *Andreas Moritz*

In *Lifting the Veil of Duality,* Andreas Moritz poignantly exposes the illusion of duality. He outlines a simple way to remove every limitation that you have imposed upon yourself during the course of living duality. You will be prompted to see yourself and the world through a new lens - the lens of clarity, discernment, and non-judgment. You will also discover that mistakes, accidents, coincidences, negativity, deception, injustice, wars, crime, and terrorism all have a deeper purpose and meaning in the larger scheme of things. So naturally, much of what you will read may conflict with the beliefs you currently hold. Yet you are not asked to change your beliefs or opinions. Instead, you are asked to have *an open mind,* for only an open mind can enjoy freedom from judgment.

Our personal views and worldviews are currently challenged by a crisis of identity. Some are being shattered altogether. The collapse of our current World Order forces humanity to deal with the most basic issues of existence. You can no longer avoid taking responsibility for the things that happen to you. When you *do* accept responsibility, you also empower and heal yourself.

Lifting the Veil of Duality shows you how you create or subdue your ability to fulfill your desires. Furthermore, you will find intriguing explanations about the mystery of time, the truth and illusion of reincarnation, the oftentimes misunderstood value of prayer, what makes relationships work, and why so often they don't. Find out why injustice is an illusion that has managed to haunt us throughout the ages.

508

Learn about our original separation from the Source of Life and what this means with regard to the current waves of instability and fear so many of us are experiencing.

Discover how to identify the angels living amongst us and why we all have light-bodies. You will have the opportunity to find the ultimate God within you and discover why a God seen as separate from yourself keeps you from being in your Divine Power and happiness. In addition, you can find out how to heal yourself at a moment's notice. Read all about the 'New Medicine' and the destiny of the old medicine, the old economy, the old religion, and the old world.

It's Time to Come Alive!
Start Using the Amazing Healing Powers of Your Body, Mind, and Spirit Today!

In this book, the author brings to light man's deep inner need for spiritual wisdom in life and helps the reader develop a new sense of reality that is based on love, power, and compassion. He describes our relationship with the natural world in detail and discusses how we can harness its tremendous powers for our personal and humanity's benefit. *Time to Come Alive* challenges some of our most commonly held beliefs and offers a way out of the emotional restrictions and physical limitations that we have created in our lives.

Topics include: What shapes our destiny, using the power of intention, secrets of defying the aging process, doubting - the cause of failure, opening the heart, material wealth and spiritual wealth, fatigue - the major cause of stress, methods of emotional transformation, techniques of primordial healing, how to increase the health of the five senses, developing spiritual wisdom, the major causes of today's earth changes, entry into the new world, twelve gateways to heaven on earth, and many more.

Cancer is Not a Disease! It's A Survival Mechanism
Discover Cancer's Hidden Purpose, Heal its Root Causes, and be Healthier Than Ever!

In *Cancer is Not a Disease*, Andreas Moritz proves the point that cancer is the physical symptom that reflects our body's final attempt to deal with life-threatening cell congestion and toxins. He claims that removing the underlying conditions that force the body to produce cancerous cells sets the preconditions for complete healing of our body, mind, and emotions.

This book confronts you with a radically new understanding of cancer - one that revolutionized the current cancer model. On the average, today's conventional 'treatments' of killing, cutting out, or burning cancerous cells offer most patients a remission rate of a mere 7%, and the majority of these survivors are 'cured' for just five years or fewer. Prominent cancer researcher and professor at the University of California at Berkeley, Dr. Hardin Jones, stated: "Patients are as well or better off untreated..." Any published success figures in cancer survival statistics are offset by equal or better scores among those receiving no treatment at all. More people are killed by cancer treatments than are saved by them.

Cancer is Not a Disease shows you why traditional cancer treatments are often fatal, what actually causes cancer, and how you can remove the obstacles that prevent the body from healing itself. Cancer is not an attempt on your life; on the contrary, this 'dread disease' is the body's final, desperate effort to save your life. Unless we change our perception of what cancer really is, it will continue to threaten the life of nearly one out of every two people. This book opens a door for those who wish to turn feelings of victimhood into empowerment and self-mastery, and disease into health.

Topics of the book include:

- Reasons the body is forced to develop cancer cells
- How to identify and remove the causes of cancer
- Why most cancers disappear by themselves, without medical intervention
- Why radiation, chemotherapy, and surgery never cure cancer
- Why some people survive cancer despite undergoing dangerously radical treatments
- The roles of fear, frustration, low self-worth, and repressed anger in the origination of cancer
- How to turn self-destructive emotions into energies that promote health and vitality
- Spiritual lessons behind cancer

Heart Disease No More!
Make Peace with Your Heart and Heal Yourself
(Excerpted from this book)

Diabetes - No More!
Discover and Heal Its True Causes
(Excerpted from this book)

Ending The AIDS Myth
It's Time To Heal The TRUE Causes!
(Excerpted from this book)

Heal Yourself with Sunlight
**Use Its Secret Medicinal Powers to Help Cure Cancer,
Heart Disease, Hypertension, Diabetes, Arthritis,
Infectious Diseases, and much more.**
(Excerpted from this book)

Hear the Whispers, Live Your Dream
A Fanfare of Inspiration

All books are available as paperback copies and electronic books
through the Ener-Chi Wellness Center

Website: http://www.ener-chi.com
Email: andmor@ener-chi.com
Toll free (1-866) 258-4006 (USA)
Local (709) 570-7401 (CanadaA)

Telephone Consultations

For a Personal Telephone Consultation or Sacred Santémony session with Andreas Moritz, please:

1. Call or send an email with your name, phone number, address, digital picture (if you have one) of your face and any other relevant information to:

E-mail: andmor@ener-chi.com

Telephone: 1 (864) 895-6285 (U.S.A)

2. Set up an appointment for the length of time you choose to spend with him. A comprehensive consultation lasts two hours or more. Shorter consultations deal with all the questions you may have and any information that is relevant to your specific health issue(s). A Sacred Santémony session usually takes half an hour.

For current fees please visit the consultation page at: http://www.ener-chi.com

INDEX

ABOUT THE AUTHOR

Andreas Moritz is a medical intuitive, a practitioner of Ayurveda, iridology, shiatsu, and vibrational medicine; a writer, and an artist. Born in southwest Germany in 1954, Moritz had to deal with several severe illnesses from an early age, which compelled him to study diet, nutrition, and various methods of natural healing while still a child.

By the age of 20, he had completed his training in iridology - the diagnostic science of eye interpretation - and dietetics. In 1981, he began studying Ayurvedic medicine in India and completed his training as a qualified practitioner of Ayurveda in New Zealand in 1991. Rather than being satisfied with merely treating the symptoms of illness, Moritz has dedicated his life's work to understanding and treating the root causes of illness. Because of this holistic approach, he has had astounding success with cases of terminal disease where conventional methods of healing proved futile.

Since 1988, he has been practicing the Japanese healing art of shiatsu, which has given him profound insights into the energy system of the body. In addition, he devoted eight years of active research into consciousness and its important role in the field of mind/body medicine.

Andreas Moritz is also the author of *The Amazing Liver and Gallbladder Flush, Lifting the Veil of Duality, Cancer Is Not a Disease, It's Time to Come Alive, Heart Disease No More, Simple Steps to Total Health, Diabetes No More, Heal Yourself with Sunlight, Hear the Whispers - Live Your Dream,* and *Ending the AIDS Myth.*

During his extensive travels throughout the world, he has consulted with heads of state and members of government in Europe, Asia, and Africa, and has lectured widely on the subject of health, mind/body medicine, and spirituality. His popular *Timeless Secrets of Health and Rejuvenation* workshops assist people in taking responsibility for their own health and well-being. Moritz has a free forum 'Ask Andreas Moritz' on the large health web site curezone.com (five million readers and increasing). Although he recently stopped writing for the forum, it contains an extensive archive or his answers to thousands of questions on nearly every health topic.

Since taking up residence in the United States in 1998, Moritz has been involved in developing a new and innovative system of healing - called *Ener-Chi Art* - that targets the root causes of many chronic illnesses. Ener-Chi Art consists of a series of light ray-encoded oil paintings that can instantly restore vital energy flow (Chi) in the organs and systems of the body. Moritz is also the founder of *Sacred Santémony - Divine Chanting for Every Occasion,* a powerful system of specially generated frequencies of sound that can transform deep-seated fears, allergies, traumas and mental or emotional blocks into useful opportunities for growth and inspiration within a matter of moments.

CPSIA information can be obtained at www.ICGtesting.com
Printed in the USA
BVOW031446200712

295783BV00001B/32/P